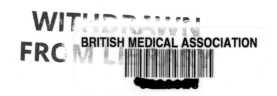

Esophageal cancer and barrett's esophagus

Esophageal cancer and barrett's esophagus

Prateek Sharma, MD

Gastroenterology, Department of Veterans Affairs Medical Center
Kansas City, MO, USA

Richard Sampliner, MD

Chief of Gastroenterology, Southern Arizona VA Health Care System
Professor of Medicine, University of Arizona Health Sciences Center, Tuscon, AZ, USA

David Ilson, MD, PHD

Gastrointestinal Oncology Service, Department of Medicine
Memorial Sloan-Kettering Cancer Center, New York, NY, USA

THIRD EDITION

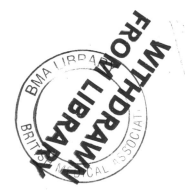

WILEY Blackwell

This edition first published 2015; © 2001, 2006, 2015 by John Wiley & Sons, Ltd

Registered office: John Wiley & Sons, Ltd, The Atrium, Southern Gate, Chichester, West Sussex, PO19 8SQ, UK

Editorial offices: 9600 Garsington Road, Oxford, OX4 2DQ, UK
　　　　　　　The Atrium, Southern Gate, Chichester, West Sussex, PO19 8SQ, UK
　　　　　　　111 River Street, Hoboken, NJ 07030-5774, USA

For details of our global editorial offices, for customer services and for information about how to apply for permission to reuse the copyright material in this book please see our website at www.wiley.com/wiley-blackwell.

Library of Congress Cataloging-in-Publication Data applied for.

ISBN: 9781118655207

A catalogue record for this book is available from the British Library.

Wiley also publishes its books in a variety of electronic formats. Some content that appears in print may not be available in electronic books.

Cover image: ©Yodiyim@gettyimages

Typeset in 8.5/12pt MeridienLTStd by SPi Global, Chennai, India
Printed and bound in Malaysia by Vivar Printing Sdn Bhd

1　2015

Contents

List of contributors

Andrea Anderloni MD, PhD
Digestive Endoscopy Unit, Division of Gastroenterology, Humanitas Research Hospital, Rozzano, Milan, Italy

Jacques J.G.H.M. Bergman MD, PhD
Department of Gastroenterology and Hepatology, Academic Medical Center, University of Amsterdam, Amsterdam, the Netherlands

Shivaram K. Bhat PhD, MRCP, MBBCh
Specialty Registrar in Gastroenterology, Altnagelvin Hospital, Western Health and Social Care Trust, Londonderry, UK

David F. Boerwinkel MD
Department of Gastroenterology and Hepatology, Academic Medical Center, University of Amsterdam, Amsterdam, the Netherlands

Marcia Irene Canto MD, MHS
Division of Gastroenterology and Hepatology, The Johns Hopkins Medical Institutions, Baltimore, MA, USA

Daniel K. Chan MD
Barrett's Esophagus Unit, Division of Gastroenterology and Hepatology, Mayo Clinic, Rochester, MN, USA

Helen G. Coleman PhD
Lecturer in Cancer Epidemiology, Centre for Public Health, Queen's University Belfast, Belfast, UK

Wouter L. Curvers MD, PhD
Department of Gastroenterology and Hepatology, Academic Medical Center, University of Amsterdam, Amsterdam, the Netherlands

Heath D. Skinner MD, PhD
Assistant Professor, Department of Radiation Oncology, The University of Texas MD Anderson Cancer Center, Houston, TX, USA

Mary Denholm MBChB (Oxon) BA (Hons)(Oxon)
Centre for Digestive Diseases, Queen Mary University of London, London, UK

Jacques Deviere MD, PhD
Department of Gastroenterology, Hepatopancreatology and Digestive Oncology, Erasme University Hospital, Brussels, Belgium

Kerry Dunbar MD, PhD
Assistant Professor of Medicine, University of Texas Southwestern Medical Center, Dallas VA Medical Center, Dallas, TX, USA

Matthias Ebert MD
Department of Medicine II, Gastroenterology, University of Mannheim, Germany

Hashem B. El-Serag MD, MPH
Professor and Chief, Section of Gastroenterology and Hepatology, Department of Medicine, Baylor College of Medicine; Clinical Epidemiology and Comparative Effectiveness Program, Houston VA HSR&D Center of Excellence, Michael E DeBakey Veterans Affairs Medical Center, Houston, TX, USA

Eun Ji Shin MD
Division of Gastroenterology and Hepatology, The Johns Hopkins Medical Institutions, Baltimore, MA, USA

Gary W. Falk MD, MS
Professor of Medicine, Division of Gastroenterology, University of Pennsylvania Perelman School of Medicine, Philadelphia, PA, USA

Rebecca Fitzgerald FMedSci
MRC Cancer Unit, Hutchison-MRC Research Centre, University of Cambridge, Cambridge, UK

John R. Goldblum MD
Professor, Cleveland Clinic Lerner College of Medicine, Chairman, Department of Anatomic Pathology, Cleveland Clinic, Cleveland, OH, USA

Takuji Gotoda MD
Division of Gastroenterology, Jichi Medical University, Shimotsuke, Tochigi, Japan

Lars Grenacher MD
Department of Diagnostic and Interventional Radiology, University of Heidelberg, Germany

Neil Gupta MD, MPH
Assistant Professor of Medicine, Division of Gastroenterology and Nutrition, Loyola University Medical Center, Maywood, IL, USA

Toshitaka Hoppo MD, PhD
Institute for the Treatment of Esophageal & Thoracic Disease, The Western Pennsylvania Hospital, Pittsburgh, PA, USA

Janusz Jankowski
Centre for Digestive Diseases, Queen Mary University of London, London, UK

Blair A. Jobe MD, FACS
Chief, Department of Surgery; Director, Institute for the Treatment of Esophageal & Thoracic Disease, The Western Pennsylvania Hospital, Pittsburgh, PA, USA

Manol Jovani MD
Digestive Endoscopy Unit, Division of Gastroenterology Humanitas Research Hospital, Rozzano, Milan, Italy

Peter Kahrilas MD
Division of Gastroenterology, Northwestern University Feinberg School of Medicine, Chicago, IL, USA

Arne Kandulski
Department of Gastroenterology, Hepatology and Infectious Diseases, Otto-von-Guericke University Hospital, Magdeburg, Germany

Ralf Kiesslich
Department of Medicine, St. Marienkrankenhaus, Katharina-Kasper gGmbH, Frankfurt am Main, Germany

Bernd-Joachim Krause MD
Department of Nuclear Medicine, University of Rostock, Germany

Kumar Krishnan
Division of Gastroenterology, Northwestern University Feinberg School of Medicine, Chicago, IL, USA

Geoffrey Y. Ku MD
Gastrointestinal Oncology Service, Department of Medicine, Memorial Sloan-Kettering Cancer Center, New York, NY, USA

Cadman L. Leggett MD
Barrett's Esophagus Unit, Division of Gastroenterology and Hepatology, Mayo Clinic, Rochester, MN, USA

Mark A. Lewis MD
Assistant Professor, General Oncology, The University of Texas MD Anderson Cancer Center, Houston, TX, USA

Florian Lordick MD
Director of the University Cancer Center Leipzig (UCCL), University Clinic Leipzig, Leipzig, Germany

Kristle Lee Lynch MD
Division of Gastroenterology and Hepatology, The Johns Hopkins Medical Institutions, Baltimore, MA, USA

Peter Malfertheiner MD
Department of Gastroenterology, Hepatology and Infectious Diseases, Otto-von-Guericke University Hospital, Magdeburg, Germany

Bruce D. Minsky MD
Professor and Deputy Division Head, Department of Radiation Oncology, The University of Texas MD Anderson Cancer Center, Houston, TX, USA

Liam J. Murray MFPHM, MD, MRCGP, MBBCh
Professor in Cancer Epidemiology, Centre for Public Health, Queen's University Belfast, Belfast, UK

Mariam Naveed MD
Fellow, Division of Gastroenterology and Hepatology, University of Texas Southwestern Medical Center, Dallas, TX, USA

Mariam Naveed MD
Fellow, Division of Gastroenterology and Hepatology, University of Texas Southwestern Medical Center, Dallas, TX, USA

Helmut Neumann
Department of Medicine I, University of Erlangen-Nuremberg, Germany

Ayesha Noorani
MRC Cancer Unit, Hutchison-MRC Research Centre, University of Cambridge, Cambridge, UK

Katja Ott MD
Department of Surgery, University of Heidelberg, Germany

Tsuneo Oyama MD
Division of Gastroenterology, Jichi Medical University, Shimotsuke, Tochigi, Japan

John E. Pandolfino
Division of Gastroenterology, Northwestern University Feinberg School of Medicine, Chicago, IL, USA

Deepa T. Patil MD
Assistant Professor, Cleveland Clinic Lerner College of Medicine, Staff Pathologist, Department of Anatomic Pathology, Cleveland Clinic, Cleveland, OH, USA

Oliver Pech MD, PhD
Department of Gastroenterology and interventional Endoscopy, St. John of God Hospital, Teaching Hospital of the University of Regensburg, Germany

Krish Ragunath MD, FRCP, FASGE
Professor & Head of GI Endoscopy, Nottingham Digestive Diseases Centre, NIHR Biomedical Research Unit, Queens Medical Centre, Nottingham University Hospitals NHS Trust, Nottingham, UK

Alessandro Repici MD
Digestive Endoscopy Unit, Division of Gastroenterology Humanitas Research Hospital, Rozzano, Milan, Italy

Nabil Rizk
Department of Surgery, Memorial Sloan Kettering Cancer Center, New York, NY, USA

Mohammad H. Shakhatreh MD
Gastroenterology Clinical Research Fellow, Section of Gastroenterology and Hepatology, Department of Medicine, Baylor College of Medicine and Houston VA HSR&D Center of Excellence, Michael E DeBakey Veterans Affairs Medical Center, Houston, TX, USA

Aaron J. Small MD
Division of Gastroenterology, University of Pennsylvania Perelman School of Medicine, Philadelphia, PA, USA

A. Samad Soudagar MD
Fellow, Division of Gastroenterology and Nutrition, Loyola University Medical Center, Maywood, IL, USA

Stuart Jon Spechler MD
Professor of Medicine, Berta M. and Cecil O. Patterson Chair in Gastroenterology, UT Southwestern Medical Center at Dallas; Chief, Division of Gastroenterology, VA North Texas Healthcare System, Dallas VA Medical Center, Dallas, TX, USA

Marino Venerito
Department of Gastroenterology, Hepatology and Infectious Diseases, Otto-von-Guericke University Hospital, Magdeburg, Germany

Kenneth Wang MD
Barrett's Esophagus Unit, Division of Gastroenterology and Hepatology, Mayo Clinic, Rochester, MN, USA

Sachin Wani MD
Assistant Professor of Medicine, Division of Gastroenterology and Hepatology, University of Colorado Anschutz Medical Center, Veterans Affairs Medical Center, Denver, Aurora, CO, USA

Christian Wittekind MD
Institute of Pathology, University Clinic Leipzig, Germany

Hironori Yamamoto MD, PhD
Professor of Medicine, Division of Gastroenterology, Jichi Medical University, Shimotsuke, Tochigi, Japan

Harry H. Yoon MD, MHS
Consultant, Medical Oncology, Mayo Clinic, Rochester, MN, USA

Preface

Many advances have occurred in the past few decades in the diagnosis and management of Barrett's esophagus and early esophageal adenocarcinoma. We have attempted to capture the salient features of these lesions in several chapters written by international experts in the field.

Highlights of this book include the recognition of the lower neoplastic progression of Barrett's esophagus (0.2–0.4 % per year), in spite of the rising incidence in younger age groups. Also, the risk factors for esophageal adenocarcinoma are detailed by epidemiology: age, gender and ethnicity. There is a complex interplay of inherited predispositions, environmental exposures and tissue responses that lead to neoplastic progression. Unfortunately, the advances in molecular biology have failed to yield a simple documented approach to the risk stratification of patients. Multiple mutations have been identified and analyzed, with sophisticated statistical techniques, without a clear clinically useful result. Histologic dysplasia remains the "standard" biomarker for the progression of Barrett's esophagus to esophageal adenocarcinoma. Therefore, careful surveillance biopsies remain necessary. A high-quality white light endoscopy examination, using high definition endoscopes, is still the best method to target biopsy the high-risk appearing areas of Barrett's esophagus.

Unfortunately, advanced esophageal adenocarcinoma is often found at the first recognition of BE. If nodular-appearing mucosa are identified in the Barrett's segment, then endoscopic resection of the most abnormal appearing area is essential for proper T staging. Endoscopic ablation therapy is the primary treatment of high-grade dysplasia and T1a esophageal adenocarcinoma. Accompanying endoscopic ultrasound and body imaging are needed for disease deeper than T1a; such disease requires surgical intervention. With limited distal esophageal cancer, a local resection may be possible. For more extensive disease, chemoradiation may be appropriate, followed by definitive surgery. Medical therapy controlling gastroesophageal reflux symptoms with proton pump inhibitors is the background for the above interventions. An ideal approach to neoplasia in Barrett's esophagus would be chemoprevention but, unfortunately, no intervention has yet been documented to be effective in a large clinical trial.

Ultimately, better risk stratification, more effective biomarker predictability of progression to neoplasia, and effective chemoprevention remain key goals for patients with esophageal cancer and Barrett's esophagus.

As editors, we hope that you will find this book comprehensive, intellectually stimulating and helpful in the clinical care of patients with this disease.

Prateek Sharma
Richard Sampliner
David Ilson

CHAPTER 1

Epidemiology of esophageal carcinoma

Mohammad H. Shakhatreh & Hashem B El-Serag

Section of Gastroenterology and Hepatology, Department of Medicine, Baylor College of Medicine and Houston VA HSR&D Center of Excellence, Michael E DeBakey Veterans Affairs Medical Center, Houston, TX, USA

1.1 The incidence and mortality related to esophageal cancer

Esophageal cancer is the sixth most common cancer among men and the ninth among women, affecting more than 450,000 people globally each year. Approximately 90% of cases of esophageal cancer are squamous cell carcinoma (ESCC) [1], and the rest are adenocarcinoma (EA). The highest reported incidence and mortality rates for ESCC occur in Jiashan, China, with an age-adjusted incidence rate of 14.6 cases per 100,000 (Figure 1.1). The highest age-adjusted incidence rates of EA occur in Scotland (6.6 per 100,000) and in other parts of the United Kingdom [2]. In the United States, the age-adjusted rate of esophageal cancer in 2009 was 4.1 per 100,000; EA alone had 2.7 cancers per 100,000, a sharp increase from the 1973 rate of 0.4 cancers per 100,000 [3] (Figure 1.2)

Although EA is the fastest-rising malignancy among white men in the United States, its increase may be slowing [4]. The US average annual percentage change in incidence was 8.4 (95% CI 7.7–9.1) before 1997, but it decreased to 1.6 (95% CI 0.0–3.3) from 1998 to 2009 [5]. In Scandinavia, the average annual percentage change has continued to increase [6].

In addition to geographic differences in the distribution of EA, there are remarkable variations in the demographics of persons affected by this cancer. The incidence of EA increases with age and peaks in the eighth decade of life. Independent of age, however, people born in more recent years have a higher incidence of EA [7]. EA incidence is five-fold higher among non-Hispanic whites than among blacks, while ESCC incidence rates among black men are four times higher than for white men [8]. Finally, most esophageal cancer cases (77.7%) affect men [6].

The incidence of EA is 7–10 times higher in men, while the incidence of ESCC is only 2–3 times higher in men than in women, according to numerous cancer registries around the world [9, 10]. This sex discrepancy varies among different races; for example, in the 50–59 age group, the highest male-to-female ratio was 20.5 in Hispanics, followed by 10.8 in whites and then 7.0 in blacks. With EA, male predominance is evident globally (Figure 1.1). Whether the difference in incidence rates among men and women or between whites and blacks is due to less gastroesophageal reflux disease (GERD) and/or Barrett's Esophagus (BE) prevalence, or to a less progressive form of these diseases, is unknown. Despite an equal distribution of GERD between men and women [11, 12], men seem to have a more severe form of the disease, with a higher complication rate [13].

With ESCC, some areas (e.g. South Karachi, Pakistan; West Midlands, UK; Oman; Penang, Malaysia; South Australia; Kuwait) have a higher age-adjusted incidence rate among women than among men [2] (Figure 1.1).

Work partly funded by NIH grants K24DK078154 and T32DK083266 and by the VA Houston HSR&D Center of Excellence (HFP90-020).
DISCLAIMER: The views expressed in this article are those of the authors and do not necessarily reflect the position or policy of the Department of Veterans Affairs, the US government, Baylor College of Medicine or the National Institutes of Health.

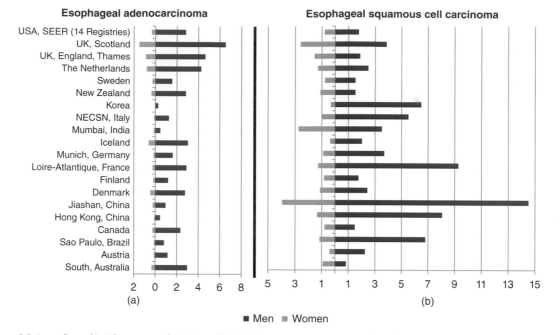

Figure 1.1 Age-adjusted incidence rates of EA (a) and ESCC (b) in 1998-2002 using world standard population (2000). EA: Esophageal adenocarcinoma. ESCC: Esophageal squamous cell carcinoma. CI5-IX: *Cancer Incidence in Five Continents*, volume 9. IARC: International Agency for Research on Cancer. SEER: Surveillance, epidemiology and end results. NECSN: North East Cancer Surveillance Network. Data from CI5-IX (2007), IARC.

The reason behind this is unknown. The main risk factors for ESCC, which show broad regional variation, include heavy alcohol consumption, tobacco smoking and human papilloma virus infection, as well as few rare disorders, such as achalasia of the cardia, and tylosis. These will not be discussed further in this review.

1.2   Mortality

Esophageal cancer is a highly fatal disease. The overall five-year relative survival for patients diagnosed with esophageal cancer in the United States was approximately 17.3% between 2003 and 2009 (Figure 1.2). The disease stage at time of diagnosis impacts survival greatly, as the age-adjusted five-year relative survival of 38.6% in localized disease declines to 3.5% in disease associated with distant spread. However, the overall survival over the past two decades has slightly, but significantly, improved. Despite the use of screening endoscopy in high-risk groups, about 35% of EA cases between 2004 and 2010 were diagnosed at an advanced

stage [14]. A higher mortality rate for nonwhite Hispanics and blacks mostly has been attributed to the decreased receipt of cancer-directed surgery, indicating possible ethnic disparities in treatment application or availability [15].

1.2.1   Progression of BE to EA

A summary of published annual EA-risk data of nondysplastic BE ranges from 0.12–0.50% to 0.33–0.70% in population-based studies and meta-analyses, respectively [16]. Recent studies have indicated that the risk of progression from BE to EA is lower than previously reported [17]. The risk in a Dutch study of 42,207 patients was 0.4% [18]; in an Irish study of 8,522 patients, it was 0.22% per year (95% CI 0.19–0.26%) [19]; and in a Danish study of 11,028 patients, it was 0.12% (95% CI 0.09–0.15) [20].

1.3   Risk factors for EA

Risk factors for esophageal adenocarcinoma are outlined in Table 1.1.

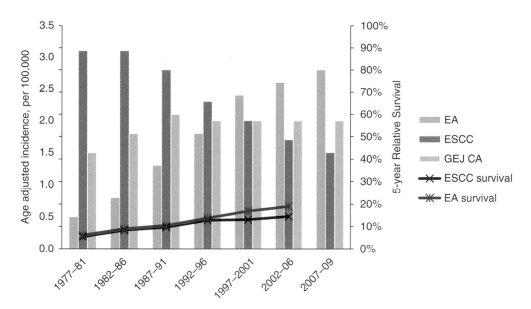

Figure 1.2 Trends in incidence and five-year relative survival of EA, ESCC, GEJ-CA. Data from SEER 9 Regs research data, Nov 2011 sub, vintage 2009 pops (1973–2009) <Katrina/Rita Population adjustment> – linked to county attributes – Total US, 1969–2010 counties, National Cancer Institute, DCCPS, Surveillance Research Program, Surveillance Systems Branch, released April 2012, based on the November 2011 submission. SEER: Surveillance, epidemiology, and end results. EA: Esophageal adenocarcinoma. ESCC: Esophageal squamous cell carcinoma. GEJ CA: Gastro-esophageal junction carcinoma.

Table 1.1 Summary of risk factors for the development of esophageal adenocarcinoma.

Degree of confidence	Risk factor(s)
Definite risk	
Increased	BE
	Obesity
	Central obesity
	Smoking
	GERD
	Family history of BE or EA
Decreased	*H. pylori*
	Aspirin/NSAIDs
No change	Alcohol
Possible risk	
Increased	Bisphosphonates
Decreased	PPI
	Statins

GERD: Gastroesophageal reflux disease. EA: Esophageal adenocarcinoma. *H. pylori*: *Helicobacter pylori*. NSAIDs: Non-steroidal anti-inflammatory drugs. PPI: Proton pump inhibitor.

1.3.1 GERD

Several population-based case control studies have established a strong association, including a dose-response relationship between GERD symptoms and EA (and adenocarcinoma of the gastric cardia), but not ESCC [21, 22]. In a meta-analysis of five population-based studies, the presence of at least weekly GERD symptoms was associated with an odds ratio (OR) for developing EA of 4.92 (95% CI 3.90–6.22), which increased to 7.4 (95% CI 4.94–11.10) when the symptoms occurred on a daily basis, compared with asymptomatic controls or those with less frequent symptoms [23]. However, up to 40% of the patients with EA may not report bothersome GERD symptoms.

1.3.2 Tobacco smoking

A pooled analysis of individual data from ten case-control and two cohort studies from Australia, Canada, Ireland, the United Kingdom and the United States, including 1242 EA cases, 1263 gastroesopheageal junction cancer (GEJ-CA) cases, 954 ESCC cases and 7053 controls without cancer [24], reported an increased risk of both types of esophageal cancer with history of tobacco smoking. The calculated OR of EA increased from 1.66 (95% CI 1.1–2.4) with 1–29 pack-years of smoking to 2.77 (95% CI 1.4–5.6) with

>60 pack-years smoking history, with a statistically significant trend ($p < 0.01$). The same study concluded that, for equal pack-years of smoking, more cigarettes per day for shorter duration was less deleterious than fewer cigarettes per day for longer duration. For example:

Previous smokers have in EA, when comparing those with equal pack-years of smoking, patients who smoked 10–19 cigarettes/day had an increased risk compared with those who smoked more than 40 cigarettes/day (p for trend = 0.40). Previous smokers have a lower risk of developing EA or ESCC than current smokers, but slightly higher than those who have never smoked [25]. Tobacco smoking does not seem to play a major role in developing BE [26]; however, in patients with established BE, the risk of EA increases with the magnitude and duration of smoking history [27]. Some studies indicate that the effect of smoking is stronger for ESCC than for EA [28]. Lastly, based on the risk estimates and the prevalence of smoking in the population, elimination of smoking would potentially prevent 39.7% of EA cases and 56.9% of ESCC cases [29].

1.3.3 Alcohol consumption

Large population-based studies consistently show a lack of association between alcohol consumption and EA [30–36]. For example, in an Irish study [34], no associations were found between total alcohol consumption in the preceding five years and reflux esophagitis, BE or EA (OR, 1.26, 95% CI 0.78–2.05; OR, 0.72, 95% CI 0.43–1.21; and OR, 0.75, 95% CI 0.46–1.22, respectively). Similarly, in a prospective evaluation of BE patients, a study found no increased risk of progressing to EA with increasing number of drinks per day or with the type of alcoholic beverage consumed [27]. However, with both alcohol consumption and current smoking, there is an eight-fold increased risk of developing ESCC [25].

The relationship between wine consumption and risk of BE or EA seems to follow a J-shaped curve, with both very low and very high intake associated with increased risk. An Australian study [36] found that those who drank modest levels of wine (<50–90 g/week) or port or spirits (<10–20 g/week) had significantly lower risks of EA, ESCC and GEJ CA than non-drinkers; higher consumption was associated with increased risks of ESCC only with a significant linear effect (OR, 1.03; 95% CI, 1.02–1.05 per 10 g alcohol/week). Where to draw the cut-offs for the transitions in this curve is unclear.

Although these findings are suggestive of a protective effect of modest intake of wine with regard to the risk of developing BE or EA, there are several biases that make it important to maintain a healthy skepticism [37].

1.3.4 Obesity

The association between obesity and EA has been corroborated in large and population-based case control studies conducted in the United States, Europe and Australia. These studies showed a strong association between increasing body mass index (BMI) and risk of developing this cancer [32, 38–47]. The association between BMI and EA has also been supported by prospective cohort studies [33, 48–54].

For example, a nested case control study from the UK General Practitioners Research Database (287 patients with EA and 10,000 randomly selected controls) found a positive association between BMI > 25 and EA (OR 1.7; 95% CI 1.2–2.3) [33]. In a cohort study from the Netherlands, including 120,852 participants, the relative risk of EA was 4.0 (95% CI 2.3–6.9) for obese individuals (BMI $\geq$ 30) compared with persons of normal weight (BMI 18.5–25.0) [50]. Abnet *et al.* found that, in a cohort of approximately 500,000 individuals from the United States, a BMI of 35 or more was associated with an EA hazard ratio [HR] of 2.3; (95% CI 1.4–3.6) compared with a normal BMI (18.5–25.0) [52].

Similarly, several meta-analyses confirmed the association between obesity and increased risk of EA. One calculated a pooled, adjusted OR of 1.52 in overweight patients and 2.78 in obese patients from nine case control studies (eight were population-based) [55], and another meta-analysis of 14 studies (two were cohort studies, eight were population-based studies, and four were hospital-based case control studies) calculated a pooled, adjusted OR of 1.9 for overweight patients and 2.4 for obese patients [56]. More recently, a larger meta-analysis that examined ten population-based case control and eight cohort studies found similar results for overweight (relative risk [RR] 1.87, 95% CI 1.61–2.17) and obese (RR 2.73, 95% CI 2.16–3.46) groups [57]. They also reported a summary RR for increments of five kg/m^2 of BMI of 1.13, 95% CI 1.11–1.16. Most data indicate that the strength of the association between obesity and EA is similar between sexes, or slightly more pronounced in men; however, data on women are limited.

The association between BMI and EA, combined with the strong male and white race predominance of this cancer, have prompted research into the influence of body fat distribution typically found in white men (predominantly abdominal adiposity) in the development of EA (and BE). Abdominal fat distribution might promote and exacerbate GERD, the main risk factor for EA, by elevating intra-abdominal and, consequently, intragastric pressure which, in turn, promotes transient relaxation of the lower esophageal sphincter and separation of the crural diaphragm from the GE junction [58]. In addition, obese individuals are more likely to have metabolic dysfunction, and there are at least three main mechanisms via which abdominal obesity may predispose to BE. These include alterations in the levels of adipokines (both proinflammatory (leptin) and anti-inflammatory (adiponectin)), cytokines and chemokines; hyperinsulinemeia and insulin resistance; and alterations in the insulin/Insulin-like Growth Factor (IGF) pathway. These reflux-independent effects of central adiposity have not been comprehensively examined [59].

That abdominal adiposity seems to confer additional increased risk of EA (to that of BMI) has some support from prospective studies [53, 54, 60, 61]. In a cohort study of 41,295 individuals in whom body fat distribution was measured using bioelectrical impedance tests, 30 patients with esophageal or gastric cardia adenocarcinomas were identified. The HR per 10 cm increase in waist circumference was 1.5 (95% CI 1.1–2.0) [60]. Steffen *et al.* identified 88 patients with EA in a prospective European study of 346,554 individuals and showed that, among several anthropometric measures (including BMI, waist circumference and waist-to-hip ratio [WHR]), the risk of EA correlated most strongly with waist circumference [54].

A nested case control study within a cohort of 206,974 US individuals, in which 101 patients with EA were identified, found that abdominal diameter equal to 25 cm (versus < 20 cm) was strongly associated with risk of developing EA (OR 3.5; 95% CI 1.3–9.3) [53]. Moreover, an Irish study comparing computerized tomography-measured abdominal fat composition showed that EA patients ($n = 110$) had greater intra-abdominal visceral adiposity than those with ESCC ($n = 46$), gastric adenocarcinoma ($n = 38$), or controls ($n = 90$) [62]. Similar to the findings from individual studies, a meta-analysis of five studies (one hospital, one population-based case-control and three cohort studies), examining the effect of central obesity

on the risk of EA, found more than a two-fold increase in risk compared with those with normal body habitus (OR 2.51, 95% CI 1.56–4.04) [63]. This association was also present when examining BMI as the risk factor (OR 2.45, 95% CI 1.84–3.28).

It is unclear whether obesity increases the risk of BE and, consequently, EA, or increases the risk of EA in people who already have BE. Hardikar *et al.* found no significant increase in risk of developing EA among BE patients when evaluating BMI or WHR, in both genders [27]. Similarly, in a meta-analysis of 11 studies, BMI was borderline significant for increasing the risk of BE (OR 1.24, 95% CI 1.02–1.52) [63]. However, central obesity almost doubled the risk of BE (OR 1.98, 95% CI 1.52–2.57), and this effect persisted after adjusting for the effect of BMI (OR 1.88, 95% CI 1.20–2.95).

1.3.5 Diet

Non-starchy vegetables, fruits, and foods containing beta-carotene and/or vitamin C or folates probably have a protective effect against esophageal cancer [64]. A meta-analysis of mainly case control studies reported an inverse associations of vitamin C and β-carotene/vitamin A intake with EA with an OR of 0.49 (95% CI 0.39–0.62) and 0.46 (95% CI 0.36–0.59), respectively, when comparing those in the highest quartile of intake to those in the lowest quartile [65]. Three studies reported on the association between vitamin E and risk of EA, but the summary OR did not reach statistical significance (0.80, 95% CI 0.63–1.03). Most studies have found a decrease in risk of developing EA with increased dietary intake of these antioxidants, but not from vitamin supplementation [66]. Even while controlling for GERD symptoms, fruit intake was significantly associated with a decreased risk of EA (OR 0.50, 95% CI 0.30–0.86) [45]. A meta-analysis of studies assessing the association of folate intake and esophageal cancer reported a summary OR of 0.50 (95% CI 0.39–0.65) among three case control studies examining the risk of EA [67].

In a population-based case control study examining fiber intake with EA, a statistically significant inverse association, mainly driven by a higher intake of cereal fibers, was found with GEJ-CA, but not EA (OR 0.3, 95% CI 0.2–0.5 and 0.7, 95% CI 0.4–1.2, respectively) [68]. No significant association between vegetable and fruit fibers with EA or GEJ-CA was found. The authors speculated that vegetables containing high levels of nitrates nullify the effect of the fibers and, thus, show no association with risk of EA or GEJ-CA. Interestingly, in a study comparing BE patients with GERD patients and population controls [10], total fiber intake was associated with decreased risk of developing BE (OR 0.34, 95% CI 0.15–0.76, comparing highest with lowest quartiles). However, when examining the sources of fiber, the association was found to be significant only with vegetable and fruit fibers, but not cereal fibers (OR 0.47, 95% CI 0.25–0.88 and 0.73, 95% CI 0.36–1.45, respectively). This highlights the problem of examining quartiles of dietary intake (g/day) among different studies. The Swedish study [68] used 3.3 g/day and 3.6 g/day for the highest quartiles of fruit and vegetable intake, respectively. However, in the US study [10], the highest quartile for fruits and vegetables was 13.2 g/day, about a four-fold difference.

Conflicting results regarding intake of red meat, fat and dairy products with EA have been reported [69]. A meta-analysis of 35 studies examined the effects of fish, and red, white and processed meat on the risk of esophageal cancer; four of these were cohort and 31 were case control studies [70]. Of these studies, 14 examined ESCC only, five focused on EA, and three reported separate results for the two cancers, while 13 did not distinguish between EA and ESCC. When stratified by type of cancer, red meat was weakly associated with increased risk of ESCC (OR 1.63, 95% CI 1.00–2.63), but not associated with EA (OR 1.19, 95% CI 0.98–1.44). However, pooling the six studies that evaluated processed meat showed a significant association with increased EA risk (OR 1.37, 95% CI 1.05–1.78), but not ESCC (OR 1.17, 95% CI 0.90–1.51). White meat, poultry and fish did not have significant associations with risk of EA or ESCC.

In their review, Kubo et al [71] reported on six studies evaluating carbohydrate intake with risk of developing EA. All were case control studies; three reported decreased risk of EA (OR ranging from 0.34 to 0.39), while the other three reported non-significant associations.

1.3.6 Proton Pump Inhibitors (PPIs)

In the United States alone, 139 million prescriptions of PPIs were dispensed in 2008. This number continues to rise, and in 2012 there were 157 million dispensed prescriptions [72]. Since BE and EA are thought to develop from continued esophageal acid exposure,

using PPIs to decrease this exposure may reduce risk of esophageal neoplasia. However, on the other hand, unimpeded nonacid reflux in the presence of PPIs use may increase risk of neoplasia.

Several observational, non-population-based cohort studies from the United States, Australia and the Netherlands have reported a significant decrease in the risk of high-grade dysplasia (HGD)/EA associated with PPI use among BE patients [73–75]. A prospective cohort study done in Australia on 328 patients with BE concluded that delaying PPI therapy for more than two years after the diagnosis of BE increased the risk of HGD/EA 20-fold (adjusted for age, sex, non-steroidal anti-inflammatory drug [NSAID]/aspirin use). A retrospective cohort study of 344 US veterans with BE, with 2,620 patient-years of follow-up, of whom 67.2% were on PPI, determined that the risk of HGD/EA was significantly lower among the PPI users (HR 0.39, 95% CI 0.19–0.80, adjusting for gender, age at BE diagnosis, and BE length).

A multi-center prospective cohort study in 540 BE patients in the Netherlands, with a median follow-up of 5.2 years, in whom regular endoscopic surveillance was performed, found that PPIs were prescribed in 85% of patients at inclusion in the study, for a median duration of 4.0 years. The use of PPIs at inclusion was associated with reduced risk of neoplastic progression (HR 0.43; 95% CI 0.21–0.88); but after adjustment for age, gender, time of BE diagnosis, BE length, esophagitis, histology and use of other medications, the risk reduction became non-significant (HR 0.47; 95% CI 0.19–1.18). In a hospital-based, case control study of 87 EA cases and 244 BE controls without dysplasia or cancer, the OR for HGD/EA in patients using PPIs for more than six months, based on information collected by questionnaires, was 0.05 (95% CI 0.02–0.1), adjusting for age, sex, educational level, smoking status, alcohol use and reflux symptoms [76].

These studies were limited by selection bias related to the referral setting; ascertainment bias, in which patients not on PPIs may undergo more frequent endoscopy; and limited adjustment for possible confounders, such as obesity or Helicobacter pylori status. Confounding by indication is also of major concern in all these studies, even after excluding patients that started on PPIs within six months or one year before diagnosis.

There is no evidence for an effect of PPI or fundoplication [77, 78] on EA development among patients with GERD but without BE. On the contrary, most studies show that PPI use is more common among patients who develop EA, but none of the studies found an effect for PPI independent of GERD symptoms (i.e. PPI are a marker of GERD, which is the EA risk factor). In a nested case control study done in the United Kingdom [79], in which 287 cases of EA were identified and 10,000 controls were randomly sampled from the general practice research database, current use of PPI was associated with a higher, but non-significant, risk of EA – adjusted OR 1.51 (95% CI 0.91–2.50). With inclusion of GERD, peptic ulcer disease and dyspepsia in the model, the point estimate decreased to 0.84 (95% CI 0.48–1.50). Moreover, PPI was not associated with EA among patients whose main symptoms were dyspepsia or ulcer.

1.3.7 Aspirin and NSAIDs

Several observational studies have examined the use of aspirin and/or NSAIDs and their association with esophageal cancer. A meta-analysis of nine observational studies published through 2001[80] (two cohort and seven case control studies, of which five were population-based) evaluated this association among 1,813 cases of esophageal cancer and reported a 43% reduction in the odds of developing esophageal cancer in patients with a history of any use of aspirin/NSAIDs (adjusted OR 0.57, 95% CI 0.47–0.71). However, only four studies stratified their analysis by histologic subtype (EA vs. ESCC) and reported that patients taking aspirin/NSAIDs had a 33% (95% CI 13–49%) and 42% (95% CI 22–57%) reduction in odds of developing EA and ESCC, respectively.

In a subsequent meta-analysis of ten observational studies published through 2008 (one cohort, one hospital-based and seven population-based case-control, of which two were included in the previously mentioned meta-analysis) that looked specifically at EA risk associated with use of aspirin or NSAIDs, the summary OR for the use of aspirin was 0.64 (95% CI 0.52–0.79) and that for NSAIDs was 0.65 (95% CI 0.50–0.85) [81]. Nine of the ten studies showed significant negative associations, and only one did not.

In a pooled individual-level analysis of six studies (five population-based case control and one cohort) within the BEACON (Barrett's and Esophageal Adenocarcinoma Consortium), with 1266 EA cases and 5314 controls, compared with nonusers, NSAIDs users had an OR of 0.68 (95% CI 0.56–0.83). Results were similar when combining aspirin or non-aspirin NSAIDs [82]. This study also reported a decreasing risk of EA with increasing frequency of overall NSAID use, with an OR of 0.66 for occasional use and 0.56 for daily or greater use (p trend < 0.001).

In conclusion, despite the different methods used or populations studied, there seems to be a consistent negative association (approximately 40–50% risk reduction) between the use of aspirin or NSAIDs and both subtypes of esophageal cancer. Less is known about the level of protection (i.e., BE prevention or BE progression) or the type, dose or duration required, or the subgroups that are more likely to benefit.

Translating the findings from observational studies into a meaningful intervention remains elusive. One randomized trial of daily celecoxib (vs. placebo) failed to show EA risk reduction among patients with BE and low- or high-grade dysplasia after 48 weeks of randomization [83]. There is an ongoing randomized, double-blinded trial to evaluate the role of esomeprazole, with or without aspirin, in preventing EA in patients with BE "AsPECT" (clinicaltrials.gov identifier NCT00357682). However, given the additional cancer-reducing benefits of aspirin and NSAIDs, there has been a recent shift toward recommending these medications for general cancer (rather than organ-specific) chemoprevention in high-risk groups [84].

1.3.8 Statins

Experimental studies have shown that statins inhibit proliferation and angiogenesis, induce apoptosis and possibly also limit metastatic potential of cancer, especially colorectal cancer [85].

A meta-analysis of human studies published through August 2012 identified 13 studies (seven case controls, five cohorts and one post hoc analysis of 22 randomized controlled trials) [86]. These studies examined 9285 esophageal cancer cases among 1,132,969 patients. Pooled, adjusted OR for statin use and esophageal cancer was 0.72 (95% CI 0.60–0.86), and OR of 0.70 (95% CI 0.56–0.88) from the seven high-quality studies. Of these studies, six reported a significant inverse association between statin use and the risk of esophageal cancer (two from United States, three from Europe and one from Asia), and seven studies reported no significant association. Of the cohort studies, only one reported a significant association.

In patients with known BE (five studies, 312 EA cases among 2125 BE patients), statin use was associated with an adjusted OR for EA of 0.59 (95% CI 0.45–0.78). Three of the five studies reported a significant inverse association between the use of statins and the risk of EA and/or HGD (one cohort and two case-control studies), and the other two cohort studies reported a non-significant association. Several studies lacked adjustment for a potentially important confounder, such as smoking or BMI [87, 88].

Apart from the modest and somewhat inconsistent significant association among studies, the other aspects of a causal association between statins and EA are either weak or not examined. Only two studies reported the relationship between the duration of statin use and risk of esophageal cancer [88, 89]. There was no clear duration-response relationship. Furthermore, the effect of dose or type of statin is not clear.

1.3.9 Bisphosphonates

Bisphosphonates have been linked to esophageal injury [90]. The interest in bisphosphonates and esophageal cancer increased after reports of persistent mucosal abnormalities were noted in some patients who developed esophagitis secondary to use of these medications [91].Twenty-three cases were submitted to the FDA's Adverse Event Reporting System of esophageal cancer in bisphosphonate users during 1995–2008 [92]. Histological analysis showed EA in seven patients and ESCC in one patient. An additional 34 cases of esophageal cancer among bisphosphonate users were also reported from Europe and Japan. Histological analysis showed EA in six patients and ESCC in five patients. One patient from the United States and three patients from Europe and Japan concomitantly carried a diagnosis of BE. All cases reported in the United States and most cases in Europe and Japan involved alendronate as the suspect bisphosphonate.

However, subsequent population-based studies examining the association between bisphosphonate use and EA have arrived at conflicting results [93–96]. Similarly, two meta-analyses published within a few months of each other [97, 98] examined the risk of esophageal cancer in patients using bisphosphonates and reported conflicting results. One meta-analysis examined four observational studies (one prospective cohort and three nested case control studies) conducted in the United Kingdom, Denmark, Taiwan and the United States [97].

In this meta-analysis, 19,320 cases of esophageal cancer developed in 589,755 people, with a slightly elevated and significant pooled OR of 1.74 (95% CI 1.19–2.25) for exposure to any oral bisphosphonate. Only the US study examined this association among patients with BE [87]. When stratified by bisphosphonate type, alendronate use had insignificant ORs, ranging from 0.73 to 1.26, depending on which overlapping studies were included, while etidronate had a significant OR of 1.58 (95% CI 1.12–2.24) when pooling the two studies that reported on this medication.

The second meta-analysis [98] included four cohort studies and three nested case control studies. This meta-analysis included studies with overlapping study populations (two used the UK General Practice Research Database [93, 94], two used the Taiwanese National Health Insurance Research Database [99, 100] and two used the Danish national prescription and discharge registries [96, 101]). The pooled RR for development of esophageal cancer in the cohort studies was 1.23 (95% CI 0.79–1.92), while the pooled OR in the case control studies was 1.24 (95% CI 0.98–1.57). Three studies examined the duration of bisphosphonate exposure. There was increased risk in both short- and long-term use (OR 1.37 (95% CI 0.77–2.39) and 2.32 (95% CI 1.57–3.43), respectively), although long-term use had the only statistically significant association.

Given the inconsistent findings, lack of distinction between EA and ESCC, and inadequate adjustment for important confounders (such as GERD), the association between bisphosphonates and increased EA risk while possible is not definite.

1.3.10 *H. pylori* gastric infection

H. pylori increases the risk of gastric adenocarcinoma by about six-fold, with a population-attributable risk of 75–90% of cancer cases [102]. However, its association with EA has been studied; and results have shown a different type of relationship.

A meta-analysis of ten epidemiological studies (two cohort; two nested case control; two hospital-based and four population-based case control studies) published through 2/2007, found a two-fold reduction in risk of EA among people infected with *H. pylori*, with a summary OR of 0.52 (95% CI 0.31–0.82). This risk reduction was similar in cag-A positive strains [103]. The authors also looked into the association between *H. pylori* and BE (seven studies; one population-based and six hospital-based case control studies) and found similar results, with a summary OR of 0.64 (95% CI 0.43–0.94) and a more protective estimate for cag-A positive strains (OR 0.39, 95% CI 0.21–0.76).

In a more recent analysis, 13 studies (seven hospital-based, four population-based, two nested case control studies), six of which were included in the previous meta-analysis, were evaluated to examine the association between EA/HGD and *H. pylori* [104]. This study reported a summary OR for *H. pylori* in EA/HGD of 0.56 (95% CI 0.46–0.68), and an even slightly lower OR for cag-A strains of 0.41 (95% CI 0.28–0.62).

Despite the heterogeneity of studies looking into *H. pylori* and its association with EA and BE, in terms of methods of *H. pylori* detection and selection of control groups, there appears to be a consistently convincing protective association between these two factors. This effect is postulated, but not proven, to be due to the decreased acid production resulting from gastric atrophy, leading to decreased esophageal exposure to these acidic contents and, thus, a decrease in risk of BE and EA [104–106].

1.3.11 Genetics and familial factors

There are several case reports of familial GERD, BE and EA [107, 108]. For example, EA in one report developed in three members of a family that had six men, over three generations, with BE [109]. Another report identified a patient with EA with six family members who were diagnosed with BE or EA [110]. The largest study to examine familial predisposition of BE reported 20 families with multiple family members affected with BE or EA [111]. One study found a significantly higher yield of BE (40.7%) on endoscopic screening in families with familial BE (defined by one or more family member with BE or EA) than in families with sporadic cases (5.7%), although the study was small, with only 62 family members receiving endoscopy [112]. In a similar study, family members of patients with EA or HGD were invited for screening endoscopy; and 27.7% of them had confirmed BE [113]. In probands diagnosed with long-segment BE, EA or GEJ-CA, 7.3% of their first- or second-degree family members were identified as being affected by one of these three conditions [114].

Researchers have attempted to identify genetic foci related to the development of EA (and BE). A genome-wide combined linkage-association analysis, followed by an independent genome-wide

single-nucleotide polymorphism (SNP)-based case control validation, found germline mutations in 11% of BE and/or EA patients, in three candidate genes, MSR1, ASCC1 and CTHRC1 [115]. The mutation in MSR1 is associated with overexpression of cyclin D1, resulting in alteration of the cell cycle progression, which can potentially contribute to tumorigenesis [116]. The other two gene mutations involve inflammatory and tissue-repair pathways.

Several gene-association studies found associations between EA and polymorphisms of single or few genes including IL-18 [117], matrix metalloproteinase genes (MMP1 and MMP2) [118], epidermal growth factor [119], insulin-like growth factor axis [120] and vascular endothelial growth factor (VEGF) [121]. In the study evaluating MMP1 and MMP2, an increased risk of EA was found only in those who had GERD, and the study of VEGF polymorphism increased the risk only in tobacco smokers, indicating an environment-gene interaction. In a systematic review of association studies published through 2007 [122], evaluating phase I and II enzyme polymorphisms, the minor allele for GSTP1 was found to increase the risk of EA (OR 1.20, 95% I 0.94–1.54). GSTM1 null, GSTT1 null, and CYP1A Val(462) SNPs did not convey an excess risk for BE and/or EA.

In conclusion, there seems to be convincing data to support a familial tendency to develop BE and EA. No single genetic mutation has been identified as the culprit for the familiality of BE and EA, but SNPs within candidate genes that might confer the increased risk have been found by several studies. It is likely that there is a component of genetic susceptibility or environment-gene interactions towards the development of EA and its precursor, BE, but the attributable risk of specific genetic factors is unclear and likely to be small.

References

1 Boyle P, Levin B (2008). *Cancer, International Agency for Research on*. World cancer report, 2008. IARC Press.

2 Curado M, Edwards B, Shin H, Storm H, Ferlay J, Heanue M, *et al*. (2007). *Cancer Incidence in Five Continents*, Vol. **IX**. IARC Scientific Publications No. 160, Lyon, IARC.

3 SEER 9 Regs Research Data, Nov 2011 Sub, Vintage 2009 Pops (1973–2009). <Katrina/Rita Population Adjustment> – Linked To County Attributes – Total U.S., 1969–2010 Counties, National Cancer Institute, DCCPS, Surveillance

Research Program, Surveillance Systems Branch, released April 2012, based on the November 2011 submission.

4 Thrift AP, Whiteman DC (2012). The incidence of esophageal adenocarcinoma continues to rise: analysis of period and birth cohort effects on recent trends. *Annals of Oncology* **23**(12), 3155–3162.

5 Hur C, Miller M, Kong CY, Dowling EC, Nattinger KJ, Dunn M, *et al.* (2013). Trends in esophageal adenocarcinoma incidence and mortality. *Cancer* **119**(6), 1149–1158.

6 Edgren G, Adami HO, Weiderpass E, Nyren O (2013). A global assessment of the oesophageal adenocarcinoma epidemic. *Gut* **62**(10), 1406–14.

7 el-Serag HB (2002). The epidemic of esophageal adenocarcinoma. *Gastroenterology Clinics of North America* **31**(2), 421–40, viii.

8 Cook MB, Chow WH, Devesa SS (2009). Oesophageal cancer incidence in the United States by race, sex, and histologic type, 1977–2005. *British Journal of Cancer* **101**(5), 855–859.

9 Vizcaino AP, Moreno V, Lambert R, Parkin DM (2002). Time trends incidence of both major histologic types of esophageal carcinomas in selected countries, 1973–1995. *International Journal of Cancer* **99**(6), 860–868.

10 Kubo A, Block G, Quesenberry CP,Jr, Buffler P, Corley DA (2009). Effects of dietary fiber, fats, and meat intakes on the risk of Barrett's esophagus. *Nutrition and Cancer* **61**(5), 607–616.

11 El-Serag HB, Petersen NJ, Carter J, Graham DY, Richardson P, Genta RM, *et al.* (2004). Gastroesophageal reflux among different racial groups in the United States. *Gastroenterology* **126**(7), 1692–1699.

12 Dent J, El-Serag HB, Wallander MA, Johansson S (2005). Epidemiology of gastro-oesophageal reflux disease: a systematic review. *Gut* **54**(5), 710–717.

13 Cook MB, Wild CP, Forman D (2005). A systematic review and meta-analysis of the sex ratio for Barrett's esophagus, erosive reflux disease, and nonerosive reflux disease. *American Journal of Epidemiology* **162**(11), 1050–1061.

14 Surveillance, Epidemiology, and End Results (SEER). Program (www.seer.cancer.gov) SEER*Stat Database: Incidence – SEER 18 Regs Research Data + Hurricane Katrina Impacted Louisiana Cases, Nov 2012 Sub (2000–2010) – Linked To County Attributes – Total U.S., 1969–2011 Counties, National Cancer Institute, DCCPS, Surveillance Research Program, Surveillance Systems Branch, released April 2013, based on the November 2012 submission.

15 Revels SL, Morris AM, Reddy RM, Akateh C, Wong SL (2013). Racial disparities in esophageal cancer outcomes. *Annals of Surgical Oncology* **20**(4), 1136–1141.

16 Lenglinger J, Riegler M, Cosentini E, Asari R, Mesteri I, Wrba F, *et al.* (2012). Review on the annual cancer risk of Barrett's esophagus in persons with symptoms of gastroesophageal reflux disease. *AntiCancer Research* **32**(12), 5465–5473.

17 Lagergren J, Lagergren P (2013). Recent developments in esophageal adenocarcinoma. *CA: A Cancer Journal for Clinicians* **63**(4), 232–248.

18 de Jonge PJ, van Blankenstein M, Looman CW, Casparie MK, Meijer GA, Kuipers EJ (2010). Risk of malignant progression in patients with Barrett's oesophagus: a Dutch nationwide cohort study. *Gut* **59**(8), 1030–1036.

19 Bhat S, Coleman HG, Yousef F, Johnston BT, McManus DT, Gavin AT, *et al.* (2011). Risk of malignant progression in Barrett's esophagus patients: results from a large population-based study. *Journal of the National Cancer Institute* **103**(13), 1049–1057.

20 Hvid-Jensen F, Pedersen L, Drewes AM, Sorensen HT, Funch-Jensen P (2011). Incidence of adenocarcinoma among patients with Barrett's esophagus. *New England Journal of Medicine* **365**(15), 1375–1383.

21 Chow WH, Finkle WD, McLaughlin JK, Frankl H, Ziel HK, Fraumeni JF, Jr. (1995). The relation of gastroesophageal reflux disease and its treatment to adenocarcinomas of the esophagus and gastric cardia. *JAMA* **274**(6), 474–477.

22 Lagergren J, Bergstrom R, Lindgren A, Nyren O (1999). Symptomatic gastroesophageal reflux as a risk factor for esophageal adenocarcinoma. *New England Journal of Medicine* **340**(11), 825–831.

23 Rubenstein JH, Taylor JB (2010). Meta-analysis: the association of oesophageal adenocarcinoma with symptoms of gastro-oesophageal reflux. *Alimentary Pharmacology & Therapeutics* **32**(10), 1222–1227.

24 Lubin JH, Cook MB, Pandeya N, Vaughan TL, Abnet CC, Giffen C, *et al.* (2012). The importance of exposure rate on odds ratios by cigarette smoking and alcohol consumption for esophageal adenocarcinoma and squamous cell carcinoma in the Barrett's Esophagus and Esophageal Adenocarcinoma Consortium. *Cancer Epidemiology* **36**(3), 306–316.

25 Steevens J, Schouten LJ, Goldbohm RA, van den Brandt PA (2010). Alcohol consumption, cigarette smoking and risk of subtypes of oesophageal and gastric cancer: a prospective cohort study. *Gut* **59**(1), 39–48.

26 Steevens J, Schouten LJ, Driessen AL, Huysentruyt CJ, Keulemans YC, Goldbohm RA, *et al.* (2011). A prospective cohort study on overweight, smoking, alcohol consumption, and risk of Barrett's esophagus. *Cancer Epidemiology, Biomarkers & Prevention* **20**(2), 345–358.

27 Hardikar S, Onstad L, Blount PL, Odze RD, Reid BJ, Vaughan TL (2013). The role of tobacco, alcohol, and obesity in neoplastic progression to esophageal adenocarcinoma: a prospective study of Barrett's esophagus. *PLoS One* **8**(1), e52192.

28 Vaughan TL, Davis S, Kristal A, Thomas DB (1995). Obesity, alcohol, and tobacco as risk factors for cancers of the esophagus and gastric cardia: adenocarcinoma versus squamous cell carcinoma. *Cancer Epidemiology, Biomarkers & Prevention* **4**(2), 85–92.

29 Engel LS, Chow WH, Vaughan TL, Gammon MD, Risch HA, Stanford JL, *et al.* (2003). Population attributable risks of esophageal and gastric cancers. *Journal of the National Cancer Institute* **95**(18), 1404–1413.

30 Gammon MD, Schoenberg JB, Ahsan H, Risch HA, Vaughan TL, Chow WH, *et al.* (1997). Tobacco, alcohol, and socioeconomic status and adenocarcinomas of the esophagus and gastric cardia. *Journal of the National Cancer Institute* **89**(17), 1277–1284.

31 Lagergren J, Bergstrom R, Lindgren A, Nyren O (2000). The role of tobacco, snuff and alcohol use in the aetiology of cancer of the oesophagus and gastric cardia. *International Journal of Cancer* **85**(3), 340–346.

32 Wu AH, Wan P, Bernstein L. A multiethnic population-based study of smoking, alcohol and body size and risk of adenocarcinomas of the stomach and esophagus (United States). *Cancer Causes and Control* (2001). **12**(8), 721–732.

33 Lindblad M, Rodriguez LA, Lagergren J (2005). Body mass, tobacco and alcohol and risk of esophageal, gastric cardia, and gastric non-cardia adenocarcinoma among men and women in a nested case-control study. *Cancer Causes and Control* **16**(3), 285–294.

34 Anderson LA, Cantwell MM, Watson RG, Johnston BT, Murphy SJ, Ferguson HR, *et al.* (2009). The association between alcohol and reflux esophagitis, Barrett's esophagus, and esophageal adenocarcinoma. *Gastroenterology* **136**(3), 799–805.

35 Kubo A, Levin TR, Block G, Rumore GJ, Quesenberry CP, , Buffler P, *et al.* (2009). Alcohol types and sociodemographic characteristics as risk factors for Barrett's esophagus. *Gastroenterology* **136**(3), 806–815.

36 Pandeya N, Williams G, Green AC, Webb PM, Whiteman DC, (2009). Australian Cancer Study. Alcohol consumption and the risks of adenocarcinoma and squamous cell carcinoma of the esophagus. *Gastroenterology* **136**(4), 1215–24, e1–2.

37 El-Serag HB, Lagergren J (2009). Alcohol drinking and the risk of Barrett's esophagus and esophageal adenocarcinoma. *Gastroenterology* **136**(4), 1155–1157.

38 Brown LM, Swanson CA, Gridley G, Swanson GM, Schoenberg JB, Greenberg RS, (1995). *et al.* Adenocarcinoma of the esophagus: role of obesity and diet. *Journal of the National Cancer Institute* **87**(2), 104–109.

39 Chow WH, Blot WJ, Vaughan TL, Risch HA, Gammon MD, Stanford JL, *et al.* (1998). Body mass index and risk of adenocarcinomas of the esophagus and gastric cardia. *Journal of the National Cancer Institute* **90**(2), 150–155.

40 Lagergren J, Bergstrom R, Nyren O (1999). Association between body mass and adenocarcinoma of the esophagus and gastric cardia. *Annals of Internal Medicine* **130**(11), 883–890.

41 Cheng KK, Sharp L, McKinney PA, Logan RF, Chilvers CE, Cook-Mozaffari P, *et al.* (2000). A case-control study of oesophageal adenocarcinoma in women: a preventable disease. *British Journal of Cancer* **83**(1), 127–132.

42 Bollschweiler E, Wolfgarten E, Nowroth T, Rosendahl U, Monig SP, Holscher AH (2002). Vitamin intake and risk of subtypes of esophageal cancer in Germany. *Journal of Cancer Research and Clinical Oncology* **128**(10), 575–580.

43 Ryan AM, Rowley SP, Fitzgerald AP, Ravi N, Reynolds JV (2006). Adenocarcinoma of the oesophagus and gastric cardia: male preponderance in association with obesity. *European Journal of Cancer* **42**(8), 1151–1158.

44 Veugelers PJ, Porter GA, Guernsey DL, Casson AG (2006). Obesity and lifestyle risk factors for gastroesophageal reflux disease, Barrett esophagus and esophageal adenocarcinoma. *Diseases of the Esophagus* **19**(5), 321–328.

45 Anderson LA, Watson RG, Murphy SJ, Johnston BT, Comber H, Mc Guigan J, *et al.* (2007). Risk factors for Barrett's oesophagus and oesophageal adenocarcinoma: results from the FINBAR study. *World Journal of Gastroenterology* **13**(10), 1585–1594.

46 Lofdahl HE, Lu Y, Lagergren J (2008). Sex-specific risk factor profile in oesophageal adenocarcinoma. *British Journal of Cancer* **99**(9), 1506–1510.

47 Whiteman DC, Sadeghi S, Pandeya N, Smithers BM, Gotley DC, Bain CJ, *et al.* (2008). Combined effects of obesity, acid reflux and smoking on the risk of adenocarcinomas of the oesophagus. *Gut* **57**(2), 173–180.

48 Engeland A, Tretli S, Bjorge T (2004). Height and body mass index in relation to esophageal cancer; 23-year follow-up of two million Norwegian men and women. *Cancer Causes and Control* **15**(8), 837–843.

49 Samanic C, Chow WH, Gridley G, Jarvholm B, Fraumeni JF, Jr. (2006). Relation of body mass index to cancer risk in 362,552 Swedish men. *Cancer Causes and Control* **17**(7), 901–909.

50 Merry AH, Schouten LJ, Goldbohm RA, van den Brandt PA (2007). Body mass index, height and risk of adenocarcinoma of the oesophagus and gastric cardia: a prospective cohort study. *Gut* **56**(11), 1503–1511.

51 Reeves GK, Pirie K, Beral V, Green J, Spencer E, Bull D, *et al.* (2007). Cancer incidence and mortality in relation to body mass index in the Million Women Study: cohort study. *BMJ* **335**(7630), 1134.

52 Abnet CC, Freedman ND, Hollenbeck AR, Fraumeni JF, Jr, Leitzmann M, Schatzkin A (2008). A prospective study of BMI and risk of oesophageal and gastric adenocarcinoma. *European Journal of Cancer* **44**(3), 465–471.

53 Corley DA, Kubo A, Zhao W (2008). Abdominal obesity and the risk of esophageal and gastric cardia carcinomas. *Cancer Epidemiology, Biomarkers & Prevention* **17**(2), 352–358.

54 Steffen A, Schulze MB, Pischon T, Dietrich T, Molina E, Chirlaque MD, *et al.* (2009). Anthropometry and esophageal cancer risk in the European prospective investigation into cancer and nutrition. *Cancer Epidemiology, Biomarkers & Prevention* **18**(7), 2079–2089.

55 Hampel H, Abraham NS, El-Serag HB (2005). Meta-analysis: obesity and the risk for gastroesophageal reflux

disease and its complications. *Annals of Internal Medicine* **143**(3), 199–211.

56 Kubo A, Corley DA (2006). Body mass index and adenocarcinomas of the esophagus or gastric cardia: a systematic review and meta-analysis. *Cancer Epidemiology, Biomarkers & Prevention* **15**(5), 872–878.

57 Turati F, Tramacere I, La Vecchia C, Negri E (2013). A meta-analysis of body mass index and esophageal and gastric cardia adenocarcinoma. *Annals of Oncology* **24**(3), 609–617.

58 El-Serag H (2008). Role of obesity in GORD-related disorders. *Gut* **57**(3), 281–284.

59 Akiyama T, Yoneda M, Maeda S, Nakajima A, Koyama S, Inamori M (2011). Visceral obesity and the risk of Barrett's esophagus. *Digestion* **83**(3), 142–145.

60 MacInnis RJ, English DR, Hopper JL, Giles GG (2006). Body size and composition and the risk of gastric and oesophageal adenocarcinoma. *International Journal of Cancer* **118**(10), 2628–2631.

61 O'Doherty MG, Freedman ND, Hollenbeck AR, Schatzkin A, Abnet CC (2012). A prospective cohort study of obesity and risk of oesophageal and gastric adenocarcinoma in the NIH-AARP Diet and Health Study. *Gut* **61**(9), 1261–1268.

62 Beddy P, Howard J, McMahon C, Knox M, de Blacam C, Ravi N, *et al.* (2010). Association of visceral adiposity with oesophageal and junctional adenocarcinomas. *British Journal of Surgery* **97**(7), 1028–1034.

63 Singh S, Sharma AN, Murad MH, Buttar NS, El-Serag HB, Katzka DA, *et al.* (2013). Central Adiposity is Associated with Increased Risk of Esophageal Inflammation, Metaplasia, and Adenocarcinoma: a Systematic Review and Meta-Analysis. *Clinical Gastroenterology and Hepatology* **11**(11), 1399–1412.

64 World *Cancer Research* Fund/American Institute for Cancer Research (2007). *Food, Nutrition, Physical Activity, and the Prevention of Cancer: a Global Perspective*. Washington DC. AICR.

65 Kubo A, Corley DA (2007). Meta-analysis of antioxidant intake and the risk of esophageal and gastric cardia adenocarcinoma. *American Journal of Gastroenterology* **102**(10), 2323–30; quiz 2331.

66 Bjelakovic G, Nikolova D, Simonetti RG, Gluud C (2008). Systematic review: primary and secondary prevention of gastrointestinal cancers with antioxidant supplements. *Alimentary Pharmacology & Therapeutics* **28**(6), 689–703.

67 Larsson SC, Giovannucci E, Wolk A (2006). Folate intake, MTHFR polymorphisms, and risk of esophageal, gastric, and pancreatic cancer: a meta-analysis. *Gastroenterology* **131**(4), 1271–1283.

68 Terry P, Lagergren J, Ye W, Wolk A, Nyren O (2001). Inverse association between intake of cereal fiber and risk of gastric cardia cancer. *Gastroenterology* **120**(2), 387–391.

69 De Ceglie A, Fisher DA, Filiberti R, Blanchi S, Conio M (2011). Barrett's esophagus, esophageal and esophagogastric junction adenocarcinomas: the role

of diet. *Clinics and Research in Hepatology and Gastroenterology* **35**(1), 7–16.

70 Salehi M, Moradi-Lakeh M, Salehi MH, Nojomi M, Kolahdooz F (2013). Meat, fish, and esophageal cancer risk: a systematic review and dose-response meta-analysis. *Nutrition Reviews* **71**(5), 257–267.

71 Kubo A, Corley DA, Jensen CD, Kaur R (2010). Dietary factors and the risks of oesophageal adenocarcinoma and Barrett's oesophagus. *Nutrition Research Reviews* **23**(2), 230–246.

72 Aitken M, Kleinrock M (2012). *Declining Medicine Use and Costs: For Better or Worse? A Review of the Use of Medicines in the United States in 2012*. IMS Institute for Healthcare Informatics.

73 Nguyen DM, El-Serag HB, Henderson L, Stein D, Bhattacharyya A, Sampliner RE (2009). Medication usage and the risk of neoplasia in patients with Barrett's esophagus. *Clinical Gastroenterology and Hepatology* **7**(12), 1299–1304.

74 Hillman LC, Chiragakis L, Shadbolt B, Kaye GL, Clarke AC (2004). Proton-pump inhibitor therapy and the development of dysplasia in patients with Barrett's oesophagus. *Medical Journal of Australia* **180**(8), 387–391.

75 Kastelein F, Spaander MC, Steyerberg EW, Biermann K, Valkhoff VE, Kuipers EJ, *et al.* (2013). Proton pump inhibitors reduce the risk of neoplastic progression in patients with Barrett's esophagus. *Clinical Gastroenterology and Hepatology* **11**(4), 382–388.

76 de Jonge PJ, Steyerberg EW, Kuipers EJ, Honkoop P, Wolters LM, Kerkhof M, *et al.* (2006). Risk factors for the development of esophageal adenocarcinoma in Barrett's esophagus. *American Journal of Gastroenterology* **101**(7), 1421–1429.

77 Ye W, Chow WH, Lagergren J, Yin L, Nyren O (2001). Risk of adenocarcinomas of the esophagus and gastric cardia in patients with gastroesophageal reflux diseases and after antireflux surgery. *Gastroenterology* **121**(6), 1286–1293.

78 Tran T, Spechler SJ, Richardson P, El-Serag HB (2005). Fundoplication and the risk of esophageal cancer in gastroesophageal reflux disease: a Veterans Affairs cohort study. *American Journal of Gastroenterology* **100**(5), 1002–1008.

79 Garcia Rodriguez LA, Lagergren J, Lindblad M (2006). Gastric acid suppression and risk of oesophageal and gastric adenocarcinoma: a nested case control study in the UK. *Gut* **55**(11), 1538–1544.

80 Corley DA, Kerlikowske K, Verma R, Buffler P (2003). Protective association of aspirin/NSAIDs and esophageal cancer: a systematic review and meta-analysis. *Gastroenterology* **124**(1), 47–56.

81 Abnet CC, Freedman ND, Kamangar F, Leitzmann MF, Hollenbeck AR, Schatzkin A (2009). Non-steroidal anti-inflammatory drugs and risk of gastric and oesophageal adenocarcinomas: results from a cohort study and a meta-analysis. *British Journal of Cancer* **100**(3), 551–557.

82 Liao LM, Vaughan TL, Corley DA, Cook MB, Casson AG, Kamangar F, *et al.* (2012). Nonsteroidal anti-inflammatory drug use reduces risk of adenocarcinomas of the esophagus and esophagogastric junction in a pooled analysis. *Gastroenterology* **142**(3), 442–452.e5; quiz e22–3.

83 Heath EI, Canto MI, Piantadosi S, Montgomery E, Weinstein WM, Herman JG, *et al.* (2007). Secondary chemoprevention of Barrett's esophagus with celecoxib: results of a randomized trial. *Journal of the National Cancer Institute* **99**(7), 545–557.

84 Chan AT, Detering E (2013). An emerging role for anti-inflammatory agents for chemoprevention. *Recent Results in Cancer Research* **191**, 1–5.

85 Alexandre L, Clark AB, Cheong E, Lewis MP, Hart AR (2012). Systematic review: potential preventive effects of statins against oesophageal adenocarcinoma. *Alimentary Pharmacology & Therapeutics* **36**(4), 301–311.

86 Singh S, Singh AG, Singh PP, Murad MH, Iyer PG (2013). Statins are associated with reduced risk of esophageal cancer, particularly in patients with Barrett's esophagus: a systematic review and meta-analysis. *Clinical Gastroenterology and Hepatology* **11**(6), 620–629.

87 Nguyen DM, Richardson P, El-Serag HB (2010). Medications (NSAIDs, statins, proton pump inhibitors) and the risk of esophageal adenocarcinoma in patients with Barrett's esophagus. *Gastroenterology* **138**(7), 2260–2266.

88 Kastelein F, Spaander MC, Biermann K, Steyerberg EW, Kuipers EJ, Bruno MJ, *et al.* (2011). Nonsteroidal anti-inflammatory drugs and statins have chemopreventative effects in patients with Barrett's esophagus. *Gastroenterology* **141**(6), (2000)-8; quiz e13–4.

89 Beales IL, Vardi I, Dearman L, Broughton T (2012). Statin use is associated with a reduction in the incidence of esophageal adenocarcinoma: a case control study. *Diseases of the Esophagus* **26**(8), 838–46.

90 de Groen PC, Lubbe DF, Hirsch LJ, Daifotis A, Stephenson W, Freedholm D, *et al.* (1996). Esophagitis associated with the use of alendronate. *New England Journal of Medicine* **335**(14), 1016–1021.

91 Ribeiro A, DeVault KR, Wolfe JT, 3rd, Stark ME (1998). Alendronate-associated esophagitis: endoscopic and pathologic features. *Gastrointestinal Endoscopy* **47**(6), 525–528.

92 Wysowski DK (2009). Reports of esophageal cancer with oral bisphosphonate use. *New England Journal of Medicine* **360**(1), 89–90.

93 Green J, Czanner G, Reeves G, Watson J, Wise L, Beral V (2010). Oral bisphosphonates and risk of cancer of oesophagus, stomach, and colorectum: case-control analysis within a UK primary care cohort. *BMJ* **341**, c4444.

94 Cardwell CR, Abnet CC, Cantwell MM, Murray LJ (2010). Exposure to oral bisphosphonates and risk of esophageal cancer. *JAMA* **304**(6), 657–663.

95 Ho YF, Lin JT, Wu CY (2012). Oral bisphosphonates and risk of esophageal cancer: a dose-intensity analysis in a nationwide population. *Cancer Epidemiology, Biomarkers & Prevention* **21**(6), 993–995.

96 Abrahamsen B, Pazianas M, Eiken P, Russell RG, Eastell R (2012). Esophageal and gastric cancer incidence and mortality in alendronate users. *Journal of Bone and Mineral Research* **27**(3), 679–686.

97 Andrici J, Tio M, Eslick GD (2012). Meta-analysis: oral bisphosphonates and the risk of oesophageal cancer. *Alimentary Pharmacology & Therapeutics* **36**(8), 708–716.

98 Sun K, Liu JM, Sun HX, Lu N, Ning G (2013). Bisphosphonate treatment and risk of esophageal cancer: a meta-analysis of observational studies. *Osteoporosis International* **24**(1), 279–286.

99 Chen YM, Chen DY, Chen LK, Tsai YW, Chang LC, Huang WF, *et al.* (2011). Alendronate and risk of esophageal cancer: a nationwide population-based study in Taiwan. *Journal of the American Geriatrics Society* **59**(12), 2379–2381.

100 Chiang CH, Huang CC, Chan WL, Huang PH, Chen TJ, Chung CM, *et al.* (2012). Oral alendronate use and risk of cancer in postmenopausal women with osteoporosis: A nationwide study. *Journal of Bone and Mineral Research* **27**(9), 1951–1958.

101 Vestergaard P (2011). Occurrence of gastrointestinal cancer in users of bisphosphonates and other antiresorptive drugs against osteoporosis. *Calcified Tissue International* **89**(6), 434–441.

102 de Martel C, Ferlay J, Franceschi S, Vignat J, Bray F, Forman D, *et al.* (2012). Global burden of cancers attributable to infections in 2008 – a review and synthetic analysis. *The Lancet Oncology* **13**(6), 607–615.

103 Rokkas T, Pistiolas D, Sechopoulos P, Robotis I, Margantinis G (2007). Relationship between Helicobacter pylori infection and esophageal neoplasia: a meta-analysis. *Clinical Gastroenterology and Hepatology* **5**(12), 1413–7, 1417.e1–2.

104 Islami F, Kamangar F (2008). Helicobacter pylori and esophageal cancer risk: a meta-analysis. *Cancer Prevention Research (Phila)* **1**(5), 329–338.

105 Blaser MJ (2008). Disappearing microbiota: *Helicobacter pylori* protection against esophageal adenocarcinoma. *Cancer Prevention Research (Phila)* **1**(5), 308–311.

106 Whiteman DC, Parmar P, Fahey P, Moore SP, Stark M, Zhao ZZ, *et al.* (2010). Association of *Helicobacter pylori* infection with reduced risk for esophageal cancer is independent of environmental and genetic modifiers. *Gastroenterology* **139**(1), 73–83; quiz e11–2.

107 Gelfand MD (1983). Barrett esophagus in sexagenarian identical twins. *Journal of Clinical Gastroenterology* **5**(3), 251–253.

108 Prior A, Whorwell PJ (1986). Familial Barrett's oesophagus? *Hepato-Gastroenterology* **33**(2), 86–87.

109 Jochem VJ, Fuerst PA, Fromkes JJ (1992). Familial Barrett's esophagus associated with adenocarcinoma. *Gastroenterology* **102**(4, pt 1), 1400–1402.

110 Eng C, Spechler SJ, Ruben R, Li FP (1993). Familial Barrett esophagus and adenocarcinoma of the gastroesophageal junction. *Cancer Epidemiology, Biomarkers & Prevention* **2**(4), 397–399.

111 Sappati Biyyani RS, Chessler L, McCain E, Nelson K, Fahmy N, King J (2007). Familial trends of inheritance in gastro esophageal reflux disease, Barrett's esophagus and Barrett's adenocarcinoma: 20 families. *Diseases of the Esophagus* **20**(1), 53–57.

112 Chak A, Faulx A, Kinnard M, Brock W, Willis J, Wiesner GL, et al. (2004). Identification of Barrett's esophagus in relatives by endoscopic screening. *American Journal of Gastroenterology* **99**(11), 2107–2114.

113 Juhasz A, Mittal SK, Lee TH, Deng C, Chak A, Lynch HT (2011). Prevalence of Barrett esophagus in first-degree relatives of patients with esophageal adenocarcinoma. *Journal of Clinical Gastroenterology* **45**(10), 867–871.

114 Chak A, Ochs-Balcom H, Falk G, Grady WM, Kinnard M, Willis JE, et al. (2006). Familiality in Barrett's esophagus, adenocarcinoma of the esophagus, and adenocarcinoma of the gastroesophageal junction. *Cancer Epidemiology, Biomarkers & Prevention* **15**(9), 1668–1673.

115 Orloff M, Peterson C, He X, Ganapathi S, Heald B, Yang YR, et al. (2011). Germline mutations in MSR1, ASCC1, and CTHRC1 in patients with Barrett esophagus and esophageal adenocarcinoma. *JAMA* **306**(4), 410–419.

116 Shan J, Zhao W, Gu W (2009). Suppression of cancer cell growth by promoting cyclin D1 degradation. *Molecular Cell* **36**(3), 469–476.

117 Babar M, Ryan AW, Anderson LA, Segurado R, Turner G, Murray LJ, et al. (2012). Genes of the interleukin-18 pathway are associated with susceptibility to Barrett's esophagus and esophageal adenocarcinoma. *American Journal of Gastroenterology* **107**(9), 1331–1341.

118 Cheung WY, Zhai R, Bradbury P, Hopkins J, Kulke MH, Heist RS, et al. (2012). Single nucleotide polymorphisms in the matrix metalloproteinase gene family and the frequency and duration of gastroesophageal reflux disease influence the risk of esophageal adenocarcinoma. *International Journal of Cancer* **131**(11), 2478–2486.

119 Menke V, Pot RG, Moons LM, van Zoest KP, Hansen B, van Dekken H, et al. (2012). Functional single-nucleotide polymorphism of epidermal growth factor is associated with the development of Barrett's esophagus and esophageal adenocarcinoma. *Journal of Human Genetics* **57**(1), 26–32.

120 McElholm AR, McKnight AJ, Patterson CC, Johnston BT, Hardie LJ, Murray LJ, et al. (2010). A population-based study of IGF axis polymorphisms and the esophageal inflammation, metaplasia, adenocarcinoma sequence. *Gastroenterology* **139**(1), 204–12.e3.

121 Zhai R, Liu G, Asomaning K, Su L, Kulke MH, Heist RS, et al. (2008). Genetic polymorphisms of VEGF, interactions with cigarette smoking exposure and esophageal adenocarcinoma risk. *Carcinogenesis* **29**(12), 2330–2334.

122 Bull LM, White DL, Bray M, Nurgalieva Z, El-Serag HB (2009). Phase I and II enzyme polymorphisms as risk factors for Barrett's esophagus and esophageal adenocarcinoma: a systematic review and meta-analysis. *Diseases of the Esophagus* **22**(7), 571–587.

CHAPTER 2

Barrett's esophagus: definition and diagnosis

Stuart Jon Spechler

Department of Gastroenterology, UT Southwestern Medical Center at Dallas; and Division of Gastroenterology, Dallas VA Medical Center, VA North Texas Healthcare System, Dallas, TX, USA

2.1 Introduction

Stratified squamous epithelium lines virtually the entire normal esophagus. The metaplastic columnar epithelium that lines Barrett's esophagus is the precursor of esophageal adenocarcinoma, a deadly cancer whose frequency has increased more than 600% over the past several decades [1]. It has been estimated that Barrett's esophagus affects approximately 2% to 7% of adults in the general population of Western countries [2, 3]. Despite the great frequency and clinical importance of the condition, however, there has not been universal consensus regarding the definition of Barrett's esophagus. Even today, there are substantial disagreements among major medical societies regarding the definition and diagnostic criteria for Barrett's esophagus [4, 5]. To appreciate why the very definition of this common disorder has been such a contentious issue requires some knowledge of the relatively brief but turbulent history of the condition.

2.2 Early history of Barrett's esophagus

Barrett's esophagus is named for Norman Rupert Barrett, a thoracic surgeon born in Adelaide, Australia, in 1903 [6]. Barrett worked as a consultant surgeon at St. Thomas' Hospital in London, and he drew attention to the condition that now bears his name in a report that he published in 1950 [7]. Barrett served for more than 25 years as the editor of *Thorax* and, by all accounts, he was an excellent and charismatic surgeon, scholar, and teacher. Norman Barrett was not the first to describe the columnar-lined esophagus, however.

In 1906, Tileston, a pathologist, described several patients who had "peptic ulcer of the oesophagus" and noted "the close resemblance of the mucous membrane about the ulcer to that normally found in the stomach" [8]. Subsequently, but still before Barrett, a number of investigators also described patients with peptic ulcerations in an esophagus lined by a gastric-type columnar mucosa [9–15]. Some of those investigators argued that the ulcerated, columnar-lined organ was not esophagus at all, but rather a tubular segment of stomach that had been tethered within the chest by a congenitally short, squamous-lined esophagus [15]. Barrett supported this view in his 1950 publication, contending that the esophagus should be defined as "that part of the foregut, distal to the cricopharyngeal sphincter, which is lined by squamous epithelium" [7]. By Barrett's original definition, therefore, the columnar-lined organ that we now call "Barrett's esophagus" is misnamed, because he defined the esophagus by its squamous lining.

Although early authorities disagreed about whether the columnar-lined, intrathoracic organ was esophagus or stomach, they did agree that the organ was lined by gastric-type columnar mucosa. For example, Lyall wrote that the columnar-lined esophagus had "a resemblance to that normally found towards the pyloric end of the stomach, the glands being fairly short and wide. Oxyntic cells were present but were comparatively few in number" [11]. None of those early authorities, including Norman Barrett himself, described a columnar lining with intestinal features that included goblet cells. In 1951, Bosher and Taylor described a woman with a long esophageal segment lined by "gastric mucosa composed of glands which contained goblet cells, but no parietal cells" [16]. In 1952, Morson and Belcher also described goblet cells in their report of a patient with

Esophageal Cancer and Barrett's Esophagus, Third Edition. Edited by Prateek Sharma, Richard Sampliner and David Ilson.
© 2015 John Wiley & Sons, Ltd. Published 2015 by John Wiley & Sons, Ltd.

adenocarcinoma in an esophageal mucosa exhibiting "atrophic changes with a tendency towards intestinal type containing many goblet cells" [17].

In 1953, Allison and Johnstone disagreed with Barrett, arguing convincingly that the columnar-lined thoracic organ must be esophagus because, unlike the stomach, it lacked a peritoneal covering, and it had esophageal-type muscularis propria and submucosal glands [18]. In 1957, Barrett finally agreed that the organ was in fact esophagus, and not stomach, and suggested that the condition should be called "lower esophagus lined by columnar epithelium" [19]. Nevertheless, the term "Barrett's esophagus" has persisted, and it is now firmly entrenched in medical jargon, literature and practice.

The pathogenesis of the columnar-lined esophagus was disputed throughout the 1950s. Although Barrett and Allison recognized that the condition was associated with hiatal hernia and severe reflux esophagitis, they assumed, nevertheless, that the esophageal columnar lining was congenital in origin [18]. In 1959, Moersch contended that the columnar lining was acquired as a consequence of reflux esophagitis. Since then, virtually all investigators have agreed that Barrett's esophagus is an acquired condition [20, 21].

In 1961, the Australian surgeon John Hayward contended that the normal distal esophagus must be lined by a short segment of mucus-secreting, junctional-type epithelium, in order to protect the organ from the peptic digestion that would result if an acid-secreting gastric epithelium joined the acid-sensitive esophageal squamous epithelium directly [22]. Although Hayward's contention was based far more on opinion than on data, many authorities accepted his proposal that the very distal esophagus is normally lined by columnar epithelium.

2.3 Early reports on the histology of Barrett's esophagus

Ever since Norman Barrett's description of the condition, the histology of Barrett's esophagus has been a controversial issue. In biopsy specimens from the columnar-lined esophagus, some early investigators found the junctional-type epithelium proposed as normal by Hayward [23], while some found an acid-secreting, gastric fundic-type of epithelium

[14, 25], and others described an intestinal type of epithelium with prominent goblet cells [25–27].

In 1976, Paull et al. described 11 patients with Barrett's esophagus who had biopsy specimens taken using manometric guidance to ensure that the specimens came from the esophagus proximal to the lower esophageal sphincter (LES) [28]. Those patients were found to have one, or a combination, of three types of columnar epithelia lining the distal esophagus:

1 junctional-type epithelium (also known as cardiac epithelium), comprised almost exclusively of mucus-secreting cells;

2 an atrophic gastric fundic-type epithelium (also called oxyntocardiac epithelium) that contained acid-secreting parietal cells;

3 an incomplete form of intestinal metaplasia that the investigators called specialized columnar epithelium (also known as specialized intestinal metaplasia). This specialized intestinal metaplasia was readily identified by its prominent goblet cells.

The three epithelial types were noted to occupy different zones in the esophagus, with specialized intestinal metaplasia found adjacent to squamous epithelium in the most proximal segment of the columnar-lined esophagus, followed by junctional-type and, most distally, by atrophic gastric fundic-type epithelium. For a number of years following the publication of these findings, the demonstration of any one or combination of these three columnar epithelial types in the esophagus was accepted as evidence of Barrett's esophagus.

2.4 Identification of the gastroesophageal junction

Identification of the gastroesophageal junction (GEJ) is another contentious issue that has confounded investigations on Barrett's esophagus. To recognize that the esophagus is lined by columnar epithelium, endoscopists first must identify the GEJ, then ascertain that columnar epithelium extends proximal to that junction. Conceptually, the GEJ is the line at which the esophagus ends and the stomach begins. Practically, there are no universally accepted and clearly reproducible landmarks that identify the GEJ with great precision. This lack of precise landmarks can result in both false-positive and false-negative diagnoses for Barrett's esophagus.

In Western countries, endoscopists generally identify the GEJ as the most proximal extent of the gastric folds. This landmark was proposed in 1987 in a report of a study that included only four "normal" controls, so identified because they had "no clinical evidence of esophageal disease" [29]. This study can be criticized both for the small number of control subjects and for the lack of documentation that the controls were, indeed, normal. In fact, the report described hiatal hernias in three of the four control subjects, and one had reflux esophagitis. Even if one ignores the numerous flaws of this report, the GEJ, defined by the proximal extent of gastric folds, is a dynamic structure that cannot be localized with great precision. The location of the proximal extent of gastric folds is affected by respiration, by gut motor activity and by the degree of distention of the esophagus and stomach, all of which change from moment to moment during an endoscopic examination.

In a number of Asian countries like Japan, endoscopists do not accept the proximal extent of the gastric folds as the endoscopic landmark for the GEJ. Instead, they define the GEJ as the distal extent of the palisade vessels, which are fine, longitudinal veins located in the lamina propria of the distal esophagus [30, 31]. Unfortunately, this landmark also has substantial shortcomings as a marker for the GEJ. The palisade vessels can be obscured by esophagitis, and their level of termination can be irregular and difficult to localize with precision. Even in autopsy studies in which blood vessels of the GEJ region are injected with resins that provide exquisite detail of the venous structures, it can be difficult to identify precisely the termination of the palisade vessels [31]. Conceptually, furthermore, it is not clear why the distal end of the palisade vessels should be considered the end of the esophagus. Thus, the scientific validity of the two most widely used landmarks for the GEJ is dubious. Inter-observer agreement among endoscopists in identifying the GEJ using either landmark is poor, and the two landmarks often do not coincide in location [32].

The issue of the "best" landmark for the GEJ is likely to remain controversial indefinitely because, with no clear-cut "gold standard", the choice of any such landmark ultimately must be arbitrary. The majority of published studies on Barrett's esophagus conducted over the past 20 years have used the proximal extent of the gastric folds as the landmark for the GEJ and, in the absence of compelling data for the use of alternative markers, it seems reasonable to use this landmark, despite its shortcomings.

2.5 Recognition of short segment Barrett's esophagus

Large hiatal hernias and severe reflux esophagitis can obscure endoscopic features of the distal esophagus and can thus make it especially difficult to identify the GEJ with precision. If an endoscopist mistakenly localizes the GEJ within a hiatal hernia, the result is a false-positive diagnosis of columnar-lined esophagus. Even if the GEJ could be identified with great precision, Hayward had contended that the esophagus normally could be lined by up to 2 cm of junctional-type epithelium [22]. This feature also might lead to false-positive diagnoses of Barrett's esophagus if this "normal" junctional epithelium were interpreted as metaplastic.

In the 1980s, investigators intent on avoiding the problem of false-positive diagnoses established arbitrary criteria for the extent of esophageal columnar lining needed to include patients in studies on Barrett's esophagus [29, 33, 34]. Those arbitrary investigative criteria, which ranged from 2–5 cm and were designed to minimize false-positive diagnoses of Barrett's esophagus, became adopted by clinicians. As a result, endoscopists in the 1980s often ignored columnar mucosa limited to the distal few centimeters of the esophagus, dismissing it as normal. In their efforts to avoid false-positive diagnoses, investigators and clinicians had created a potentially larger problem of false-negative diagnoses.

In 1994, Spechler *et al.* reported the results of a study in which consecutive patients having elective endoscopic examinations in a general endoscopy unit had biopsy specimens taken at the squamo-columnar junction in the distal esophagus, irrespective of its appearance and location [35]. Among 142 patients who had columnar epithelium involving < 3 cm of the distal esophagus, 26 (18%) were found to have specialized intestinal metaplasia typical of Barrett's esophagus in the biopsy specimens. The metaplastic epithelium in those patients would have gone unrecognized if the study protocol had not mandated the procurement of biopsy specimens from a normal-appearing distal esophagus (i.e. these would have been false-negative diagnoses).

A number of subsequent studies have confirmed this observation that intestinal metaplasia is present frequently in short segments of columnar epithelium in the distal esophagus, even in patients without symptoms or endoscopic signs of GERD [36]. Since the description by Spechler *et al.*, clinicians have called this condition "short-segment Barrett's esophagus" [37].

2.6   Intestinal metaplasia and adenocarcinoma of the esophagus

The association between adenocarcinoma and Barrett's esophagus had been well established by the 1970s [38–40]. In patients found to have Barrett's cancers, the columnar epithelium surrounding the tumors almost invariably contained specialized intestinal metaplasia that often exhibited dysplastic features [41]. By the late 1980s, it had become widely accepted that intestinal metaplasia was the epithelial type especially associated with neoplasia in Barrett's esophagus [42, 43].

Since specialized intestinal metaplasia was the most frequent and (with its prominent goblet cells) the most distinctive of the epithelial types, the type that was clearly abnormal (unlike the cardiac and atrophic gastric fundic types) and the type most clearly associated with cancer, a number of investigators chose to define Barrett's esophagus by the presence of intestinal metaplasia [44, 45]. Those investigators rejected the diagnosis of Barrett's for patients with only cardiac and atrophic gastric fundic-type epithelia in the esophagus, arguing that it was too difficult to exclude the possibility that the endoscopist had inadvertently taken those biopsy specimens from the stomach – and that, without specialized intestinal metaplasia, the condition had no cancer risk and, therefore, no clinical importance. This requirement for intestinal metaplasia to define Barrett's esophagus, which was based more on convenience than on scientific concerns, was also embraced by clinicians and adopted widely into clinical practice.

2.7   The problem of cardiac mucosa

By the early 1990s, the demonstration of specialized intestinal metaplasia in esophageal biopsy specimens had become virtually a *sine qua non* for the diagnosis of Barrett's esophagus. Since then, however, there have been challenges to the validity of this practice, because of observations regarding the nature and importance of cardiac mucosa. Chandrasoma was the first to suggest that cardiac (junctional) mucosa was not a normal epithelial type, as per the traditional teaching, but was, rather, a metaplastic epithelium acquired as a consequence of reflux esophagitis [46]. According to this unproved hypothesis, the normal epithelial junction at the end of the esophagus is one between esophageal squamous epithelium and gastric oxyntic (acid producing) epithelium, and the finding of squamous epithelium abutting cardiac epithelium defines the presence of GERD [47]. In addition, although cardiac mucosa lacks the goblet cells characteristic of specialized intestinal metaplasia, cardiac mucosa expresses molecular markers of intestinal differentiation (e.g. villin, CDX2) and exhibits genetic abnormalities similar to those described in specialized intestinal metaplasia [48, 49].

Some clinical studies have suggested that cardiac epithelium has increased malignant potential. One study of 141 patients who had endoscopic mucosal resections of small esophageal adenocarcinomas found that 71% had cardiac epithelium, not intestinal metaplasia, adjacent to the cancer [50]. Another retrospective study of 712 patients in one hospital, who had endoscopic biopsy specimens taken from esophageal columnar epithelium, found no significant difference in the rate of esophageal adenocarcinoma development between patients with and without intestinal metaplasia (4.5% vs. 3.6% rate of cancer development, respectively) during a median follow-up interval of 12 years [51].

For these reasons, some authorities have proposed that cardiac epithelium in the esophagus should be considered a form of Barrett's esophagus [52] and, in 2005, the British Society of Gastroenterology defined Barrett's esophagus as one "in which any portion of the normal squamous lining has been replaced by a metaplastic columnar epithelium which is visible macroscopically" [5]. This definition includes patients with cardiac epithelium in the esophagus.

Today, the importance of cardiac epithelium in the esophagus remains disputed. However, the debate about whether patients who have only cardiac epithelium lining the distal esophagus have "Barrett's esophagus" is primarily a semantic issue. Norman Barrett himself did not mention either intestinal metaplasia or cardiac epithelium in his original report of the condition that now bears his name [7]. The columnar-lined esophagus has clinical importance only because it predisposes to the development of esophageal cancer. The great majority of studies on the risk of cancer in Barrett's esophagus have included patients with specialized intestinal metaplasia, either primarily or exclusively [4]. Although the data mentioned above suggest that cardiac epithelium might also predispose to malignancy, the magnitude of that risk is not clear. Furthermore, some more recent reports suggest that the risk of cancer in cardiac epithelium is minimal [53].

2.8 Definition of Barrett's esophagus

The definition of Barrett's esophagus has undergone substantial evolution since Norman Barrett's original report in 1950. Since Barrett did not describe intestinal metaplasia or cardiac mucosa in any of his patients, they might not be recognized as "Barrett's esophagus" by many modern authorities. Some have argued that the very term "Barrett's esophagus" should be discarded, because the condition has been defined so variably by different investigators who have imposed arbitrary criteria to fit their personal perspectives [20]. Nevertheless, the term is so firmly entrenched in the medical literature and in clinical practice that it is unlikely to be abandoned.

Recently, the authors of the American Gastroenterological Association's medical position statement on Barrett's esophagus made a distinction between the conceptual definition of Barrett's esophagus and its diagnostic criteria [4]. They defined Barrett's esophagus conceptually as, "the condition in which any extent of metaplastic columnar epithelium that predisposes to cancer development replaces the stratified squamous epithelium that normally lines the distal esophagus." The authors also wrote that, "Presently, intestinal metaplasia (with goblet cells) is required for the diagnosis of Barrett's esophagus, because intestinal metaplasia is the only type of esophageal columnar epithelium that clearly predisposes to malignancy." That statement remains valid to date.

This distinction between the conceptual definition of Barrett's esophagus and its diagnostic criteria might seem trivial, but I contend that it has useful, practical implications. If future studies confirm a malignant predisposition for cardiac mucosa, the conceptual definition of Barrett's esophagus will not change, but the diagnostic criteria for the condition can be altered to include cardiac mucosa. Future refinements in endoscopic or histological techniques might alter our diagnostic criteria, but they will not alter the concept that Barrett's esophagus is a medical condition only because it predisposes to cancer.

2.9 Diagnostic criteria for Barrett's esophagus

Establishment of the diagnosis of Barrett's esophagus requires endoscopic examination with esophageal biopsy, and two diagnostic criteria must be fulfilled:

1 The endoscopist must document that columnar epithelium extends above the GEJ to line the distal esophagus.
2 Biopsy specimens of the esophageal columnar epithelium must reveal intestinal metaplasia.

To document that columnar epithelium lines the esophagus, the endoscopist must identify both the squamocolumnar junction (SCJ) and the GEJ (Figure 2.1).

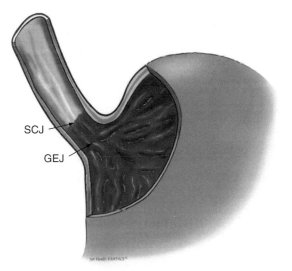

SCJ

GEJ

Figure 2.1 Endoscopic landmarks that define a columnar-lined esophagus. The squamocolumnar junction (SCJ, also called the Z-line) is the visible line formed by the juxtaposition of squamous and columnar epithelia. The gastroesophageal junction (GEJ) is recognized as the most proximal extent of the gastric folds. When the SCJ is located proximal to the GEJ, then the region between the two landmarks is a columnar-lined segment of esophagus. Source: Spechler, 2004 [56]. Adapted by permission of Elsevier.

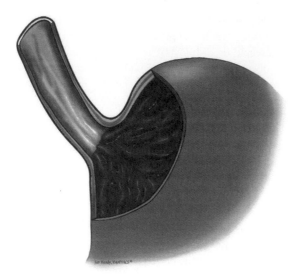

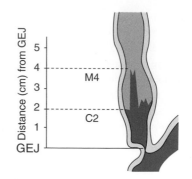

Figure 2.3 Prague C and M criteria. Cartoon shows C2M4 Barrett's esophagus. C = extent of circumferential metaplasia; M = maximal extent of the metaplasia; GEJ = gastroesophageal junction. Source: Sharma *et al.*, 2006 [54]. Reproduced by permission of Elsevier.

Figure 2.2 The SCJ and GEJ coincide. In this situation, the entire esophagus is lined by squamous epithelium. Source: Spechler, 2004 [56]. Adapted by permission of Elsevier.

Columnar epithelium has a reddish color and a velvet-like texture on endoscopic examination, whereas squamous epithelium has a pale, glossy appearance. The juxtaposition of those epithelia at the SCJ forms a visible, typically jagged line called the Z-line. The GEJ is recognized endoscopically as the level of the most proximal extent of the gastric folds [29]. When the SCJ is proximal to the GEJ, then there is a columnar-lined segment of esophagus. When the SCJ and GEJ coincide (Figure 2.2), then the entire esophagus is lined by squamous epithelium. If biopsy specimens from the columnar-lined esophagus show specialized intestinal metaplasia, then the diagnosis of Barrett's esophagus is confirmed. There is long-segment Barrett's esophagus if the distance between the Z-line and the GEJ is ≥ 3 cm, and short-segment Barrett's esophagus if that distance is < 3 cm [37].

The "Prague C and M criteria" is a modern system used to describe the endoscopic appearance of Barrett's esophagus by evaluating both the circumferential (C) and the maximum (M) extent of Barrett's metaplasia above the GEJ (Figure 2.3) [54]. The Prague C and M system has been found to have excellent reproducibility among endoscopists for a number of features of Barrett's esophagus. The notable exception is short-segment Barrett's with metaplasia that extends <1 cm above the GEJ, for which interobserver agreement is poor.

2.10   Intestinal metaplasia at the GEJ

As discussed above, chronic reflux esophagitis leads to the development of intestinal metaplasia in the esophagus (Barrett's esophagus). Intestinal metaplasia also occurs commonly in the stomach as a consequence of chronic gastritis caused by infection with *Helicobacter pylori* [55]. On histological examination, intestinal metaplasia in the stomach and esophagus can be indistinguishable. Since the GEJ cannot be identified with great precision, it can be difficult to determine whether short segments of intestinal metaplasia found in the GEJ region are lining the esophagus (i.e. short-segment Barrett's esophagus) or the proximal stomach (i.e. intestinal metaplasia of the gastric cardia).

The term "intestinal metaplasia at the GEJ" has been used to describe the condition in which intestinal metaplasia is found at a Z-line that appears to coincide precisely with the GEJ [56]. Intestinal metaplasia at the GEJ almost certainly represents either very short-segment Barrett's esophagus or intestinal metaplasia of the gastric cardia; however, for technical reasons, it is difficult to distinguish those two conditions.

For clinical purposes, it might be important to distinguish short-segment Barrett's esophagus from intestinal metaplasia of the gastric cardia, because the former condition appears to have a substantially higher risk of malignancy. For example, one study found dysplasia (the precursor of malignancy) in 20 of 177 patients (11.3%) with short-segment Barrett's esophagus, but in only 1 of 76 patients (1.3%) with intestinal metaplasia in the gastric cardia [57]. Authorities recommend endoscopic cancer surveillance routinely for patients with Barrett's esophagus, but not for patients with intestinal metaplasia in the stomach [58].

A number of histochemical and immunological biomarkers have been proposed to differentiate intestinal metaplasia of the cardia from short-segment Barrett's esophagus, including cytokeratin staining patterns [59–62], immunoreactivity for mAb Das-1 (a monoclonal antibody raised against colonic epithelial cells) [63], and mucosal expression of colonic-type sulfomucins [56]. However, the utility of biomarkers in distinguishing short-segment Barrett's esophagus from intestinal metaplasia of the gastric cardia has not been established, and it has been recommended that clinical decisions should not be based on the presence of these biomarkers [64].

It is not recommended that endoscopists take biopsy specimens from a normal-appearing Z-line. When such biopsies are taken, and patients are found to have intestinal metaplasia at the GEJ, management is disputed. The cancer risk for these patients appears to be very low [65]. In the absence of definitive data and clear societal guidelines, however, a conservative approach is to assume a worst-case scenario in which the condition is short-segment Barrett's esophagus, and to manage patients according to established guidelines for Barrett's esophagus.

References

1 Pohl H, Sirovich B, Welch HG (2010). Esophageal adenocarcinoma incidence: are we reaching the peak? *Cancer Epidemiology, Biomarkers & Prevention* **19**, 1468–70.

2 Rex DK, Cummings OW, Shaw M, Cumings MD, Wong RK, Vasudeva RS, Dunne D, Rahmani EY, Helper DJ (2003). Screening for Barrett's esophagus in colonoscopy patients with and without heartburn. *Gastroenterology* **125**, 1670–7.

3 Ronkainen J, Aro P, Storskrubb T, Johansson SE, Lind T, Bolling-Sternevald E, Vieth M, Stolte M, Talley NJ, Agreus L (2005). Prevalence of Barrett's esophagus in the general population: an endoscopic study. *Gastroenterology* **129**, 1825–31.

4 Spechler SJ, Sharma P, Souza RF, Inadomi JM, Shaheen NJ (2011). American Gastroenterological Association technical review on the management of Barrett's esophagus. *Gastroenterology* **140**, e18–52.

5 British Society of Gastroenterology (2005). Guidelines for the diagnosis and management of Barrett's columnar-lined oesophagus. A Report of the working party of the British Society of Gastroenterology. August http://www.bsg.org.uk.

6 Lord RV (1999). Norman Barrett, "doyen of esophageal surgery". *Annals of Surgery* **229**, 428–39.

7 Barrett NR (1950). Chronic peptic ulcer of the oesophagus and "oesophagitis." *British Journal of Surgery* **38**, 175–82.

8 Tileston W (1906). Peptic ulcer of the esophagus. *American Journal of the Medical Sciences* **132**, 240–65.

9 Stewart MJ, Hartfall SJ (1929). Chronic peptic ulcer of the esophagus. *J Path Bact* **32**, 9–14.

10 Jackson C (1929). Peptic ulcer of the esophagus. *JAMA* **92**, 369–72.

11 Lyall A (1937). Chronic peptic ulcer of the esophagus: a report of eight cases. *British Journal of Surgery* **24**, 534–47.

12 Chamberlin DT. Peptic ulcer of esophagus. *American Journal of Digestive Diseases* (1939). **5**, 725–30.

13 Dick RCS, Hurst A (1942). Chronic peptic ulcer of oesophagus and its association with congenitally short oesophagus and diaphragmatic hernia. *Quarterly Journal of Medicine* **11**, 105–20.

14 Allison PR (1948). Peptic ulcer of oesophagus. *Thorax* **3**, 20–42.

15 Frindlay L, Kelley AB (1931). Congenital shortening of the esophagus and the thoracic stomach results therefrom. *Proceedings of the Royal Society of Medicine* **24**, 1561–78.

16 Bosher LH, Taylor FH (1951). Heterotopic gastric mucosa in the esophagus with ulceration and stricture formation. *Journal of Thoracic Surgery* **21**, 306–12.

17 Morson BC, Belcher JR (1952). Adenocarcinoma of the esophagus and ectopic gastric mucosa. *British Journal of Cancer* **6**, 127–30.

18 Allison PR, Johnstone AS (1953). The oesophagus lined with gastric mucous membrane. *Thorax* **8**, 87–101.

19 Barrett NR (1957). The lower esophagus lined by columnar epithelium. *Surgery* **41**, 881–94.

20 Moersch RN, Ellis FH, McDonald JR (1959). Pathologic changes occurring in severe reflux esophagitis. *Surgery, Gynecology & Obstetrics* **108**, 476.

21 Spechler SJ, Goyal RK (1996). The columnar lined esophagus, intestinal metaplasia, and Norman Barrett. *Gastroenterology* **110**, 614–21.

22 Hayward J (1961). The lower end of the oesophagus. *Thorax* **16**, 36–41.

23 Pedersen SA, Hage E, Nielsen PA, Sorensen HR (1971). Barrett's syndrome: morphological and physiological characteristics. *Scandinavian Journal of Thoracic and Cardiovascular Surgery* **6**, 191–205.

24 Burgess JN, Payne WS, Andersen HA, Weiland LH, Carlson HC (1971). Barrett esophagus: the columnar-epithelial-lined lower esophagus. *Mayo Clinic Proceedings* **46**, 728–34.

25 Abrams L, Heath D (1965). Lower oesophagus lined with intestinal and gastric epithelia. *Thorax* **20**, 66–72.

26 Trier JS (1970). Morphology of the epithelium of the distal esophagus in patients with midesophageal peptic strictures. *Gastroenterology* **58**, 444–61.

27 Berenson MM, Herbst JJ, Freston JW (1974). Enzyme and ultrastructural characteristics of esophageal columnar epithelium. *American Journal of Digestive Diseases* **19**, 895–907.

28 Paull A, Trier JS, Dalton MD, Camp RC, Loeb P, Goyal RK (1976). The histologic spectrum of Barrett's esophagus. *New England Journal of Medicine* **295**, 476–80.

29 McClave SA, Boyce HW Jr.,, Gottfried MR (1987). Early diagnosis of columnar-lined esophagus: a new endoscopic criterion. *Gastrointestinal Endoscopy* **33**, 413–416.

30 Choi do W, Oh SN, Baek SJ, Ahn SH, Chang YJ, Jeong WS, Kim HJ, Yeon JE, Park JJ, Kim JS, Byun KS, Bak YT, Lee CH (2002). Endoscopically observed lower esophageal capillary patterns. *Korean Journal of Internal Medicine* **17**, 245–8.

31 Vianna A, Hayes PC, Moscoso G, Driver M, Portmann B, Westaby D, William R (1987). Normal venous circulation of the gastroesophageal junction. A route to understanding varices. *Gastroenterology* **93**, 876–89.

32 Ishimura N, Amano Y, Kinoshita Y (2009). Endoscopic definition of esophagogastric junction for diagnosis of Barrett's esophagus: importance of systematic education and training. *Digestive Endoscopy* **21**, 213–8.

33 Skinner DB, Walther BC, Riddell RH, Schmidt H, Iascone C, DeMeester TR (1983). Barrett's esophagus: comparison of benign and malignant cases. *Annals of Surgery* **198**, 554–65.

34 Rothery GA, Patterson JE, Stoddard CJ, Day DW (1986). Histological and histochemical changes in the columnar lined (Barrett's) oesophagus. *Gut* **27**, 1062–8.

35 Spechler SJ, Zeroogian JM, Antonioli DA, Wang HH, Goyal RK (1994). Prevalence of metaplasia at the gastro-oesophageal junction. *Lancet* **344**, 1533–1536.

36 Spechler SJ (1997). The columnar lined oesophagus: a riddle wrapped in a mystery inside an enigma. *Gut* **41**, 710–711.

37 Sharma P, Morales TG, Sampliner RE (1998). Short segment Barrett's esophagus. *The need for standardization of the definition and of endoscopic criteria. American Journal of Gastroenterology* **93**, 1033–6.

38 Adler RH (1963). The lower esophagus lined by columnar epithelium: its association with hiatal hernia, ulcer, stricture, and tumor. *Journal of Thoracic and Cardiovascular Surgery* **45**, 13–32.

39 Hawe A, Payne WS, Weiland LH (1973). Adenocarcinoma in the columnar epithelial lined lower (Barrett) esophagus. *Thorax* **28**, 511–4.

40 Haggitt RC, Tryzelaar J, Ellis FH, Colcher H (1978). Adenocarcinoma complicating columnar epithelium-lined (Barrett's) esophagus. *American Journal of Clinical Pathology* **70**, 1–5.

41 Haggitt RC, Dean PJ (1985). Adenocarcinoma in Barrett's epithelium. In: Spechler SJ, Goyal RK, eds. *Barrett's esophagus: pathophysiology, diagnosis, and management.* pp. 153–66. New York: Elsevier Science Publishing Co., Inc.

42 Reid BJ, Weinstein WM, Lewin KJ, Haggitt RC, VanDeventer G, DenBesten L, Rubin CE (1988). Endoscopic biopsy can detect high-grade dysplasia or early adenocarcinoma in Barrett's esophagus without grossly recognizable neoplastic lesions. *Gastroenterology* **94**, 81–90.

43 Reid BJ, Weinstein WM (1987). Barrett's esophagus and adenocarcinoma. *Annual Review of Medicine* **38**, 477–92.

44 Reid BJ (1991). Barrett's esophagus and esophageal adenocarcinoma. *Gastroenterology Clinics of North America* **20**, 817–834.

45 Weinstein WM, Ippoliti AF (1996). The diagnosis of Barrett's esophagus: goblets, goblets, goblets. *Gastrointestinal Endoscopy* **44**, 91–95.

46 Chandrasoma P (1997). Pathophysiology of Barrett's esophagus. *Seminars in Thoracic and Cardiovascular Surgery* **9**, 270–278.

47 Chandrasoma PT (2013). Histologic definition of gastroesophageal reflux disease. *Current Opinion in Gastroenterology* **29**, 460–7.

48 Hahn HP, Blount PL, Ayub K, Das KM, Souza R, Spechler S, Odze RD (2009). Intestinal differentiation in metaplastic, nongoblet columnar epithelium in the esophagus. *American Journal of Surgical Pathology* **33**, 1006–15.

49 Liu W, Hahn H, Odze RD, Goyal RK (2009). Metaplastic esophageal columnar epithelium without goblet cells shows DNA content abnormalities similar to goblet cell-containing epithelium. *American Journal of Gastroenterology* **104**, 816–24.

50 Takubo K, Aida J, Naomoto Y, Sawabe M, Arai T, Shiraishi H, Matsuura M, Ell C, May A, Pech O, Stolte M, Vieth M (2009). Cardiac rather than intestinal-type background in endoscopic resection specimens of minute Barrett adenocarcinoma. *Human Pathology* **40**, 65–74.

51 Kelty CJ, Gough MD, Van Wyk Q, Stephenson TJ, Ackroyd R (2007). Barrett's oesophagus: intestinal metaplasia is not essential for cancer risk. *Scandinavian Journal of Gastroenterology* **42**, 1271–4.

52 Riddell RH, Odze RD (2009). Definition of Barrett's esophagus: time for a rethink – is intestinal metaplasia dead? *American Journal of Gastroenterology* **104**, 2588–94.

53 Westerhoff M, Hovan L, Lee C, Hart J (2012). Effects of dropping the requirement for goblet cells from the diagnosis of Barrett's esophagus. *Clinical Gastroenterology and Hepatology* **10**, 1232–6.

54 Sharma P, Dent J, Armstrong D, Bergman JJ, Gossner L, Hoshihara Y, Jankowski JA, Junghard O, Lundell L, Tytgat GN, Vieth M (2006). The development and validation of an endoscopic grading system for Barrett's esophagus: the Prague C & M criteria. *Gastroenterology* **131**, 1392–9.

55 Correa P (1995). Helicobacter pylori and gastric carcinogenesis. *American Journal of Surgical Pathology* **19**(Suppl 1), S37–S43.

56 Spechler SJ (2004). Intestinal metaplasia at the gastroesophageal junction. *Gastroenterology* **126**, 567–75.

57 Sharma P, Weston AP, Morales, T, Topalovski M, Mayo MS, Sampliner RE (2000). Relative risk of dysplasia for patients with intestinal metaplasia in the distal oesophagus and in the gastric cardia. *Gut* **46**, 9–13.

58 Fennerty MB (2003). Gastric intestinal metaplasia on routine endoscopic biopsy. *Gastroenterology* **125**, 586–90.

59 Ormsby AH, Goldblum JR, Rice TW, Richter JE, Falk GW, Vaezi MF, Gramlich TL (1999). Cytokeratin subsets can reliably distinguish Barrett's esophagus from intestinal metaplasia of the stomach. *Human Pathology* **30**, 288–94.

60 Jovanovic I, Tzardi M, Mouzas IA, Micev M, Pesko P, Milosavljevic T, Zois M, Sganzos M, Delides G, Kanavaros P (2002). Changing pattern of cytokeratin 7 and 20 expression from normal epithelium to intestinal metaplasia of the gastric mucosa and gastroesophageal junction. *Histology and Histopathology* **17**, 445–54.

61 Glickman JN, Wang H, Das KM, Goyal RK, Spechler SJ, Antonioli D, Odze RD (2001). Phenotype of Barrett's esophagus and intestinal metaplasia of the distal esophagus and gastroesophageal junction. An immunohistochemical study of cytokeratins 7 and 20, Das-1 and 45 MI. *American Journal of Surgical Pathology* **25**, 87–94.

62 El-Zimaity HMT, Graham DY (2001). Cytokeratin subsets for distinguishing Barrett's esophagus from intestinal metaplasia in the cardia using endoscopic biopsy specimens. *American Journal of Gastroenterology* **96**, 1378–82.

63 Das KM, Prasad I, Garla S, Amenta PS (1994). Detection of a shared colon epithelial epitope on Barrett epithelium by a novel monoclonal antibody. *Annals of Internal Medicine* **120**, 753–6.

64 Morales CP, Spechler SJ (2003) Intestinal metaplasia at the gastroesophageal junction: Barrett's, bacteria, and biomarkers. *American Journal of Gastroenterology* **98**, 759–62.

65 Jung KW, Talley NJ, Romero Y, Katzka DA, Schleck CD, Zinsmeister AR, Dunagan KT, Lutzke LS, Wu TT, Wang KK, Frederickson M, Geno DM, Locke GR, Prasad GA (2011). Epidemiology and natural history of intestinal metaplasia of the gastroesophageal junction and Barrett's esophagus: a population-based study. *American Journal of Gastroenterology* **106**, 1447–55.

CHAPTER 3

Epidemiology and prevalence of Barrett's esophagus

Helen G. Coleman[1], Shivaram K. Bhat[2] & Liam J. Murray[1]

[1] Centre for Public Health, Institute of Clinical Sciences, Queen's University Belfast, Belfast, UK
[2] Department of Gastroenterology, Altnagelvin Hospital, Western Health and Social Care Trust, Londonderry, UK

3.1 Introduction

The well-documented rise in esophageal adenocarcinoma (EAC) incidence [1–4] has primed a wealth of research in Barrett's esophagus (BE) epidemiology. However, understanding the epidemiology of BE is challenging for a number of reasons. Firstly, many cases of BE may remain undiagnosed in the population, making it very difficult to gain a true perspective of BE prevalence and incidence. As such, published data on BE rates must be interpreted with the knowledge that they are likely to represent only a small proportion of existing cases.

Secondly, temporal and geographic differences in the definition of BE can make it difficult to compare rates over time and between regions. Where research findings are presented in this chapter, we have used the term "BE" to refer to specialized intestinal metaplasia (SIM) of the esophagus. Otherwise, we have specified if columnar-lined epithelium (CLE) was the definition used.

Finally, variations in BE incidence and prevalence rates may reflect changes in endoscopic practice, recognition and/or reporting of BE, rather than true trends of the disease. This last consideration is probably the most challenging to address in research study designs.

Identifying accurate estimates of BE prevalence and incidence in the population is important for planning suitable management of patients and at-risk populations and ultimately preventing, or improving outcomes for, EAC. This chapter seeks to clarify the evidence to date on BE epidemiology by summarizing key studies of prevalence and incidence estimates, and by describing trends in different sub-groups of the population. A summary of key risk factors for BE development and risk of neoplastic progression is also provided.

3.2 BE prevalence

Prevalence refers to the total number of existing cases in a population or region at a given time-point. Uncertainty remains as to the prevalence of BE in the population, since its diagnosis requires endoscopy (although less invasive diagnostic procedures [5] are being trialed) and no population-based screening programs are currently in place. Accurately determining BE prevalence is necessary for evaluating effectiveness and cost-effectiveness of potential screening programs [6]. In clinical settings, only those patients experiencing symptoms are likely to undergo endoscopic investigation, while in research settings, only those who are willing to volunteer for such investigations will be included in prevalence estimates. In both settings, these individuals are unlikely to be representative of the general population at risk for BE, thus introducing referral and selection biases into estimates of BE prevalence.

There has been progress in the past decade to overcome these issues. Several studies have now estimated the overall prevalence of *diagnosed* BE in the general population, or representative samples of the population, rather than in a single-center or hospital/institution. Studies of the latter design were historically informative, but are prone to the aforementioned biases and tend to include small numbers of cases with little information on the population catchment area. Population-based

Esophageal Cancer and Barrett's Esophagus, Third Edition. Edited by Prateek Sharma, Richard Sampliner and David Ilson.
© 2015 John Wiley & Sons, Ltd. Published 2015 by John Wiley & Sons, Ltd.

Table 3.1 Summary of population-based or representative studies of diagnosed BE prevalence per 100,000 population.

Author/ publication year	Country/ region	Population sampled	BE definition	Number of BE cases	Year	Sex	Prevalence (per 100,000 population)
Alcedo, 2009 [8]	Zaragoza region, Spain	Patients undergoing upper gastrointestinal endoscopy	Visible CLE plus histologically confirmed SIM	386	1985	Males and Females	6.5
					2001	Males and Females	76
					2001	Males	123
					2001	Females	30
Alexandropoulou, 2013 [7]	UK	General Practice Research Database	Codes for CLE, BE and Barrett's ulcer	5,860	1996	Males	22
					1996	Females	12
					2005	Males	171
					2005	Females	86
Conio, 2001; Jung, 2011 [10, 11]	Olmsted County, USA	Review of upper gastrointestinal endoscopy records	Visible CLE plus histologically confirmed SIM	77	1987	Males and Females	23
					1998	Males and Females	83
					1998	Males	148
					1998	Females	36
				401*	2007	Males and Females	220
					2007	Males	320
					2007	Females	129
Corley, 2009 [9]	Northern California, USA	Kaiser Permanente Health system database	ICD/SNOMED codes for BE, corrected for expected incidence of SIM from previous validation study	4,205	2006	Males and Females	131
Musana, 2008 [12]	Marshfield region, Wisconsin, USA	Patients undergoing upper gastrointestinal endoscopy	SNOMED codes for BE, esophageal ulcers and SIM plus histologically confirmed SIM	216	2002	Males and Females	262
					2002	Males	398
					2002	Females	142

*Estimates from 2007 included n=48 BE patients with prevalent HGD or EAC. Separate estimates for BE without prevalent HGD/EAC were not available.

studies are less prone to such biases, and a summary of those that have published on BE prevalence in unselected population groups [7–12] is presented in Table 3.1. Where studies provided prevalence estimates for multiple years, only data from the first and last years of the study have been extracted to illustrate any temporal changes.

As shown in Table 3.1, the earliest estimates suggested a population prevalence of diagnosed BE of 6.5–23 per 100,000 population in the 1980s (equivalent to 0.07–0.23% of the population), with the highest prevalence reported among a mid-Western US population in 2002 (262 per 100,000 population,

equivalent to 2.6% of the population). Overall, BE is being diagnosed more often in recent years. Studies using codes to identify BE (including CLE) cases from electronic databases [7, 9] tended to have slightly more modest prevalence estimates, compared with studies reviewing patients from endoscopy reports or clinics at comparable time points.

However, while useful, these studies do not provide insight into the prevalence of *undiagnosed* BE in the population. In a widely cited study, Ronkainen and colleagues attempted to capture the prevalence of undetected BE within a random sample of 1,000 adults from Northern Sweden who underwent upper gastrointestinal endoscopy [13]. They found that 103 patients had suspected CLE, of whom 16 patients had BE (1.6%).

These estimates would suggest true population BE prevalence rates of less than 2%. This is lower than computer simulation model estimates, based upon US SEER data of EAC natural history, which suggested BE prevalence of approximately 5.6% [14]. One potential explanation for these different estimates are the different risk factor profiles in European and US populations, and varying prevalence in symptomatic and asymptomatic groups, which is discussed later in this chapter.

3.2.1 Segment length

There are conflicting reports with respect to the breakdown of BE prevalence by segment length. Some studies report the majority of BE cases to be of short-segment length (traditionally less than 3 cm) [13, 15, 16], while others have detected a predominance of long-segment BE [8, 12]. It is likely that some of the increased prevalence of BE in recent years can be attributed to increased recognition and reporting of short-segment BE [8].

3.2.2 Age and sex distribution

As shown in Table 3.1, males have a consistently higher prevalence of BE than females. The ratio of this male dominance ranges from approximately 2–4 : 1. The mean age of BE diagnosis is reported at 57–64 years in most studies [7–12], although this masks a gender disparity in BE diagnostic age. Females are commonly reported to be 5–10 years older than males at the time of their BE diagnosis, with the males being diagnosed in their early-mid 50s, on average [8, 13].

3.2.3 Racial, ethnic and geographic variation

The best examples of racial/ethnic variation in BE epidemiology are found in data from the USA [17–21]. In these studies, BE prevalence amongst black, Hispanic or Asian/pacific islander population groups is consistently lower than that seen in white counterparts, ranging from 0.8–4% of individuals undergoing endoscopy [17–21]. Corley and colleagues have estimated that BE prevalence in non-Hispanic whites is double that of Hispanic counterparts (247 v. 135 per 100,000 person-years), and approximately five times greater

than that of black (49 per 100,000 person-years) or Asian populations (65 per 100,000 person-years) in 2006 [9].

Several studies of BE prevalence have also emerged from Asian countries in recent years, most of which are from single-centers [22–27]. although multi-center estimates have been reported from Korea [28, 29]. BE prevalence estimates ranged from 0.2–2% in Chinese, Taiwanese and Korean studies [24–29]. However, much higher prevalence estimates of 20–37% have been reported from a Japanese university hospital [22, 23], which may be due to the inclusion of ultra-short segment BE [30].

Data from other global regions is extremely sparse. BE has been reported as a rare finding in a Turkish study, affecting less than 2% of patients attending an endoscopy clinic [31]. A small study from Brazil has estimated BE prevalence to be approximately 4% in a patient group undergoing endoscopy [32]. Higher BE prevalence rates of 7.3% were observed in an Egyptian study; however, these patients had chronic gastro-esophageal reflux symptoms [33].

The overwhelming majority of BE cases in the studies of non-Western populations were of short-segment length. Therefore, BE does not appear to be a major public health problem in regions outside of North America and Europe, although better quality population-based data is required to confirm this. Notably, the racial and geographic variations described here for BE epidemiology are very similar to patterns noted for gastro-esophageal reflux disease in general [34]. Further studies, comparing risk factors and genetic profiles between regions and racial groups, could provide a useful insight into BE etiology.

3.2.4 BE prevalence in symptomatic v. asymptomatic patients

As stated above, Ronkainen and colleagues identified a BE prevalence of 1.6% in an asymptomatic Swedish population, giving a rare insight into true prevalence in the population [35]. Other studies have attempted to compare BE prevalence in asymptomatic and symptomatic individuals by performing upper gastrointestinal endoscopy on patients undergoing colonoscopy. In one such study from the USA, Rex *et al.* reported the prevalence of BE as 5.6% in asymptomatic patients, and 8.3% in those with heartburn [36]. Higher BE prevalence among symptomatic, compared with asymptomatic, individuals is a well-described phenomenon, [15, 37–39] but rates in the latter group are certainly not negligible. Indeed, a smaller US study that recruited individuals undergoing sigmoidoscopy for colorectal cancer screening reported a BE prevalence of 25% in asymptomatic subjects [40].

The variability in the reported prevalence of BE may be due to a number of factors. Selection bias, sample size and risk factors present in the studied cohorts may all have influenced the estimated prevalence. Regardless of the perception of symptom, it is clear that BE affects a substantial number of patients, even if the lowest estimates of population prevalence are assumed to be the most accurate. Since symptoms are subjective, any future BE screening programs should probably reach out to individuals on the basis of other risk factors.

3.3   BE incidence

Incidence refers to the number of new cases of BE that occur in a specified time period, in a region, and are usually presented as annual estimates. Assessing BE incidence is extremely important for predicting future trends in BE and EAC, and for allowing health providers to plan appropriate patient management strategies. A number of studies [7–10, 41–45] have reported temporal increases in the incidence of diagnosed BE, as shown in Table 3.2. However, it must be borne in mind that trends in diagnosed BE may not necessarily reflect true trends in incidence.

Dramatic increases in BE are seen in those studies comparing diagnoses in the 1990s–2000s with much earlier estimates [8, 10, 44]. These are highly likely to reflect increased recognition and reporting of the disease, although it is possible that they partially explain the recent EAC rise also [1–4].

3.3.1   Segment length
Although studies tend to have observed a steady increase in long-segment BE over time, at least two reports have noted much sharper increases in short-segment BE that may account for the majority of overall temporal changes in BE incidence [8, 10]. Again, this would suggest that the increasing BE incidence can be attributed to improved reporting of short-segment BE, to some extent.

3.3.2   Age and sex distribution
BE incidence is consistently higher in males compared with females, although similar proportional increases in incidence have been observed in both sexes (Table 3.2). Peak BE incidence generally occurs in the 55–64 year age group [7], although suggestions of increasingly younger age at diagnosis over time have been noted by some [46]. Indeed, the documented increase in BE/CLE incidence in Northern Ireland, and BE incidence in The Netherlands, was particularly evident in younger individuals, aged 60 years or less [41, 43]. This was observed for both sexes; however, the most marked increases were noted in males aged under 40 years [41].

3.3.3   Racial, ethnic and geographic variation
Little is known about trends in BE incidence among varying racial groups, or in geographic regions outside of North America and Europe. Incidence estimates would be welcome to ensure that any changes to the low BE prevalence seen in these populations can be evaluated.

3.3.4   Is BE incidence related to corresponding endoscopy and biopsy rates?
Several reports have noted a correlation between BE incidence and the total number of endoscopies performed in a population, thus concluding that any changes are a result of endoscopic practice changes [10, 11, 42]. Very few studies have attempted to analyze the crucial issue of interpreting BE incidence in the context of changing endoscopy rates or biopsy rates. In the Northern Ireland BE register, the increase in BE/CLE incidence over a 13-year period (160% rise) exceeded corresponding increases in endoscopy and esophageal biopsy rates in the general population (which rose by 35% and 46%, respectively) [41]. Furthermore, data linkage revealed that BE incidence per 100 endoscopies performed had risen by 93%, and by 79% per 100 esophageal biopsies performed [41].

Post *et al.* also demonstrated a 25–33% rise in the proportion of esophageal biopsies that detected BE, but did not have access to endoscopy data in their Dutch population [43]. These data suggest a true rise in the incidence of BE in Western populations, but cannot entirely rule out better targeting of patients and recognition of the disease as underlying reasons for the observed trends [44].

Table 3.2 Summary of population-based studies publishing on temporal trends in diagnosed BE incidence.

Author/ publication year	Country/ region	Population sampled	BE definition	Number of BE cases	Time periods for comparison	Sex	Incidence (per 100,000 population)	Corresponding % increase
Alcedo, 2009 [8]	Spain	Patients undergoing upper gastrointestinal endoscopy	Visible CLE, plus histologically confirmed SIM	386	1995–2001 v 1976–82	Males and Females	10 v 0.7	1,329
Alexandropoulou, 2013 [7]	UK	General Practice Research Database	Codes for CLE, BE and Barrett's ulcer	5,860	2005 v 1996	Males Females	24 v 11 11 v 6	118 83
Coleman, 2011 [41]	Northern Ireland	Review of esophageal biopsy reports	BE, including CLE or SIM	9,329	2002–05 v 1993–97	Males and Females Males Females	62 v 24 76 v 30 45 v 19	160 150 135
Conio, 2001 [10]	Olmsted County, USA	Record review of upper gastrointestinal endoscopy records	Visible CLE, plus histologically confirmed SIM	117	1995–97 v 1965–69	Males and Females	11 v 0.4	2,650
Corley, 2009 [9]	Northern California, USA	Kaiser Permanente Health system database	ICD/SNOMED codes for BE, corrected for expected SIM incidence from prior validation study	4,205	2006 v 1998	Males and Females	24 v 15	60
Hurschler, 2003 [42]	St Gallen-Appenzell, Switzerland	Review of esophageal biopsy reports	BE, including CLE or SIM	742	1994–98 v 1989–93	Males and Females	16 v 9	78
Post, 2007 [43]	The Netherlands	Review of esophageal biopsy reports	Histologically confirmed SIM	35,365*	2003–05 v 1992–1995	Males Females	18 v 13 9 v 7	38 29
Prach, 1997 [44]	Tayside region, Scotland	Patients undergoing upper gastrointestinal endoscopy	BE, not stated	961	1993 v 1980	Males and Females Males and Females	48 v 1	4,700
van Soest, 2005 [45]	The Netherlands	Integrated primary care database	Codes for CLE, Barrett and SIM	260	2003 v 1996	Males and Females	23 v 11	109

*Included n=1,952 BE patients with prevalent EAC. Separate estimates for BE without prevalent EAC were not available.

3.4 Etiology and risk factors for BE

Since BE is found to be highly prevalent in individuals with chronic gastro-esophageal reflux symptoms, injury of the esophageal mucosa from acid reflux is likely to be a key factor in BE development [47, 48]. The prevailing hypothesis is that metaplasia of the normal epithelium occurs as a reparative response to injury. Pluripotent stem cells are thought to be triggered to undergo differentiation along an intestinal type of cell lineage. The cells then undergo a clonal expansion to form the abnormal mucosa of BE [47]. Indeed, meta-analyses of high-quality studies indicates that experiencing gastro-esophageal reflux symptoms is associated with a three-fold increased risk of BE, and is particularly predictive for long-segment BE [49].

Factors other than simple acid reflux have been shown to play a role in the development of BE. Bile acids, known to be present in the gastro-esophageal refluxate, have also been linked with esophageal injury and metaplasia development [50], most likely acting via oxidative stress or DNA damage [51–53]. On the other hand, Fletcher *et al.* demonstrated that the distal esophagus can be chronically exposed to acid reflux, with no evidence of the development of Barrett's metaplasia [54]. It is clear that other factors are likely to be involved in the development of BE, either by inducing acid/bile reflux and/or via alternative pathways [55].

Well-established risk factors for BE development tend to mirror known risk factors for EAC, such as advanced age, male sex, and white race [56–58]. Additional metabolic factors have been postulated to increase the risk of BE, such as excess body weight [58–60], particularly central adiposity [61–63] and Type 2 diabetes mellitus [64]. There is also strong evidence that tobacco smoking is directly associated with BE development; however, alcohol consumption does not appear to increase the risk of BE [58, 65]. Previous observations of inverse associations between wine consumption and BE risk have been attributed to confounding by socio-economic status [66].

Other modifiable factors linked with reduced risks of BE include dietary aspects, such as fruit and vegetable intake, fiber, iron and antioxidant intakes [60, 67–71]. In contrast, high intakes of meat and fat are associated with greater risks of BE [70–72]. Medication use, particularly the use of non-steroidal anti-inflammatory drugs

and aspirin, may be protective against BE development [73, 74]. A robust meta-analysis of 49 studies, four of which were deemed to have low risk of selection or information biases, determined that *Helicobacter pylori* infection was also protective against BE [75]. More recently, genetic factors have been implicated in BE etiology as a result of consortial analyses [76, 77], building upon findings from previous smaller studies and thus providing a promising platform for future research in this area.

It should be noted that study design is a general limitation in most investigations of modifiable risk factors for BE, as most evidence originates from case-control studies that may be subject to recall and selection bias. The future replication of these analyses in prospective studies is warranted. In addition, these studies do not incorporate undiagnosed BE cases, so investigation of risk factors in screening studies therefore would be useful.

3.5 Neoplastic progression risk in BE

Since evidence suggests rising prevalence and incidence rates of BE, the appropriate clinical management of this burgeoning patient group becomes even more pertinent. The ultimate importance of a diagnosis of BE lies in its relationship with EAC. Transition of BE is likely to occur in steps, progressing through states of low and high grade dysplasia (HGD), before finally developing into EAC [78].

Early studies examining neoplastic progression in BE reported HGD/EAC risks as high as 3% per year [79, 80]. Subsequent meta-analyses and large population-based studies would suggest more modest risks of cancer progression of approximately 0.4% per year [56, 80], which may be even lower in short-segment BE [56, 81]. A number of reasons have been suggested for variation in the reported risk of progression between historic and recent studies, including referral bias, publication bias and the failure to exclude prevalent HGD or early incident cancers in earlier studies [79, 80]. The lower, more precise, estimates of neoplastic progression risk have important implications with respect to the management of BE patients. Ideally, patients with the highest risk of progression would be identified, and surveillance intervals determined according to progression risk. This would hopefully aid detection of early neoplasia, while providing a cost-effective health service that is acceptable to the patient.

3.6   Conclusions

BE incidence and prevalence rates appear to be rising in Caucasians residing in Western regions. Smaller but notable proportions of other racial groups living in Western countries are affected by BE. Other geographic regions have very low BE prevalence, with the possible exception of Japan, and the majority of cases are short-segment BE. BE is consistently male-predominant and is most often diagnosed in individuals aged 50–64 years, although rising incidence in younger age groups is of concern.

Overall, the proportion of diagnosed BE cases, who are therefore undergoing endoscopic surveillance, is likely to underestimate true BE prevalence in the population. Although BE is a pre-cancerous condition, neoplastic progression risk is low. Clinicians and researchers are now challenged with the dilemma of detecting BE in the general population, while balancing appropriate clinical management that would allow for early detection of neoplasms without overburdening health services.

Developing evidence-based advice to reduce the risk of BE and future neoplastic progression, identifying those patients at highest risk of progression, and ultimately developing personalized surveillance protocols, remain urgent priorities in BE epidemiology.

References

1 Edgren G, Adami HO, Weiderpass E, Nyren O (2013). A global assessment of the oesophageal adenocarcinoma epidemic. *Gut* **62**(10), 1406–14.

2 Cook MB, Chow W, Devesa SS (2009). Oesophageal cancer incidence in the United States by race, sex, and histologic type, 1977–2005. *British Journal of Cancer* **101**(5), 855–859.

3 Devesa SS, Blot WJ, Fraumeni JF, Jr. (1998). Changing patterns in the incidence of esophageal and gastric carcinoma in the United States. *Cancer* **83**(10), 2049–2053.

4 Bosetti C, Levi F, Ferlay J, Garavello W, Lucchini F, Bertuccio P, *et al.* (2008). Trends in oesophageal cancer incidence and mortality in Europe. *International Journal of Cancer* **122**(5), 1118–1129.

5 Kadri SR, Lao-Sirieix P, O'Donovan M, Debiram I, Das M, Blazeby JM, *et al.* (2010). Acceptability and accuracy of a non-endoscopic screening test for Barrett's oesophagus in primary care: cohort study. *BMJ* **341**, c4372.

6 Benaglia T, Sharples LD, Fitzgerald RC, Lyratzopoulos G (2013). Health benefits and cost effectiveness of endoscopic and nonendoscopic cytosponge screening for Barrett's esophagus. *Gastroenterology* **144**(1), 62–73.e6.

7 Alexandropoulou K, van Vlymen J, Reid F, Poullis A, Kang JY (2013). Temporal trends of Barrett's oesophagus and gastro-oesophageal reflux and related oesophageal cancer over a 10-year period in England and Wales and associated proton pump inhibitor and H2RA prescriptions: a GPRD study. *European Journal of Gastroenterology & Hepatology* **25**(1), 15–21.

8 Alcedo J, Ferrandez A, Arenas J, Sopena F, Ortego J, Sainz R, *et al.* (2009). Trends in Barrett's esophagus diagnosis in Southern Europe: implications for surveillance. *Diseases of the Esophagus* **22**(3), 239–248.

9 Corley DA, Kubo A, Levin TR, Block G, Habel L, Rumore G, *et al.* (2009). Race, ethnicity, sex and temporal differences in Barrett's oesophagus diagnosis: a large community-based study, 1994–2006. *Gut* **58**(2), 182–188.

10 Conio M, Cameron AJ, Romero Y, Branch CD, Schleck CD, Burgart LJ, *et al.* (2001). Secular trends in the epidemiology and outcome of Barrett's oesophagus in Olmsted County, Minnesota. *Gut* **48**(3), 304–309.

11 Jung KW, Talley NJ, Romero Y, Katzka DA, Schleck CD, Zinsmeister AR, *et al.* (2011). Epidemiology and Natural History of Intestinal Metaplasia of the Gastroesophageal Junction and Barrett's Esophagus: A Population-Based Study. *American Journal of Gastroenterology* **106**(8), 1447–55.

12 Musana AK, Resnick JM, Torbey CF, Mukesh BN, Greenlee RT (2008). Barrett's esophagus: incidence and prevalence estimates in a rural Mid-Western population. *American Journal of Gastroenterology* **103**(3), 516–524.

13 Ronkainen J, Aro P, Storskrubb T, Johansson SE, Lind T, Bolling-Sternevald E, *et al.* (2005). Prevalence of Barrett's esophagus in the general population: an endoscopic study. *Gastroenterology* **129**(6), 1825–1831.

14 Hayeck TJ, Kong CY, Spechler SJ, Gazelle GS, Hur C (2010). The prevalence of Barrett's esophagus in the US: estimates from a simulation model confirmed by SEER data. *Diseases of the Esophagus* **23**(6), 451–457.

15 Zagari RM, Fuccio L, Wallander MA, Johansson S, Fiocca R, Casanova S, *et al.* (2008). Gastro-oesophageal reflux symptoms, oesophagitis and Barrett's oesophagus in the general population: the Loiano-Monghidoro study. *Gut* **57**(10), 1354–1359.

16 Csendes A, Smok G, Burdiles P, Quesada F, Huertas C, Rojas J, *et al.* (2000). Prevalence of Barrett's esophagus by endoscopy and histologic studies: a prospective evaluation of 306 control subjects and 376 patients with symptoms of gastroesophageal reflux. *Diseases of the Esophagus* **13**(1), 5–11.

17 Abrams JA, Fields S, Lightdale CJ, Neugut AI (2008). Racial and ethnic disparities in the prevalence of Barrett's

esophagus among patients who undergo upper endoscopy. *Clinical Gastroenterology and Hepatology* **6**(1), 30–34.

18 Fan X, Snyder N (2009). Prevalence of Barrett's esophagus in patients with or without GERD symptoms: role of race, age, and gender. *Digestive Diseases and Sciences* **54**(3), 572–577.

19 Khoury JE, Chisholm S, Jamal MM, Palacio C, Pudhota S, Vega KJ (2012). African Americans with Barrett's esophagus are less likely to have dysplasia at biopsy. *Digestive Diseases and Sciences* **57**(2), 419–423.

20 Lam KD, Phan JT, Garcia RT, Trinh H, Nguyen H, Nguyen K, *et al.* (2008). Low proportion of Barrett's esophagus in Asian Americans. *American Journal of Gastroenterology* **103**(7), 1625–1630.

21 Wang A, Mattek NC, Holub JL, Lieberman DA, Eisen GM (2009). Prevalence of complicated gastroesophageal reflux disease and Barrett's esophagus among racial groups in a multi-center consortium. *Digestive Diseases and Sciences* **54**(5), 964–971.

22 Amano Y, Kushiyama Y, Yuki T, Takahashi Y, Moriyama I, Fukuhara H, *et al.* (2006). Prevalence of and risk factors for Barrett's esophagus with intestinal predominant mucin phenotype. *Scandinavian Journal of Gastroenterology* **41**(8), 873–879.

23 Okita K, Amano Y, Takahashi Y, Mishima Y, Moriyama N, Ishimura N, *et al.* (2008). Barrett's esophagus in Japanese patients: its prevalence, form, and elongation. *Journal of Gastroenterology* **43**(12), 928–934.

24 Zhang M, Fan XS, Zou XP (2012). The prevalence of Barrett's esophagus remains low in Eastern China. Single-center 7-year descriptive study. *Saudi Medical Journal* **33**(12), 1324–1329.

25 Tseng PH, Lee YC, Chiu HM, Huang SP, Liao WC, Chen CC, *et al.* (2008). Prevalence and clinical characteristics of Barrett's esophagus in a Chinese general population. *Journal of Clinical Gastroenterology* **42**(10), 1074–1079.

26 Chen MJ, Lee YC, Chiu HM, Wu MS, Wang HP, Lin JT (2010). Time trends of endoscopic and pathological diagnoses related to gastroesophageal reflux disease in a Chinese population: eight years single institution experience. *Diseases of the Esophagus* **23**(3), 201–207.

27 Xiong LS, Cui Y, Wang JP, Wang JH, Xue L, Hu PJ, *et al.* (2010). Prevalence and risk factors of Barrett's esophagus in patients undergoing endoscopy for upper gastrointestinal symptoms. *Journal of Digestive Diseases* **11**(2), 83–87.

28 Lee IS, Choi SC, Shim KN, Jee SR, Huh KC, Lee JH, *et al.* (2010). Prevalence of Barrett's esophagus remains low in the Korean population: nationwide cross-sectional prospective multicenter study. *Digestive Diseases and Sciences* **55**(7), 1932–1939.

29 Park JJ, Kim JW, Kim HJ, Chung MG, Park SM, Baik GH, *et al.* (2009). The prevalence of and risk factors for Barrett's esophagus in a Korean population: A nationwide multicenter prospective study. *Journal of Clinical Gastroenterology* **43**(10), 907–914.

30 Akiyama T, Sekino Y, Iida H, Koyama S, Gotoh E, Maeda S, *et al.* (2012). Endoscopic diagnosis of Barrett's esophagus. *World Journal of Gastroenterology* **18**(26), 3477–3478.

31 Bayrakci B, Kasap E, Kitapcioglu G, Bor S (2008). Low prevalence of erosive esophagitis and Barrett esophagus in a tertiary referral center in Turkey. *Turkish Journal of Gastroenterology* **19**(3), 145–151.

32 Freitas MC, Moretzsohn LD, Coelho LG (2008). Prevalence of Barrett's esophagus in individuals without typical symptoms of gastroesophageal reflux disease. *Arquivos de Gastroenterologia* **45**(1), 46–49.

33 Fouad YM, Makhlouf MM, Tawfik HM, el-Amin H, Ghany WA, el-Khayat HR (2009). Barrett's esophagus: prevalence and risk factors in patients with chronic GERD in Upper Egypt. *World Journal of Gastroenterology* **15**(28), 3511–3515.

34 Sharma P, Wani S, Romero Y, Johnson D, Hamilton F (2008). Racial and geographic issues in gastroesophageal reflux disease. *American Journal of Gastroenterology* **103**(11), 2669–2680.

35 Ronkainen J, Aro P, Storskrubb T, Johansson SE, Lind T, Bolling-Sternevald E, *et al.* (2005). High prevalence of gastroesophageal reflux symptoms and esophagitis with or without symptoms in the general adult Swedish population: a Kalixanda study report. *Scandinavian Journal of Gastroenterology* **40**(3), 275–285.

36 Rex DK, Cummings OW, Shaw M, Cumings MD, Wong RK, Vasudeva RS, *et al.* (2003). Screening for Barrett's esophagus in colonoscopy patients with and without heartburn. *Gastroenterology* **125**(6), 1670–1677.

37 Balasubramanian G, Singh M, Gupta N, Gaddam S, Giacchino M, Wani SB, *et al.* (2012). Prevalence and predictors of columnar lined esophagus in gastroesophageal reflux disease (GERD) patients undergoing upper endoscopy. *American Journal of Gastroenterology* **107**(11), 1655–1661.

38 Veldhuyzen van Zanten SJ, Thomson AB, Barkun AN, Armstrong D, Chiba N, White RJ, *et al.* (2006). The prevalence of Barrett's ocsophagus in a cohort of 1040 Canadian primary care patients with uninvestigated dyspepsia undergoing prompt endoscopy. *Alimentary Pharmacology & Therapeutics* **23**(5), 595–599.

39 Ward EM, Devault KR, Bouras EP, Stark ME, Wolfsen HC, Davis DM, *et al.* (2004). Successful oesophageal pH monitoring with a catheter-free system. *Alimentary Pharmacology & Therapeutics* **19**(4), 449–454.

40 Gerson LB, Shetler K, Triadafilopoulos G (2002). Prevalence of Barrett's esophagus in asymptomatic individuals. *Gastroenterology* **123**(2), 461–467.

41 Coleman HG, Bhat S, Murray LJ, McManus D, Gavin AT, Johnston BT (2011). Increasing incidence of Barrett's oesophagus: a population-based study. *European Journal of Epidemiology* **26**(9), 739–45.

42 Hurschler D, Borovicka J, Neuweiler J, Oehlschlegel C, Sagmeister M, Meyenberger C, *et al.* (2003). Increased detection rates of Barrett's oesophagus without rise in

incidence of oesophageal adenocarcinoma. *Swiss Medical Weekly* **133**(37–38), 507–514.

43 Post PN, Siersema PD, Van Dekken H (2007). Rising incidence of clinically evident Barrett's oesophagus in The Netherlands: a nation-wide registry of pathology reports. *Scandinavian Journal of Gastroenterology* **42**(1), 17–22.

44 Prach AT, MacDonald TA, Hopwood DA, Johnston DA (1997). Increasing incidence of Barrett's oesophagus: education, enthusiasm, or epidemiology? *Lancet* **350**(9082), 933.

45 van Soest EM, Dieleman JP, Siersema PD, Sturkenboom MC, Kuipers EJ (2005). Increasing incidence of Barrett's oesophagus in the general population. *Gut* **54**(8), 1062–1066.

46 Wall CM, Charlett A, Caygill CP, Gatenby PA, Ramus JR, Winslet MC, *et al.* (2009). Are newly diagnosed columnar-lined oesophagus patients getting younger? *European Journal of Gastroenterology & Hepatology* **21**(10), 1127–1131.

47 Fitzgerald RC (2005). Barrett's oesophagus and oesophageal adenocarcinoma: how does acid interfere with cell proliferation and differentiation? *Gut* **54**(Suppl 1), i21–6.

48 British Society of Gastroenterology (2005). *Guidelines for the diagnosis and management of Barrett's columnar-lined oesophagus*, p. 28.

49 Taylor JB, Rubenstein JH (2010). Meta-analyses of the effect of symptoms of gastroesophageal reflux on the risk of Barrett's esophagus. *American Journal of Gastroenterology* **105**(8), 1729, 1730–7; quiz 1738.

50 Souza RF, Krishnan K, Spechler SJ (2008). Acid, bile, and CDX: the ABCs of making Barrett's metaplasia. *American Journal of Physiology – Gastrointestinal and Liver Physiology* **295**(2), G211–8.

51 Bernstein H, Bernstein C, Payne CM, Dvorak K (2009). Bile acids as endogenous etiologic agents in gastrointestinal cancer. *World Journal of Gastroenterology* **15**(27), 3329–3340.

52 Dvorak K, Payne CM, Chavarria M, Ramsey L, Dvorakova B, Bernstein H, *et al.* (2007). Bile acids in combination with low pH induce oxidative stress and oxidative DNA damage: relevance to the pathogenesis of Barrett's oesophagus. *Gut* **56**(6), 763–771.

53 Agarwal A, Polineni R, Hussein Z, Vigoda I, Bhagat TD, Bhattacharyya S, *et al.* (2012). Role of epigenetic alterations in the pathogenesis of Barrett's esophagus and esophageal adenocarcinoma. *International Journal of Clinical and Experimental Pathology* **5**(5), 382–396.

54 Fletcher J, Wirz A, Henry E, McColl KE (2004). Studies of acid exposure immediately above the gastro-oesophageal squamocolumnar junction: evidence of short segment reflux. *Gut* **53**(2), 168–173.

55 Wild CP, Hardie LJ (2003). Reflux, Barrett's oesophagus and adenocarcinoma: Burning questions. *Nature Reviews Cancer* **3**(9), 676–684.

56 Bhat S, Coleman HG, Yousef F, Johnston BT, McManus D, Murray LJ (2011). Risk of Malignant Progression in Barrett's Esophagus Patients: Results from a Large Population-Based Study. *JNCI* **103**(13), 1049–57.

57 Edelstein ZR, Bronner MP, Rosen SN, Vaughan TL (2009). Risk factors for Barrett's esophagus among patients with gastroesophageal reflux disease: a community clinic-based case-control study. *American Journal of Gastroenterology* **104**(4), 834–842.

58 Steevens J, Schouten LJ, Driessen AL, Huysentruyt CJ, Keulemans YC, Goldbohm RA, *et al.* (2011). A prospective cohort study on overweight, smoking, alcohol consumption, and risk of Barrett's esophagus. *Cancer Epidemiology, Biomarkers & Prevention* **20**(2), 345–358.

59 Seidel D, Muangpaisan W, Hiro H, Mathew A, Lyratzopoulos G (2009). The association between body mass index and Barrett's esophagus: a systematic review. *Diseases of the Esophagus* **22**(7), 564–570.

60 Anderson LA, Watson RG, Murphy SJ, Johnston BT, Comber H, Mc Guigan J, *et al.* (2007). Risk factors for Barrett's oesophagus and oesophageal adenocarcinoma: results from the FINBAR study. *World Journal of Gastroenterology* **13**(10), 1585–1594.

61 Ryan AM, Healy LA, Power DG, Byrne M, Murphy S, Byrne PJ, *et al.* (2008). Barrett esophagus: prevalence of central adiposity, metabolic syndrome, and a proinflammatory state. *Annals of Surgery* **247**(6), 909–915.

62 Edelstein ZR, Farrow DC, Bronner MP, Rosen SN, Vaughan TL (2007). Central adiposity and risk of Barrett's esophagus. *Gastroenterology* **133**(2), 403–411.

63 Jacobson BC, Chan AT, Giovannucci EL, Fuchs CS (2009). Body mass index and Barrett's oesophagus in women. *Gut* **58**(11), 1460–1466.

64 Iyer PG, Borah BJ, Heien HC, Das A, Cooper GS, Chak A (2013). Association of Barrett's Esophagus With Type II Diabetes Mellitus: Results From a Large Population-Based Case-Control Study. *Clinical Gastroenterology and Hepatology* **11**(9), 1108–1114.e5.

65 Anderson LA, Cantwell MM, Watson RG, Johnston BT, Murphy SJ, Ferguson HR, *et al.* (2009). The association between alcohol and reflux esophagitis, Barrett's esophagus, and esophageal adenocarcinoma. *Gastroenterology* **136**(3), 799–805.

66 Kubo A, Levin TR, Block G, Rumore GJ, Quesenberry CP, Jr, Buffler P, *et al.* (2009). Alcohol types and sociodemographic characteristics as risk factors for Barrett's esophagus. *Gastroenterology* **136**(3), 806–815.

67 Mulholland HG, Cantwell MM, Anderson LA, Johnston BT, Watson RG, Murphy SJ, *et al.* (2009). Glycemic index, carbohydrate and fiber intakes and risk of reflux esophagitis, Barrett's esophagus, and esophageal adenocarcinoma. *Cancer Causes and Control* **20**(3), 279–288.

68 O'Doherty MG, Abnet CC, Murray LJ, Woodside JV, Anderson LA, Brockman JD, *et al.* (2010). Iron intake and markers of iron status and risk of Barrett's esophagus and esophageal adenocarcinoma. *Cancer Causes and Control* **21**(12), 2269–79.

69 Kubo A, Levin TR, Block G, Rumore GJ, Quesenberry CP, Jr, Buffler P, *et al.* (2008). Dietary antioxidants, fruits, and vegetables and the risk of Barrett's esophagus. *American Journal of Gastroenterology* **103**(7), 1614–23; quiz 1624.

70 Kubo A, Corley DA, Jensen CD, Kaur R (2010). Dietary factors and the risks of oesophageal adenocarcinoma and Barrett's oesophagus. *Nutrition Research Reviews* **23**(2), 230–246.

71 Kubo A, Block G, Quesenberry CP, Jr., Buffler P, Corley DA (2009). Effects of Dietary Fiber, Fats, and Meat Intakes on the Risk of Barrett's Esophagus. *Nutrition and Cancer – an International Journal* **61**(5), 607–616.

72 O'Doherty MG, Cantwell MM, Murray LJ, Anderson LA, Abnet CC, FINBAR Study Group (2011). Dietary fat and meat intakes and risk of reflux esophagitis, Barrett's esophagus and esophageal adenocarcinoma. *International Journal of Cancer* **129**(6), 1493–1502.

73 Anderson LA, Johnston BT, Watson RG, Murphy SJ, Ferguson HR, Comber H, *et al.* (2006). Nonsteroidal anti-inflammatory drugs and the esophageal inflammation-metaplasia-adenocarcinoma sequence. *Cancer Research* **66**(9), 4975–4982.

74 Omer ZB, Ananthakrishnan AN, Nattinger KJ, Cole EB, Lin JJ, Kong CY, *et al.* (2012). Aspirin protects against Barrett's esophagus in a multivariate logistic regression analysis. *Clinical Gastroenterology and Hepatology* **10**(7), 722–727.

75 Fischbach LA, Nordenstedt H, Kramer JR, Gandhi S, Dick-Onuoha S, Lewis A, *et al.* (2012). The association between Barrett's esophagus and Helicobacter pylori infection: a meta-analysis. *Helicobacter* **17**(3), 163–175.

76 Ochs-Balcom HM, Falk G, Grady WM, Kinnard M, Willis J, Elston R, *et al.* (2007). Consortium approach to identifying genes for Barrett's esophagus and esophageal adenocarcinoma. *Translational Research* **150**(1), 3–17.

77 Su Z, Gay LJ, Strange A, Palles C, Band G, Whiteman DC, *et al.* (2012). Common variants at the MHC locus and at chromosome 16q24.1 predispose to Barrett's esophagus. *Nature Genetics* **44**(10), 1131–1136.

78 Flejou JF (2005). Barrett's oesophagus: from metaplasia to dysplasia and cancer. *Gut* **54**(Suppl 1), i6–12.

79 Shaheen NJ, Crosby MA, Bozymski EM, Sandler RS (2000). Is there publication bias in the reporting of cancer risk in Barrett's esophagus? *Gastroenterology* **119**(2), 333–338.

80 Yousef F, Cardwell C, Cantwell MM, Galway K, Johnston BT, Murray L (2008). The incidence of esophageal cancer and high-grade dysplasia in Barrett's esophagus: a systematic review and meta-analysis. *American Journal of Epidemiology* **168**(3), 237–249.

81 Hvid-Jensen F, Pedersen L, Drewes AM, Sorensen HT, Funch-Jensen P (2011). Incidence of adenocarcinoma among patients with Barrett's esophagus. *New England Journal of Medicine* **365**(15), 1375–1383.

CHAPTER 4

Esophageal adenocarcinoma: risk factors

Mariam Naveed & Kerry B. Dunbar

Division of Gastroenterology and Hepatology, University of Texas Southwestern Medical Center, Dallas VA Medical Center, Dallas, TX, USA

4.1 Introduction

The incidence of esophageal adenocarcinoma (EAC) has been steadily rising over the last three decades, with population-based cohort studies suggestive of a 300–500% increase during this time [1]. This dramatic rise was initially attributed to anatomic reclassifications of tumors, advances in diagnostic capabilities, and over-diagnosis secondary to increased screening efforts. However, the idea has since been dismissed, as studies have shown this increase to represent a true increase in disease burden [2, 3].

While the exact cause remains uncertain, a large body of evidence implicates changes in prevalence of several risk factors as a plausible explanation for the observed increase in EAC. In one population-based case-control study, smoking, a body mass index (BMI) higher than the lowest quartile, gastroesophageal reflux disease (GERD), and a diet low in fruits and vegetables accounted for almost 80% of cases of EAC in the United States [4]. Here, we further discuss the known and suspected risk factors for developing esophageal adenocarcinoma (summarized in Table 4.1).

4.2 Gastroesophageal reflux disease (GERD)

GERD causes esophageal inflammation and can lead to conversion of the esophageal mucosa to a more protective intestinal columnar mucosa, known as Barrett's esophagus (BE) [5]. The specialized epithelium of BE is more resistant to acid damage than the native squamous epithelium, partly due to mucous production by goblet cells [6]. Unfortunately, BE is predisposed to

carcinogenesis and is a risk factor for the development of EAC [5, 7–10].

GERD is recognized as an independent risk factor for the development of EAC [11–14]. In a recent meta-analysis by Rubenstein *et al.*, patients with weekly symptoms of GERD had five times greater risk of developing EAC than the control group [15]. Several studies using large population databases have estimated the risk of EAC in GERD. The relative risk (RR) of EAC with GERD is 1.7–3.0, and this increases when erosive esophagitis is present (RR 4.5–6.9), with the highest risk when BE is present (RR 30) [7, 16, 17].

Numerous studies have estimated the odds ratio (OR) of developing EAC in the backdrop of GERD to be between 2.5 to greater than 40, depending on duration and symptom severity [11, 18–20]. Other studies have confirmed the dose response relationship, also noting that a history of hiatal hernia was associated with increased risk of EAC [21, 22].

Despite the aforementioned alarming statistics, the absolute risk of an individual with GERD or esophagitis developing EAC is low. It has been estimated that in a population of 100,000, over 10,000 subjects would be expected to have reflux symptoms, with a corresponding incidence of EAC of only about 2.3/100,000 per year [23]. It has been suggested that among 50 year old men with symptoms of GERD, one-time screening endoscopy for BE and EAC would be cost-effective [24]. Another study calculated that if the risk of EAC with GERD were assumed to be 20 times the normal population risk, 1400 men over the age of 50 would have to be screened each year to identify one case of EAC [11].

Several medical societies have recommendations for which GERD patients to screen for BE and EAC,

Esophageal Cancer and Barrett's Esophagus, Third Edition. Edited by Prateek Sharma, Richard Sampliner and David Ilson.
© 2015 John Wiley & Sons, Ltd. Published 2015 by John Wiley & Sons, Ltd.

Table 4.1 Risk factors and protective factors for development of esophageal adenocarcinoma.

Risk factors	Magnitude of effect
Barrett's esophagus – without or with dysplasia	+++
GERD	+++
Central obesity and elevated BMI	+++
Smoking	++
Male gender	++
White race	+
Increasing age	+
High fat diet	+

Protective factors	Magnitude of effect
High intake of fruits, vegetables and antioxidants	+++
H Pylori infection	++
Dietary fiber	++
Aspirin and NSAIDs	+
Proton pump Inhibitors	+
Statins	+

+ low, ++ moderate, +++ high

including patients with long-standing GERD symptoms, age 50 years or older, male sex, white race, a history of hiatal hernia, elevated BMI, and intra-abdominal distribution of body fat [25–28]. Several cohort studies have shown patients enrolled in surveillance endoscopy programs have asymptomatic cancers detected at an earlier stage and longer survival. However, some of this apparent benefit may be due to lead time and length time bias [29, 30]. In addition, several studies have shown that 40% of individuals who develop cancer never experience reflux symptoms [11, 31]. The decision to pursue screening endoscopy in a GERD patient should be made after discussion with the patient of the risk and benefits of screening endoscopy.

4.3 Barrett's esophagus (BE)

The majority of esophageal adenocarcinomas arise from a backdrop of BE [1, 5, 32, 33]. The prevalence of BE has been estimated at 3–7% in patients with frequent reflux symptoms undergoing endoscopy, while the prevalence in asymptomatic individuals or those undergoing endoscopy for any clinical indication is approximately 1% [34]. The prevalence and incidence of BE have increased over time, parallel to the increase in frequency of EAC. An increase in the incidence of GERD during the same period of time may be to blame [5].

There are various estimates (ranging from 0.1–2.0%) of the annual rate of progression from BE to cancer [9, 35–38]. In a recent meta-analysis of 50 studies with nearly 14,000 patients and 62,000 person-years follow-up, the pooled estimate for EAC incidence in BE was 5.0 per 1000 person years [39]. Recent data is notable for lower rates of EAC, with incidence rates ranging from 1.2 to 1.4 cases per 1000-person years [36–38].

Risk factors for progression from BE to EAC include age, male gender, smoking, decreased intake of fruit and vegetables, obesity, increasing length of BE, and the presence of dysplasia [40–42]. The degree of dysplasia is one of the most predictive factors for the development of EAC. There is considerable variation in the reported rates at which non-dysplastic BE, low grade dysplasia (LGD) and HGD progress to cancer. Referral bias, inclusion of patients with prevalent cancers, endoscopic sampling variability, and inter-observer variability during histopathological interpretation, have been reported as plausible explanations for the considerable variation in reported estimates [43–45].

Based on recent data, incidence of progression to EAC in patients with non-dysplastic metaplasia is reported as being anywhere from 1.0 to 3.9 cases per 1000 person-years. Patients with LGD were reported to have anywhere from 5.1 to 7.7 cases per 1000 person-years [36, 46]. A recent meta-analysis reported that the incidence of EAC in patients with HGD was approximately 6.58% annually [47].

There is still debate concerning the relationship between length of BE and risk of EAC, suggesting that the risk of EAC is higher with long-segment BE (LSBE) than with short-segment BE (SSBE), with one study showing LSBE had a 2.7-fold higher OR of developing cancer or HGD than SSBE [41]. It has been estimated that for every 1 cm increase in BE length, the risk of HGD and EAC increases by 19% [41]. In contrast, a recent meta-analysis did not find a statistically significant decreased cancer risk for SSBE, compared to LSBE [48]. At this time, patients with short- and long-segment BE are managed similarly.

Familial and genetic factors have also been implicated in contributing to the development of EAC in a subset of patients with BE. Of patients with BE, 6.2% have a first or second degree relative with BE, while 9.5% of patients with EAC have a relative with BE [49, 50]. Patients with a family history of BE may develop EAC at a younger age and lower BMI compared with sporadic EAC cases. Familial and genetic factors may represent a risk factor for development of EAC in a small subset of patients, and further studies are required in order to determine the magnitude of risk.

While the risk of developing EAC in patients who have Barrett's esophagus is increased almost 30-fold above that of the general population, the absolute risk is low, with an annual incidence reported as low as 0.12% [36]. Furthermore, studies have shown that the majority of patients with BE are more likely to die of other causes than EAC [51]. In one study, mortality incidence was 3.0 per 1000 person-years due to esophageal adenocarcinoma, and 37.1 per 1000 person-years due to other causes [39].

4.4 Obesity

Global obesity rates have doubled since the 1980s [52]. Recent national data from the US Centers for Disease Control and Prevention show that more than one-third of adults and almost 17% of children and adolescents are obese [53]. Worldwide, more than 1.4 billion adults are overweight (defined as BMI $\geq$ 25), with over 200 million men and nearly 300 million women who are obese (defined as BMI $\geq$ 30). Epidemiological studies have shown that obesity is associated with increased risk of several cancers, including esophageal cancer [54]. A large body of evidence has examined the relationship between increased BMI and EAC, with a relative risk of EAC of 1.7 in overweight patients and 2.3 in obese patients [55–57]. Pooled analysis of data from 12 studies detected a strong linear relationship between increased BMI and risk of EAC, with a BMI > 40 associated with nearly a five-fold increased risk of EAC, compared with those with BMI $\leq$ 25 [58].

The relationship between EAC and abdominal (central) obesity is stronger than with simple obesity or increased BMI [59]. Three case control studies have shown increased risk of BE, thought to be mediated predominantly by intra-abdominal adipose tissue [60–62]. The association was noted predominantly in men, regardless of the presence or absence of GERD,

and may also contribute to the gender disparities seen in EAC [61].

There are several proposed mechanisms by which obesity increases the risk of EAC. Individuals with a higher BMI, especially those with central obesity, have an increased intra-gastric pressure, which subsequently relaxes the lower esophageal sphincter, facilitating esophageal reflux [56, 63]. Obese patients experience 48% more reflux episodes than patients with a normal BMI [64]. Other studies have also shown the prevalence of GERD to increase with increasing BMI [56, 65]. The increase in abdominal pressure also increases the risk of developing a hiatal hernia, which is associated with the development of GERD (OR 3.62) [41]. Therefore, obesity may increase the risk of EAC through a mechanical pathway, by increasing the risk of hiatal hernia and GERD, which would increase the risk of BE, the precursor lesion for EAC [66].

Non-mechanical factors may also lead to an increased risk of EAC in obesity. In a meta-analysis by Hoyo *et al.*, the association between increasing BMI and EAC was only minimally attenuated by the absence of reflux symptoms, suggesting that an indirect pathway for EAC development may also exist [58]. Obesity alters circulating levels of proliferative (i.e. insulin-like growth factors and leptin) and anti-proliferative hormones (i.e. adiponectin), providing a mechanism by which obesity plays a role in carcinogenesis independent of reflux [67].

4.5 Smoking

Smoking has been identified as a risk factor for EAC, with a 55% increased risk of EAC in smokers [68]. In smokers, the risk of progression from non-dysplastic BE to HGD or EAC is two to four times higher than non-smokers [41, 69, 70]. A multi-center, population-based, case control study by Gammon *et al.* showed the risk of EAC to be more than doubled in smokers, with higher risk seen with increased intensity and duration of smoking [71]. Unlike squamous cell carcinoma of the esophagus (SCC), the risk of EAC remained elevated up to 30 years after quitting. In addition, pooled data from the Barrett's Esophagus and Esophageal Adenocarcinoma Consortium (BEACON) noted strong associations between cigarette smoking and EAC in white patients (OR of 1.96). A dose response relationship was seen, and the risk was reduced after smoking cessation, although not to the level of the non-smokers [70].

While the exact mechanism by which smoking increases the risk of EAC is unknown, reduction in lower esophageal sphincter tone and increased reflux is one proposed theory [71]. Others have suggested a genetic component, with increased susceptibility to the presence of an active allele of the glutathione S-transferase M1 and T1 genes, which modulate susceptibility to EAC [72].

4.6 Alcohol

Multiple epidemiologic studies have examined the relationship between alcohol intake and EAC, with mixed results [68, 73]. Gammon *et al.* found the risk of EAC was unrelated to beer or liquor consumption, and significantly lessened with wine consumption (OR 0.6) [71]. A recent meta-analysis on alcohol and risk of esophageal and gastric cardiac adenocarcinoma including 5500 cases found no association between alcohol and EAC, regardless of degree of consumption [74].

4.7 Dietary factors

There has been much discussion in the last few years on the role of diet and risk of EAC. Investigators have proposed that increased intake of foods high in nitrates could be contributing to the increased incidence of EAC, with conversion of dietary nitrates to potentially carcinogenic compounds [75, 76]. Nitrates are found in many foods, including high levels in green leafy vegetables, beets, celery and radishes. While the majority of ingested nitrate is absorbed by the small bowel and excreted unchanged in the urine, 25% is concentrated by the salivary glands and reduced to nitrite. Nitrites are converted to nitrous oxide (NO) in the presence of gastric acid, and diffusion of NO into the esophageal epithelial compartment can then lead to production of potentially carcinogenic N-nitroso products [77].

Epidemiologic studies examining the relationship between dietary nitrates and EAC have produced mixed results. One study found a non-significant positive association between EAC and nitrite intake, while other studies have suggested no association with nitrite intake [78, 79]. Keszei *et al.* found that while N-nitroso

compounds may influence the risk of esophageal SCC in men, no clear associations for other esophageal and gastric cancer subtypes was noted [80]. At this time, prospective long term studies are needed to confirm the role of N-nitroso compounds in esophageal carcinogenesis.

Vegetable and fruit intake may also impact the risk of EAC. Several studies have shown an inverse association between fruit intake, vegetable intake and combined fruit and vegetable intake, and the risk of BE and EAC [41, 78, 81, 82]. In a multi-center, population-based, case control study, Engel *et al.* found the population attributable risk of low fruit and vegetable consumption on development of EAC to be 15.3% [4]. Conversely, a recent prospective study found no association between total fruit and vegetable intake and the incidence of EAC [83]. These authors suggest that fruit and vegetable intake may be a surrogate for other markers of health, such as smoking or socioeconomic status (SES) [83]. Intake of fruits and vegetables may also be a proxy for antioxidant intake. Several studies, including a recent meta-analysis, have shown a higher intake of antioxidants to be inversely associated with risk of EAC [84, 85].

Diets high in calories, fat, cholesterol, and animal protein and a low intake of dietary fiber have been shown to increase the risk of EAC. Frequent red meat intake and high fat dairy product intake are associated with an increased risk of EAC [78]. High intake of cereal fiber was associated with a moderately decreased risk of esophageal adenocarcinoma, which may be due to wheat fiber's ability to act neutralize nitrites under acidic conditions [82].

4.8 Medication use

Due to poor long-term survival rates for EAC, there has been increased focus on primary and secondary prevention strategies, including chemoprevention. Studies have shown the use of aspirin (ASA) and non-steroidal anti-inflammatory drugs (NSAIDs) to be protective against the development of esophageal cancer, with approximately 50–90% reduction in risk [86–88]. Vaughn *et al.* reported a lower risk of progression to EAC in patients with HGD who reported current use of NSAIDs [86]. The majority of the studies examining the relationship between ASA, NSAIDS and

EAC are observational studies, so ASA and NSAID users may have other behaviors that reduce their risk of EAC, as suggested by Mehta *et al.* [89]. A prospective randomized study of aspirin and PPI in patients with BE is ongoing [90].

Recent observational studies have also suggested statins may have a protective effect on development of cancers, including EAC [87, 91]. Several studies have examined the role of acid suppression, such as that produced by proton pump inhibitors (PPI) in modifying the clinical course of GERD. Four retrospective cohort studies have shown an association of PPI use and a reduced risk of dysplasia in patients with BE [92–95].

4.9 *H. pylori*

Multiple studies have examined the relationship between *H. pylori* and EAC, suggesting that colonization with *H. pylori* may be protective against EAC, possibly by leading to gastric atrophy and reduced esophageal acid exposure [96–98]. A similar inverse relationship between *H. pylori* infection and Barrett's esophagus has been seen [99]. There is speculation that the increasing incidence of EAC may be partly attributable to the decreasing prevalence of *H. pylori* infection in the Western world [100]. This hypothesis is supported by the observation that EAC rates are still low in most developing countries, where *H. pylori* is still common in the population [101].

Additional details regarding the association between H. pylori and esophageal neoplasia will be discussed in Chapter 8.

4.10 Demographics

The epidemiological characteristics of EAC differ from those of SCC of the esophagus. A key feature of EAC is its male preponderance, with male-to-female ratios of around 7 : 1 [2, 18, 19]. In a recent study by Pohl *et al.*, male gender more than doubled the risk for GERD patients to develop BE, and doubled the risk for Barrett's patients to develop EAC or high-grade dysplasia (HGD) [41]. BE may develop at an earlier age in men, allowing for more time to develop dysplasia and EAC with fewer competing causes of mortality, which could potentially explain some of the gender disparity [102]. Differences

in parietal cell mass, lower esophageal sphincter function, and higher BMI in males, have also been proposed as contributing to the gender disparity [103].

There are also clear ethnic imbalances, with increased incidence of EAC in white Americans compared to any other race, although increases have been reported across all races. In 1973, the incidence of EAC in white males was 0.8 per 100,000, and in 2002 it was 5.4 per 100,000, a mean annual increase of 8 % [104]. An analysis of the SEER cancer registry data found that the average annual incidence rate for EAC for white men was double that of Hispanic men and four times higher than in African-Americans, Asians/Pacific Islanders and Native Americans. Similar patterns were seen in women, although the rates of EAC for women of all ethnicities were lower than those encountered among men [105].

Along with male sex and white ethnicity, studies have consistently shown older age to be a risk factor. Data from the SEER program demonstrated an increased incidence of EAC with age until rates peak for males between the age of 77 and 79 and for females between 80 and 84, with decline in risk thereafter [106, 107]. Other studies have verified this, with a two-fold increase in incidence seen in men under the age of 65, compared with a three-to-four-fold increase in those over the age of 65 [108]. A "birth cohort effect" phenomenon has also been suggested, in which higher incidence rates of a disease are seen among cohorts of subjects born more recently; for each five-year increase in age, the odds of EAC were noted to have increased by 6.6 % [106].

While low socioeconomic status (SES) has been associated with a higher risk of SCC, this effect is not as strong for EAC [32]. Conversely, other studies have suggested increased risk of EAC in persons of higher SES, thought to be related to increased incidence of BE [109].

4.11 Summary

The incidence of EAC has increased rapidly in Western countries. This steep increase has led to considerable attention being paid to EAC risk factors, in the hope of identifying areas of prevention. GERD and BE are associated with EAC. Other risk factors include male gender, increasing BMI, abdominal obesity, white race, and increasing age. Although fruits, cereal fibers and vegetable intake have a protective effect, there is limited evidence at this time that dietary interventions prevent EAC. Avoidance of smoking, weight loss, and chemoprevention could potentially help reduce the risk of developing EAC.

References

1 Shaheen N, Ransohoff DF (2002). Gastroesophageal reflux, Barrett esophagus, and esophageal cancer: clinical applications. *JAMA* **287**(15), 1982–6.

2 Blot WJ, McLaughlin JK (1999). The changing epidemiology of esophageal cancer. *Seminars in Oncology* **26**(5 Suppl 15), 2–8.

3 Pohl, H, Welch HG (2005). The role of overdiagnosis and reclassification in the marked increase of esophageal adenocarcinoma incidence. *Journal of the National Cancer Institute* **97**(2), 142–6.

4 Engel LS, Chow WH, Vaughan TL, *et al.* (2003). Population attributable risks of esophageal and gastric cancers. *Journal of the National Cancer Institute* **95**(18), 1404–13.

5 Spechler SJ (2002). Clinical practice. Barrett's Esophagus. *New England Journal of Medicine* **346**(11), 836–42.

6 Chai J, Jamal MM (2012). Esophageal malignancy: a growing concern. *World Journal of Gastroenterology* **18**(45), 6521–6.

7 Solaymani-Dodaran M, Logan RF, West J, Card T, Coupland C. (2004). Risk of extra-oesophageal malignancies and colorectal cancer in Barrett's oesophagus and gastro-oesophageal reflux. *Scandinavian Journal of Gastroenterology* **39**(7), 680–5.

8 Cameron AJ, Ott, BJ, Payne WS (1985). The incidence of adenocarcinoma in columnar-lined (Barrett's) esophagus. *New England Journal of Medicine* **313**(14), 857–9.

9 Drewitz DJ, Sampliner RE, Garewal HS (1997). The incidence of adenocarcinoma in Barrett's esophagus: a prospective study of 170 patients followed 4.8 years. *American Journal of Gastroenterology* **92**(2), 212–5.

10 O'Connor JB, Falk GW, Richter JE (1999). The incidence of adenocarcinoma and dysplasia in Barrett's esophagus: report on the Cleveland Clinic Barrett's Esophagus Registry. *American Journal of Gastroenterology* **94**(8), 2037–42.

11 Lagergren J, Bergström R, Lindgren A, Nyrén O (1999). Symptomatic gastroesophageal reflux as a risk factor for esophageal adenocarcinoma. *New England Journal of Medicine* **340**(11), 825–31.

12 Lassen A, Hallas J, de Muckadell OB (2006). Esophagitis: incidence and risk of esophageal adenocarcinoma – a population-based cohort study. *American Journal of Gastroenterology* **101**(6), 1193–9.

13 Chow WH, Finkle WD, McLaughlin JK, Frankl H, Ziel HK, Fraumeni JF, Jr. (1995). The relation of gastroesophageal reflux disease and its treatment to adenocarcinomas of the esophagus and gastric cardia. *JAMA* **274**(6), 474–7.

14 Theisen J, Peters JH, Stein HJ (2003). Experimental evidence for mutagenic potential of duodenogastric juice on Barrett's esophagus. *World Journal of Surgery* **27**(9), 1018–20.

15 Rubenstein JH, Taylor JB (2010). Meta-analysis: the association of oesophageal adenocarcinoma with symptoms of gastro-oesophageal reflux. *Alimentary Pharmacology & Therapeutics* **32**(10), 1222–7.

16 Ruigómez A, García Rodríguez LA, Wallander MA, Johansson S, Graffner H, Dent J (2004). Natural history of gastro-oesophageal reflux disease diagnosed in general practice. *Alimentary Pharmacology & Therapeutics* **20**(7), 751–60.

17 García Rodríguez LA, Lagergren J, Lindblad M (2006). Gastric acid suppression and risk of oesophageal and gastric adenocarcinoma: a nested case control study in the UK. *Gut* **55**(11), 1538–44.

18 Lagergren J (2005). Adenocarcinoma of oesophagus: what exactly is the size of the problem and who is at risk? *Gut* **54**(Suppl 1), i1–5.

19 Pera M, Manterola C, Vidal O, Grande L (2005). Epidemiology of esophageal adenocarcinoma. *Journal of Surgical Oncology* **92**(3), 151–9.

20 Shaheen N, Ransohoff DF (2002). Gastroesophageal reflux, barrett esophagus, and esophageal cancer: scientific review. *JAMA* **287**(15), 1972–81.

21 Wu AH, Tseng CC, Bernstein L (2003). Hiatal hernia, reflux symptoms, body size, and risk of esophageal and gastric adenocarcinoma. *Cancer* **98**(5), 940–8.

22 Whiteman DC, Sadeghi S, Pandeya N, *et al.* (2008). Combined effects of obesity, acid reflux and smoking on the risk of adenocarcinomas of the oesophagus. *Gut* **57**(2), 173–80.

23 Cameron AJ, Romero Y (2000). Symptomatic gastro-oesophageal reflux as a risk factor for oesophageal adenocarcinoma. *Gut* **46**(6), 754–5.

24 Inadomi JM, Sampliner R, Lagergren J, Lieberman D, Fendrick AM, Vakil N (2003). Screening and surveillance for Barrett esophagus in high-risk groups: a cost-utility analysis. *Annals of Internal Medicine* **138**(3), 176–86.

25 Spechler SJ, Sharma P, Souza RF, Inadomi JM, Shaheen NJ (2011). American Gastroenterological Association medical position statement on the management of Barrett's esophagus. *Gastroenterology* **140**(3), 1084–91.

26 Katz PO, Gerson LB, Vela MF (2013). Guidelines for the diagnosis and management of gastroesophageal reflux disease. *American Journal of Gastroenterology* **108**(3), 308–28; quiz 329.

27 Shaheen NJ, Weinberg DS, Denberg TD, Chou R, Qaseem A, Shekelle P (2012). Upper endoscopy for gastroesophageal reflux disease: best practice advice from the clinical guidelines committee of the American College of Physicians. *Annals of Internal Medicine* **157**(11), 808–16.

28 Spechler SJ, Sharma P, Souza RF, Inadomi JM, Shaheen NJ (2011). American Gastroenterological Association

technical review on the management of Barrett's esophagus. *Gastroenterology* **140**(3), e18–52; quiz e13.

29 Streitz JM, Jr., Andrews CW, Jr., Ellis FH, Jr. (1993). Endoscopic surveillance of Barrett's esophagus. Does it help? *Journal of Thoracic and Cardiovascular Surgery.* **105**(3), 383–7; discussion 387–8.

30 Wong T, Tian J, Nagar AB (2010). Barrett's surveillance identifies patients with early esophageal adenocarcinoma. *American Journal of Medicine* **123**(5), 462–7.

31 Bytzer P, Christensen PB, Damkier P, Vinding K, Seersholm N (1999). Adenocarcinoma of the esophagus and Barrett's esophagus: a population-based study. *American Journal of Gastroenterology* **94**(1), 86–91.

32 Brown LM, Devesa SS (2002). Epidemiologic trends in esophageal and gastric cancer in the United States. *Surgical Oncology Clinics of North America* **11**(2), 235–56.

33 Spechler SJ, Fitzgerald RC, Prasad GA, Wang KK (2010). History, molecular mechanisms, and endoscopic treatment of Barrett's esophagus. *Gastroenterology* **138**(3), 854–69.

34 Ronkainen J, Aro P, Storskrubb T, *et al.* (2005). Prevalence of Barrett's esophagus in the general population: an endoscopic study. *Gastroenterology* **129**(6), 1825–31.

35 Shaheen NJ, Crosby MA, Bozymski EM, Sandler RS (2000). Is there publication bias in the reporting of cancer risk in Barrett's esophagus? *Gastroenterology* **119**(2), 333–8.

36 Hvid-Jensen F, Pedersen L, Drewes AM, Sørensen HT, Funch-Jensen P (2011). Incidence of adenocarcinoma among patients with Barrett's esophagus. *New England Journal of Medicine* **365**(15), 1375–83.

37 de Jonge PJ, van Blankenstein M, Looman CW, Casparie MK, Meijer GA, Kuipers EJ (2010). Risk of malignant progression in patients with Barrett's oesophagus: a Dutch nationwide cohort study. *Gut* **59**(8), 1030–6.

38 Bhat S, Coleman HG, Yousef F, *et al.* (2011). Risk of malignant progression in Barrett's esophagus patients: results from a large population-based study. *Journal of the National Cancer Institute* **103**(13), 1049–57.

39 Sikkema M, de Jonge PJ, Steyerberg EW, Kuipers EJ (2010). Risk of esophageal adenocarcinoma and mortality in patients with Barrett's esophagus: a systematic review and meta-analysis. *Clinical Gastroenterology and Hepatology* **8**(3), 235–44; quiz e32.

40 Prasad GA, Bansal A, Sharma P, Wang KK (2010). Predictors of progression in Barrett's esophagus: current knowledge and future directions. *American Journal of Gastroenterology* **105**(7), 1490–1502.

41 Pohl H, Wrobel K, Bojarski C, *et al.* (2013). Risk factors in the development of esophageal adenocarcinoma. *American Journal of Gastroenterology* **108**(2), 200–7.

42 van Blankenstein M, Looman CW, Johnston BJ, Caygill CP (2005). Age and sex distribution of the prevalence of Barrett's esophagus found in a primary referral endoscopy center. *American Journal of Gastroenterology* **100**(3), 568–76.

43 Schnell TG, Sontag SJ, Chejfec G, *et al.* (2001). Long-term nonsurgical management of Barrett's esophagus with high-grade dysplasia. *Gastroenterology* **120**(7), 1607–19.

44 Montgomery E, Bronner MP, Goldblum JR, *et al.* (2001). Reproducibility of the diagnosis of dysplasia in Barrett esophagus: a reaffirmation. *Human Pathology* **32**(4), 368–78.

45 Falk GW, Rice TW, Goldblum JR, Richter JE (1999). Jumbo biopsy forceps protocol still misses unsuspected cancer in Barrett's esophagus with high-grade dysplasia. *Gastrointestinal Endoscopy* **49**(2), 170–6.

46 Sharma P, Falk GW, Weston AP, Reker D, Johnston M, Sampliner RE (2006). Dysplasia and cancer in a large multicenter cohort of patients with Barrett's esophagus. *Clinical Gastroenterology and Hepatology* **4**(5), 566–72.

47 Rastogi A, Puli S, El-Serag HB, Bansal A, Wani S, Sharma P (2008). Incidence of esophageal adenocarcinoma in patients with Barrett's esophagus and high-grade dysplasia: a meta-analysis. *Gastrointestinal Endoscopy* **67**(3), 394–8.

48 Thomas T, Abrams KR, De Caestecker JS, Robinson RJ (2007). Meta analysis: Cancer risk in Barrett's oesophagus. *Alimentary Pharmacology & Therapeutics* **26**(11–12), 1465–77.

49 Chak A, Ochs-Balcom H, Falk G, *et al.* (2006). Familiality in Barrett's esophagus, adenocarcinoma of the esophagus, and adenocarcinoma of the gastroesophageal junction. *Cancer Epidemiology, Biomarkers & Prevention* **15**(9), 1668–73.

50 Chak A, Chen Y, Vengoechea J, *et al.* (2012). Variation in age at cancer diagnosis in familial versus nonfamilial Barrett's esophagus. *Cancer Epidemiology, Biomarkers & Prevention* **21**(2), 376–83.

51 van der Burgh A, Dees J, Hop WC, van Blankenstein M (1996). Oesophageal cancer is an uncommon cause of death in patients with Barrett's oesophagus. *Gut* **39**(1), 5–8.

52 Finucane MM, Stevens GA, Cowan MJ, *et al.* (2011). National, regional, and global trends in body-mass index since 1980: systematic analysis of health examination surveys and epidemiological studies with 960 country-years and 9.1 million participants. *Lancet* **377**(9765), 557–67.

53 Ogden CL, Carroll MD, Kit BK, Flegal KM (2012). Prevalence of obesity in the United States 2009–2010. *NCHS Data Brief* **82**, pp. 1–8.

54 Vucenik I, Stains JP (2012). Obesity and cancer risk: evidence, mechanisms, and recommendations. *Annals of the New York Academy of Sciences* **1271**, 37–43.

55 Turati F, Tramacere I, La Vecchia C, Negri E (2013). A meta-analysis of body mass index and esophageal and gastric cardia adenocarcinoma. *Annals of Oncology* **24**(3), 609–17.

56 Corley DA, Kubo A (2006). Body mass index and gastroesophageal reflux disease: a systematic review and meta-analysis. *American Journal of Gastroenterology* **101**(11), 2619–28.

57 Lagergren J (2011). Influence of obesity on the risk of esophageal disorders. *Nature Reviews Gastroenterology & Hepatology* **8**(6), 340–7.

58 Hoyo C, Cook MB, Kamangar F, *et al.* (2012). Body mass index in relation to oesophageal and oesophagogastric junction adenocarcinomas: a pooled analysis from the International BEACON Consortium. *International Journal of Epidemiology* **41**(6), 1706–18.

59 Corley DA, Kubo A, Zhao W (2008). Abdominal obesity and the risk of esophageal and gastric cardia carcinomas. *Cancer Epidemiology, Biomarkers & Prevention* **17**(2), 352–8.

60 Corley DA, Kubo A, Levin TR, *et al.* (2007). Abdominal obesity and body mass index as risk factors for Barrett's esophagus. *Gastroenterology* **133**(1), 34–41; quiz 311.

61 Kendall BJ, Macdonald GA, Hayward NK, *et al.* (2013). The risk of Barrett's esophagus associated with abdominal obesity in males and females. *International Journal of Cancer* **132**(9), 2192–9.

62 O'Doherty MG, Freedman ND, Hollenbeck AR, Schatzkin A, Abnet CC (2012). A prospective cohort study of obesity and risk of oesophageal and gastric adenocarcinoma in the NIH-AARP Diet and Health Study. *Gut* **61**(9), 1261–8.

63 Barak N, Ehrenpreis ED, Harrison JR, Sitrin MD (2002). Gastro-oesophageal reflux disease in obesity: pathophysiological and therapeutic considerations. *Obesity Reviews* **3**(1), 9–15.

64 El-Serag HB, Ergun GA, Pandolfino J, Fitzgerald S, Tran T, Kramer JR (2007). Obesity increases oesophageal acid exposure. *Gut* **56**(6), 749–55.

65 Friedenberg FK, Xanthopoulos M, Foster GD, Richter JE (2008). The association between gastroesophageal reflux disease and obesity. *American Journal of Gastroenterology* **103**(8), 2111–22.

66 Brown LM, Swanson CA, Gridley G, *et al.* (1995). Adenocarcinoma of the esophagus: role of obesity and diet. *Journal of the National Cancer Institute* **87**(2), 104–9.

67 Frystyk J, Skjaerbaek C, Vestbo E, Fisker S, Orskov H (1999). Circulating levels of free insulin-like growth factors in obese subjects: the impact of type 2 diabetes. *Diabetes/Metabolism Research and Reviews* **15**(5), 314–22.

68 Freedman ND, Abnet CC, Leitzmann MF, *et al.* (2007). A prospective study of tobacco, alcohol, and the risk of esophageal and gastric cancer subtypes. *American Journal of Epidemiology* **165**(12), 1424–33.

69 Coleman HG, Bhat S, Johnston BT, McManus D, Gavin AT, Murray LJ (2012). Tobacco smoking increases the risk of high-grade dysplasia and cancer among patients with Barrett's esophagus. *Gastroenterology* **142**(2), 233–40.

70 Cook MB, Kamangar F, Whiteman DC, *et al.* (2010). Cigarette smoking and adenocarcinomas of the esophagus and esophagogastric junction: a pooled analysis from the international BEACON consortium. *Journal of the National Cancer Institute* **102**(17), 1344–53.

71 Gammon MD, Schoenberg JB, Ahsan H, *et al.* (1997). Tobacco, alcohol, and socioeconomic status and adenocarcinomas of the esophagus and gastric cardia. *Journal of the National Cancer Institute* **89**(17), 1277–84.

72 Casson AG, Zheng Z, Porter GA, Guernsey DL (2006). Genetic polymorphisms of microsomal epoxide hydroxylase and glutathione S-transferases M1, T1 and P1, interactions with smoking, and risk for esophageal (Barrett) adenocarcinoma. *Cancer Detection and Prevention* **30**(5), 423–31.

73 Lindblad M, Rodriguez LA, Lagergren J (2005). Body mass, tobacco and alcohol and risk of esophageal, gastric cardia, and gastric non-cardia adenocarcinoma among men and women in a nested case-control study. *Cancer Causes and Control* **16**(3), 285–94.

74 Tramacere I, Pelucchi C, Bagnardi V, *et al.* (2012). A meta-analysis on alcohol drinking and esophageal and gastric cardia adenocarcinoma risk. *Annals of Oncology* **23**(2), 287–97.

75 Iijima K , Henry E, Moriya A, *et al.* (2002). Dietary nitrate generates potentially mutagenic concentrations of nitric oxide at the gastroesophageal junction. *Gastroenterology* **122**(5), 1248–57.

76 Spechler SJ (2002). Carcinogenesis at the gastroesophageal junction: free radicals at the frontier. *Gastroenterology* **122**(5), 1518–20.

77 Iijima K, Grant J, McElroy K, *et al.* (2003). Novel mechanism of nitrosative stress from dietary nitrate with relevance to gastro-oesophageal junction cancers. *Carcinogenesis* **24**(12), 1951–60.

78 Mayne ST, Risch HA, Dubrow R, *et al.* (2001). Nutrient intake and risk of subtypes of esophageal and gastric cancer. *Cancer Epidemiology, Biomarkers & Prevention* **10**(10), 1055–62.

79 Rogers MA, Vaughan TL, Davis S, Thomas DB (1995). Consumption of nitrate, nitrite, and nitrosodimethylamine and the risk of upper aerodigestive tract cancer. *Cancer Epidemiology, Biomarkers & Prevention* **4**(1), 29–36.

80 Keszei AP, Goldbohm RA, Schouten LJ, Jakszyn P, van den Brandt PA (2013). Dietary N-nitroso compounds, endogenous nitrosation, and the risk of esophageal and gastric cancer subtypes in the Netherlands Cohort Study. *American Journal of Clinical Nutrition* **97**(1), 135–46.

81 Kubo A, Levin TR, Block G, *et al.* (2008). Dietary antioxidants, fruits, and vegetables and the risk of Barrett's esophagus. *American Journal of Gastroenterology* **103**(7), 1614–23; quiz 1624.

82 Terry P, Lagergren J, Ye W, Wolk A, Nyrén O (2001). Inverse association between intake of cereal fiber and risk of gastric cardia cancer. *Gastroenterology* **120**(2), 387–91.

83 Freedman ND, Park Y, Subar AF, *et al.* (2007). Fruit and vegetable intake and esophageal cancer in a large prospective cohort study. *International Journal of Cancer* **121**(12), 2753–60.

84 Murphy SJ, Anderson LA, Ferguson HR, *et al.* (2010). Dietary antioxidant and mineral intake in humans is associated with reduced risk of esophageal adenocarcinoma

but not reflux esophagitis or Barrett's esophagus. *Journal of Nutrition* **140**(10), 1757–63.

85 Kubo A, Corley DA (2007). Meta-analysis of antioxidant intake and the risk of esophageal and gastric cardia adenocarcinoma. *American Journal of Gastroenterology* **102**(10), 2323–30; quiz 2331.

86 Vaughan TL, Dong LM, Blount PL, *et al.* (2005). Non-steroidal anti-inflammatory drugs and risk of neoplastic progression in Barrett's oesophagus: a prospective study. *The Lancet Oncology* **6**(12), 945–52.

87 Nguyen DM, Richardson P, El-Serag HB (2010). Medications (NSAIDs, statins, proton pump inhibitors) and the risk of esophageal adenocarcinoma in patients with Barrett's esophagus. *Gastroenterology* **138**(7), 2260–6.

88 Sivarasan N, Smith G (2013). Role of aspirin in chemoprevention of esophageal adenocarcinoma: a meta-analysis. *Journal of Digestive Diseases* **14**(5), 222–30.

89 Mehta S, Johnson IT, Rhodes M (2005). Systematic review: the chemoprevention of oesophageal adenocarcinoma. *Alimentary Pharmacology & Therapeutics* **22**(9), 759–68.

90 Das D, Chilton AP, Jankowski JA (2009). Chemoprevention of oesophageal cancer and the AspECT trial. *Recent Results in Cancer Research* **181**, 161–9.

91 Karp I, Behlouli H, Lelorier J, Pilote L (2008). Statins and cancer risk. *American Journal of Medicine* **121**(4), 302–9.

92 El-Serag HB, Aguirre TV, Davis S, Kuebeler M, Bhattacharyya A, Sampliner RE (2004). Proton pump inhibitors are associated with reduced incidence of dysplasia in Barrett's esophagus. *American Journal of Gastroenterology* **99**(10), 1877–83.

93 Hillman LC, Chiragakis L, Shadbolt B, Kaye GL, Clarke AC (2008). Effect of proton pump inhibitors on markers of risk for high-grade dysplasia and oesophageal cancer in Barrett's oesophagus. *Alimentary Pharmacology & Therapeutics* **27**(4), 321–6.

94 Hillman LC, Chiragakis L, Shadbolt B, Kaye GL, Clarke AC (2004). Proton-pump inhibitor therapy and the development of dysplasia in patients with Barrett's oesophagus. *Medical Journal of Australia* **180**(8), 387–91.

95 Nguyen DM, El-Serag HB, Henderson L, Stein D, Bhattacharyya A, Sampliner RE (2009). Medication usage and the risk of neoplasia in patients with Barrett's esophagus. *Clinical Gastroenterology and Hepatology* **7**(12), 1299–304.

96 Islami F, Kamangar F (2008). *Helicobacter pylori* and esophageal cancer risk: a meta-analysis. *Cancer Prevention Research (Phila)* **1**(5), 329–38.

97 Rokkas T, Pistiolas D, Sechopoulos P, Robotis I, Margantinis G (2007). Relationship between *Helicobacter pylori* infection and esophageal neoplasia: a meta-analysis. *Clinical Gastroenterology and Hepatology* **5**(12), 1413–7, 1417 e1–2.

98 Chow WH, Blaser MJ, Blot WJ, *et al.* (1998). An inverse relation between cagA+ strains of *Helicobacter pylori* infection and risk of esophageal and gastric cardia adenocarcinoma. *Cancer Research* **58**(4), 588–90.

99 Sonnenberg A, Lash RH, Genta RM (2010). A national study of *Helicobactor pylori* infection in gastric biopsy specimens. *Gastroenterology* **139**(6), 1894–1901 e2; quiz e12.

100 McColl KE, Watabe H, Derakhshan MH (2008). Role of gastric atrophy in mediating negative association between *Helicobacter pylori* infection and reflux oesophagitis, Barrett's oesophagus and oesophageal adenocarcinoma. *Gut* **57**(6), 721–3.

101 Islami F, Kamangar F, Aghcheli K, *et al.* (2004). Epidemiologic features of upper gastrointestinal tract cancers in Northeastern Iran. *British Journal of Cancer* **90**(7), 1402–6.

102 Anderson LA, Murray LJ, Murphy SJ, *et al.* (2003). Mortality in Barrett's oesophagus: results from a population based study. *Gut* **52**(8), 1081–1084.

103 Adeniyi KO (1991). Gastric acid secretion and parietal cell mass: effect of sex hormones. *Gastroenterology* **101**(1), 66–69.

104 Holmes RS, Vaughan TL (2007). Epidemiology and pathogenesis of esophageal cancer. *Seminars in Radiation Oncology* **17**(1), 2–9.

105 Kubo A, Corley DA (2004). Marked multi-ethnic variation of esophageal and gastric cardia carcinomas within the United States. *American Journal of Gastroenterology* **99**(4), 582–8.

106 El-Serag HB, Mason AC, Petersen N, Key CR (2002). Epidemiological differences between adenocarcinoma of the oesophagus and adenocarcinoma of the gastric cardia in the USA. *Gut* **50**(3), 368–72.

107 van Blankenstein M, Looman CW, Hop WC, Bytzer P (2005). The incidence of adenocarcinoma and squamous cell carcinoma of the esophagus: Barrett's esophagus makes a difference. *American Journal of Gastroenterology* **100**(4), 766–74.

108 Devesa SS, Blot WJ, Fraumeni JF, Jr (1998). Changing patterns in the incidence of esophageal and gastric carcinoma in the United States. *Cancer* **83**(10), 2049–53.

109 Kabat GC, Ng SK, Wynder EL (1993). Tobacco, alcohol intake, and diet in relation to adenocarcinoma of the esophagus and gastric cardia. *Cancer Causes and Control* **4**(2), 123–32.

CHAPTER 5

Esophageal motility abnormalities in Barrett's esophagus

Kumar Krishnan, John E. Pandolfino & Peter J. Kahrilas

Division of Gastroenterology, Department of Medicine, Northwestern University's, Feinberg School of Medicine, Chicago, IL, USA

5.1 Introduction

Although the etiology of Barrett's esophagus (BE) is uncertain, it is clearly associated with gastroesophageal reflux disease (GERD) [1]. Early studies quantifying gastroesophageal reflux in BE and GERD patients concluded that BE patients represented an extreme end of the spectrum [2–4]. When studies were controlled for the grade of esophagitis, it became evident that acid exposure was increased in BE, compared with patients with non-erosive GERD and mild to moderate esophagitis, but that the differences in acid exposure between patients with severe esophagitis and BE were insignificant [5]. However, despite the general agreement that esophageal acid exposure is increased with BE, there is less certainty as to whether or not there are unique motor abnormalities in BE, distinct from the GERD population in general.

Greater acid exposure in BE is a consequence of both an increased frequency of reflux events and impaired esophageal acid clearance. Given the similarities between the acid exposure profile of severe esophagitis and BE, it is not surprising that the motility abnormalities are also comparable. Unfortunately, there are a paucity of data focused specifically on motor abnormalities in BE and, consequently, motility abnormalities in BE will be discussed within the context of those associated with severe esophagitis. Owing to their importance in the pathogenesis of acid induced mucosal damage, abnormalities of the anti-reflux barrier, esophageal clearance, and gastric function will each be reviewed. Particular emphasis will be given to the discussion of the motility abnormalities associated with hiatal hernia, because of the strong association of this condition with BE.

5.2 Antireflux barrier

A prerequisite for the development of GERD is reflux of gastric contents into the esophagus, an event indicative of dysfunction of the esophagogastric junction (EGJ). The EGJ is a complex anatomic zone, whose functional integrity is attributable to both the intrinsic lower esophageal sphincter (LES) pressure and extrinsic compression of the LES by the crural diaphragm. Loss of EGJ integrity occurs by three dominant mechanisms:

1 Transient lower esophageal sphincter relaxation (TLESRs);
2 LES hypotension; or
3 anatomic disruption of the EGJ, inclusive of, but not limited to, hiatal hernia [6, 7].

Transient LES relaxations are the dominant mechanism of reflux in patients with mild to moderate GERD [6]. Patients with severe GERD differ from those with mild to moderate reflux, in that a greater proportion of their reflux occurs in the context of decreased LES pressure and a coexistent hiatal hernia [8, 9]. Given that patients with Barrett's esophagus have comparable acid exposure to patients with severe GERD, it is not

This work was supported by grant RO1 DK056033 (PJK) from the Public Health Service and RO1 DK079902 (JEP) from the Public Health Service.

surprising that Barrett's esophagus is usually associated with decreased LES pressure [10–12] and hiatal hernia [13–16].

5.3 Lower esophageal sphincter

The LES is a short segment of tonically contracted smooth muscle at the distal esophagus. Resting LES tone varies among normal individuals from 10–30 mm Hg relative to intragastric pressure, and continuous pressure monitoring reveals considerable temporal variation. Large fluctuations of LES pressure occur with the migrating motor complex; during phase III, LES pressure may exceed 80 mm Hg. Lesser fluctuations occur throughout the day with pressure decreasing in the post-cibal state and increasing during sleep [17]. The genesis of LES tone is a property of both the smooth muscle itself and its extrinsic innervation [18]. At any instant, LES pressure is affected by myogenic factors, intra-abdominal pressure, gastric distention, peptides, hormones, various foods, and many medications.

Early reports indicated that patients with BE had lower LES pressures, compared with either control subjects or patients with reflux disease [3, 19]. However, in 1987, Gillen reported no difference in LES pressure between patients with BE and those with esophagitis [2]. However, that study included a high proportion of patients with severe esophagitis (16 of 25 patients with grade 3–4 esophagitis). Given these conflicting results, subsequent investigations measured the LES pressure in patients with stratified grades of esophagitis and BE [5, 20, 21]. These studies reported that LES pressure in patients with BE were decreased to the same degree as seen with severe esophagitis. Furthermore, analogous to the situation with esophageal acid exposure, patients with BE and esophagitis had lower LES pressure than BE patients without esophagitis [20].

Treated achalasia is another relevant group to study. In a cohort of 331 patients with achalasia, with a mean follow-up of 67 months after pneumatic dilation, 27 developed BE and median LES pressures decreased from 30 to 13.5 mm Hg [22]. These data suggest that LES pressure, along with delayed acid clearance, is a key mechanism for reflux induced esophageal metaplasia.

Gastroesophageal reflux can occur in the context of low LES pressure, either by abdominal straining or free reflux. Manometric studies suggest that strain-induced reflux or free reflux are unlikely unless the LES pressure is less than 10 mm Hg and 4 mm Hg, respectively [23]. They are also rare in patients without hiatus hernia [24]. Free reflux is characterized by a fall in intra-esophageal pH without an identifiable change in either intragastric pressure or LES pressure. A wide-open or patulous hiatus will predispose to free reflux, as both the intrinsic and extrinsic sphincter are compromised. From the above discussion, it is apparent that many patients with BE are at risk for strain-induced or free reflux.

Compelling evidence exists that transient LES relaxations (TLESRs) are the most frequent mechanism for reflux during periods of normal LES pressure (>10 mm Hg). Transient LES relaxations occur independently of swallowing, are not accompanied by peristalsis, are accompanied by crural diaphragm inhibition, and persist for longer periods than do swallow-induced LES relaxations (>10 seconds) [25, 26]. Of note, prolonged manometric recordings have not consistently demonstrated an increased frequency of TLESRs in GERD patients, compared with normal controls [27]. However, the frequency of acid reflux (as opposed to gas reflux) during TLESRs has been consistently reported to be greater in GERD patients [27, 28]. Similar to patients with severe esophagitis and large hiatus hernias, BE patients are also subject to TLESRs. Patel studied seven patients with BE, using concurrent manometry and pH monitoring, and reported that TLESRs accounted for 64% of reflux events [29]. This is similar to the frequency of TLESRs found in patients with severe esophagitis and hiatus hernia, and further supports the hypothesis that both groups have a similar compromise of EGJ function [24, 26, 30].

5.4 Diaphragmatic sphincter and hiatal hernia

Most patients with severe esophagitis have a hiatal hernia and, consequently, there is a high prevalence of hiatal hernia in BE. Cameron reported finding a 2 cm hernia in 96% of patients with BE and 72 % of patients with short segment BE [13]. Furthermore, the presence of hiatal hernia is an independent risk factor for the presence of BE in patients with GERD symptoms [31]. The role that hiatal hernia plays in compromising the anti-reflux barrier is multifactorial. From an anatomical perspective, hiatal hernia may be associated with widening of the diaphragmatic hiatus, limiting the ability of the right crus to function as a sphincter. In addition to this anatomical consideration, the physiologic function of the crural diaphragm may be compromised by its dissociation from the LES.

Evidence of a specialized role of the crural diaphragm in preventing reflux begins with the observation that the costal and crural diaphragm function independently. During the LES relaxation associated with vomiting, electrical activity is absent in the crural diaphragm but active in the costal diaphragm [32]. A similar pattern is evident during TLESR and belching [26]. Additional evidence of the sphincteric role of the hiatus are manometric data from patients after oncologically prompted removal of the distal esophagus [33]. These patients still exhibit a high-pressure zone within the hiatal canal.

In addition to contributing to basal pressure, the crural diaphragm augments the EGJ during activities associated with increased intra-abdominal pressure. The importance of this function was evident in studies in which gastroesophageal reflux was elicited by straining maneuvers in individuals with graded severity of hiatus hernia [8]. Of several physiologic and anatomical variables tested, the size of the hiatal hernia was shown to have the highest correlation with the susceptibility to strain-induced reflux. The implication of this observation is that patients with hiatus hernia exhibit progressive impairment of the EGJ proportional to the length of axial herniation.

The patulous hiatal canal associated with large hiatal hernias also affects the antireflux barrier during swallowing. One of the differences between a swallow-induced LES relaxation and a TLESR is the crural inhibition, which occurs only with the latter [26]. In the presence of a large hiatal hernia, as is often the case in BE patients, the hiatal canal is distorted to the point where it becomes a patulous orifice, incapable of achieving luminal closure during inspiration. Under these circumstances, deglutitive LES relaxation, which is usually accompanied by continued respiratory contraction, becomes indistinguishable from a TLESR. As a result, the EGJ opens at the onset of any LES relaxation, including deglutitive relaxation, thereby broadening the set of circumstances associated with reflux.

Yet another effect that hiatal hernia exerts on the antireflux barrier pertains to diminishing both the length and intrinsic pressure of the LES. Relevant animal experiments revealed that simulating the effect of hiatal hernia by severing the phrenoesophageal ligament reduced the LES pressure, and that the subsequent repair of the ligament restored the LES pressure to levels similar to baseline [34]. Similarly, manometric studies in humans, using a topographic representation of the EGJ high pressure zone of hiatal hernia patients, revealed a distinct intrinsic sphincter and hiatal canal pressure components, each of which was of lower magnitude than the EGJ pressure of a comparator group of normal controls [35]. However, simulating reduction of the hernia, by arithmetically repositioning the intrinsic sphincter back within the hiatal canal, resulted in calculated EGJ pressures that were practically indistinguishable from those of the control subjects.

These and previous studies also demonstrated that hiatus hernia may also affect the overall length of the LES high pressure zone [36]. Combined manometric and fluoroscopic studies found that both peak EGJ pressure and length correlated negatively with hiatal hernia size. This is likely due to disruption of the EGJ segment distal to the squamocolumnar junction attributable to the gastroesophageal flap valve [37].

5.5 Mechanical properties of the relaxed EGJ

For reflux to occur in the setting of a relaxed or hypotensive sphincter, it is necessary for the relaxed sphincter to open. Recent physiologic studies exploring the role of compliance in GERD reported that GERD patients without and particularly with hiatus hernia had increased compliance at the EGJ, compared with normal subjects [38] and patients with fundoplication [39]. These experiments utilized a combination of barostat-controlled distention, manometry, and fluoroscopy to directly measure the compliance of the EGJ. Several parameters of EGJ compliance were shown to be increased in hiatus hernia patients with GERD:

1 the EGJ opened at lower distention pressure;
2 the relaxed EGJ opened at distention pressures that were at or near resting intra-gastric pressure;
3 for a given distention pressure the EGJ opened about 0.5 cm wider.

Still significant, but lesser, compliance-related changes were demonstrated in the non-hernia GERD patients. These alterations of EGJ mechanics are likely to be secondary to a disrupted, distensible crural aperture and may be the root causes of the physiological aberrations associated with GERD.

Increased EGJ compliance may help explain why patients with hiatus hernia have a distinct mechanistic reflux profile, compared with patients without hiatus hernia [24]. Anatomical alterations, such as hiatal hernia, dilatation of the diaphragmatic hiatus, and disruption of the gastroesophageal flap valve, may alter the elastic characteristics of the hiatus, such that this factor is no longer protective in preventing gastroesophageal reflux. In that setting, reflux no longer requires "two hits" to the EGJ, because the extrinsic sphincteric mechanism is chronically disrupted. Thus, the only prerequisite for reflux becomes LES relaxation – be that in the setting of swallow-induced relaxation, TLESR, or a period of prolonged LES hypotension. Patients with BE will likely have abnormal compliance at the EGJ secondary to the high prevalence of hiatus hernia. Whether EGJ compliance is altered to a greater extent in BE patients versus GERD patients with severe esophagitis, with and without hiatus hernia, is unclear.

5.6 Esophageal clearance

Following reflux, the period that the esophageal mucosa remains at a pH < 4 is defined as the acid clearance time. Acid clearance begins with emptying of the refluxed fluid from the esophagus by peristalsis and is completed by the titration of residual acid by the buffering effect of swallowed saliva [40]. Prolongation of esophageal clearance among patients with esophagitis was demonstrated along with the initial description of an acid clearance test. Subsequent studies suggest that about 50% of patients with GERD exhibit prolonged esophageal acid clearance [1]. Clinical data from patients with BE also suggest prolonged acid clearance. Scintigraphic studies demonstrated impaired esophageal emptying in 50–80% of BE patients [41, 42]. Ambulatory pH studies subsequently confirmed prolonged acid clearance in BE patients, and added further insight by stratifying the esophagitis patients by severity.

Gillen reported that, after selecting the patients with severe esophagitis and comparing them to patients with BE, there was no significant difference in acid clearance [2]. Several other reports have subsequently confirmed this observation, and it is now generally accepted that patients with severe esophagitis and BE have similar defects in esophageal clearance [5, 20]. Investigations also confirm the additive effect of esophagitis and BE on impairment of acid clearance, with the combination being worse than either entity alone [5]. In addition, it appears that patients with long segment BE have prolonged clearance, compared with patients with short segment disease [43]. Ambulatory pH monitoring studies suggest that the heterogeneity within the GERD population, with respect to acid clearance, is at least partially attributed to hiatus hernia, as these individuals tended to have the most prolonged supine acid clearance [44].

5.6.1 Hiatal hernia and esophageal clearance

Although hiatal hernia is probably not an independent risk factor for developing BE, it is an important contributor to the underlying pathogenesis of increased acid exposure, both by compromising the antireflux barrier as discussed above and by impairing the process of acid clearance. Concurrent pH recording and scintigraphic scanning over the EGJ showed that impaired clearance was caused by reflux of fluid from the hernia during swallowing [45]. This observation was subsequently confirmed radiographically when Sloan *et al.* analyzed esophageal emptying in patients with reducing and non-reducing hiatal hernias [46]. The efficacy of emptying was significantly diminished in both hernia groups when compared to normal controls. Emptying was particularly impaired in the non-reducing hiatal hernia patients, who exhibited complete emptying with only one third of test swallows. These patients with non-reducing hernias were the only group that exhibited retrograde flow of fluid from the hernia during deglutitive relaxation, consistent with the scintigraphic studies.

The mechanism of impaired esophageal emptying is evident from an analysis of esophageal emptying in the normal patient [47]. Typically, LES relaxation occurs within three seconds of the swallow, but LES opening does not occur until the bolus reaches the distal esophagus. In order for the LES to open, pressure acting on the lumen of the sphincter must overcome the pressure acting extrinsic to the lumen. Since the normal position of the distal esophagus is intraabdominal, the intragastric pressure acting to open the distal esophagus is negated by external pressure of equal magnitude.

However, once the distal esophagus is positioned above the diaphragm, the extrinsic pressure at the LES is reduced, more reflective of intrathoracic pressure. This leads to LES opening at the time of relaxation, and early retrograde flow of gastric contents from the stomach into the low-pressure esophagus. Hiatal hernia also impairs the function of the crural diaphragm as a one-way valve during distal esophageal emptying, owing to the persistence of a gastric pouch above the diaphragm. Both of these effects are particularly evident while in a recumbent posture.

5.7 Peristaltic dysfunction

Peristaltic dysfunction in esophagitis has been described by a number of investigators. Failed peristalsis and hypotensive contractions (<30 mm Hg), which result in incomplete emptying, are of particular significance [48]. As esophagitis increases in severity, so does the incidence of failed peristalsis and hypotensive contractions [49]. More recent investigations of peristaltic function has labeled this "ineffective esophageal motility", defined by the occurrence of > 30% of hypotensive or failed contractions. Applying this definition, a significant increase in recumbent esophageal acid exposure time, compared with patients with normal motility, esophageal spasm, nutcracker esophagus and hypertensive LES, was reported [50]. With respect to the reversibility of peristaltic dysfunction, recent studies show no improvement after healing of esophagitis by acid inhibition [51], or by antireflux surgery [52].

Although early investigations reported normal peristaltic function in BE [53, 54], these studies can be criticized on methodological grounds, and more recent data reveal that peristaltic dysfunction is prevalent in BE patients. Similar to the case of esophagitis patients, patients with BE exhibit both failed and ineffective contractions when compared with controls. Parilla reported that BE patients had a higher incidence of failed peristalsis than both controls and patients with mild esophagitis [20]; there was no difference when he compared BE patients to patients with severe esophagitis. However, when he separated the BE population into those with esophagitis and without esophagitis, there was a significant difference, such that patients with concomitant esophagitis and BE had failed peristalsis 23% of the time, compared with 1.7% in patients without esophagitis. This suggests that the increased peristaltic dysfunction is more dependent on chronic inflammation than on metaplasia.

Esophageal contractility is impaired in a qualitatively similar way in patients with BE and patients with severe esophagitis. Mean peristaltic amplitude is lower than in either controls [4] or patients with mild esophagitis [5]. Furthermore, patients with severe esophagitis and BE both exhibit ineffective esophageal motility, as previously defined [55]. Two studies evaluating peristaltic amplitude in BE patients with and without esophagitis found no difference between the two groups [5, 20]. However, Mason compared the esophageal contractility of patients with extensive BE (>5cm) to patients with more limited BE (3–5 cm) and found that patients with extensive disease exhibited a significant decrease in peristaltic amplitude [56]. Adding to the controversy, Loughney compared patients with long (>3 cm) and short segment (<3 cm) BE, and showed no difference in peristaltic contraction between the two groups [57]. However, the patients with long segment BE did have significantly reduced peristaltic amplitude, compared with normal subjects, raising the issue of a type II error in this investigation.

5.8 Gastric emptying and duodenogastroesophageal reflux

Gastric emptying may be impaired in 41–57% of patients with GERD [58]. Defects in gastric emptying may exacerbate reflux by increasing the gastroesophageal pressure gradient, thereby promoting reflux, or by increasing TLESR frequency as a result of increased gastric distention. However, contrary to what one would expect, patients with BE have been shown to have relatively normal gastric emptying, and two published series revealed no difference in either solid or liquid phase gastric emptying [59, 60]. Probably of more interest, given the recent description of an unbuffered acid pocket after meals, are potential abnormalities in proximal stomach acid pooling [61].

Normal gastric emptying in BE is also surprising, given the recent interest in duodenogastroesophageal reflux as a possible pathogenic mechanism in the development and progression of BE. Studies suggest that duodenal contents may act synergistically with acid to damage the esophageal epithelium [62]. Studies specifically quantifying bile reflux have reported that it is more common in patients with BE, compared with GERD patients without BE [63]. The motility abnormalities that promote duodenogastroesophageal reflux have not been defined, although impaired gastric emptying does not appear to be a major mechanism. Studies of transpyloric flow and antroduodenal motility in patients with GERD similarly have revealed no functional abnormalities [64].

5.9 Therapy of motor abnormalities in Barrett's esophagus

5.9.1 Medical management

Most investigations of the effect of antireflux therapy on motor function suggest that no improvement is demonstrable after healing esophagitis [42, 51]. The focus of medical management beyond acid suppression has been centered on improving clearance mechanisms via promotility agents, and by decreasing reflux events by inhibiting TLESRs. Given the likely irreversibility of reflux-related motor dysfunction, treatment with motility modifying agents may seem appropriate. Unfortunately, the therapeutic efficacy of available drugs is disappointing. The two most widely used promotility drugs in reflux are metoclopramide and cisapride.

Metoclopramide has been shown to increase LES pressure via increased release of acetylcholine in the enteric nervous system, but this has not been shown to have a beneficial impact on reflux [65]. Whether or not metoclopramide improves esophageal peristalsis is controversial. An early study suggested a 39% increase in peristaltic amplitude after intravenous metoclopramide [66], but two more recent randomized, controlled, double-blinded studies in GERD patients failed to show any improvement [67, 68].

Similar to the data with metoclopramide, cisapride has proven ineffective at augmenting LES pressure or esophageal peristalsis. Cisapride is a mixed serotonergic agent with 5HT-3 antagonist and 5HT-4 agonist properties, which also enhances the release of acetylcholine from postganglionic fibers in the myenteric plexus. Several studies have reported minor increases in LES pressure and peristaltic amplitude with cisapride therapy but, as with metoclopramide, these effects were not clinically relevant [65].

Several studies have investigated the role of γ-aminobutyric acid B-type receptor agonist, the most common being baclofen. Short and long term studies have demonstrated the efficacy of baclofen in reducing TLESRs and improving GERD symptoms [69–71]. Unfortunately, the side-effect profile of baclofen makes it undesirable as an adjunct to acid suppressive therapy. Hence, the best available clinical evidence suggests that promotility cannot be strongly recommended for the treatment of GERD. The minimal increases in LES pressure observed are insignificant in patients with severely compromised lower esophageal sphincters. Similarly, the mild increase in peristaltic amplitude is unlikely to improve esophageal clearance.

Other than hiatus hernia, failed peristalsis is the more important mechanism of impaired esophageal emptying and, unfortunately, neither metoclopramide nor cisapride impact that feature of peristaltic dysfunction. Baclofen, while able to decrease TLESRs in patients with GERD, is less relevant in the setting of very low LES pressure and hiatal hernia. In summary, poor efficacy and a poor side effect profile make these agents unsuitable for treatment of motility abnormalities in BE.

5.9.2 Surgical treatment

Antireflux surgery improves the antireflux barrier in patients with GERD, with several studies demonstrating a significant increase in EGJ pressure after fundoplication [3, 72, 73]. Along with improved EGJ pressure, the anatomic defect of hiatal hernia is also repaired. A more controversial and debated question is whether or not fundoplication improves esophageal peristalsis in patients with esophagitis and BE. A number of studies suggest that antireflux surgery increases peristaltic amplitude [73, 74]. However, even if real, and not a methodological artifact attributable to the operation, these changes would be unlikely to improve impaired clearance, which is largely attributable to failed peristalsis. No study has shown a reduction in the frequency of failed peristalsis, or restoration of peristalsis, in an aperistaltic patient as a result of antireflux surgery.

5.10 Conclusion

Barrett's epithelium is a result of increased esophageal acid exposure, similar to that seen with severe esophagitis. Thus, it is not surprising that these two groups of reflux patients have similar motility abnormalities, with both patient populations exhibiting a compromised antireflux barrier and prolonged esophageal acid clearance. Central to the mechanism of these defects is the association of both BE and severe esophagitis with hiatal hernia. Why some patients with severe esophagitis develop BE, while some do not, remains to be determined; however, the epidemiological literature suggests that this is at least partially a function of genetic predisposition. Other factors, such as the role of duodenogastroesophageal reflux, are being explored. Neither medical nor surgical therapy corrects the peristaltic defect associated with BE, although antireflux therapy clearly creates an effective antireflux barrier.

References

1 Lidums I, Holloway R (1997). Motility abnormalities in the columnar-lined esophagus. *Gastroenterology Clinics of North America* **26**(3), 519–31.

2 Gillen P, Keeling P, Byrne PJ, Hennessy TP (1987). Barrett's oesophagus: pH profile. *British Journal of Surgery* **74**(9), 774–6.

3 Iascone C, DeMeester TR, Little AG, Skinner DB (1983). Barrett's esophagus. Functional assessment, proposed pathogenesis, and surgical therapy. *Archives of Surgery* **118**(5), 543–9.

4 Singh P, Taylor RH, Colin-Jones DG (1994). Esophageal motor dysfunction and acid exposure in reflux esophagitis are more severe if Barrett's metaplasia is present. *American Journal of Gastroenterology* **89**(3), 349–56.

5 Coenraad M, Masclee AA, Straathof JW, Ganesh S, Griffioen G, Lamers CB (1998). Is Barrett's esophagus characterized by more pronounced acid reflux than severe esophagitis? *American Journal of Gastroenterology* **93**(7), 1068–72.

6 Dodds WJ, Dent J, Hogan WJ, Helm JF, Hauser R, Patel GK, *et al.* (1982). Mechanisms of gastroesophageal reflux in patients with reflux esophagitis. *New England Journal of Medicine* **307**(25), 1547–52.

7 Kahrilas PJ (1998). GERD revisited: advances in pathogenesis. *Hepato-Gastroenterology* **45**(23), 1301–7.

8 Sloan S, Rademaker AW, Kahrilas PJ (1992). Determinants of gastroesophageal junction incompetence: hiatal hernia, lower esophageal sphincter, or both? *Annals of Internal Medicine* **117**(12), 977–82.

9 Barham CP, Gotley DC, Mills A, Alderson D (1995). Precipitating causes of acid reflux episodes in ambulant patients with gastro-oesophageal reflux disease. *Gut* **36**(4), 505–10.

10 Brandt MG, Darling GE, Miller L (2004). Symptoms, acid exposure and motility in patients with Barrett's esophagus. *Canadian Journal of Surgery* **47**(1), 47–51.

11 Zentilin P, Reglioni S, Savarino V (2003). Pathophysiological characteristics of long- and short-segment Barrett's oesophagus. *Scandinavian Journal of Gastroenterology Suppl* **239**, 40–3.

12 Oberg S, DeMeester TR, Peters JH, Hagen JA, Nigro JJ, DeMeester SR, *et al.* (1999). The extent of Barrett's esophagus depends on the status of the lower esophageal sphincter and the degree of esophageal acid exposure. *Journal of Thoracic and Cardiovascular Surgery* **117**(3), 572–80.

13 Cameron AJ (1999). Barrett's esophagus: prevalence and size of hiatal hernia. *American Journal of Gastroenterology* **94**(8), 2054–9.

14 Avidan B, Sonnenberg A, Schnell TG, Sontag SJ (2002). Hiatal hernia and acid reflux frequency predict presence and length of Barrett's esophagus. *Digestive Diseases and Sciences* **47**(2), 256–64.

15 Avidan B, Sonnenberg A, Schnell TG, Chejfec G, Metz A, Sontag SJ (2002). Hiatal hernia size, Barrett's length, and severity of acid reflux are all risk factors for esophageal adenocarcinoma. *American Journal of Gastroenterology* **97**(8), 1930–6.

16 Wakelin DE, Al-Mutawa T, Wendel C, Green C, Garewal HS, Fass R (2003). A predictive model for length of Barrett's esophagus with hiatal hernia length and duration of esophageal acid exposure. *Gastrointestinal Endoscopy* **58**(3), 350–5.

17 Dent J, Dodds WJ, Friedman RH, Sekiguchi T, Hogan WJ, Arndorfer RC, *et al.* (1980). Mechanism of gastroesophageal reflux in recumbent asymptomatic human subjects. *Journal of Clinical Investigation* **65**(2), 256–67.

18 Goyal RK, Rattan S (1976). Genesis of basal sphincter pressure: effect of tetrodotoxin on lower esophageal sphincter pressure in opossum *in vivo*. *Gastroenterology* **71**(1), 62–7.

19 Heitmann P, Csendes A, Strauszer T (1971). Esophageal strictures and lower esophagus lined with columnar epithelium. Functional and morphologic studies. *American Journal of Digestive Diseases* **16**(4), 307–20.

20 Parrilla P, Ortiz A, Martinez de Haro LF, Aguayo JL, Ramirez P (1990). Evaluation of the magnitude of gastro-oesophageal reflux in Barrett's oesophagus. *Gut* **31**(9), 964–7.

21 Frazzoni M, Manno M, De Micheli E, Savarino V (2006). Pathophysiological characteristics of the various forms of gastro-oesophageal reflux disease. Spectrum disease or distinct phenotypic presentations? *Digestive and Liver Disease: official journal of the Italian Society of Gastroenterology and the Italian Association for the Study of the Liver* **38**(9), 643–8. Epub 2006/04/22.

22 Leeuwenburgh I, Scholten P, Calje TJ, Vaessen RJ, Tilanus HW, Hansen BE, *et al.* (2013). Barrett's Esophagus and Esophageal Adenocarcinoma Are Common After Treatment for Achalasia. *Digestive Diseases and Sciences* **58**(1), 244–52. Epub 2012/11/28.

23 Kahrilas PJ (1997). Anatomy and physiology of the gastroesophageal junction. *Gastroenterology Clinics of North America* **26**(3), 467–86.

24 van Herwaarden MA, Samsom M, Smout AJ (2000). Excess gastroesophageal reflux in patients with hiatus hernia is caused by mechanisms other than transient LES relaxations. *Gastroenterology* **119**(6), 1439–46.

25 Holloway RH, Penagini R, Ireland AC (1995). Criteria for objective definition of transient lower esophageal sphincter relaxation. *American Journal of Physiology* **268**(1, Pt 1), G128–33.

26 Mittal RK, Holloway RH, Penagini R, Blackshaw LA, Dent J (1995). Transient lower esophageal sphincter relaxation. *Gastroenterology* **109**(2), 601–10.

27 Sifrim D, Holloway R (2001). Transient lower esophageal sphincter relaxations: how many or how harmful? *American Journal of Gastroenterology* **96**(9), 2529–32.

28 Sifrim D, Holloway R, Silny J, Xin Z, Tack J, Lerut A, *et al.* (2001). Acid, nonacid, and gas reflux in patients with gastroesophageal reflux disease during ambulatory 24-hour pH-impedance recordings. *Gastroenterology* **120**(7), 1588–98.

29 Patel GK, Clift SA, Read RC (1982). Mechanisms of gastroesophageal reflux in patients with Barrett's esophagus. *Gastroenterology* **82**, A1146.

30 Dent J, Holloway RH, Toouli J, Dodds WJ (1988). Mechanisms of lower oesophageal sphincter incompetence in patients with symptomatic gastrooesophageal reflux. *Gut* **29**(8), 1020–8.

31 Balasubramanian G, Singh M, Gupta N, Gaddam S, Giacchino M, Wani SB, *et al.* (2012). Prevalence and predictors of columnar lined esophagus in gastroesophageal reflux disease (GERD) patients undergoing upper endoscopy. *American Journal of Gastroenterology* **107**(11), 1655–61. Epub (2012)/10/04.

32 Monges H, Salducci J, Naudy B (1978). Dissociation between the electrical activity of the diaphragmatic dome and crura muscular fibers during esophageal distension, vomiting and eructation. An electromyographic study in the dog. *Journal of Physiology (Paris)* **74**(6), 541–54.

33 Klein WA, Parkman HP, Dempsey DT, Fisher RS (1993). Sphincterlike thoracoabdominal high pressure zone after esophagogastrectomy. *Gastroenterology* **105**(5), 1362–9.

34 Friedland GW (1978). Historical review of the changing concepts of the lower esophageal anatomy: 430 BC–1977. *American Journal of Roentgenology* **131**, 373–88.

35 Kahrilas PJ, Lin S, Manka M, Shi G, Joehl RJ (2000). Esophagogastric junction pressure topography after fundoplication. *Surgery* **127**(2), 200–8.

36 Kahrilas PJ, Lin S, Chen J, Manka M (1999). The effect of hiatus hernia on gastro-oesophageal junction pressure. *Gut* **44**(4), 476–82.

37 Hill LD, Kozarek RA, Kraemer SJ, Aye RW, Mercer CD, Low DE, *et al.* (1996). The gastroesophageal flap valve: *in vitro* and *in vivo* observations. *Gastrointestinal Endoscopy* **44**(5), 541–7.

38 Pandolfino JE, Shi G, Trueworthy B, Kahrilas PJ (2003). Esophagogastric junction opening during relaxation distinguishes nonhernia reflux patients, hernia patients, and normal subjects. *Gastroenterology* **125**(4), 1018–24.

39 Curry J, Shi G, Pandolfino JE, Joehl RJ, Brasseur JG, Kahrilas PJ (2001). Mechanical characteristics of the EGJ after fundoplication compared to normal subjects and GERD patients. *Gastroenterology* **120**, A112.

40 Helm JF (1989). Role of saliva in esophageal function and disease. *Dysphagia* **4**(2), 76–84.

41 Karvelis KC, Drane WE, Johnson DA, Silverman ED (1987). Barrett esophagus: decreased esophageal clearance shown by radionuclide esophageal scintigraphy. *Radiology* **162**(1, Pt 1), 97–9.

42 Singh P, Adamopoulos A, Taylor RH, Colin-Jones DG (1992). Oesophageal motor function before and after healing of oesophagitis. *Gut* **33**(12), 1590–6.

43 Savarino E, Zentilin P, Frazzoni M, Cuoco DL, Pohl D, Dulbecco P, *et al.* (2010). Characteristics of gastro-esophageal reflux episodes in Barrett's esophagus, erosive esophagitis and healthy volunteers. *Neurogastroenterology and Motility : the official journal of the European Gastrointestinal Motility Society* **22**(10), 1061-e280. Epub (2010)/06/19.

44 Johnson LF (1980). 24-hour pH monitoring in the study of gastroesophageal reflux. *Journal of Clinical Gastroenterology* **2**(4), 387–99.

45 Mittal RK, Lange RC, McCallum RW (1987). Identification and mechanism of delayed esophageal acid clearance in subjects with hiatus hernia. *Gastroenterology* **92**(1), 130–5.

46 Sloan S, Kahrilas PJ (1991). Impairment of esophageal emptying with hiatal hernia. *Gastroenterology* **100**(3), 596–605.

47 Lin S, Brasseur JG, Pouderoux P, Kahrilas PJ (1995). The phrenic ampulla: distal esophagus or potential hiatal hernia? *American Journal of Physiology* **268**(2, Pt 1), G320–7.

48 Kahrilas PJ, Dodds WJ, Hogan WJ (1988). Effect of peristaltic dysfunction on esophageal volume clearance. *Gastroenterology* **94**(1), 73–80.

49 Kahrilas PJ, Dodds WJ, Hogan WJ, Kern M, Arndorfer RC, Reece A (1986). Esophageal peristaltic dysfunction in peptic esophagitis. *Gastroenterology* **91**(4), 897–904.

50 Leite LP, Johnston BT, Barrett J, Castell JA, Castell DO (1997). Ineffective esophageal motility (IEM) the primary finding in patients with nonspecific esophageal motility disorder. *Digestive Diseases and Sciences* **42**(9), 1859–65.

51 Timmer R, Breumelhof R, Nadorp JH, Smout AJ (1994). Oesophageal motility and gastro-oesophageal reflux before and after healing of reflux oesophagitis. A study using 24 hour ambulatory pH and pressure monitoring. *Gut* **35**(11), 1519–22.

52 Rydberg L, Ruth M, Lundell L (1997). Does oesophageal motor function improve with time after successful antireflux surgery? Results of a prospective, randomised clinical study. *Gut* **41**(1), 82–6.

53 Burgess JN, Payne WS, Andersen HA, Weiland LH, Carlson HC (1971). Barrett esophagus: the columnar-epithelial-lined lower esophagus. *Mayo Clinic Proceedings* **46**(11), 728–34.

54 Robbins AH, Hermos JA, Schimmel EM, Friedlander DM, Messian RA (1977). The columnar-lined esophagus – analysis of 26 cases. *Radiology* **123**(1), 1–7.

55 Stein HJ, Eypasch EP, DeMeester TR, Smyrk TC, Attwood SE (1990). Circadian esophageal motor function in patients with gastroesophageal reflux disease. *Surgery* **108**(4), 769–77; discussion 77–8.

56 Mason RJ, Bremner CC (1993). Motility differences between long-segment and short-segment Barrett's esophagus. *American Journal of Surgery* **165**(6), 686–9.

57 Loughney T, Maydonovitch CL, Wong RK (1998). Esophageal manometry and ambulatory 24-hour pH monitoring in patients with short and long segment Barrett's esophagus. *American Journal of Gastroenterology* **93**(6), 916–9.

58 McCallum RW (1990). Gastric emptying in gastroesophageal reflux and the therapeutic role of prokinetic agents. *Gastroenterology Clinics of North America* **19**(3), 551–64.

59 Johnson DA, Winters C, Drane WE, Cattau EL, Jr., Karvelis KC, Silverman ED, *et al.* (1986). Solid-phase gastric emptying in patients with Barrett's esophagus. *Digestive Diseases and Sciences* **31**(11), 1217–20.

60 Kogan FJ, Kotler J, Sampliner R (1985). Normal gastric emptying in Barrett's esophagus. *Gastroenterology* **88**, 1451A.

61 Fletcher J, Wirz A, Young J, Vallance R, McColl KE (2001). Unbuffered highly acidic gastric juice exists at the gastroesophageal junction after a meal. *Gastroenterology* **121**(4), 775–83.

62 Vaezi MF, Richter JE (1999). Importance of duodeno-gastroesophageal reflux in the medical outpatient practice. *Hepato-Gastroenterology* **46**(25), 40–7.

63 Lord RV, DeMeester SR, Peters JH, Hagen JA, Elyssnia D, Sheth CT, *et al.* (2009). Hiatal hernia, lower esophageal sphincter incompetence, and effectiveness of Nissen fundoplication in the spectrum of gastroesophageal reflux disease. *Journal of Gastrointestinal Surgery : official journal of the Society for Surgery of the Alimentary Tract* **13**(4), 602–10. Epub 2008/12/04.

64 King PM, Pryde A, Heading RC (1987). Transpyloric fluid movement and antroduodenal motility in patients with gastro-oesophageal reflux. *Gut* **28**(5), 545–8.

65 Pandolfino JE, Howden CW, Kahrilas PJ (2000). Motility-modifying agents and management of disorders of gastrointestinal motility. *Gastroenterology* **118**(2, Suppl 1), S32–47.

66 DiPalma JA, Perucca PJ, Martin DF, Pierson WP, Meyer GW (1987). Metoclopramide effect on esophageal peristalsis in normal human volunteers. *American Journal of Gastroenterology* **82**(4), 307–10.

67 Grande L, Lacima G, Ros E, Garcia-Valdecasas JC, Fuster J, Visa J, *et al.* (1992). Lack of effect of metoclopramide and domperidone on esophageal peristalsis and esophageal acid clearance in reflux esophagitis. A randomized, double-blind study. *Digestive Diseases and Sciences* **37**(4), 583–8.

68 McCallum RW, Fink SM, Winnan GR, Avella J, Callachan C (1984). Metoclopramide in gastroesophageal reflux disease: rationale for its use and results of a double-blind trial. *American Journal of Gastroenterology* **79**(3), 165–72.

69 Zhang Q, Lehmann A, Rigda R, Dent J, Holloway RH (2002). Control of transient lower oesophageal sphincter relaxations and reflux by the GABA(B) agonist baclofen in patients with gastro-oesophageal reflux disease. *Gut* **50**(1), 19–24. Epub 2002/01/05.

70 Vela MF, Tutuian R, Katz PO, Castell DO (2003). Baclofen decreases acid and non-acid post-prandial gastro-oesophageal reflux measured by combined multichannel intraluminal impedance and pH. *Alimentary Pharmacology & Therapeutics* **17**(2), 243–51. Epub 2003/01/22.

71 Ciccaglione AF, Marzio L (2003). Effect of acute and chronic administration of the GABA B agonist baclofen on 24 hour pH metry and symptoms in control subjects and in patients with gastro-oesophageal reflux disease. *Gut* **52**(4), 464–70. Epub 2003/03/13.

72 Sagor G (1982). Hiatus hernia: slip sliding away. *Nursing Mirror* **154**(13), 39–41.

73 Ortiz Escandell A, Martinez de Haro LF, Parrilla Paricio P, Aguayo Albasini JL, Garcia Marcilla JA, Morales Cuenca G (1991). Surgery improves defective oesophageal peristalsis in patients with gastro-oesophageal reflux. *British Journal of Surgery* **78**(9), 1095–7.

74 Wetscher GJ, Glaser K, Gadenstaetter M, Profanter C, Hinder RA (1999). The effect of medical therapy and antireflux surgery on dysphagia in patients with gastroesophageal reflux disease without esophageal stricture. *American Journal of Surgery* **177**(3), 189–92.

CHAPTER 6

Molecular biology of Barrett's esophagus and esophageal adenocarcinoma

Ayesha Noorani & Rebecca C. Fitzgerald

MRC Cancer Unit, University of Cambridge, UK

Abbreviations used in this chapter

HGD High Grade Dysplasia
LGD Low Grade Dysplasia
BE Barrett's Esophagus
EAC Esophageal Adenocarcinoma
WGS Whole Genome Sequencing
WES Whole Exome Sequencing

6.1 Introduction

This chapter focuses on the hallmark molecular changes that define Barrett's Esophagus (BE) and esophageal adenocarcinoma (EAC) and mark the transition from pre-invasive to invasive disease. The molecular biology of BE is of broad interest, as it serves as a model of the evolution to cancer that, in many respects, can be applied to other cancers. In addition, research into identifying key events in the dysplasia-adenocarcinoma sequence has been extensive, with the hope of identifying ideal diagnostic and therapeutic checkpoints to halt the advancement of the disease.

The current body of evidence supports the theory that there is an accumulation of molecular changes occurring in the context of chronic inflammation, which results in the development of BE. This appears to be random, with variation between patients, rather than supporting a precise sequence of events. Furthermore, it is becoming apparent that the bulk of these molecular alterations may not be relevant for the progression to cancer that occurs in a minority of patients. The challenge remains to identify the patients who will most likely progress to adenocarcinoma and, hence, may benefit from early intervention.

Until recently, our knowledge has been dependent on a hypothesis-driven search for molecular alterations. However, the revolution in evaluation of genome-wide changes has now enabled us to get an overview of the plethora of alterations occurring at the level of DNA, DNA and mRNA regulators, transcription and protein. The critical question is how to interpret this wealth of knowledge to help us understand the crucial steps for malignant progression, with the goal of providing clinically applicable solutions for early detection and surveillance of BE, and treatment and monitoring for esophageal adenocarcinoma (EAC). After providing a general overview of the biology of both BE and EAC, this chapter focuses on the role that next generation technologies may play in further deciphering the key genomic events in BE and EAC, as displayed in Figure 6.1.

6.2 Genetic and host susceptibility

Familial BE is present in 7.3% of patients presenting with BE and EAC. In addition, endoscopy screening studies have identified Barrett's in first-degree relatives of affected individuals within familial BE more frequently than in first-degree relatives of isolated cases [1]. Twin studies of GERD indicate a heritability of 30–40%, although Mendelian inheritance remains unlikely, as concordance rates are less than 50%, with recent data striving to identify low penetrance susceptibility loci [2].

Esophageal Cancer and Barrett's Esophagus, Third Edition. Edited by Prateek Sharma, Richard Sampliner and David Ilson.
© 2015 John Wiley & Sons, Ltd. Published 2015 by John Wiley & Sons, Ltd.

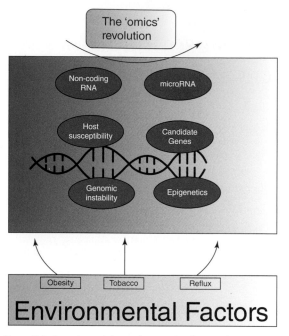

Figure 6.1 Overview of the pathogenesis of BE and EAC.

There has been a recent wave of genome-wide association studies, which have been informative in identifying susceptibility loci for BE and EAC. Levine *et al.* compared 2390 EAC cases and 3175 precancerous BE cases, with 10120 controls [3]. This study identified three susceptibility loci involved in BE and EAC carcinogenesis: 19p13 (rs10419226, $p = 3.6 \times 10^{-10}$) in CRTC1 (encodes CREB-regulated transcription co-activator); 9q22 (rs11789015, $p = 1.0 \times 10^{-9}$) in the transcription factor BARX1, which is involved in esophageal differentiation; and 3p14 (rs2687201, $p = 5.5 \times 10^{-9}$) near the transcription factor FOXP1, which regulates esophageal development.

Ek *et al.* used genome-wide association data to employ all known single-nucleotide polymorphisms (SNPS) in a method to investigate the genetic variance and correlation in GERD, BE and EAC [4]. The genetic correlation between BE and EA was found to be high ($rq = 1$, SE = 0.37), and there was also a statistically significant polygenic overlap between BE and EAC (one-sided $p = 1 \times 10^{-6}$), which suggests that shared genes underlie the development of BE and EAC. There were no genetic correlation traits observed for GERD.

Candidate gene approaches have been used to identify inherited gene variants in pathways such as DNA

Repair, xenobiotic metabolism, and inflammation that might alter the risk of developing BE or EAC. A population based study on 1181 patients examined the relative risk of EAC in relation to five SNPs in the DNA repair gene MGMT. Among patients who reported frequent episodes of GERD, a substantially increased relative risk was observed for those homozygous for the minor allele at the intronic locus rs12268840 (OR-15.5, 95% CI = 48–42) [5].

Variants in the NAD(P)H:quinone oxireductase 1(NQ01) gene, which encodes a detoxifying enzyme of common dietary compounds, have also been evaluated in various studies. There is evidence to support that NQ01 TT genotypes may offer protection from complications of GERD, and cases with the TT genotype were less common than expected in BE and EAC, resulting in a 4.5-fold decreased risk of developing BE and a 6.2-fold decreased risk of EAC [6].

Kala *et al.* showed that flutathione S-transferase GSTP1 B allele carriers were more frequent among BE patients than in individuals affected by esophagitis and control subjects (OR 2.1, 95% CI 0.99–4.44 and OR 2.56, 95% CI 1.3–5.05, respectively) [7]. In contrast, Murphy *et al.* did not demonstrate a correlation between polymorphisms at the level of this enzyme and the development of BE [8]. GSTM1 and GSTT1 (glutathione S-transferase) were also found to be increased in smokers with an associated risk to develop EAC, with an OR of 7.9 (95% CI 1.1.3–5476) and 3.2 (95% CI 1.23–8.35) respectively [9]

As a result of a single base polymorphism (G870A) of Cyclin D1 (CCND1), alternative gene splicing is thought to give rise to two functional transcripts. The normal gene transcript (cyclin D1a) interacts with and activates G1 CDK4 and CDK6. The resulting complex phosphorylates the Retinoblastoma (RB1) tumor suppression gene, thereby resulting in cell cycle progression to S phase. The variant transcript cyclin D1b, the result of the polymorphic A allele, encodes a truncated protein isoform with an altered C terminal domain that has been implicated in progression to cancer. Individuals with the CCND1 A/A genotype have been shown to be at an increased risk for GERD, BE and EAC, supporting the hypothesis that this polymorphism confers individual susceptibility in the molecular progression of EAC [10, 11] .

Cox 2 (also known as PTGS2) is another candidate gene that has been thought to confer susceptibility in BE and EAC. Variants in the promoter region of COX2 have been observed to increase the risk of EAC [12, 13]. This is interesting, as there is evidence to suggest the protective effect of NSAIDs in the development of EAC [14, 15]

6.3 Environmental factors contributing to the development of BE

Reflux, abdominal obesity and cigarette smoking have all been shown to be important etiological factors in the development of BE and the progression to EAC. The common pathway seems to be secondary to chronic inflammation.

6.3.1 Role of the inflammatory environment

The telomere length of leukocytes in BE has been implicated as a surrogate marker of inflammation and oxidative damage [16]. Analysis of baseline blood samples in patients with BE revealed that shorter overall telomere length, as well as shortened 17p and 12q telomere lengths, was associated with increased risk of progression to EAC [18]

NF-kβ is a major transcription factor involved in the regulation of genes responsible for both innate and adaptive immune response. High levels of NF-kβ are found in EAC, but are undetectable in the normal esophagus. There is a gradual increase in interleukins involved in the NF-kβ pathway in reflux esophagitis, BE and EAC, in particular of IL-1β, IL-16, IL-8, and TNFα. NF-kβ activation also results in up-regulation of COX-2 and nitric oxide synthase (iNOS). Elevation in NF-kβ expression has also been noted to occur, following the progression from low-grade dysplasia to high-grade dysplasia in BE and EAC. Jenkins *et al.* demonstrated that bile and stomach acids can induce NF-kβ and NF-kβ linked genes such as IL-8.

6.3.2 Obesity

A cross-sectional analysis of baseline data from a cohort study of BE was amongst the first to suggest that fat deposition was more important than weight in predicting risk [20]. Recent results from case control studies strongly suggest that abdominal adiposity, rather than BMI, may be the defining characteristic which places persons at increased risk of BE and subsequent EAC [21].

As overweight men tend to have more visceral fat than overweight women, these studies suggest a possible explanation for the marked preponderance of men with EAC and BE.

Obesity was originally believed to increase reflux by increasing intra-gastric pressure, though the situation now appears to be more complex, with both direct and indirect mechanisms pertaining. High levels of serum leptin produced by visceral fat may promote carcinogenesis, and this is associated with an increased risk of BE, particularly among males.

Obesity can also increase concentration of IGF-1 and insulin, growth factors that promote cellular proliferation and reduce apoptosis, as well as affecting downstream signaling pathways involved in cell growth. IGF-1 serum levels were measured in BE, EAC and control patients. These were shown to be highest in EAC patients ($p < 0.01$) and higher in viscerally obese patients ($P < 0.05$). In resected EAC, increased expression, as determined by immunohistochemistry, was observed in the tumor and the invasive edge, as opposed to the stroma, which was associated with increased CD68 cells in stromal tissue surrounding the invasive tumor edge [23].

Abdominal obesity promotes reflux, but also contributes independently to the pathogenesis of BE and EAC. It induces low-level systemic inflammation, marked by increased plasma levels of pro-inflammatory cytokines and receptors such as IL-7, TNF-α and TNF-alpha receptor 2, CRP and leptin [24].

6.3.3 Tobacco

Cook *et al.* analyzed data from five case control studies included in the International Barrett's and Esophageal Adenocarcinoma Consortium. Data were compared from 1059 BE subjects, with 1332 GERD controls and 1143 population based controls. Patients with BE were significantly more likely to have ever smoked cigarettes than the population based controls (OR = 1.67, 95% CI: 1.04–2.67) or GERD controls (OR = 1.61, 95% CI: 1.33–1.96). Increasing pack-years of smoking also increased the risk for BE until 20 pack years, where this association levels out. Smoking was also shown to have a synergistic effect with GERD [25].

Similarly Coleman *et al.* used the Northern Ireland Cancer Registry to identify BE subjects diagnosed between 1993 and 2005 with intestinal metaplasia (3167 subjects), that were followed up for progression to HGD and EAC. By 2008, 117 of these patients had developed HGD or EAC [26]. Tobacco smoking significantly increased risk of progression (hazard ratio 2.03, 95% CI, 12.9–3.18), compared with those who had never smoked. Andrici *et al.* confirmed the potential association of smoking and development of GE in a meta-analysis of 7069 patients, where it was demonstrated that being an ever-smoker increased the risk of BE [27].

6.4 Genomic instability mutations and copy number changes in candidate genes

6.4.1 Genomic instability

What are the key changes in cancer related genes within the BE and EAC tissues, irrespective of the inherited and environmental susceptibility factors? Genomic instability refers to a high frequency of mutations within the genome of a cellular lineage. These mutations can include chromosomal rearrangements, aneuploidy, and changes in nucleic acid sequences which have been evaluated using techniques such as flow cytometry, cytogenetics, loss of heterozygosity (LOH) studies, CGH array and SNP arrays. The Human Hap 300 SNP array of 23 cases of EAC demonstrated 97 copy number changes, of varying sizes, spanning this cohort of cancers, with copy gain, copy loss and copy neutral loss of heterozygosity (LOH) occupying on average 13 Mb, 18 Mb and 23 Mb of the genome [28].

Microsatellite instability, arising for deficiency in DNA mismatch repair enzymes, is relatively less important in progression to EAC, and is estimated to account for 5% cases, compared to other cancers, such as colon cancer, where it is present in up to 15% of cases [29].

6.4.2 Aneuploidy

Aneuploidy (or abnormal cell nuclear DNA content) in BE has been shown to be associated with a risk of progression to malignancy, with the degree of aneuploidy being proportional to the extent of tissue dysplasia [30, 31].

Various studies employing flow cytometry to determine ploidy in BE have demonstrated that patients without HGD at baseline accompanied by a diploid cell population have a low risk of progressing to EAC. Certain ploidy variables predict cancer progression, in particular aneuploidy content greater than 2.7 N and a 4 N fraction greater than 6% [32, 33].

Flow cytometry is also used to study cell cycle kinetics including an estimate of the S phase fraction. The S phase fraction has been shown by univariate analysis to be a predictor of cancer risk, but was not a significant independent risk factor in a multivariate model incorporating aneuploidy and dysplasia [33].

6.4.3 Tumor suppressor genes

Genetic alterations in the tumor suppressor genes p53 and p16 occur prior to the development of invasive cancer. When followed by loss of cell cycle checkpoints, these abnormalities result in ongoing genomic instability, making the tissue more cancer-prone.

The p16 gene (MTS1, CDKN2a) encodes a 16kdA protein which interacts with cyclin-dependent kinases and, hence, regulates cell cycle growth. This locus (9p21) is frequently subjected to allelic loss in EAC, and it is almost always lost early and precedes the loss of p53. Promoter methylation (with or without p16 LOH) is a common mechanism of p16 inactivation during neoplastic progression in BE, and can also be present in non-dysplastic premalignant BE [34, 35].

TP53 is located on chromosome 17p13, and encodes a 53 kDA polypeptide that responds to DNA damage by cell cycle arrest. Specifically, it induces expression of CKN1A that attracts a number of cyclin-dependent kinases (CDKs) that negotiate both G1 and G2/M arrest. Cells that lack functional p53 proceed inappropriately to the S-phase and are predisposed to genomic instability in EAC. Point mutations leading to a loss of function of p53 are common and, in addition, more than 90% of these mutations occur within the conserved DNA binding domain (exons 5–8). A prospective study of surgically resected EAC over the course of ten years demonstrated that TP53 mutations were associated with poor tumor differentiation and reduced cancer-free and overall survival [36].

LOH is commonly responsible for the loss of the second TP53 allele. In a Phase 4 study of 325 patients with BE, 17p LOH was present in 6% in non-dysplastic Barrett's, compared with 57% in high-grade dysplasia, and was a significant independent predictor of progression to esophageal adenocarcinoma [37]. In the subset of patients who progressed to EAC, only three lacked 17p LOH. 17p LOH was also increased with tetraploidy, HGD and aneuploidy.

Maley *et al.* assayed for LOH and microsatellite shifts in p16, p53 and methylation of the p16 promoter from biopsies taken at 2 cm intervals in Barrett's segments, In particular, 'selective sweeps' were identified, which were events that encompassed large expanses of BE in a wave of initial clonal expansion, compared with smaller hitchhiker or bystander events. P16 LOH, promoter methylation and sequence mutations were shown to occur early, whereas second events in p16 and p53 were associated with later selective sweeps. All other expansions, including microsatellite shifts, could be explained as hitchhikers on an initial clonal expansion of cells with a p16 abnormality [38] . This work, using a candidate approach, provided an early indication that changes critical for actual malignant progression were relatively uncommon, compared with the associated "noise" or non-critical mutations. This will be revisited in the discussion of the new and emerging data from genome-wide technologies.

Loss of functional TP53 commonly leads to stabilization of the protein that can be detected immunohistochemically. The prevalence of P53 protein immunostaining in EAC ranges from 53–87% [39, 40]. This has been demonstrated to increase incrementally in correlation with the histological severity; 5% of patients with non- dysplastic Barrett's epithelium showed p53 overexpression, compared with 15% of those with indefinite or low-grade dysplasia, 45% of those with high-grade dysplasia and 53% of those with Barrett's adenocarcinoma [41].

Flejou et al. demonstrated that p53 overexpression was present only in EAC and HGD, suggesting that this was a late event in the progression to adenocarcinoma [42]. There remains, however, a subset of patients that have p53 overexpression but who do not proceed to invasive cancer and, similarly, a cohort of patients with BE who will undergo malignant transformation despite a lack of immunostaining for p53 protein [43] although, subsequently, loss of p53 staining (when compared with wild-type) was also recognized to be abnormal.

Kastelein et al. evaluated the value of abnormal p53 immunostaining for predicting neoplastic progression in a prospective cohort of 720 patients with BE, including over 12,000 biopsies in which 8% of patients progressed to HGD and EAC [44]. P53 overexpression was associated with an increased risk of malignant progression, after adjusting for other variables such as gender, age, Barrett's length and esophagitis (adjusted relative risks RR 5.6; 95% CI 3.1–10.3). Loss of p53 expression (RR 14.0; 95% CI 5.3–37.2) was associated

with an even higher risk of neoplastic progression. The positive predictive value for progression to HGD and EAC increased from 15% with histological diagnosis of LGD, to 33% in patients with LGD who also had p53 over-expression. Hence, p53 immunohistochemistry was superior to histology alone for predicting neoplastic progression in BE.

As a consequence of these observations, in the newest edition of the British Society of Gastroenterology guidelines, p53 immunostaining is considered for the first time as an adjunct to routine histopathological diagnosis to improve the diagnosis of dysplasia in BE [45]. Evidence for p53 as a biomarker for BE and risk of progression to invasive disease is summarized in Table 6.1.

6.4.4 Proto-oncogenes

Receptor tyrosine kinases (RTKs) are high-affinity cell surface receptors for cytokines, hormones and growth factors. They are involved in regulating normal cellular processors and have also been implicated in many cancers.

A number of tyrosine receptor kinases are dysregulated in EAC and have attracted attention as therapeutic targets. Al-Kasspooles et al. demonstrated that up to 30% of EAC and Barrett's had amplified Epidermal Growth Factor Receptor (EGFR), but that there was no direct correlation with this and the level of EGFR expression by immunohistochemistry [52]. The c-erb2 proto-oncogene encodes a transmembrane tyrosine receptor kinase receptor highly homologous to EGF with intrinsic tyrosine kinase activity. C-erbB2 protein expression or amplification of the c-erbB2 receptor gene occurs in 23% of esophageal adenocarcinomas [53].

Overexpression of c-erbB2 is not demonstrated in dysplastic BE, suggesting that it is a late event in the dysplasia-adenocarcinoma sequence [42]. Overexpression of c-erbB2 correlates with tumor invasion, lymph node involvement, distant metastasis and status of residual tumor after resection [54]. The precise timing of receptor tyrosine kinase (RTK) up-regulation has been better characterized recently. Patersen et al. performed immunohistochemistry on the RTK panel (EGFR, erbB2, ErbB3, Met and FGFR2) in patients with pre-invasive disease ($n = 201$) and invasive disease ($n = 367$) [55]. 51% of esophageal adenocarcinomas overexpressed at least one of the RTK panel, with 21% of these overexpressing multiple receptors. Up-regulation of RTK expression was an early event

Table 6.1 Role of p53 as a biomarker for progression of BE to HGD and EAC.

Study	Study Design	Results	Cohort Details
Bani-Hani *et al.*, 2005 [46]	Retrospective nested case control study	OR = 2.99 (95% CI, 0.57–15.76; $p = 0.197$)	11 cases, 41 controls
Bird Lieberman *et al.*, 2012 [47]	Population-based nested case control study	OR = 1.95 (95% CI,1.04–3.67; $p = 0.02$) for progression from BE to cancer	89 cases, 291 controls
Weston *et al.*, 2001 [48]	Prospective cohort study	Kaplan-Meier estimates of progression of LGD differed significantly between p53-positive and p53-negative patents ($p < 0.002$)	5 progressors, 43 non-progressors
Skacel *et al.*, 2002 [49]	Retrospective case control study	P53 positivity – sensitivity 88% and specificity 75% for progression of LGD to HGD or EAC; ($p = 0.017$)	8 progressors, 8 non-progressors
Murray *et al.*, 2006 [50]	Retrospective nested case control study	OR = 8.42 (95% CI, 2.37–30.0)	35 progressors, 175 non-progressors
Sikkema *et al.*, 2009 [51]	Retrospective case control study	HR = 6.5 (95% CI, 2.5–17.1; $p < 0.001$)	27 progressors, 27 non-progressors
Kastelein *et al.*, 2012 [44]	Case control study within a prospective cohort. *Included p53 overexpression and complete loss*	P53 protein overexpression. RR = 5.6 (95% CI, 3.1–10.3); loss of p53 expression; RR = 14 (95% CI, 5.3–37.2)	49 progressors, 586 non-progressors.

that corresponded with low-grade dysplasia development ($p < 0.001$). Progression of BE was marked by an increasing trend of concomitant overexpression in multiple receptors 7–10% from IM to LGD, 10–19% in LGD to HGD ($p = 0.06$ and 0.24 respectively).

The precise receptor which was up-regulated varied between cases. ErbB3 overexpression was rare in both BE and EAC, FGFR, erbB2 and Met overexpression was predominant in dysplastic BE, and EGFR overexpression was strongest in EAC. This study suggested that the early dysregulation of receptor kinases in esophageal carcinogenesis may support a role targeting receptor kinases for inhibition in pre-invasive disease.

Transforming Growth Factor (TGF-β) is expressed in both non-dysplastic BE and EAC [56]. During the initial stages of Barrett's carcinogenesis, Onweugbusi *et al.* demonstrated that a reduction in activity of the TGF-β signaling cascade occurred through down-regulation of SMAD4, with subsequent impairment of TGF-β dependent growth suppression [57]. In later stages of tumor development, increased expression of TGFβ1 at the margins of the tumor may mediate epithelial to mesenchymal transition and enable the development of a more invasive phenotype. Recent data from Dulak *et al.* employed whole exome and genome sequencing to detect somatic mutations in EAC [58]. This supports the role of the TGFβ/SMAD signaling in invasive disease, and this pathway was shown to be mutated in 18% of EAC tumors. The most recurrently mutated gene in this pathway was SMAD4. This is discussed in more detail below, in whole genome and exome sequencing.

The Ras family encodes proteins that are essential components in division and differentiation of normal cells. H-ras mutations have been shown to be associated with dysplastic Barrett's and EAC but have not been found in non-dysplastic Barrett's metaplasia. Increased expression of H-ras and amplification of the K-ras gene in esophageal adenocarcinoma have been reported [59, 60]. The overall involvement of the ras family of genes in EAC appears to be minimal, compared with other cancers.

C-myc is located on chromosome 8q24 and encodes a nuclear protein thought to regulate the transcription of other genes essential for cell growth. Hetero-dimerization of myc and max is required for myc transformation, and c-myc has been shown to be essential for the transition from the G0/G1 to S phase of the cell cycle by regulating cyclin-dependent kinase (CDK) complexes. *In situ* hybridization experiments [60], using biotinylated complimentary DNA probes, found enhanced c-myc expression in dysplastic BE and adenocarcinoma, but not in non-dysplastic Barrett's mucosa. Schmidt *et al.* demonstrated that c-myc was overexpressed in 37% cases of BE without dysplasia, 46% BE with dysplasia and 73% of EAC cases [61]. It remains unclear whether amplification or mutation of c-myc is the primary mechanism for dysregulation of this gene in BE.

6.5 The advent of next generation sequencing

6.5.1 Whole-Genome and exome sequencing

The advent of genome-wide analyses has provided an invaluable opportunity to understand the pathogenesis of BE and EAC. Whole-genome sequencing (targeting the entire genome) and exome sequencing (targeting the coding region alone) enable us to adopt an unbiased approach to identifying key single nucleotide variants (mutations affecting a single base), small insertions and deletions (indels) and structural rearrangements (larger-scale chromosomal aberrations) which may be involved in the carcinogenesis of BE and EAC. Compared with exome sequencing, whole-genome sequencing provides us more information on structural variations, which are typically chromosomal rearrangements that affect a sequence length about 1 Kb to 3 Mb and include deletions, duplications, copy number variants, insertions, inversion and translocations.

The summary of findings from these recent sequencing studies are displayed in Table 6.2. In future, studies BE should ideally be sampled at earlier time points, and in spatially distinct locations, in order for definite conclusions about progression to be drawn.

Agrawal *et al.* performed exome sequencing in EAC and demonstrated that the majority of mutations in two different tumors were also present in adjacent BE [66].

Dulak *et al.* performed whole exome sequencing of 149 EAC tumor-normal pairs, 15 of which had also undergone whole genome sequencing (WGS) [58]. The authors identified a mutational signature defined by a high prevalence of A > C transversions at AA dinucleotides, which was previously described by Weaver *et al.* [67]. Their analyses revealed 26 significantly mutated genes, of which five (TP53, CDKNA1a, SMAD4, ARID1a and PIK3CA) have already been implicated in EAC in various studies.

Genes with mutations occurring above that expected by chance, which had not been implicated in this disease previously, included chromatin modifying factors such as ARID1a, SPG20, TLR4, ELMO1 and DOCK2. Further functional work demonstrated that the RAC1 pathway may play an important role in the development of EAC. The RAC1 gene encodes for a 21kDA signaling GTPase protein, which is a member of the larger Rho Family of GTPases. It is involved, along with other genes in this superfamily, in the regulation of cell growth, cytoskeleton integrity, cell-cell motility and adhesion and epithelial differentiation. The authors performed functional analyses to assess the role of increased invasion, decreased apoptosis and increased cell survival in the RAC pathway, but did not investigate the role of proliferation. Future studies will, hopefully, identify how chromatin modifying factors and the RAC1 pathway may potentially influence disease progression.

Streppel *et al.* performed whole-genome sequencing of snap-frozen samples from a single BE 'progressor' case with a matched normal, BE and EAC endoscopic biopsies to identify genes that may be involved in the dysplasia-neoplasia sequence for EAC [64]. The overwhelming majority of SNVs detected were found in both BE and EAC, supporting the notion that, despite being a precancerous lesion, BE is highly mutated. Nonsense mutations were also found in ARID1A which, as mentioned earlier, is a member of the SWI/SNF family, whose members have helicase and ATPase activities, and are thought to regulate transcription of certain genes by altering the chromatic structure round these genes. Immunohistochemistry for ARID1A was also performed to elucidate the protein expression of ARID 1a in a independent retrospective cohort; this demonstrated ARID1a protein loss in 0%, 4.9%, 14.3%, 16%, 12.2%, 6.5% of normal squamous epithelium, BE, LGD, HGD EAC and lymph node metastases, respectively.

Although there will be an increase in the number of cases analyzed through The Cancer Genome Atlas and the International Cancer Genome Consortium (ICGC), so far these studies have suggested that there is a significant degree of heterogeneity between different

Table 6.2 Table summarizing next generation sequencing advances in EAC.

Name of study	Type of analysis	Platform	Cohort details	Genes identified
Streppel et al., 2013 [64]	Genome	WGS	1 patient with BE and EAC	ARID1a
Dulak et al., 2012 [65]	Genome	SNP array	186 chemo naïve EAC at surgery (FF)	RUNX1
Agrawal et al., 2012 [66]	Genome	WES	11 chemo-naive EAC	ARID1a
Weaver et al., 2012 [67]	Genome	WGS	22 EAC (chemo treated and chemo-naïve patients)	ARID1A, SMARCA4, MYO18B, SMAD4, ABCB1
Dulak et al., 2013 [58]	Genome	WGS, WES	15 WGS, 149 WES in chemo-naïve EAC from surgery	ELMO1, DOCK1, TLR4, ARID1A, SMARCA4, SYNE1, SMAD4, CTNAP5
Goh et al., 2011 [68]	Transcriptome, Genome	Microarray and aCGH	56 fresh frozen surgically resected EAC	NEIL2, WT1, MTMR9
Alvarez et al., 2011 [69]	Transcriptome, Genome	aCGH	19 LGD, 38 HGD, 80 EAC	GATA6, CXCL1, CDKN2B
Kim et al., 2010 [70]	Transcriptome	Microarray	64 EAC endoscopy samples from patients undergoing surgery and chemoradiation. Validated in 52 patients	SPARC, SPP1
Schauer et al., 2010 [71]	Transcriptome	Microarray	47 T3N+ (advanced EAC) patients	EPHB3
Lagarde et al., 2008 [72]	Transcriptome	Microarray	77 patients (55 no lymph node metastases, 22 lymph node metastases)	ASS1

aCGH – array Comparative Genome Hybridization; WGS – Whole Genome Sequencing; WES – Whole Exome Sequencing; SNP – Single Nucleotide Polymorphism.

cases of EAC (http://icgc.org/icgc/cgp/72/508/70708, tcga-data.nci.nih.gov). Only TP53 is mutated in greater than half of the cases. This is echoed in other epithelial cancers, in which the majority of recurrent mutations seem to be found in only a small percentage of tumors, and only a few genes are mutated in a large proportion of cases of a given cancer type.

6.5.2   Microbiome

There has recently been an increased interest in the microbiome and its role in malignancy. Yang et al. demonstrated changes in the microbiota in BE compared to the normal esophagus. [73]. Two main microbiome profiles were found, the type 1 microbiome was more closely associated with the normal esophagus (11/12 cases = 91.7%), while the type 2 microbiome was more likely to be associated with either esophagitis

(7/12 = 58.3%, odds ratio 15.4) or BE (6/10 = 60%, odd ratio 16.5) than normal epithelium. Overall, Gram-negative bacteria comprised only 14.9% of the type 1 microbiome, compared with 53.4% of the type 2 microbiome. The significance of these findings remains to be determined.

6.5.3   Non-Coding RNAs and microRNAs

Non-coding regions in the human genome refer to RNAs that are transcribed into RNA but not translated to protein. These are present throughout the genomic DNA, and are comprised of long non-coding RNAs (lncRNAs) more than 200 nucleotides in length, and microRNAs (miRNAs), which are numerous (in excess of 21,000 documented in 2012 MiRBase) small, well conserved, non-coding RNAS of 20–24 nucleotides that regulate the translation of RNAs. MiRNAs serve as potential biomarkers in the clinical setting, since they are relatively stable because of their small size and stability in blood.

Yang *et al.* compared samples from BE patients with LGD, HGD and EAC [74]. 24 miRNAs showed altered expression (14 up-regulated in disease tissues and ten down-regulated in disease tissues) in HGD and EAC, compared with normal tissue. Several studies have examined the role of miRNAs in disease progression from Barrett's to EAC. These have been extensively reviewed by Sakai *et al.* [76]. Kan *et al.* studied 22 normal, 24 BE and 22 EAC samples, and identified three miRNAs that were up-regulated and four miRNAs that were down-regulated in BE and EAC, compared with normal tissue [77]. Feber *et al.* reported the sequential up-regulation of miRNAs-192, 194, 21 and 93 marked the progression from NE to BE to EAC [78]. Leidner *et al.* investigated the expression of candidate miRNAs as identified from the literature, and identified that 23 out of 26 of these were deregulated in LGD. As a result of their work, they proposed that miR-33 and miR-374 constitute part of the genetic changes that mark the progression of BE to EAC [79].

6.5.4 Epigenetics

Epigenetics is increasingly recognized to be important for regulation of gene expression [81]. Several studies have employed a candidate approach of selecting potential methylation targets from other cancers, namely promoters of genes of interest, and investigated their methylation in BE and EAC using methylation-specific PCR.

Jin *et al.* examined MAL promoter hypermethylation in 260 esophageal specimens, using real-time quantitative methylation specific PCR (qMSP) [82]. Myelin and Lymphocte protein (MAL) is a 17 kDA hydrophobic membrane protein which is widely expressed in a variety of cell types, playing an essential role in apical transport which is required for the normal functioning of epithelial cells. MAL methylation frequency and normalized methylation value (NMV) were significantly higher in BE, dysplastic BE, and EAC than in normal squamous epithelium. In addition, methylation of MAL correlated with segment length of BE.

Jin *et al.* previously demonstrated hypermethylation of tachykinin-1 (TAC-1) as a potential biomarker in esophageal cancer [83]. Frequencies and NMVs of TACI in tissue methylation were higher in non-dysplastic BE,

dysplastic BE and EAC compared to normal epithelium ($P < 0.01$). The frequency of TAC1 hypermethylation increased during neoplastic progression from 7.5% in normal esophagus to 55.6% in non-dysplastic BE, 57.5% in dysplastic BE and 61.2% in EAC. There was no significant association between TAC1 hypermethylation in EAC and patient survival. Mean NMV and frequency of TAC1 hypermethylation in plasma samples was significantly higher in EAC patients, suggesting that circulating methylated TAC1 promoter DNA may be a potential biomarker for diagnosis of EAC.

Tischoff *et al.* investigated the methylation of suppressors of cytokine signaling (SOCS), as methylation of SOCS-3 has previously been implicated in hepatocellular carcinoma [84]. In non-dysplastic BE, SOCS-3 was methylated in 13% of cases, whereas SOCS-1 was unmethylated. A hypermethylated SOCS-3 promoter was found in 74% of EAC, and 69% of HGD and 22% of LGD. SOCS-1 promoter hypermethylation occurred in 52% of EAC, and 21% of HGD and 4% of LGD. Subsequent transcript down-regulation of SOCS-3 and, to a lesser extent, SOCS-1 was also demonstrated to be involved in BE carcinogenesis.

Alvi *et al.* tested DNA methylation using methylation arrays to test whether methylation could predict dysplasia and early stage neoplasia. Four genes (PIGR, SLC22A18, GJA12 and RIN2) were taken forward in a methylation panel to stratify patients into three risk groups in a prospective patient cohort, based on the number of genes methylated (low risk < 2 genes, intermediate 2, and high > 2). This panel has potential use in clinical practice, especially as an adjunct to conventional histopathology, which is often ambiguous in detecting prevalent, inconspicuous dysplasia and early stage neoplasia in BE [85].

6.6 Future directions and conclusions

The molecular biology of BE and EAC is a complex interplay of inherited pre-disposition, environmental exposures and tissue responses. No single molecular event has been identified as being solely responsible for marking the progression of BE to EAC, which appears to be a complex and heterogeneous process.

The advent of genome-wide analyses will no doubt contribute enormously to our understanding of both BE and OA and, more importantly, the progression sequence from precancerous lesion to malignancy. Studies at present employ both candidate and unbiased genome-wide approaches, and have started to shed light on the relative role of point mutations and epigenetic modifications in the progression of BE. With the opportunity to incorporate methylation into genome-wide sequencing experiments, and integrate data from DNA and RNA sequences obtained from the same patients, it is hoped to gain further biological insights into the pathogenesis of this disease.

The challenge will be to introduce these technologies in a clinically applicable setting, so that patients with BE can be monitored and surveillance performed in a realistic time scale, with practical alterations in treatment pathways. This, hopefully, will lead to improved patient risk stratification and, potentially, earlier therapeutic intervention.

References

1 Chak A, Ochs-Balcom H, Falk G, Grady WM, Kinnard M, Willis JE, *et al.* (2006). Familiality in Barrett's esophagus, adenocarcinoma of the esophagus, and adenocarcinoma of the gastroesophageal junction. *Cancer Epidemiology, Biomarkers & Prevention* **15**, 1668–73.

2 Romero Y, Cameron AJ, Schaid DJ, McDonnell SK, Burgart LJ, Hardtke CL, *et al.* (2002). Barrett's esophagus: prevalence in symptomatic relatives. *American Journal of Gastroenterology* **97**, 1127–32.

3 Levine DM, Ek WE, Zhang R, Liu X, Onstad L, Sather C, *et al.* (2013). A genome-wide association study identifies new susceptibility loci for esophageal adenocarcinoma and Barrett's esophagus. *Nature Genetics* **45**(12), 1487–93.

4 Ek WE, Levine DM, D'Amato M, Pedersen NL, Magnusson PKE, Bresso F, *et al.* (2013). Germline Genetic Contributions to Risk for Esophageal Adenocarcinoma, Barrett's Esophagus, and Gastroesophageal Reflux. *Journal of the National Cancer Institute* **105**(22), 1711–8.

5 Doecke JD, Zhao ZZ, Stark MS, Green AC, Hayward NK, Montgomery GW, *et al.* (2008). Single nucleotide polymorphisms in obesity-related genes and the risk of esophageal cancers. *Cancer Epidemiology, Biomarkers & Prevention* **17**, 1007–12.

6 Di Martino E, Hardie LJ, Wild CP, Gong YY, Olliver JR, Gough MD, *et al.* (2007). The NAD(P)H:quinone oxidoreductase I C609T polymorphism modifies the risk of Barrett esophagus and esophageal adenocarcinoma. *Genetics in Medicine* **9**, 341–7.

7 Kala Z, Dolina J, Marek F, Izakovicova Holla L (2007). Polymorphisms of glutathione S-transferase M1, T1 and P1 in patients with reflux esophagitis and Barrett's esophagus. *Journal of Human Genetics* **52**, 527–34.

8 Murphy SJ, Hughes AE, Patterson CC, Anderson LA, Watson RGP, Johnston BT, *et al.* (2007). A population-based association study of SNPs of GSTP1, MnSOD, GPX2 and Barrett's esophagus and esophageal adenocarcinoma. *Carcinogenesis* **28**, 1323–8.

9 Casson AG, Zheng Z, Porter GA, Guernsey DL (2006). Genetic polymorphisms of microsomal epoxide hydroxylase and glutathione S-transferases M1, T1 and P1, interactions with smoking, and risk for esophageal (Barrett) adenocarcinoma. *Cancer Detection and Prevention* **30**, 423–31.

10 Casson AG, Zheng Z, Evans SC, Geldenhuys L, van Zanten SV, Veugelers PJ, *et al.* (2005). Cyclin D1 polymorphism (G870A) and risk for esophageal adenocarcinoma. *Cancer* **104**, 730–9.

11 Lu F, Gladden AB, Diehl JA (2003). An alternatively spliced cyclin D1 isoform, cyclin D1b, is a nuclear oncogene. *Cancer Research* **63**, 7056–61.

12 Moons LMG, Kuipers EJ, Rygiel AM, Groothuismink AZM, Geldof H, Bode WA, *et al.* (2007). COX-2 CA-haplotype is a risk factor for the development of esophageal adenocarcinoma. *American Journal of Gastroenterology* **102**, 2373–9.

13 Ferguson HR, Wild CP, Anderson LA, Murphy SJ, Johnston BT, Murray LJ, *et al.* (2008). Cyclooxygenase-2 and inducible nitric oxide synthase gene polymorphisms and risk of reflux esophagitis, Barrett's esophagus, and esophageal adenocarcinoma. *Cancer Epidemiology, Biomarkers & Prevention* **17**, 727–31.

14 Anderson LA, Johnston BT, Watson RGP, Murphy SJ, Ferguson HR, Comber H, *et al.* (2006). Nonsteroidal anti-inflammatory drugs and the esophageal inflammation-metaplasia-adenocarcinoma sequence. *Cancer Research* **66**, 4975–82.

15 Galipeau PC, Li X, Blount PL, Maley CC, Sanchez CA, Odze RD, *et al.* (2007). NSAIDs modulate CDKN2A, TP53, and DNA content risk for progression to esophageal adenocarcinoma. *PLoS Medicine* **4**, e67.

16 Risques RA, Vaughan TL, Li X, Odze RD, Blount PL, Ayub K, *et al.* (2007). Leukocyte telomere length predicts cancer risk in Barrett's esophagus. *Cancer Epidemiology, Biomarkers & Prevention* **16**, 2649–55.

17 Kim S, Parks CG, DeRoo LA, Chen H, Taylor JA, Cawthon RM, *et al.* (2009). Obesity and weight gain in adulthood and telomere length. *Cancer Epidemiology, Biomarkers & Prevention* **18**, 816–20.

18 Xing J, Ajani JA, Chen M, Izzo J, Lin J, Chen Z, *et al.* (2009). Constitutive short telomere length of chromosome 17p and 12q but not 11q and 2p is associated with an increased risk for esophageal cancer. *Cancer Prevention Research (Phila)* **2**, 459–65.

19 McAdam E, Haboubi HN, Forrester G, Eltahir Z, Spencer-Harty S, Davies C, *et al.* (2012). Inducible Nitric Oxide Synthase (iNOS) and Nitric Oxide (NO) are Important Mediators of Reflux-induced Cell Signalling in Esophageal Cells. *Carcinogenesis* **33**, 2035–43.

20 Vaughan TL, Kristal AR, Blount PL, Levine DS, Galipeau PC, Prevo LJ, *et al.* (2002). Nonsteroidal anti-inflammatory drug use, body mass index, and anthropometry in relation to genetic and flow cytometric abnormalities in Barrett's esophagus. *Cancer Epidemiology, Biomarkers & Prevention* **11**, 745–52.

21 Edelstein ZR, Farrow DC, Bronner MP, Rosen SN, Vaughan TL (2007). Central adiposity and risk of Barrett's esophagus. *Gastroenterology* **133**, 403–11.

22 El-Serag HB, Graham DY, Satia JA, Rabeneck L (2005). Obesity is an independent risk factor for GERD symptoms and erosive esophagitis. *American Journal of Gastroenterology* **100**, 1243–50.

23 Doyle SL, Donohoe CL, Finn SP, Howard JM, Lithander FE, Reynolds J V, *et al.* (2012). IGF-1 and its receptor in esophageal cancer: association with adenocarcinoma and visceral obesity. *American Journal of Gastroenterology* **107**, 196–204.

24 Kendall BJ, Macdonald GA, Hayward NK, Prins JB, Brown I, Walker N, *et al.* (2008). Leptin and the risk of Barrett's oesophagus. *Gut* **57**, 448–54.

25 Cook MB, Shaheen NJ, Anderson LA, Giffen C, Chow W-H, Vaughan TL, *et al.* (2012). Cigarette smoking increases risk of Barrett's esophagus: an analysis of the Barrett's and Esophageal Adenocarcinoma Consortium. *Gastroenterology* **142**, 744–53.

26 Coleman HG, Bhat S, Johnston BT, McManus D, Gavin AT, Murray LJ (2012). Tobacco smoking increases the risk of high-grade dysplasia and cancer among patients with Barrett's esophagus. *Gastroenterology* **142**, 233–40.

27 Andrici J, Cox MR, Eslick GD (2013). Cigarette Smoking and the Risk of Barrett'S Esophagus: a Systematic Review and Meta-Analysis. *Journal of Gastroenterology and Hepatology* **28**(8), 1258–73.

28 Nancarrow DJ, Handoko HY, Smithers BM, Gotley DC, Drew PA, Watson DI, *et al.* (2008). Genome-wide copy number analysis in esophageal adenocarcinoma using high-density single-nucleotide polymorphism arrays. *Cancer Research* **68**, 4163–72.

29 Boland CR, Goel A (2010). Microsatellite instability in colorectal cancer. *Gastroenterology* **138**, 2073–2087.e3.

30 Menke-Pluymers MB, Mulder AH, Hop WC, van Blankenstein M, Tilanus HW (1994). Dysplasia and aneuploidy as markers of malignant degeneration in Barrett's oesophagus. The Rotterdam Oesophageal Tumour Study Group. *Gut* **35**, 1348–51.

31 Galipeau PC, Cowan DS, Sanchez CA, Barrett MT, Emond MJ, Levine DS, *et al.* (1996). 17p (p53) allelic losses, 4N (G2/tetraploid) populations, and progression to aneuploidy in Barrett's esophagus. *Proceedings of the National Academy of Sciences of the United States of America* **93**, 7081–4.

32 Reid BJ, Sanchez CA, Blount PL, Levine DS (1993). Barrett's esophagus: cell cycle abnormalities in advancing stages of neoplastic progression. *Gastroenterology* **105**, 119–29.

33 Rabinovitch PS, Longton G, Blount PL, Levine DS, Reid BJ (2001). Predictors of progression in Barrett's esophagus III: baseline flow cytometric variables. *American Journal of Gastroenterology* **96**, 3071–83.

34 Klump B, Hsieh CJ, Holzmann K, Gregor M, Porschen R (1998). Hypermethylation of the CDKN2/p16 promoter during neoplastic progression in Barrett's esophagus. *Gastroenterology* **115**, 1381–6.

35 Wong DJ, Barrett MT, Stöger R, Emond MJ, Reid BJ (1997). p16INK4a promoter is hypermethylated at a high frequency in esophageal adenocarcinomas. *Cancer Research* **57**, 2619–22.

36 Casson AG, Evans SC, Gillis A, Porter GA, Veugelers P, Darnton SJ, *et al.* (2003). Clinical implications of p53 tumor suppressor gene mutation and protein expression in esophageal adenocarcinomas: results of a ten-year prospective study. *Journal of Thoracic and Cardiovascular Surgery* **125**, 1121–31.

37 Reid BJ, Prevo LJ, Galipeau PC, Sanchez CA, Longton G, Levine DS, *et al.* (2001). Predictors of progression in Barrett's esophagus II: baseline 17p (p53) loss of heterozygosity identifies a patient subset at increased risk for neoplastic progression. *American Journal of Gastroenterology* **96**, 2839–48.

38 Maley CC, Galipeau PC, Li X, Sanchez CA, Paulson TG, Blount PL, *et al.* (2004). The combination of genetic instability and clonal expansion predicts progression to esophageal adenocarcinoma. *Cancer Research* **64**, 7629–33.

39 Rice TW, Goldblum JR, Falk GW, Tubbs RR, Kirby TJ, Casey G (1994). p53 immunoreactivity in Barrett's metaplasia, dysplasia, and carcinoma. *Journal of Thoracic and Cardiovascular Surgery* **108**, 1132 7.

40 Krishnadath KK, Tilanus HW, van Blankenstein M, Bosman FT, Mulder AH (1995). Accumulation of p53 protein in normal, dysplastic, and neoplastic Barrett's oesophagus. *Journal of Pathology* **175**, 175–80.

41 Younes M, Lebovitz RM, Lechago L V, Lechago J (1993). p53 protein accumulation in Barrett's metaplasia, dysplasia, and carcinoma: a follow-up study. *Gastroenterology* **105**, 1637–42.

42 Fléjou JF, Muzeau F, Potet F, Lepelletier F, Fékété F, Hénin D (1994). Overexpression of the p53 tumor suppressor gene product in esophageal and gastric carcinomas. *Pathology, Research and Practice* **190**, 1141–8.

43 Coggi G, Bosari S, Roncalli M, Graziani D, Bossi P, Viale G, *et al.* (1997). p53 protein accumulation and p53 gene mutation in esophageal carcinoma. *A molecular and immunohistochemical study with clinicopathologic correlations. Cancer* **79**, 425–32.

44 Kastelein F, Biermann K, Steyerberg EW, Verheij J, Kalisvaart M, Looijenga LH, *et al.* (2012). Aberrant p53 protein expression is associated with an increased risk of neoplastic progression in patients with Barrett's oesophagus. *Gut* **62**(12), 1676–83.

45 Fitzgerald RC, di Pietro M, Ragunath K, Ang Y, Kang J-Y, Watson P, *et al.* (2014). British Society of Gastroenterology guidelines on the diagnosis and management of Barrett's oesophagus. *Gut* **63**(1), 7–42.

46 Bani-Hani KE, Bani-Hani BK, Martin IG (2005). Characteristics of patients with columnar-lined Barrett's esophagus and risk factors for progression to esophageal adenocarcinoma. *World Journal of Gastroenterology* **11**, 6807–14.

47 Bird-Lieberman EL, Dunn JM, Coleman HG, Lao-Sirieix P, Oukrif D, Moore CE, *et al.* (2012). Population-based study reveals new risk-stratification biomarker panel for Barrett's esophagus. *Gastroenterology* **143**(4), 927–35.

48 Weston AP, Banerjee SK, Sharma P, Tran TM, Richards R, Cherian R (2001). p53 protein overexpression in low grade dysplasia (LGD) in Barrett's esophagus: immunohistochemical marker predictive of progression. *American Journal of Gastroenterology* **96**, 1355–62.

49 Skacel M, Petras RE, Rybicki LA, Gramlich TL, Richter JE, Falk GW, *et al.* (2002). p53 expression in low grade dysplasia in Barrett's esophagus: correlation with interobserver agreement and disease progression. *American Journal of Gastroenterology* **97**, 2508–13.

50 Murray L, Sedo A, Scott M, McManus D, Sloan JM, Hardie LJ, *et al.* (2006). TP53 and progression from Barrett's metaplasia to oesophageal adenocarcinoma in a UK population cohort. *Gut* **55**, 1390–7.

51 Sikkema M, Kerkhof M, Steyerberg EW, Kusters JG, van Strien PMH, Looman CWN, *et al.* (2009). Aneuploidy and overexpression of Ki67 and p53 as markers for neoplastic progression in Barrett's esophagus: a case-control study. *American Journal of Gastroenterology* **104**, 2673–80.

52 al-Kasspooles M, Moore JH, Orringer MB, Beer DG (1993). Amplification and over-expression of the EGFR and erbB-2 genes in human esophageal adenocarcinomas. *International Journal of Cancer* **54**, 213–9.

53 Hardwick RH, Barham CP, Ozua P, Newcomb PV, Savage P, Powell R, *et al.* (1997). Immunohistochemical detection of p53 and c-erbB-2 in oesophageal carcinoma; no correlation with prognosis. *European Journal of Surgical Oncology* **23**, 30–5.

54 Polkowski W, van Lanschot JJ, Offerhaus GJ (1999). Barrett esophagus and cancer: pathogenesis, carcinogenesis, and diagnostic dilemmas. *Histology and Histopathology* **14**, 927–44.

55 Paterson AL, O'Donovan M, Provenzano E, Murray LJ, Coleman HG, Johnson BT, *et al.* (2013). Characterization of the timing and prevalence of receptor tyrosine kinase expression changes in oesophageal carcinogenesis. *Journal of Pathology* **230**(1), 118–28.

56 Triadafilopoulos G, Kaczynska M, Iwane M (1996). Esophageal mucosal eicosanoids in gastroesophageal reflux disease and Barrett's esophagus. *American Journal of Gastroenterology* **91**, 65–74.

57 Onwuegbusi BA, Rees JRE, Lao-Sirieix P, Fitzgerald RC (2007). Selective loss of TGFbeta Smad-dependent signalling prevents cell cycle arrest and promotes invasion in oesophageal adenocarcinoma cell lines. *PLoS One* **2**, e177.

58 Dulak AM, Stojanov P, Peng S, Lawrence MS, Fox C, Stewart C, *et al.* (2013). Exome and whole-genome sequencing of esophageal adenocarcinoma identifies recurrent driver events and mutational complexity. *Nature Genetics* **45**, 478–86.

59 Trautmann B, Wittekind C, Strobel D, Meixner H, Keymling J, Gossner L, *et al.* (1996). K-ras point mutations are rare events in premalignant forms of Barrett's oesophagus. *European Journal of Gastroenterology & Hepatology* **8**, 799–804.

60 Abdelatif OM, Chandler FW, Mills LR, McGuire BS, Pantazis CG, Barrett JM (1991). Differential expression of c-myc and H-ras oncogenes in Barrett's epithelium. A study using colorimetric in situ hybridization. *Archives of Pathology & Laboratory Medicine* **115**, 880–5.

61 Schmidt MK, Meurer L, Volkweis BS, Edelweiss MI, Schirmer CC, Kruel CDP, *et al.* (2007). c-Myc overexpression is strongly associated with metaplasia-dysplasia-adenocarcinoma sequence in the esophagus. *Diseases of the Esophagus* **20**, 212–6.

62 Vissers KJ, Riegman PH, Alers JC, Tilanus HW van Dekken H (2001). Involvement of cancer-activating genes on chromosomes 7 and 8 in esophageal (Barrett's) and gastric cardia adenocarcinoma. *AntiCancer Research* **21**(6A) 3813–20.

63 Jenkins RB, Qian J, Lieber MM, Bostwick DG (1997). Detection of c-myc oncogene amplification and chromosomal anomalies in metastatic prostatic carcinoma by fluorescence in situ hybridization. *Cancer Research* **57**, 524–31.

64 Streppel MM, Lata S, Delabastide M, Montgomery E a, Wang JS, Canto MI, *et al.* (2014). Next-generation sequencing of endoscopic biopsies identifies ARID1A as a tumor-suppressor gene in Barrett's esophagus. *Oncogene* **33**(3), 347–57.

65 Dulak AM, Schumacher SE, van Lieshout J, Imamura Y, Fox C, Shim B, *et al.* (2012). Gastrointestinal Adenocarcinomas of the Esophagus, Stomach, and Colon Exhibit Distinct Patterns of Genome Instability and Oncogenesis. *Cancer Research* **2**(17), 4383–93.

66 Agrawal N, Jiao Y, Bettegowda C, Hutfless SM, Wang Y, David S, *et al.* (2012). Comparative genomic analysis of esophageal adenocarcinoma and squamous cell carcinoma. *Cancer Discovery* **2**(10), 899–905.

67 Weaver JMJ, Shannon NB, Smith M, Dunning M, Ong CA, Ross-Innes C, Underwood T, Lynch A, Eldridge M, Caldas C, Edwards PAW, Tavaré S & Fitzgerald RC (2012). Defining the genetic landscape of esophageal adenocarcinoma by next generation sequencing. *Gut* **61**, A3–A4.

68 Goh XY, Rees JRE, Paterson AL, Chin SF, Marioni JC, Save V, *et al.* (2011). Integrative analysis of array-comparative genomic hybridisation and matched gene expression profiling data reveals novel genes with prognostic significance in oesophageal adenocarcinoma. *Gut* **60**, 1317–26.

69 Alvarez H, Opalinska J, Zhou L, Sohal D, Fazzari MJ, Yu Y, *et al.* (2011). Widespread hypomethylation occurs early and synergizes with gene amplification during esophageal carcinogenesis. *PLoS Genetics* **7**(3), e1001356.

70 Kim SM, Park Y-Y, Park ES, Cho JY, Izzo JG, Zhang D, *et al.* (2010). Prognostic biomarkers for esophageal

adenocarcinoma identified by analysis of tumor transcriptome. *PLoS One* **5**, e15074.

71 Schauer M, Janssen K-P, Rimkus C, Raggi M, Feith M, Friess H, *et al.* (2010). Microarray-based response prediction in esophageal adenocarcinoma. *Clinical Cancer Research* **16**, 330–7.

72 Lagarde SM, Ver Loren van Themaat PE, Moerland PD, Gilhuijs-Pederson LA, Ten Kate FJW, Reitsma PH, *et al.* (2008). Analysis of gene expression identifies differentially expressed genes and pathways associated with lymphatic dissemination in patients with adenocarcinoma of the esophagus. *Annals of Surgical Oncology* **15**, 3459–70.

73 Yang L, Lu X, Nossa CW, Francois F, Peek RM, Pei Z (2009). Inflammation and intestinal metaplasia of the distal esophagus are associated with alterations in the microbiome. *Gastroenterology* **137**, 588–97.

74 Yang H, Gu J, Wang KK, Zhang W, Xing J, Chen Z, *et al.* (2009). MicroRNA expression signatures in Barrett's esophagus and esophageal adenocarcinoma. *Clinical Cancer Research* **15**(18), 5744–52.

75 Ali S, Almhanna K, Chen W, Philip PA, Sarkar FH (2010). Differentially expressed miRNAs in the plasma may provide a molecular signature for aggressive pancreatic cancer. *American Journal of Translational Research* **3**, 28–47.

76 Sakai NS, Samia-Aly E, Barbera M, Fitzgerald RC (2013). A review of the current understanding and clinical utility of miRNAs in esophageal cancer. *Seminars in Cancer Biology* **23**(6, pt B), 512–21.

77 Kan T, Sato F, Ito T, Matsumura N, David S, Cheng Y, *et al.* (2009). The miR-106b-25 polycistron, activated by genomic amplification, functions as an oncogene by suppressing p21 and Bim. *Gastroenterology* **136**, 1689–700.

78 Feber A, Xi L, Luketich JD, Pennathur A, Landreneau RJ, Wu M, *et al.* (2008). MicroRNA expression profiles of esophageal cancer. *Journal of Thoracic and Cardiovascular Surgery* **135**, 255–260; discussion 260.

79 Leidner RS, Ravi L, Leahy P, Chen Y, Bednarchik B, Streppel M, *et al.* (2012). The microRNAs, MiR-31 and MiR-375, as candidate markers in Barrett's esophageal carcinogenesis. *Genes, Chromosomes and Cancer* **51**, 473–9.

80 Hu Y, Correa AM, Hoque A, Guan B, Ye F, Huang J, *et al.* (2011). Prognostic significance of differentially expressed miRNAs in esophageal cancer. *International Journal of Cancer* **128**, 132–43.

81 Jin Z, Cheng Y, Gu W, Zheng Y, Sato F, Mori Y, *et al.* (2009). A multicenter, double-blinded validation study of methylation biomarkers for progression prediction in Barrett's esophagus. *Cancer Research* **69**, 4112–5.

82 Jin Z, Wang L, Zhang Y, Cheng Y, Gao Y, Feng X, Dong M, Cao Z, Chen S, Yu H, Zhao Z, Zhang X, Liu J, Mori Y, Fan XMS (2013). MAL hypermethylation is a tissue-specific event that correlates with MAL mRNA expression in esophageal carcinoma. *Scientific Reports* **3**, 2838.

83 Jin Z, Olaru A, Yang J, Sato F, Cheng Y, Kan T, *et al.* (2007). Hypermethylation of tachykinin-1 is a potential biomarker in human esophageal cancer. *Clinical Cancer Research* **13**, 6293–300.

84 Tischoff I, Hengge UR, Vieth M, Ell C, Stolte M, Weber A, *et al.* (2007). Methylation of SOCS-3 and SOCS-1 in the carcinogenesis of Barrett's adenocarcinoma. *Gut* **56**, 1047–53.

85 Alvi M a, Liu X, O'Donovan M, Newton R, Wernisch L, Shannon NB, *et al.* (2013). DNA methylation as an adjunct to histopathology to detect prevalent, inconspicuous dysplasia and early-stage neoplasia in Barrett's esophagus. *Clinical Cancer Research* **19**, 878–88.

CHAPTER 7

Histology of Barrett's esophagus: metaplasia and dysplasia

Deepa T. Patil & John R. Goldblum

Department of Anatomic Pathology, Cleveland Clinic, Cleveland, OH, USA

7.1 Introduction

Although there have been several definitions of Barrett's esophagus since its original description almost 100 years ago [1], all have shared two features in common – an alteration of the esophageal mucosa, visible endoscopically, and a corresponding histologic abnormality. The endoscopic landmarks used to identify the esophagogastric junction (EGJ) are reviewed in greater detail elsewhere in this book but, given that the definition of Barrett's esophagus depends upon this anatomic landmark, a brief review of the macroscopic and microscopic anatomy of this region is in order.

7.2 Normal anatomy and histology

In the region where the esophagus joins the stomach, two anatomic landmarks are visible at the time of endoscopy – the muscular EGJ and the mucosal EGJ, also known as the squamocolumnar junction (SCJ), Z line or ora serrata. The muscular EGJ is the point at which the distal most portion of the tubular esophagus meets the saccular stomach. Although the EGJ may be approximated by the most proximal extent of the gastric folds, precise anatomic localization remains difficult in many cases, particularly in the setting of a hiatal hernia [2]. The mucosal EGJ is also identifiable at endoscopy by differences in color and texture of the mucosal lining. Normally, the mucosal and muscular EGJ coincide but, in many adult patients, the SCJ lies 1–2 cm proximal to the muscular EGJ, presumably secondary to reflux of gastric contents into the distal esophagus.

Traditionally, the narrow segment of mucus-secreting columnar mucosa distal to the squamous esophageal mucosa, but proximal to acid-secreting oxyntic gastric mucosa, has been termed the gastric cardia. In recent years, the existence of the gastric cardia as a native structure has been called into question by some authors, who believe that cardiac-type mucosa is always metaplastic, most likely in response to gastroesophageal reflux [3, 4]. While metaplastic cardiac-type mucosa undoubtedly is frequently identified in the distal esophagus, evidence from detailed studies of the anatomy and histology of the EGJ, including pediatric autopsy series, supports the notion that the gastric cardia is a native structure [5–7]. Thus, there is sufficient evidence to support the presence of a small zone of native cardiac mucosa in the most proximal stomach and, in many individuals, metaplastic cardiac-type mucosa of variable length in the distal esophagus.

7.3 Histology of Barrett's esophagus

Although the existence of a columnar-lined organ within the thorax had been documented for nearly 50 years prior to Dr. Norman Barrett's influential paper in 1957 [8], his description affirmed that this structure was, indeed the esophagus, and not the stomach. In 1976, Paull *et al.* reported that columnar metaplasia of esophagus (or columnar-line esophagus, CLE) is a mosaic of three different types of epithelia:

a. fundic type (with oxyntic glands);

b. junctional type (with cardiac type glands); and

c. specialized type (with goblet cells) [9].

Esophageal Cancer and Barrett's Esophagus, Third Edition. Edited by Prateek Sharma, Richard Sampliner and David Ilson.
© 2015 John Wiley & Sons, Ltd. Published 2015 by John Wiley & Sons, Ltd.

Barrett's esophagus was synonymous with CLE and was classified into these three histologic subtypes. However, following multiple studies that documented that adenocarcinoma only arises in CLE with intestinal metaplasia, we now diagnose BE based on the 2008 American College of Gastroenterology Practice Parameters Committee Guidelines [10] and the recent Position Statement issued by the American Gastroenterological Association [11, 12]. BE is defined as "change in the distal esophageal epithelium of any length that can be recognized as columnar-type mucosa at endoscopy and is confirmed to have intestinal metaplasia by biopsy of the tubular esophagus." [11]. Thus, the definition consists of a two-pronged approach – an endoscopically visible mucosal change/abnormality and a histologic correlate, characterized by the identification of goblet cells.

This definition, however, is not universally accepted. In fact, the British Society of Gastroenterology does not require the presence of intestinal metaplasia to diagnose BE [13]. Similarly, the Japanese simply require the documentation of columnar-lined esophagus, with or without goblet cells [14]. Additional details regarding evolving definition of Barrett's esophagus can be found in Chapter 2.

Specialized columnar epithelium most closely resembles slightly distorted gastric mucosa with glands and foveolae, but it may take on a more villiform appearance in some cases. In addition to goblet cells, gastric foveolar-type cells (incomplete intestinal metaplasia), and intestinal absorptive- type cells (complete intestinal metaplasia), the metaplastic glands may also contain Paneth cells, neuroendocrine cells, and even pancreatic acinar cells. The lamina propria surrounding the glands contains variable numbers of inflammatory cells and fibroblasts.

Goblet cells are best identified by virtue of their shape and the chemical composition of intracytoplasmic mucin. Because they are rich in acidic mucins (predominantly sialomucins, admixed with lesser quantities of sulfated mucins), they acquire a basophilic cytoplasmic blush that is readily recognized on a routine hematoxylin and eosin-stained tissue section [15]. Histochemical stains for acidic mucins, such as Alcian blue at pH 2.5, show intense dark-blue/magenta staining for this combination of sialomucins and sulfated mucins, which contrasts with the predominantly periodic acid-Schiff (PAS)-positive neutral mucins found within

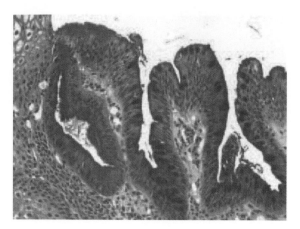

Figure 7.1 Periodic acid-Schiff (PAS)/Alcian blue at pH 2.5 demonstrates incomplete intestinal metaplasia. Goblet cells containing acid mucin stain intensely blue with Alcian blue (right), while the adjacent columnar cells containing neutral mucin stain with PAS (left). *(See insert for color representation of this figure.)*

the adjacent gastric foveolar-type cells (Figure 7.1: see also Plate 7.1).

On occasion, markedly distended foveolar epithelial cells may mimic goblet cells ("pseudogoblet cells") and cause diagnostic confusion. These are usually distributed in a continuous fashion compared to true goblet cells, which tend to be dispersed sporadically throughout the metaplastic epithelium. Additionally, they stain pale eosinophilic on hematoxylin-eosin stain, and contain neutral mucin that does not react with Alcian blue at pH 2.5. Caution must be exercised when interpreting histochemical stains for detecting goblet cells. The columnar cells located between the goblet cells contain small quantities of acidic mucin and may show some Alcian blue positivity (so-called "columnar blues"). In the absence of goblet cell metaplasia, the identification of these cells does not fulfill the criteria for a definitive diagnosis of Barrett's esophagus.

If the endoscopic impression is clearly that of Barrett's esophagus, then the absence of intestinal metaplasia may simply be a function of sampling error. Studies have shown that columnar-lined esophagus is a heterogeneous mucosa that demonstrates considerable variability in the distribution of goblet cells, including a distinct gradient, with the proximal segment containing a higher density of goblet cells, compared to the distal segment [16]. A retrospective study has shown that at least eight biopsy specimens are required to adequately assess intestinal metaplasia. In addition, the yield of intestinal metaplasia is lower in the presence of short-segment BE [17]

7.4 Intestinal metaplasia of the EGJ

The finding of intestinal metaplasia in biopsies obtained from the EGJ raises two diagnostic possibilities: ultra-short segment BE, or chronic carditis with intestinal metaplasia (CIM). Unfortunately, clinical, endoscopic, or pathologic findings do not allow one to distinguish accurately between these two entities. There is clear evidence that CIM carries a lower risk of neoplastic progression than either short or long segment Barrett's esophagus [18–22]. In a recent study, Srivastava *et al.* [23] showed that, in a mucosal biopsy from EGJ, the presence of the following features was significantly associated with a diagnosis of BE over CIM:

1 Crypt disarray and atrophy.
2 Incomplete and diffuse IM.
3 Multi-layered epithelium.
4 Squamous epithelium overlying columnar crypts with IM.
5 Hybrid glands.
6 Esophageal glands/ducts.

The expression of *CDX2*, a caudal homeobox gene expressed during development, is specific evidence of intestinal differentiation [24], and several studies have shown that *CDX2* is expressed in Barrett's esophagus-related intestinal metaplasia [25–27]. To date, no direct comparisons have been published with regard to potential expression differences between CIM and short segment Barrett's esophagus. Several other markers evaluated for this purpose include Das1, MUC1, MUC2, MUC 5AC, MUC6 and CD10. These studies are hampered by differences in endoscopic biopsy protocols, and study populations that contribute to apparent discrepancies in their results and lack of reproducibility. Thus, the clinical utility of evaluating intestinal metaplasia of the EGJ using these various biomarkers has not yet been established.

7.5 Barrett's esophagus-related dysplasia

All patients with Barrett's esophagus are at risk of developing esophageal adenocarcinoma [28]. The vast majority of adenocarcinomas arise through a metaplasia-dysplasia-carcinoma sequence. Mapping studies have documented epithelial dysplasia in mucosa adjacent to most adenocarcinomas in resection specimens, supporting a dysplasia-carcinoma sequence [29]. In addition, there are also studies that have reported patients progressing from dysplasia to adenocarcinoma in serial endoscopic biopsies [30, 31]. Epithelial dysplasia, particularly high-grade dysplasia, has come to be considered one of the most important risk factors for both synchronous and metachronous esophageal adenocarcinoma [32–34]. Therefore, its identification is an integral part of cancer screening and surveillance programs, as well as a trigger point for therapeutic intervention.

Dysplasia is defined as neoplastic change of the epithelium that remains confined within the basement membrane of the gland from which it arises (i.e. intraepithelial neoplasia) [35]. Grossly, dysplastic epithelium may demonstrate a spectrum of mucosal changes, ranging from ulcers to flat or elevated/polypoid lesions. This morphologic spectrum forms the basis of the Paris classification used by many gastroenterologists [36]. On occasion, dysplastic mucosa may be indistinguishable from adjacent non-dysplastic mucosa. The most widely accepted histologic grading scheme for Barrett's-related dysplasia has been adapted from the classification system used for idiopathic inflammatory bowel disease-related dysplasia, and is discussed below [35].

7.5.1 Negative for dysplasia

One of the unique features of metaplastic Barrett's mucosa is that there is a certain degree of "baseline atypia", which is most pronounced within the regenerative glandular compartment at the base of the mucosa. Importantly, these nuclear changes do not involve the surface epithelial cells (surface maturation) and, as such, these biopsies are classified as negative for dysplasia.

Active inflammation, and its attendant neutrophil-mediated epithelial cell injury, is capable of producing profound cytologic alterations that overlap with those of Barrett's-related dysplasia. Distinguishing reactive cytologic atypia from dysplasia is frequently very difficult, if not impossible. The appearance from low-magnification is critical in this evaluation, because truly dysplastic epithelium usually appears darker (hyperchromatic) than normal at this power. Confirmation of these changes is required at higher magnification, and reveals nuclear enlargement, hyperchromasia, crowding, and irregular nuclear contours. In addition, inspection at higher power enables one to determine whether these changes extend onto the mucosal surface. Accurate assessment of the changes involving the mucosal surface is more difficult when faced with a tangentially sectioned biopsy specimen.

In contrast to dysplasia, reactive atypia has a more uniform appearance among the cells in question, whereas dysplastic nuclei are pleomorphic and, thus, vary considerably from one cell to the next. While cell size does not discriminate between a reactive cell and a dysplastic cell, the nuclear : cytoplasmic (N : C) ratio is increased in the setting of dysplasia when compared with reactive cells. The chromatin distribution pattern is also helpful, as reactive nuclei have a more open chromatin pattern, with prominent nucleoli, which contrasts with the more condensed chromatin pattern seen in dysplastic nuclei. In practice, one needs to weigh all of these features together when deciding whether or not the changes qualify as dysplasia.

7.5.2 Indefinite for dysplasia

The diagnosis of indefinite for dysplasia should be reserved for cases where:

1 the cytologic and glandular architectural changes exceed the so-called "baseline atypia" of metaplastic specialized columnar epithelium, but fall short of low-grade dysplasia;

2 co-existing inflammation or ulceration is associated with striking cytologic atypia, precluding a definitive distinction between regenerative atypia and dysplasia;

3 there is marked glandular distortion in the absence of surface nuclear changes which would be diagnostic of dysplasia.

7.5.3 Low-grade dysplasia

The glandular architecture is mildly distorted in low-grade dysplasia, as the crypts remain parallel to one another, with minimal crypt branching or budding. The crypts are lined by cells with enlarged, hyperchromatic, and stratified nuclei with irregular nuclear membranes. These changes extend from the crypts to involve the mucosal surface (Figure 7.2). Goblet cells are often decreased in number and so-called dystrophic goblet

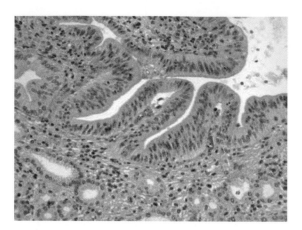

Figure 7.2 Barrett's esophagus with low-grade dysplasia. The dysplastic cells contain enlarged hyperchromatic nuclei with slightly irregular contours. The nuclear changes extend out from the base of the glands onto the mucosal surface, where there is also significant overlapping and crowding. Note the small, round nuclei of the non-dysplastic glands beneath the dysplastic epithelium.

cells, wherein the nucleus is located at the apical aspect of the cell, may also be present.

7.5.4 High-grade dysplasia

In high-grade dysplasia, both the cytologic atypia and architectural complexity are more pronounced. The crypts are crowded and show a "back-to-back" or cribriform arrangement. The nuclei show full-thickness stratification, with marked hyperchromasia and prominent nucleoli. Loss of nuclear polarity, where the long axis of the nucleus is no longer perpendicular to the basement membrane, is a frequent finding (Figure 7.3).

7.6 Intramucosal adenocarcinoma (IMC)

Intramucosal adenocarcinoma is defined by the presence of lamina propria or muscularis mucosae invasion. In addition to demonstrating invasion of single cells within the lamina propria, a diagnosis of IMC is also rendered, based on architectural features. These features include the presence of sheets of dysplastic glands replacing the lamina propria (with very little intervening lamina propria), small, angulated, abortive glandular profiles infiltrating the lamina propria, and a "never-ending" glandular pattern [37]. Although

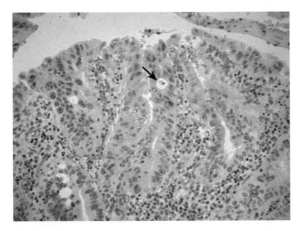

Figure 7.3 Barrett's esophagus with high-grade dysplasia. This focus of high-grade dysplasia is characterized by severe cytologic atypia, including markedly enlarged, irregular nuclei with coarse chromatin and small nucleoli. There is also an area of cribriform growth (arrowhead).

establishing a diagnosis of IMC may be relevant, due to the small, but finite, risk of lymph node metastasis, as endoscopic mucosal resection is the therapeutic procedure of choice for both HGD and IMC, its distinction from HGD is less important in biopsy specimens.

7.7 Submucosal adenocarcinoma

Submucosal adenocarcinoma is defined by the presence of dysplastic glands surrounded by desmoplastic stromal response. A diagnosis of submucosal adenocarcinoma can be challenging on biopsy specimens, in part due to the superficial nature of endoscopic biopsies that do not typically sample the submucosa. Additionally, Barrett's mucosa is associated with duplication of muscularis mucosae, which can pose diagnostic difficulty [38]. In this unique musculo-fibrous anomaly of Barrett's mucosa, there is development of a new inner layer of muscularis mucosae, which is separated from the deeper layer of true muscularis mucosae by loose fibrovascular stroma. Thus, on mucosal biopsy samples, invasion beyond this newly developed smooth muscle layer can potentially be misdiagnosed as submucosal invasion.

7.8 Morphologic types of dysplasia

The most common form of Barrett's dysplasia is the intestinal ("adenomatous") type dysplasia. Two other

forms of dysplasia that were recently characterized include the non-adenomatous type (gastric foveolar-type) and basal crypt dysplasia.

7.8.1 Gastric foveolar-type dysplasia (non-adenomatous dysplasia)

More recently, a second type of Barrett's dysplasia – namely, the gastric foveolar type – was defined with respect to its prevalence, diagnostic criteria, and natural history [39–41]. Cumulative data shows that the overall incidence of this subtype of dysplasia ranges from 7–15% among patients with Barrett's-related dysplasia. It is more common in women than in men, and the patients are typically at least a decade older than those with intestinal-type dysplasia. Most cases of Barrett's gastric foveolar-type dysplasia are high-grade, and neoplastic progression occurs in up to 64% of patients [40].

In contrast to intestinal (adenomatous) dysplasia, Barrett's gastric foveolar-type dysplasia is characterized by a uniform monolayer of basally oriented nuclei with abundant apical cytoplasm (Figure 7.4: see also Plate 7.4). Architecturally, it is typified by full-thickness replacement of the mucosa and, in the great majority of cases, by a glandular, rather than villiform, growth pattern.

The grading system for gastric foveolar-type dysplasia is similar to intestinal (adenomatous) dysplasia

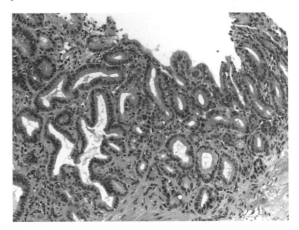

Figure 7.4 Barrett's gastric foveolar-type dysplasia, low-grade. H&E-stained section of Barrett's esophageal biopsy showing full-thickness mucosal replacement by crowded glands and non-villiform architecture. The cells demonstrate basally oriented monolayered and uniform nuclei, with abundant pale eosinophilic to mucinous cytoplasm. *(See insert for color representation of this figure.)*

(negative, indefinite, low-grade and high-grade). However, the criteria for classifying the grade of dysplasia are somewhat different. Low-grade gastric foveolar-type dysplasia is characterized by slightly crowded glands, lined by regular, non-stratified cells with nuclei that are 2–3 times the size of a small mature lymphocyte. There is mild nuclear pleomorphism. High-grade dysplasia is characterized by crowded glandular architecture and villiform growth pattern of the mucosa. The glands are lined by cells with nuclei that are 3–4 times the size of a small lymphocyte. The nuclei are still basally oriented, and nucleoli are frequently present [40].

7.8.2 Basal crypt dysplasia

Molecular evidence suggests that BE-related dysplasia begins in the crypt bases and progressively involves the upper half of the crypts and the surface epithelium (so-called basal crypt dysplasia) [42]. Morphologically, basal crypt dysplasia has all of the features of traditional low-grade dysplasia, but it is limited to the crypt bases. In their study, Lomo *et al.* found that basal crypt dysplasia was seen in biopsies devoid of acute inflammation and, in 47% of cases, there was evidence of full-thickness dysplasia elsewhere in the biopsies.

7.9 Sampling error and observer variation in Barrett's esophagus-related dysplasia

Dysplasia may extend diffusely throughout a Barrett's esophagus segment, or the changes may be focal and limited to a small area of one fragment in a patient with multiple biopsy specimens. When dysplasia is diffuse, there is a high likelihood that a rigorous biopsy protocol will detect foci of dysplasia at a high frequency; however, small foci may go unsampled. The need for thorough biopsy sampling is further emphasized by the fact that high-grade dysplasia, and even early adenocarcinoma, may not be associated with an endoscopically visible lesion [32, 43]. Given this potential for sampling error, subsequent biopsies that are negative for dysplasia, following earlier biopsies with dysplasia, should not lull the gastroenterologist into a false sense of security.

Another problem facing the pathologist, gastroenterologist, thoracic surgeon and, ultimately, the patient, is both the intra- and inter-observer variation in the diagnosis of dysplasia. Given the spectrum of changes from baseline atypia to low-grade to high-grade dysplasia, it is not surprising that this variation exists. Reid *et al.* found this variation to be most significant at the low end of the spectrum – that is, in distinguishing negative for dysplasia from low-grade dysplasia or indefinite for dysplasia [44]. This study described overall agreement in terms of a percentage, which does not take into account agreement that may occur by chance alone.

Two other studies, by Montgomery *et al.* and Downs-Kelly *et al.*, using kappa statistical analysis (which accounts for agreement occurring by chance alone), confirmed a high degree of intra- and inter-observer variation among these same diagnostic categories, even among pathologists with a special interest in gastrointestinal pathology [45]. The study performed by Downs-Kelly and colleagues showed that is it difficult to distinguish high-grade dysplasia reliably from intramucosal and submucosal adenocarcinoma on biopsy specimens. This variation underscores the need to obtain multiple opinions in challenging cases, and it further supports the AGA requirement that a diagnosis of dysplasia should be confirmed by an expert gastrointestinal pathologist.

7.10 Surrogate biomarkers for assessing risk of esophageal adenocarcinoma

Given the limitations of light microscopy, several adjunctive techniques have been proposed as having a possible role in the screening or surveillance of patients with Barrett's esophagus. For virtually every marker tested, there is an increased probability of finding an abnormality as one progresses along the dysplasia-carcinoma sequence. Certain markers are detectable early in the sequence, whereas others are found at later stages. The ideal marker would be detectable early in the metaplasia-dysplasia-carcinoma sequence, even before there is morphologic evidence of dysplasia, and capable of distinguishing progressors from non-progressors.

Numerous studies have evaluated p53 expression by immunohistochemistry, and most of these attempt to correlate the degree of p53 expression with the grade of dysplasia, or solely as a marker of increased risk of progressing to adenocarcinoma. p53 overexpression has been observed in 9–60% of cases with low-grade dysplasia, and 55–100% of cases with high-grade dysplasia [46–49]. Although some have advocated the use of p53 immunohistochemistry to confirm a diagnosis of dysplasia and/or assist in grading of dysplasia, its use has not been widely accepted. There is some discrepancy between p53 expression, as detected by immunohistochemistry, and molecular alterations detectable at the gene level [50, 51]. Also, the lack of a standardized immunohistochemical technique likely accounts for some of the discrepant data reported in the literature.

DNA content, as measured by flow cytometry, has also been evaluated in patients with Barrett's esophagus, but the results are conflicting. A prospective study found that patients with negative, indefinite, or low-grade dysplasia histology, and no evidence of aneuploidy or increased 4N fractions by flow cytometry, had a cumulative 0% five-year cancer risk, compared with a 28% risk for patients with either aneuploidy or increased 4N fractions [52]. Patients with baseline increased 4N, aneuploidy, and high-grade dysplasia had five-year cancer rates of 56%, 43%, and 59%, respectively. In contrast to the results of Reid *et al.*, Fennerty *et al.* found discordance between flow cytometric abnormalities and dysplasia in Barrett's esophagus patients [53].

Although numerous others potential individual biomarkers of neoplastic progression in Barrett's esophagus patients have also been evaluated with variable results (e.g. Ki-67, *bcl*-2, cyclin D1, *p16*, EGFR, c-*erb*B-2), microarray-based technologies are well suited for surveying genomic abnormalities on a much broader scale. These methods allow for the rapid comparison of chromosomal copy numbers, or relative expression of thousands of genes in a single assay, creating genomic profiles for the tissues tested.

Not surprisingly, earlier studies [54–56] identified a long list of chromosomal abnormalities and genes that are up- or down-regulated as one proceeds along the metaplasia-dysplasia-carcinoma sequence in Barrett's esophagus. More recent studies have documented differential expression of miRNAs and protein glycosylation products in the Barrett's carcinogenesis pathway [57]. However, much work is needed to implement these assays in large-scale high-risk population screening to identify early preneoplastic changes, and to determine whether or not they have a potential role in selecting those subset of patients who are at greatest risk of neoplastic progression.

References

1 Tileston W (1906). Peptic ulcer of the oesophagus. *American Journal of Medical Sciences* **132**, 240–65.

2 Spechler SJ, Goyal RK (1996). The columnar-lined esophagus, intestinal metaplasia, and Norman Barrett. *Gastroenterology* **110**, 614–21.

3 Chandrasoma PT, Der R, Ma Y, *et al.* (2000). Histology of the gastroesophageal junction: an autopsy study. *American Journal of Surgical Pathology* **24**, 402–9.

4 Chandrasoma PT, Lokuhetty DM, Demeester TR, *et al.* (2000). Definition of histopathologic changes in gastroesophageal reflux disease. *American Journal of Surgical Pathology* **24**, 344–51.

5 Kilgore SP, Ormsby AH, Gramlich TL, *et al.* (2000). The gastric cardia: fact or fiction? *American Journal of Gastroenterology* **95**, 921–4.

6 Zhou H, Greco MA, Daum F, *et al.* (2001). Origin of cardiac mucosa: ontogenic consideration. *Pediatric and Developmental Pathology* **4**, 358–63.

7 Derdoy JJ, Bergwerk A, Cohen H, *et al.* (2003). The gastric cardia: to be or not to be? *American Journal of Surgical Pathology* **27**, 499–504.

8 Barrett N (1957). The lower esophagus lined by columnar epithelium. *Surgery* **41**, 881–94.

9 Paull A, Trier JS, Dalton MD, *et al.* (1976). The histologic spectrum of Barrett's esophagus. *The New England Journal of Medicine* **295**, 476–80.

10 Sampliner RE. (2002). Updated guidelines for the diagnosis, surveillance, and therapy of Barrett's esophagus. *American Journal of Gastroenterology* **97**, 1888–95.

11 Wang KK, Sampliner RE (2008). Gastroenterology. PPCo-tACo. Updated guidelines 2008 for the diagnosis, surveillance and therapy of Barrett's esophagus. *American Journal of Gastroenterology* **103**, 788–97.

12 Spechler SJ, Sharma P, Souza RF, *et al.* (2011). American Gastroenterological Association medical position statement on the management of Barrett's esophagus. *Gastroenterology* **140**, 1084–91.

13 Playford RJ (2006). New British Society of *Gastroenterology* (BSG) guidelines for the diagnosis and management of Barrett's oesophagus. *Gut* **55**, 442.

14 Ogiya K, Kawano T, Ito E, *et al.* (2008). Lower esophageal palisade vessels and the definition of Barrett's esophagus. *Diseases of the Esophagus* **21**, 645–9.

15 Haggitt RC, Reid BJ, Rabinovitch PS, *et al.* (1988). Barrett's esophagus. Correlation between mucin histochemistry, flow cytometry, and histologic diagnosis for predicting increased cancer risk. *American Journal of Pathology* **131**, 53–61.

16 Chandrasoma PT, Der R, Dalton P, *et al.* (2001). Distribution and significance of epithelial types in columnar-lined esophagus. *American Journal of Surgical Pathology* **25**, 1188–93.

17 Harrison R, Perry I, Haddadin W, *et al.* (2007). Detection of intestinal metaplasia in Barrett's esophagus: an observational comparator study suggests the need for a minimum

of eight biopsies. *American Journal of Gastroenterology* **102**, 1154–61.

18 Sharma P, Weston AP, Morales T, *et al.* (2000). Relative risk of dysplasia for patients with intestinal metaplasia in the distal oesophagus and in the gastric cardia. *Gut* **46**, 9–13.

19 Morales TG, Camargo E, Bhattacharyya A, *et al.* (2000). Long-term follow-up of intestinal metaplasia of the gastric cardia. *American Journal of Gastroenterology* **95**, 1677–80.

20 Goldstein NS (2000). Gastric cardia intestinal metaplasia: biopsy follow-up of 85 patients. *Modern Pathology* **13**, 1072–9.

21 Weston AP, Krmpotich PT, Cherian R, *et al.* (1997). Prospective evaluation of intestinal metaplasia and dysplasia within the cardia of patients with Barrett's esophagus. *Digestive Diseases and Sciences* **42**, 597–602.

22 Sharma P (1999). Recent advances in Barrett's esophagus: short-segment Barrett's esophagus and cardia intestinal metaplasia. *Seminars in Gastrointestinal Disease* **10**, 93–102.

23 Srivastava A, Odze RD, Lauwers GY, *et al.* (2007). Morphologic features are useful in distinguishing Barrett esophagus from carditis with intestinal metaplasia. *American Journal of Surgical Pathology* **31**, 1733–41.

24 Suh E, Traber PG (1996). An intestine-specific homeobox gene regulates proliferation and differentiation. *Molecular and Cellular Biology* **16**, 619–25.

25 Groisman GM, Amar M, Meir A (2004). Expression of the intestinal marker Cdx2 in the columnar-lined esophagus with and without intestinal (Barrett's) metaplasia. *Modern Pathology* **17**, 1282–8.

26 Phillips RW, Frierson HF, Jr., Moskaluk CA (2003). Cdx2 as a marker of epithelial intestinal differentiation in the esophagus. *American Journal of Surgical Pathology* **27**, 1442–7.

27 Moons LM, Bax DA, Kuipers EJ, *et al.* (2004). The homeodomain protein CDX2 is an early marker of Barrett's oesophagus. *Journal of Clinical Pathology* **57**, 1063–8.

28 Haggitt RC, Tryzelaar J, Ellis FH, *et al.* (1978). Adenocarcinoma complicating columnar epithelium-lined (Barrett's) esophagus. *American Journal of Clinical Pathology* **70**, 1–5.

29 Spechler SJ, Goyal RK (1986). Barrett's esophagus. *The New England Journal of Medicine* **315**, 362–71.

30 Reid BJ, Blount PL, Rubin CE, *et al.* (1992). Flow-cytometric and histological progression to malignancy in Barrett's esophagus: prospective endoscopic surveillance of a cohort. *Gastroenterology* **102**, 1212–9.

31 Hameeteman W, Tytgat GN, Houthoff HJ, *et al.* (1989). Barrett's esophagus: development of dysplasia and adenocarcinoma. *Gastroenterology* **96**, 1249–56.

32 Reid BJ, Weinstein WM, Lewin KJ, *et al.* (1988). Endoscopic biopsy can detect high-grade dysplasia or early adenocarcinoma in Barrett's esophagus without grossly recognizable neoplastic lesions. *Gastroenterology* **94**, 81–90.

33 Schmidt HG, Riddell RH, Walther B, *et al.* (1985). Dysplasia in Barrett's esophagus. *Journal of Cancer Researchearch and Clinical Oncology* **110**, 145–52.

34 Smith RR, Hamilton SR, Boitnott JK, *et al.* (1984). The spectrum of carcinoma arising in Barrett's esophagus. A clinicopathologic study of 26 patients. *American Journal of Surgical Pathology* **8**, 563–73.

35 Riddell RH, Goldman H, Ransohoff DF, *et al.* (1983). Dysplasia in inflammatory bowel disease: standardized classification with provisional clinical applications. *Human Pathology* **14**, 931–68.

36 Endoscopic Classification Review Group (2005).Update on the Paris classification of superficial neoplastic lesions in the digestive tract. *Endoscopy* **37**, 570–8.

37 Downs-Kelly E, Mendelin JE, Bennett AE, *et al.* (2008). Poor interobserver agreement in the distinction of high-grade dysplasia and adenocarcinoma in pretreatment Barrett's esophagus biopsies. *American Journal of Gastroenterology* **103**, 2333–40; quiz 41.

38 Abraham SC, Krasinskas AM, Correa AM, *et al.* (2007). Duplication of the muscularis mucosae in Barrett esophagus: an underrecognized feature and its implication for staging of adenocarcinoma. *American Journal of Surgical Pathology* **31**, 1719–25.

39 Rucker-Schmidt RL, Sanchez CA, Blount PL, *et al.* (2009). Nonadenomatous dysplasia in barrett esophagus: a clinical, pathologic, and DNA content flow cytometric study. *American Journal of Surgical Pathology* **33**, 886–93.

40 Mahajan D, Bennett AE, Liu X, *et al.* (2010). Grading of gastric foveolar-type dysplasia in Barrett's esophagus. *Modern Pathology* **23**, 1–11.

41 Brown IS, Whiteman DC, Lauwers GY (2010). Foveolar type dysplasia in Barrett esophagus. *Modern Pathology* **23**, 834–43.

42 Lomo LC, Blount PL, Sanchez CA, *et al.* (2006). Crypt dysplasia with surface maturation: a clinical, pathologic, and molecular study of a Barrett's esophagus cohort. *American Journal of Surgical Pathology* **30**, 423–35.

43 Falk GW, Rice TW, Goldblum JR, *et al.* (1999). Jumbo biopsy forceps protocol still misses unsuspected cancer in Barrett's esophagus with high-grade dysplasia. *Gastrointestinal Endoscopy* **49**, 170–6.

44 Reid BJ, Haggitt RC, Rubin CE, *et al.* (1988). Observer variation in the diagnosis of dysplasia in Barrett's esophagus. *Human Pathology* **19**, 166–78.

45 Montgomery E, Bronner MP, Goldblum JR, *et al.* (2001). Reproducibility of the diagnosis of dysplasia in Barrett esophagus: a reaffirmation. *Human Pathology* **32**, 368–78.

46 Younes M, Lebovitz RM, Lechago LV, *et al.* (1993). p53 protein accumulation in Barrett's metaplasia, dysplasia, and carcinoma: a follow-up study. *Gastroenterology* **105**, 1637–42.

47 Krishnadath KK, Tilanus HW, van Blankenstein M, *et al.* (1995). Accumulation of p53 protein in normal, dysplastic, and neoplastic Barrett's oesophagus. *Journal of Pathology* **175**, 175–80.

48 Jones DR, Davidson AG, Summers CL, *et al.* (1994). Potential application of p53 as an intermediate biomarker in Barrett's esophagus. *Annals of Thoracic Surgery* **57**, 598–603.

49 Ramel S, Reid BJ, Sanchez CA, *et al.* (1992). Evaluation of p53 protein expression in Barrett's esophagus by two-parameter flow cytometry. *Gastroenterology* **102**, 1220–8.

50 Hamelin R, Flejou JF, Muzeau F, *et al.* (1994). TP53 gene mutations and p53 protein immunoreactivity in malignant and premalignant Barrett's esophagus. *Gastroenterology* **107**, 1012–8.

51 Coggi G, Bosari S, Roncalli M, *et al.* (1997). p53 protein accumulation and p53 gene mutation in esophageal carcinoma. A molecular and immunohistochemical study with clinicopathologic correlations. *Cancer* **79**, 425–32.

52 Reid BJ, Levine DS, Longton G, *et al.* (2000). Predictors of progression to cancer in Barrett's esophagus: baseline histology and flow cytometry identify low- and high-risk patient subsets. *American Journal of Gastroenterology* **95**, 1669–76.

53 Fennerty MB, Sampliner RE, Way D, *et al.* (1989). Discordance between flow cytometric abnormalities and dysplasia in Barrett's esophagus. *Gastroenterology* **97**, 815–20.

54 Xu Y, Selaru FM, Yin J, *et al.* (2002). Artificial neural networks and gene filtering distinguish between global gene expression profiles of Barrett's esophagus and esophageal cancer. *Cancer Research* **62**, 3493–7.

55 Brabender J, Marjoram P, Salonga D, *et al.* (2004). A multigene expression panel for the molecular diagnosis of Barrett's esophagus and Barrett's adenocarcinoma of the esophagus. *Oncogene* **23**, 4780–8.

56 Selaru FM, Zou T, Xu Y, *et al.* (2002). Global gene expression profiling in Barrett's esophagus and esophageal cancer: a comparative analysis using cDNA microarrays. *Oncogene* **21**, 475–8.

57 Shah AK, Saunders NA, Barbour AP, *et al.* (2013). Early diagnostic biomarkers for esophageal adenocarcinoma – the current state of play. *Cancer Epidemiology, Biomarkers & Prevention* **22**, 1185–209.

CHAPTER 8

Helicobacter pylori and esophageal neoplasia

Arne Kandulski, Marino Venerito & Peter Malfertheiner

Department of Gastroenterology, Hepatology and Infectious Diseases, Otto-von-Guericke University Hospital, Magdeburg, Germany

8.1 Introduction

The relationship between *H. pylori* infection and gastroesophageal reflux disease (GERD) remains an issue of debates and controversial discussions. The subject of these debates concerns whether *H. pylori* is just coincidental, protective or even aggravating GERD.

Initial suggestions for *H. pylori* as a protective factor against GERD came from studies reporting a lower prevalence of *H. pylori* infection in patients with GERD, compared to healthy controls [1, 2]. These studies showed a negative association of *H. pylori* and complicated GERD, Barrett's metaplasia and esophageal adenocarcinoma. Therefore, the concept of *H. pylori* as a protective factor for Barrett's esophagus and esophageal adenocarcinoma became extended. However, studies addressing this issue are heterogeneous, with profound biases of selection and information [3–7]. The effect of *H. pylori* has been extended on GERD symptoms, the prevalence of erosive changes of esophageal mucosa, as well. Furthermore, the influence of *H. pylori* eradication on reflux symptoms and erosive esophagitis has been addressed. Eradication therapy has been initially suggested to worsen reflux symptoms and esophagitis, but such an association was rebutted in a recent meta-analysis [8].

8.2 *H. pylori* infection – gastritis pattern and gastric physiology with impact on gastroesophageal reflux disease

H. pylori infection always causes chronic active gastritis, which may progress to peptic ulcer disease, gastric adenocarcinoma and primary gastric B-cell lymphoma (gastric MALT lymphoma). Clinical manifestations develop only in about 20% of subjects infected with the bacterium. In most cases, the infection is asymptomatic. Factors leading to a symptomatic infection are abnormalities in gastric acid regulation and mucosal infiltration of immune cells, with cytokine release leading to gastric mucosal damage [9]. *H. pylori* impairs the homeostasis of gastric acid secretion via different mechanisms, depending on the severity of gastritis and intragastric distribution patterns, defining different phenotypes of gastritis (Figure 8.1) [10].

Most infected subjects present a multifocal gastritis phenotype, characterized by mild inflammation of the gastric mucosa and only little impairment of gastric acid secretion (Figure 8.1c) [10]. In 20–40% of infected individuals, *H. pylori* infection leads to antral predominant gastritis with hypergastrinaemia and hyperchlorhydria (Figure 8.1a) [11–15].

In Western world countries, only a small subset of infected individuals develops a corpus- and fundus-predominant gastritis pattern. The chronic inflammation over time (usually decades) may lead to loss of parietal cells and gastric glands of the corpus, with development of atrophy and hypo- or achlorhydria (FGA, fundic gland atrophy), which usually is not reversible after *H. pylori* eradication therapy (Figure 8.1b) [15].

These different pattern of gastritis need to be considered for interpretation of studies from different parts of the world, with antrum predominant gastritis in Western world countries, and more frequent corpus predominant pattern with the development of FGA in Asian countries.

For the evaluation of gastric morphology, histology remains the gold standard [16]. However serum

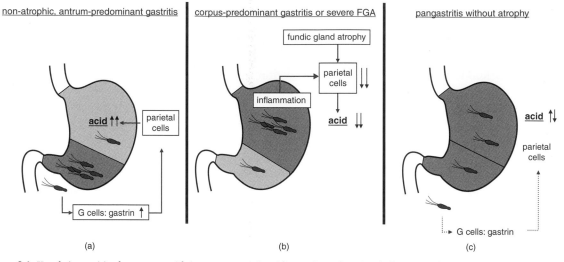

Figure 8.1 *H. pylori*, gastritis phenotypes with impact on gastric acid secretion. The critical phenotype disussed as having a protective effect on the esophagus is illustrated in (b).

pepsinogen (PG) I and II as non-invasive tools for the assessment of gastric physiology, especially for evaluation of gastric fundic gland atrophy (FGA) are increasingly used. In patients with FGA, serum PG I levels are reduced, whereas PG II levels are normal or even increased. Therefore, low serum PG I levels or a low ratio of PG I/II are used as surrogate markers for FGA [17, 18].

8.3   Epidemiological studies – GERD symptoms, erosive esophagitis and *H. pylori*

In the US, GERD represents the most frequent diagnosis by general practitioners and an enormous burden for health care systems [19, 20]. Studies on the relationship between *H. pylori* and GERD are heterogeneous, mostly due to different methodologies that were used for diagnosis of *H. pylori* infection or GERD. In epidemiological studies, GERD diagnosis is based on the presence of typical GERD-related symptoms (heartburn, regurgitation) and/or endoscopic visible esophageal erosions or the presence of Barrett's metaplasia, [21, 22]. Non-erosive reflux disease (NERD) in these studies is defined by the presence of GERD-related symptoms without esophageal erosions detectable by upper GI endoscopy [21, 22]. Indeed, studies in which NERD was diagnosed by pathologic acid exposure based during pH-metry are very rare notably with a high response rates to PPI

therapy in case of pathologic acid exposure to the distal esophagus [24–27].

Most studies on the relationship of *H. pylori* and GERD differentiate between symptoms, on the one hand, and severity of reflux esophagitis on the other hand (Table 8.1). A systematic review on the relationship of both conditions in Europe and Northern America reported a pooled odds ratio of 0.76 (0.61–0.96); 0.70 (0.55–0.9), respectively for H. pylori infection in patients with GERD. However, there is a substantial heterogeneity among studies that were published before 2001 [2]. For exclusion and inclusion criteria in this meta-analysis, GERD was defined as erosive esophagitis or pathological pH-metry in case of normal upper GI endoscopy. Information about the methods for *H. pylori* diagnosis was unavailable.

Concerning GERD symptoms, a European population-based study from 2007 selected 472 persons with GERD symptoms and 472 controls. The authors reported that *H. pylori* infection is not associated with a decreased risk for typical GERD symptoms, such as heartburn or regurgitation, irrespective of the CagA status. Analyzing confounding factors, the presence of FGA with reduced PG level was associated with less frequent GERD-related symptoms (OR 0.2 (95% CI 0.8–1.5) [28]. Due to the low prevalence of gastric atrophy (1.8% of the study cohort), the authors concluded that this observation is probably not relevant on a European population-based level.

Table 8.1 *H. pylori*, GERD symptoms and erosive esophagitis.

Author	Year, study	*H. pylori* diagnosis	GERD diagnosis	OR (95% CI) (GERD symptoms)	OR (95% CI) (erosive esophagitis)
Raghunath [2]	2003, systematic review	n. a.	endoscopy (± pH-metry)	esophagitis (and/or path. pH-metry) pooled ratio: 0.60 (0.47–0.78) Europe: 0.76 (0.61–0.96) North America: 0.70 (0.55–0.9) Far East: 0.24 (0.19–0.32)	
Nordenstedt [28]	2007, population based (n = 944)	*H. pylori* IgG Cag IgG PG I	Symptoms	GERD symptoms 1.1 (0.8–1.6) gastric atrophy (PG I): 0.2 (0.0–0.6)	
Chung [30]	2011, case controlled study	*H. pylori* IgG	endoscopy + symptoms	n. a.	esophagitis 0.44 (0.39 –0.49)
Rubenstein [29]	2013, prospective study	*H. pylori* IgG CagA IgG	symptoms + endoscopy	0.95 (0.55–1.64)	0.63 (0.37–1.08)
Minatsuki [31]	2013, cross-sectional study	*H. pylori* IgG PG I + II	symptoms + endoscopy	symptoms only* 1.0 (0.94–1.17)	0.58 (0.51–0.65) PGI/II ratio: 0.61 (0.50–0.72)

*patients with erosive esophagitis were excluded.
OR – odds ratio; CI – confidence interval; PGI – pepsinogen I; PGII – pepsinogen II; IgG – immunoglobuline G antibody; CagA [+] – studies investigating CagA sero-positivity.

Similar to the European data, a recent study from the US also demonstrated that reflux symptoms are not associated with *H. pylori* infection, irrespective of the CagA status.

In contrast to reflux-symptoms only, the prevalence of erosive esophagitis is negative associated with *H. pylori* infection, in particular with CagA positive strains (OR: 0.47 (0.21–1.03)) [29]. Potential limitations of this study are that only male gender was included, and data on gastritis pattern, including the presence of FGA, is missing.

There are recent studies from Asian countries that further underline these associations. Korea and Japan are among the countries with a high prevalence of corpus-predominant gastritis pattern and highest incidence of gastric cancer. *H. pylori*-induced corpus-predominant gastritis frequently progresses to FGA, which is associated with impairment of acid secretion. In this condition, the esophageal mucosa is less exposed to esophageal acid.

A Korean case-control study with more than 5000 patients showed an inverse correlation of *H. pylori* seroprevalence with the risk and severity of erosive esophagitis (OR: 0.44 (0.39–0.49). GERD symptoms were not investigated in this study separately, and there is also no data on gastric atrophy or gastric physiology available [30]. A large cross-sectional survey from Japan with more than 10,000 subjects differentiated erosive reflux disease (ERD) from symptomatic GERD without mucosal lesions (NERD). On the one hand, there was no association between NERD (GERD symptoms, no erosions) and *H. pylori* infection but, on the other hand, both *H. pylori* non-infection (OR 1.74) and a higher PG I/II ratio (no FGA) were positively associated with ERD (OR 1.64) [31].

8.4 *H. pylori*, Barrett's esophagus and esophageal adenocarcinoma

H. pylori infection is negatively associated with the presence of Barrett's esophagus (BE) and esophageal adenocarcinoma (EAC). The heterogeneity in all studies is high, mainly due to methodological aspects, as well as to selection and characterization of patients and controls (Table 8.2). Fischbach and El Serag included 49 studies in their meta-analysis to examine the effect of *H. pylori* on Barrett's esophagus. In one third of the studies, BE diagnosis was not exactly confirmed, neither by endoscopic description, nor by histology.

Table 8.2 Association of *H. pylori*, Barrett's esophagus and esophageal adenocarcinoma.

Author	Year, study	Barrett's Esophagus OR (95% CI)	Esophageal Adenocarcinoma OR (95% CI)
Anderson [35]	2007 prospective, case control	0.35 (0.22–0.56) CagA[+]: 0.50 (0.31–0.79) PG I/II < 3: 0.19 (0.05–0.70) PG I/II < 7: 0.11 (0.06–0.23)	0.35 (0.21–0.59) CagA[+]: 0.46 (0.27–0.76) PG I/II <3: 0.34 (0.09–1.22) PG I/II <7: 0.51 (0.29–0.89)
Rokkas [32]	2007 meta-analysis	0.64 (0.43–0.94) CagA[+]: 0.39 (0.21–0.76)	0.52 (0.37–0.73) CagA[+]: 0.51 (0.31–0.82)
Fischbach [7]	2011 meta-analysis	0.46 (0.35–0.60) (4 studies) 0.46 (0.40–0.53) (US only, 7 studies) CagA[+]: 0.39 (0.19–0.78) (7 studies)	Not applicable
Rubenstein [29]	2013 prospective, case control study	0.53 (0.29–0.97) CagA[+]:0.36 (0.14–0.90)	Not applicable

OR – odds ratio; CI – confidence interval; PGI – pepsinogen I; PGII –pepsinogen II; CagA[+] – studies investigating CagA sero-positivity.

In seven of these studies, *H. pylori* was diagnosed histologically. However, biopsies had not been taken from either gastric antrum or corpus according to the updated Sydney classification; moreover, in six of these seven studies, *H. pylori* infection was assessed in biopsies from the esophagus or gastro-esophageal junction [7].

The authors selected four methodological appropriate studies for final analysis and calculated a relative risk of 0.46 (95% CI: 0.35–0.60) for patients with *H. pylori* infection to develop BE. For studies conducted in the United States only, the relative risk was comparable, with a negative association of *H. pylori* and the prevalence of BE.

The same meta-analysis addressed the effect of CagA positivity on BE. Seven studies were included in this subgroup analysis and showed a negative correlation of the CagA status with BE (0.38; 95% CI: 0.19–0.78) [7].

In a recent prospective case control study from the US, BE was also negatively associated with *H. pylori* (OR 0.53; 95% CI: 0.29–0.97), in particular with CagA positive strains (OR: 0.36; 95% CI: 0.14–0.90). No cases of esophageal adenocarcinoma were included in this prospective study [29].

Another systematic review from Rokkas and colleagues also reported lower *H. pylori* prevalence in patients with BE, especially when infected with CagA positive strains, suggesting a protective role of *H. pylori* infection for Barrett's esophagus. This meta-analysis included 10 studies with esophageal adenocarcinoma. A significant inverse correlation of *H. pylori* prevalence and

CagA positive strains with esophageal adenocarcinoma was reported, as well (0.51 (0.31–0.82) [32].

A potential mechanism of *H. pylori* infection to "protect" the esophagus from BE and EAC development is the presence of FGA, which goes along with impaired gastric acid secretion (Figure 8.1b) [33]. For the pathogenesis of BE and EAC, esophageal exposure to acid and to bile acids arising from duodeno-gastroesophageal reflux are considered to be essential for initiation and promotion of neoplastic changes [34]. In a prospective case control study from Finland, Anderson *et al.* reported a negative association of *H. pylori* prevalence with BE and EAC in cases of FGA. In a subgroup analysis for FGA, based on serological markers (PG I/II ratio), even mild gastric atrophy (PG I/II<7) was associated with a reduced risk for developing BE [35]. Based on these findings, it is suggested, that BE and the development to EAC occurs mostly in patients with non-atrophic gastric mucosa [36].

8.5 *H. pylori* eradication and GERD

A prospective trial investigating the effect of *H. pylori* eradication on reflux symptoms and the development of erosive esophagitis found no differences between eradicated and non-eradicated patients [37]. A meta-analysis of 10 randomized controlled trials found neither the incidence of reflux symptoms (OR 0.81 (0.56–1.17), nor reflux esophagitis (OR 1.13

(0.72–1.78) to be associated with patients that received eradication therapy [8].

Other meta-analyses dealing with *H. pylori* eradication and GERD came to similar conclusions. In these studies, *H. pylori* eradication did not aggravate GERD symptoms or the prevalence of erosive esophagitis [38, 39]. A subgroup analysis of five studies with confirmed *H. pylori* eradication showed even a significant improvement of GERD symptoms after successful eradication, when compared with patients in those *H. pylori* infection persisted [8]. A study from Japan suggested a benefit after eradication therapy, in terms of negative association with GERD symptoms. The authors showed a significant improvement of GERD symptoms-related quality of life one year after eradication therapy [41].

In line with these observations, the current Maastricht guideline concluded that *H. pylori* eradication has no effects on symptoms, and does not aggravate pre-existing GERD [40].

8.6 *H. pylori* and esophageal squamous cell carcinoma

Whether *H. pylori* infection and, more specifically, the role of FGA may play a role in the pathogenesis of esophageal squamous cell carcinoma (ESCC) has been the focus of several studies. Tables 8.3 and 8.4 show most relevant studies on the association between fundic gastric atrophy and esophageal squamous cell carcinoma diagnosed by serology and histology, respectively.

Table 8.4 Association between fundic gastric atrophy diagnosed by histology and esophageal squamous cell carcinoma.

Author	Study design	Population	OR (95% CI)
Iijima *et al.*	Case control	Chinese	4.2 (1.5–11.7)*
Venerito *et al.*	Case control	German	1.91 (0.6–5.99)
De Vries *et al.*	Case cohort	Dutch	2.2 (1.8–2.6)*

*– statistically significant.
OR – odds ratio; CI – confidence interval.

In a case control study published in 2004, Ye *et al.* reported a small but significant association between FGA diagnosed by serology, and an increased risk for ESCC was also reported in a case control study conducted in the general Swedish population (OR 4.3, 95% CI 1.9–9.6) [44]. A further case control study from Japan reported similar data [45, 46]. Bacterial overgrowth due to reduced acid secretion in patients with FGA was proposed as a possible causal mechanism. The excess in production of bacterial-derived nitrites and N-nitroso compounds were suggested to increase the exposure of the esophageal mucosa to endogenous carcinogenic nitrosamines. Beyond this speculation, no other mechanistic explanation for an association between FGA and ESCC can be provided and, in particular, no increased gastroesophageal reflux has been documented in these patients.

In a case control study conducted in German patients, we found no association between FGA diagnosed either by serology or histology and ESCC [47]. These results are

Table 8.3 Association between fundic gastric atrophy diagnosed by serology and esophageal squamous cell carcinoma.

Author	Study design	Population	OR (95% CI)	Definition of FGA
Ye *et al.*	Case control	Swedish	4.3 (1.9–9.6)*	PGI < 28 µg/l
Iijima *et al.*	Case control	Japanese	8.2 (2.2–30.4)*	PGI < 25 µg/l
Kamangar *et al.***	Case control	Chinese	1.8 (0.58–5.53)	PGI/PGII ≤ 3
Venerito *et al.*	Case control	German	1.17 (0.54–2.56)	PGI<70 ng/ml or PGI/PGII ≤ 3
Ren *et al.*#	Case cohort	Chinese	1.10 (0.59– 2.04)	PGI/PGII ≤ 3

*– statistically significant.
**– patients included in this study had esophageal squamous dysplasia, not an invasive cancer.
#– Prospective case cohort study with over 15 years of follow-up.
OR – odds ratio; CI – confidence interval; PGI – pepsinogen I; PGII – pepsinogen II; FGA – fundic gastric atrophy.

in line with those from a large case cohort Chinese study nested in a prospective cohort involving 29,584 subjects with over 15 years of follow-up, in which an association between FGA and ESCC was not confirmed [48]. Methodological differences among studies, and the presence of confounding factors, may explain the discrepant results. In particular, for case control studies, the results are often dependent on the quality and the size of the control group.

The lack of association between severity of FGA and increased risk for ESCC found in a Dutch study [49] strengthened the hypothesis that the positive association between ESCC and FGA found in some studies might be related to confounding factors, rather than a direct causal association of *H. pylori* with ESCC. In fact, in a recent meta-analysis, only a low-magnitude association between ESCC and FGA (RR 1.94, CI 95% 1.48–2.55) was found [50].

As *H. pylori* infection is the principal cause of FGA, and CagA-positive *H. pylori* strains carry a further increased risk for developing FGA [51], the relationship between *H. pylori* serology and ESCC has been also investigated in different studies, and two meta-analyses have been published on this topic [32]. Rokkas included five studies investigating the association between ESCC and *H. pylori*-prevalence, and three other studies focusing on the association between ESCC and the prevalence of CagA-positive strains [51]. They found no significant relationship between ESCC and both *H. pylori* prevalence and the prevalence of CagA-positive strains (pooled OR 0.85; 95% CI, 0.55–1.33 for *H. pylori* infection and OR 1.22; 95% CI, 0.7–2.13 for CagA-positive strains, respectively).

In a subsequent meta-analysis by Islami *et al.* [50], nine studies on the association between ESCC and *H. pylori*-prevalence and four studies on the association between ESCC and the prevalence of CagA-positive strains were included. This meta-analysis included more studies and confirmed the results of the previous analysis (pooled OR 1.10; 95% CI, 0.78–1.55 for *H. pylori* infection and OR 1.01; 95% CI, 0.8-1.27 for CagA-positive strains, respectively). In conclusion, current evidence does not support a role for either *H. pylori* infection or FGA in the development of esophageal squamous cell carcinoma.

8.7 Conclusions

Due to many epidemiological studies with conflicting results, the relationship between *H. pylori*, gastroesophageal reflux disease and Barrett's esophagus remains a matter of debates. Most discrepancies have resulted from a high heterogeneity of study populations and the methods used in these studies. In the interpretation of study results, it is essential to distinguish between reflux symptoms, the prevalence of erosive esophagitis and BE. For developed countries of the Western world, there is growing evidence that there is no association of *H. pylori* infection and GERD-related symptoms. Also *H. pylori* eradication neither increases nor decreases the incidence of GERD.

Based on the literature, there is an inverse correlation of *H. pylori* infection and the presence of erosive esophagitis, BE and EAC. A possible explanation for this association is the pattern of *H. pylori*- induced gastritis with distinct characteristics of gastric acid secretion. Some studies indicate that this "protective role" of *H. pylori* infection can be explained by the development of FGA and reduced gastric acid secretion, even in cases of mild gastric atrophy [33, 52]. The impact of antrum-predominant gastritis with hypergastrinaemia and hyperchlorhydria (as predominant in developed Western populations) on the presence of BE has not been specifically investigated.

With respect to esophageal squamous cell carcinoma, the association with FGA remains controversial, and a causal relationship is lacking.

References

1 Metz DC, Kroser JA (1999). *Helicobacter pylori* and gastroesophageal reflux disease. *Gastroenterology Clinics of North America* **28**(4), 971–85, viii.

2 Raghunath A, Hungin AP, Wooff D, Childs S (2003). Prevalence of *Helicobacter pylori* in patients with gastrooesophageal reflux disease: systematic review. *BMJ* **326**(7392), 737.

3 Graham DY (2003). The changing epidemiology of GERD: geography and *Helicobacter pylori*. *American Journal of Gastroenterology* **98**(7), 1462–70.

4 El-Serag HB, Sonnenberg A, Jamal MM, Inadomi JM, Crooks LA, Feddersen RM (1999). Corpus gastritis is protective against reflux oesophagitis. *Gut* **45**(2), 181–5.

5 Sharma P, Vakil N (2003). Review article: *Helicobacter pylori* and reflux disease. *Alimentary Pharmacology & Therapeutics* **17**(3), 297–305.

6 Malfertheiner P, Dent J, Zeijlon L, Sipponen P, Veldhuyzen Van Zanten SJ, Burman CF, *et al.* (2002). Impact of *Helicobacter pylori* eradication on heartburn in patients with gastric or duodenal ulcer disease – results from a randomized trial programme. *Alimentary Pharmacology & Therapeutics* **16**(8), 1431–42.

7 Fischbach LA, Nordenstedt H, Kramer JR, Gandhi S, Dick-Onuoha S, Lewis A, *et al.* (2012). The association between Barrett's esophagus and *Helicobacter pylori* infection: a meta-analysis. *Helicobacter* **17**(3), 163–75.

8 Saad AM, Choudhary A, Bechtold ML (2012). Effect of *Helicobacter pylori* treatment on gastroesophageal reflux disease (GERD): meta-analysis of randomized controlled trials. *Scandinavian Journal of Gastroenterology* **47**(2), 129–35.

9 Tummala S, Keates S, Kelly CP (2004). Update on the immunologic basis of *Helicobacter pylori* gastritis. *Current Opinion in Gastroenterology* **20**(6), 592–7.

10 Amieva MR, El-Omar EM (2008). Host-bacterial interactions in *Helicobacter pylori* infection. *Gastroenterology* **134**(1), 306–23.

11 McColl KE, El-Omar EM, Gillen D (1997). Alterations in gastric physiology in *Helicobacter pylori* infection: causes of different diseases or all epiphenomena? *Italian Journal of Gastroenterology and Hepatology* **29**(5), 459–64.

12 Leodolter A, Wolle K, Peitz U, Ebert M, Gunther T, Kahl S, *et al.* (2003). *Helicobacter pylori* genotypes and expression of gastritis in erosive gastro-oesophageal reflux disease. *Scandinavian Journal of Gastroenterology* **38**(5), 498–502.

13 Malfertheiner P, Chan FK, McColl KE (2009). Peptic ulcer disease. *Lancet* **374**(9699), 1449–61.

14 Leodolter A, Ebert MP, Peitz U, Wolle K, Kahl S, Vieth M, *et al.* (2006). Prevalence of H pylori associated "high risk gastritis" for development of gastric cancer in patients with normal endoscopic findings. *World Journal of Gastroenterology* **12**(34), 5509–12.

15 El-Omar EM, Oien K, El-Nujumi A, Gillen D, Wirz A, Dahill S, *et al.* (1997). *Helicobacter pylori* infection and chronic gastric acid hyposecretion. *Gastroenterology* **113**(1), 15–24.

16 Dixon MF, Genta RM, Yardley JH, Correa P (1996). Classification and grading of gastritis. The updated Sydney System. International Workshop on the Histopathology of Gastritis, Houston (1994). *American Journal of Surgical Pathology* **20**(10), 1161–81.

17 Borch K, Axelsson CK, Halgreen H, Damkjaer Nielsen MD, Ledin T, Szesci PB (1989). The ratio of pepsinogen A to pepsinogen C: a sensitive test for atrophic gastritis. *Scandinavian Journal of Gastroenterology* **24**(7), 870–6.

18 Kekki M, Samloff IM, Varis K, Ihamaki T (1991). Serum pepsinogen I and serum gastrin in the screening of severe atrophic corpus gastritis. *Scandinavian Journal of Gastroenterology* Suppl **186**, 109–16.

19 Irvine EJ (2004). Quality of life assessment in gastro-oesophageal reflux disease. *Gut* **53** (Suppl 4), iv35–iv39.

20 Peery AF, Dellon ES, Lund J, Crockett SD, McGowan CE, Bulsiewicz WJ, *et al.* (2012). Burden of gastrointestinal disease in the United States: 2012 update. *Gastroenterology* **143**(5), 1179–87.

21 Vakil N, van Zanten SV, Kahrilas P, Dent J, Jones R. (2006). The Montreal definition and classification of gastroesophageal reflux disease: a global evidence-based consensus. *American Journal of Gastroenterology* **101**(8), 1900–20.

22 [No authors listed] (1999). An evidence-based appraisal of reflux disease management – the Genval Workshop Report. *Gut* **44**(Suppl 2), S1–16.

23 Numans ME, Lau J, de Wit NJ, Bonis PA (2004). Short-term treatment with proton-pump inhibitors as a test for gastroesophageal reflux disease: a meta-analysis of diagnostic test characteristics. *Annals of Internal Medicine* **140**(7), 518–27.

24 Kandulski A, Peitz U, Monkemuller K, Neumann H, Weigt J, Malfertheiner P (2013). GERD assessment including pH-metry predicts a high response rate to PPI standard therapy. *BMC Gastroenterology* **13**, 12.

25 Weigt J, Monkemuller K, Peitz U, Malfertheiner P (2007). Multichannel intraluminal impedance and pH-metry for investigation of symptomatic gastroesophageal reflux disease. *Digestive Diseases* **25**(3), 179–82.

26 Katz PO, Gerson LB, Vela MF (2013). Guidelines for the diagnosis and management of gastroesophageal reflux disease. *American Journal of Gastroenterology* **108**(3), 308–28.

27 Weijenborg PW, Cremonini F, Smout AJ, Bredenoord AJ (2012). PPI therapy is equally effective in well-defined non-erosive reflux disease and in reflux esophagitis: a meta-analysis. *Neurogastroenterology & Motility* **24**, 747–e350.

28 Nordenstedt H, Nilsson M, Johnsen R, Lagergren J, Hveem K (2007). *Helicobacter pylori* infection and gastroesophageal reflux in a population-based study (The HUNT Study). *Helicobacter* **12**(1), 16–22.

29 Rubenstein JH, Inadomi JM, Scheiman J, Schoenfeld P, Appelman H, Zhang M, *et al.* (2014). Association between *Helicobacter pylori* and Barrett's Esophagus, Erosive Esophagitis, and Gastroesophageal Reflux Symptoms. *Clinical Gastroenterology and Hepatology* **12**(2), 239–45.

30 Chung SJ, Lim SH, Choi J, Kim D, Kim YS, Park MJ, *et al.* (2011). *Helicobacter pylori* Serology Inversely Correlated With the Risk and Severity of Reflux Esophagitis in *Helicobacter pylori* Endemic Area: A Matched Case-Control Study of 5,616 Health Check-Up Koreans. *Journal of Neurogastroenterology and Motillity* **17**(3), 267–73.

31 Minatsuki C, Yamamichi N, Shimamoto T, Kakimoto H, Takahashi Y, Fujishiro M, *et al.* (2013). Background factors

of reflux esophagitis and non-erosive reflux disease: a cross-sectional study of 10,837 subjects in Japan. *PLoS One* **8**(7), e69891.

32 Rokkas T, Pistiolas D, Sechopoulos P, Robotis I, Margantinis G. (2007). Relationship between *Helicobacter pylori* infection and esophageal neoplasia: a meta-analysis. *Clinical Gastroenterology and Hepatology* **5**(12), 1413–7, 1417.

33 Abe Y, Ohara S, Koike T, Sekine H, Iijima K, Kawamura M, *et al.* (2004). The prevalence of *Helicobacter pylori* infection and the status of gastric acid secretion in patients with Barrett's esophagus in Japan. *American Journal of Gastroenterology* **99**(7), 1213–21.

34 Fitzgerald RC (2006). Molecular basis of Barrett's oesophagus and oesophageal adenocarcinoma. *Gut* **55**(12), 1810–20.

35 Anderson LA, Murphy SJ, Johnston BT, Watson RG, Ferguson HR, Bamford KB, *et al.* (2008). Relationship between *Helicobacter pylori* infection and gastric atrophy and the stages of the oesophageal inflammation, metaplasia, adenocarcinoma sequence: results from the FINBAR case-control study. *Gut* **57**(6), 734–9.

36 McColl KE, Going JJ (2010). Aetiology and classification of adenocarcinoma of the gastro-oesophageal junction/cardia. *Gut* **59**(3), 282–4.

37 Kim N, Lee SW, Kim JI, Baik GH, Kim SJ, Seo GS, *et al.* (2011). Effect of *Helicobacter pylori* Eradication on the Development of Reflux Esophagitis and Gastroesophageal Reflux Symptoms: A Nationwide Multi-Center Prospective Study. *Gut Liver* **5**(4), 437–46.

38 Qian B, Ma S, Shang L, Qian J, Zhang G (2011). Effects of *Helicobacter pylori* eradication on gastroesophageal reflux disease. *Helicobacter* **16**(4), 255–65.

39 Yaghoobi M, Farrokhyar F, Yuan Y, Hunt RH (2010). Is there an increased risk of GERD after *Helicobacter pylori* eradication?: a meta-analysis. *American Journal of Gastroenterology* **105**(5), 1007–13.

40 Malfertheiner P, Megraud F, O'Morain CA, Atherton J, Axon AT, Bazzoli F, *et al.* (2012). Management of *Helicobacter pylori* infection – the Maastricht IV/ Florence Consensus Report. *Gut* **61**(5), 646–64.

41 Hirata K, Suzuki H, Matsuzaki J, Masaoka T, Saito Y, Nishizawa T, *et al.* (2013). Improvement of reflux symptom related quality of life after *Helicobacter pylori* eradication therapy. *Journal of Clinical Biochemistry and Nutrition* **52**(2), 172–8.

42 Vannella L, Lahner E, Osborn J, Bordi C, Miglione M, Delle FG, *et al.* (2010). Risk factors for progression to gastric neoplastic lesions in patients with atrophic gastritis. *Alimentary Pharmacology & Therapeutics* **31**(9), 1042–50.

43 Helicobacter and Cancer Collaborative Group (2001). Gastric cancer and *Helicobacter pylori*: a combined analysis of 12 case control studies nested within prospective cohorts. *Gut* **49**(3), 347–53.

44 Ye W, Held M, Lagergren J, Engstrand L, Blot WJ, McLaughlin JK, *et al.* (2004). *Helicobacter pylori* infection and gastric atrophy: risk of adenocarcinoma and squamous-cell carcinoma of the esophagus and adenocarcinoma of the gastric cardia. *Journal of the National Cancer Institute* **96**(5), 388–96.

45 Iijima K, Koike T, Abe Y, Inomata Y, Sekine H, Imatani A, *et al.* (2007). Extensive gastric atrophy: an increased risk factor for superficial esophageal squamous cell carcinoma in Japan. *American Journal of Gastroenterology* **102**(8), 1603–9.

46 Kamangar F, Diaw L, Wei WQ, Abnet CC, Wang GQ, Roth MJ, *et al.* (2009). Serum pepsinogens and risk of esophageal squamous dysplasia. *International Journal of Cancer* **124**(2), 456–60.

47 Venerito M, Kohrs S, Wex T, Adolf D, Kuester D, Schubert D, *et al.* (2011). *Helicobacter pylori* infection and fundic gastric atrophy are not associated with esophageal squamous cell carcinoma: a case-control study. *European Journal of Gastroenterology & Hepatology* **23**(10), 859–64.

48 Ren JS, Kamangar F, Qiao YL, Taylor PR, Liang H, Dawsey SM, *et al.* (2009). Serum pepsinogens and risk of gastric and oesophageal cancers in the General Population Nutrition Intervention Trial cohort. *Gut* **58**(5), 636–42.

49 de Vries AC, Capelle LG, Looman CW, van BM, van Grieken NC, Casparie MK, *et al.* (2009). Increased risk of esophageal squamous cell carcinoma in patients with gastric atrophy: independent of the severity of atrophic changes. *International Journal of Cancer* **124**(9), 2135–8.

50 Islami F, Sheikhattari P, Ren JS, Kamangar F (2011). Gastric atrophy and risk of oesophageal cancer and gastric cardia adenocarcinoma – a systematic review and meta-analysis. *Annals of Oncology* **22**(4), 754–60.

51 Adamu MA, Weck MN, Rothenbacher D, Brenner H (2011). Incidence and risk factors for the development of chronic atrophic gastritis: five year follow-up of a population-based cohort study. *International Journal of Cancer* **128**(7), 1652–8.

52 Koike T, Ohara S, Sekine H, Iijima K, Kato K, Shimosegawa T, *et al.* (1999). *Helicobacter pylori* infection inhibits reflux esophagitis by inducing atrophic gastritis. *American Journal of Gastroenterology* **94**(12), 3468–72.

CHAPTER 9

Screening and surveillance

Sarmed S. Sami & Krish Ragunath

Nottingham Digestive Diseases Centre, NIHR Biomedical Research Unit, Nottingham University Hospitals NHS Trust, Nottingham, UK

9.1 Introduction

Over the last three and a half decades, the incidence of esophageal adenocarcinoma (EAC) has risen remarkably compared to other types of cancer in the west with an estimated increase of up to seven-fold [1]. This problem is compounded by the rising mortality and dismal five-year survival rates in cases diagnosed after onset of symptoms [2]. Survival rates are still influenced by early diagnosis after five years, and they are strongly dependent on the success of treatment. These facts provide the strongest impetus to attempts at screening, surveillance and early diagnosis, not least because up to 50% of patients have incurable disease at presentation, requiring palliative measures [3].

9.2 Screening

In order to assess the usefulness and potential feasibility of screening for Barrett's esophagus (BE), it is necessary to explore the rationale, the target population, the screening tests available and, finally, to identify the current challenges to screening which may inform future research.

9.2.1 The rationale for screening

Screening and early detection of EAC, might – in theory – offer curable treatment options, which may result in reducing mortality from this otherwise deadly cancer. However, the benefits have to be weighed carefully against the economical and psychological costs, because most pre-malignant lesions, if left untreated, would not actually progress to cancer [4].

Surveillance for BE is widely practiced, however cancer progression rates are much lower than previously thought (0.33% per year), and only 5% of cancers are detected during surveillance [5, 6]. The vast majority (>90%) of patients who present with EAC do not have a previous diagnosis of BE, despite its presence [7]. It is also known that the overall survival of patients with non-dysplastic Barrett's esophagus (NDBE) does not differ significantly from age- and gender-matched cohorts [8]. In fact, only 7% of BE "surveillance" patients die of EAC, whereas the majority die from other causes [9].

These data present clinicians with a dilemma; on the one hand, there is continuing rise in a lethal cancer and under-diagnosis of curable early disease while, on the other hand, there is continuing clinical diagnosis of low-risk or "benign" BE, with minimal impact on overall survival.

One explanation for the above could be that we are missing the high risk or "malignant" BE until those patients present with dysphagic symptoms and incurable cancer; hence, screening to identify the "undiagnosed" cases in the community might have an advantage. Indeed, this argument is supported, at least in part, by evidence from epidemiological and autopsy studies from Olmsted County (Minnesota, USA), which estimates that only 20–30% of patients with BE are clinically detected, while the majority (around 70%) remain undiagnosed in the community [8]. The authors noted that, despite the continuing increase in endoscopy use, the rate of increase in the incidence of both long-segment BE (LSBE) and short-segment BE (SSBE) appeared to have slowed, compared to rates reported previously from 1976 to 1996. Hence, the rising incidence of clinically diagnosed

BE is unlikely to explain the increase in incidence of EAC. It is possible that this undetected cohort may have different clinico-pathological risk profiles from the diagnosed surveillance population.

Retrospective cohort and case control studies have found that a previous diagnosis of BE was associated with early stage EAC and improved survival. A prior diagnosis of gastroesophageal reflux disease (GERD) was associated with early stage EAC, and prior endoscopy was associated with better survival from EAC [10]. All of these statistics suggest that screening to detect this condition might be worthy of consideration. Until recently, this has not been seriously considered, in part due to the lack of treatment options. Over the last decade, minimally invasive Barrett's endotherapy techniques have resulted in a paradigm shift towards providing a more economically favorable and better cancer prevention treatment options compared to esophagectomy.

9.2.2 Target population for screening

GERD is one of the strongest risk factors for BE and EAC [11]. However, it should also be noted that prevalence rates of 5.6–25% for BE have been reported in patients who were asymptomatic for GERD [12]. In one large population study, the prevalence of BE was 1.2% in those without reflux symptoms, compared with 2.3% for those with symptoms [13]. Therefore, a screening program that uses the presence of GERD as the only selection criteria may not be ideal.

Male gender, Caucasian race, age and central obesity have all been shown to be risk factors for developing BE in multiple studies [14]. The prevalence of BE increases with age, such that the typical median age of diagnosis is 60 years [15]. Visceral adiposity (waist circumference), rather than body mass index, has been implicated in the pathogenesis of BE [16]. A positive family history is also associated with an increased risk of BE, and up to 28% of first-degree relatives of patients with EAC or high-grade dysplasia (HGD) have BE [17]. A recent genome-wide association study of 5986 BE cases and 12,825 controls identified genetic variants associated with BE risk at two loci – one at chromosome 6p21, and another on chromosome 16q24 [18]. Germline mutations in the ASCC1, MSR1, and CTHRC1 genes have also been associated with the presence of BE and EAC [19].

In the largest study so far, Rubenstein *et al* [20] extracted data from a US national standardized endoscopic database established by the Clinical Outcomes Research Initiative. Overall, 9% of GERD patients were diagnosed with suspected BE on endoscopy. Analysis of 25,337 patients with histologically confirmed BE revealed 2.8% prevalence across all ages, genders and races. There was clear evidence that the prevalence of BE among white, non-Hispanic male GERD patients increased sharply from 3.3% in the fourth decade of life, to 6.3% in the fifth decade and 9.3% in the sixth decade of life, and then reached a plateau afterwards. Interestingly, authors found that older white women with GERD symptoms were no more likely to have BE than white men without GERD.

A recent modeling study estimated the symptom-, age-, and sex-specific incidences of EAC, and placed these figures in the context of other cancers for which screening is endorsed, namely colorectal and breast cancer. Results showed that the cut-off age for screening white men with weekly GERD was ≥ 60, while in those with daily GERD the corresponding age for screening was ≥ 55 [21].

Gastroenterological societies acknowledge that screening might be justified in selected high-risk individuals. Indeed, guidelines from the American and British Societies suggest that screening can be considered in patients with multiple risk factors (chronic GERD symptoms, age ≥ 50 years, white race, male sex, obesity, family history including at least one first degree relative with BE or EAC) [22–25].

These data confirm that, if screening is considered to be valuable in reducing mortality from EAC, then clinicians and policymakers should focus their efforts on targeting a white male population older than the age of 50 with chronic GERD symptoms.

9.2.3 Screening tests available

Sedated endoscopy (SE) has many limitations as a screening tool. It is performed in a hospital setting with a small but significant risk of morbidity- and mortality-related complications from conscious sedation. It also results in an increased loss of work time on the day of endoscopy, and the need for the patient to be accompanied home after the procedure. All these factors have limited the use of SE for screening purposes, because screening tests need to be simple, safe, acceptable to the population, and cost-effective. Several alternatives have been evaluated, as below:

9.2.3.1 Questionnaire-based tests

Validated symptoms questionnaires have been evaluated in two studies to examine their ability to predict the presence of BE. Gerson *et al.* used logistic regression analysis to devise a score to predict the presence of BE from demographic and symptom data in a US population [26]. The model had a sensitivity of 77% and specificity of 63% for the diagnosis of BE. Locke *et al.* developed another prediction model which had a sensitivity and specificity of 62% and 57% respectively [27].

Overall, the accuracy of these tools was suboptimal and cannot be recommended for use unless combined with more robust tests for BE. They are inexpensive and could be used as a pre-selection tool for BE screening.

9.2.3.2 Cytology-based tests

A non-endoscopically guided blind balloon cytology sampling device to collect esophageal samples has been tried, with little success. This was compared with SE and brush cytology in one study [28]. Adequate columnar epithelium was obtained in 83% of patients with balloon cytology and in 97% with brush cytology. Sensitivity of balloon cytology for HGD and EAC was 80%, but only 25% for LGD.

A non-endoscopic flexible mesh balloon catheter was designed as an alternative to SE to obtain cytology samples. Adequate specimens were obtained in only 73% of patients. The sensitivity of identifying goblet cells in those patients was 87.5% [29]. These techniques were limited by the inadequacy of sampling and poor accuracy.

Over the last few years, the Cytosponge, a novel cell collection device coupled with a biomarker, has been developed [30]. This is a capsule made of gelatin and attached to a string. Once swallowed, the capsule dissolves and expands a sponge, which can be pulled out using the attached string, while collecting cytology specimens from the esophagus. To overcome the limitation of relying on cytology alone, the sample is analyzed using immunohistochemical biomarkers in an automated method. The Cytosponge samples are analyzed for the presence of Trefoil Factor 3 (TFF3), a biomarker of columnar epithelium.

In a large primary care study involving 12 UK general practices, 504 patients with GERD symptoms underwent both the Cytosponge, followed by SE with biopsies. The test was feasible technically in 99% of patients and was well tolerated. The sensitivity and specificity of the test was 73.3% and 93.8% (Barrett's circumferential length $\geq$ 1 cm). When considering Barrett's circumferential length of $\geq$ 2 cm ("clinically relevant" BE), the sensitivity increased to 90.0%, with a specificity of 93.5% [30]. A recent economic modeling study reported that Cytosponge screening in 50-year-old men with GERD symptoms, followed by endotherapy in those with dysplasia or intra-mucosal cancer, is cost-effective and may reduce mortality from EAC, compared with no screening [31].

This technique shows promise in terms of accuracy, simplicity, cost-effectiveness and acceptability to patients. However, this is a non-endoscopic technique so, therefore, mucosal visualization is not possible. The main aim of a BE screening program is to identify patients with dysplasia and early EAC, so further information is needed regarding the ability of the Cytosponge to diagnose these two conditions. Multicentre studies are currently under way to validate these results in other UK and international centers.

9.2.3.3 Imaging-based tests

Wireless Capsule Endoscopy (WCE) is a relatively new technology to visualize the esophagus. Bhardwaj *et al.* [32] performed a meta-analysis of nine studies, comprising a total of 618 patients. The pooled sensitivity and specificity of WCE (using SE or histology as the gold standard) for the diagnosis of BE were 77% and 86%, respectively. WCE is an attractive tool for screening because it is safe, non-invasive, acceptable, does not require sedation, and it can be carried out by a single trained technician. Nevertheless, major disadvantages include low sensitivity, inability to take biopsies, and lack of cost-effectiveness compared to SE [33]. It is, therefore, not a suitable tool for BE screening at the present time.

String Capsule Endoscopy is a modified technique where a string is attached to the WCE device to allow its controlled movement up and down the esophagus. This also makes it re-usable, thus reducing the cost. The sensitivity and specificity are reportedly around 78.3% and 82.8%, respectively, when compared with SE [34]. While this technology is more promising, its accuracy remains suboptimal for use in screening.

Ultra-thin endoscopy (UE) has been evaluated in the diagnosis of BE. A meta-analysis of five studies (439 patients) was presented recently [35]. All patients underwent both UE (diameter 4–6 mm) and SE (gold standard). The pooled sensitivity and specificity of UE in detecting BE were 91% and 96%, respectively. Procedure was successful (95–100%) and well tolerated in the majority of patients.

The unsedated transnasal route is more applicable for screening, compared with the sedated technique and oral route, because the latter is still limited by costs and consequences of sedation, compared with the former. However, the need for dedicated rooms with endoscopy equipment and decontamination facilities is likely to hamper the use of currently available UE devices for population screening. More recently, The EndoSheath® transnasal esophagoscopy (Vision-Sciences Inc., Orangeburg, New York) has been used. This utilizes a disposable rubber sheath that covers the scope, and the system is compact, allowing some portability. Another promising device is the EG Scan® (Intromedic Ltd., Seoul, South Korea), which is a highly portable device with disposable probes, eliminating the need for decontamination equipment and improving access for community use. These technologies need to be comprehensively evaluated in the setting of screening for BE and EAC.

9.2.4 Challenges to screening and areas for future research

All of the gastroenterological societies agree that the evidence is currently not sufficient to recommend screening for BE in unselected GERD population [23]. This is partly due to the lack of a suitable test to replace SE. The Cytosponge and portable unsedated transnasal endoscopes are attractive tools which need further evaluation. However, a blood biomarker would represent an ideal tool which may be available in the future.

Another challenge to screening is the lack of a clearly defined high-risk target population. Up to 45% of patients with BE do not have GERD symptoms [36]. It has also been shown that approximately 40% of patients with EAC have no GERD history prior to diagnosis [37]. Therefore, focusing screening on GERD patients may still miss a significant proportion of BE patients. Moreover, the target population will be very large, because of the high prevalence of GERD in Western populations (15–20%) [38].

Any screening program is likely to result in an increased workload and costs to the healthcare system, which is difficult to justify, given the lack of direct evidence of benefit for patients. Furthermore, the

best pathway for management of screen-diagnosed patients with NDBE remains unclear, bearing in mind that the majority will not progress to cancer and that performing surveillance may potentially expose patients to unnecessary harm. Therefore, methods to detect individuals at increased risk of EAC merit serious and careful consideration. This will allow more targeted surveillance and therapy. Health economic studies broadly demonstrate that screening, followed by surveillance for BE, can be cost-effective in certain circumstances. However, the evidence remains insufficient to confidently recommend screening for BE.

9.3 Surveillance

9.3.1 Rationale for endoscopic surveillance

The aim of endoscopic surveillance is to detect cancer or pre-cancer at a stage when intervention maybe curative. Surveillance should detect cancer prior to invasion of the submucosa, when the risk of lymph node metastases increases significantly [39]. Endoscopic surveillance is widespread and recommended by European and North American GI societies (Table 9.1), despite the lack thus far of prospective randomized controlled trials comparing surveillance to no surveillance in patients with BE. Nevertheless, current evidence from case control and retrospective cohort studies suggests that surveillance-detected cancers are significantly more likely to be at an earlier stage and associated with improved survival [22]. Accurate data on survival rates from these studies are either not available, or are subject to inherent length bias and lead-time bias.

Cancer progression rate in patients with BE is one important statistic to consider when deciding whether surveillance is justified. Previous case series reported a risk of cancer progression in NDBE around 0.5% per annum, but these studies were small and subject to publication bias. Two recent large population-based studies have suggested that the true rate may be lower than previously thought. In a Northern Ireland population-based study, the incidence of cancer and HGD was estimated in 8522 patients with an endoscopic diagnosis of BE, with or without IM, with a mean follow-up of 7.0 years. The overall risk for HGD and EAC was 0.22% per year (or 0.16% per year for EAC

Table 9.1 Guidelines for surveillance of Barrett's Esophagus (BE).

	Grade of dysplasia			
	NDBE	IGD	LGD*	HGD*
AGA	Every 3–5 years	NR	Every 6–12 months	Every three months if no endoscopic therapy
ACG	Two EGDs in first year, then every three years if no dysplasia	NR	Repeat EGD in six months, then every year until no dysplasia X2	Repeat EGD in three months or endoscopic therapy. ER if mucosal irregularity
ASGE	Consider discharge or surveillance every 3–5 years. Ablation in select cases	Maximize acid suppression. Repeat EGD to clarify dysplasia status*	Repeat EGD in six months, then every year if no HGD. Consider ER or ablation	Repeat EGD three months in select patients. Consider endoscopic therapy and surgical consultation
BSG	LSBE = 3 cm = every 2–3 years. SSBE < 3 cm = every 3–5 years	Every six months with maximal acid suppression	Repeat every six months until two consecutive with no dysplasia	Endoscopic therapy
SFED	LSBE > 6 cm = every two years. LSBE 3–6 cm = every three years. SSBE < 3 cm = every five years	NR	Second EGD, if LGD confirmed, then repeat at six months, one year, and then every year. Maximize acid suppression	Second EGD, if HGD confirmed then endoscopic or surgical therapy. Maximize acid suppression

*confirmation by expert histopathologist.

AGA – American Gastroenterological Association; ACG – American College of Gastroenterology; ASGE – American Society for Gastrointestinal Endoscopy; BSG – British Society of Gastroenterology; SFED – French Society of Digestive Endoscopy; NDBE – non-dysplastic BE; IGD – Indeterminate grade of dysplasia; LGD – low grade dysplasia; HGD – high grade dysplasia; NR – not reported; EGD – Esophagogastroduodenoscopy; ER – endoscopic resection; SSBE – short segment BE; LSBE – long segment BE.

only), which increased to 0.38% per year when the analysis was restricted to those with IM [40].

Meta-analyses provide more rigorous evidence and, in the most recently published meta-analysis [41], the investigators extracted data from 57 studies that met inclusion criteria, including a total of 11,434 patients and 58,547 years of follow-up. The incidence of EAC in NDBE was 0.33% (95% CI 0.28% to 0.38%), with no evidence of publication bias.

When comparing the cancer risk in patients with BE with other conditions, even taking the most conservative study, the standardized incidence ratio (SIR) of EAC was 11.3 [37], which is 4.7-fold higher than the colon cancer risk in ulcerative colitis [42], 3.9-fold higher than primary sclerosing cholangitis [43], and nearly equal to the risk of breast cancer in first-degree relatives of BRCA1/2 mutation carrier with breast cancer [44]. Therefore, methods to detect individuals at increased risk of EAC merit serious and careful consideration. If surveillance is going to be deemed worthwhile, then it should detect earlier stage cancers and, hence, should be a reasonable predictor of longer survival.

9.3.2 Cancer risk stratification in patients with BE

The ability to predict cancer risk progression rates for individual patients with BE can result in a massive paradigm shift in the way these patients are managed. Moreover, this will likely make any future population screening and surveillance program for BE more cost-effective. A cancer risk prediction model that incorporates demographic, clinical, histological and molecular biomarkers is urgently needed. Several independent risk factors have been identified, as detailed below.

9.3.2.1 Demographic and clinical risk factors

Studies have shown that men are at increased risk for development of esophageal adenocarcinoma, compared to women. The overall risk is reportedly around 0.28% per year in men and 0.13% per year in women [40]. Data on the association of male gender and risk of progression is somewhat scarce and inconsistent, so recommendations for surveillance in both men and women are currently the same. Increasing age was associated with higher risk of malignant progression in several studies, but these results were not replicated in other large cohort studies [45]. Active tobacco smoking was associated with an increased risk of progression (hazard ratio = 2.03; 95% confidence interval, 1.29–3.17) across all classes of smoking intensity in some studies, but not all [46]. Alcohol consumption is not related to risk of progression. Increased waist to hip ratio, but not BMI, is associated with risk of aneuploidy, 9p loss of heterozygosity (LOH) and 17p LOH, suggesting that visceral adipose tissue may be a biomarker of malignant progression [45].

There is now overwhelming evidence that the length of BE segment is strongly associated with the risk of cancer although, in a few studies, the association was not statistically significant [22]. The majority of studies used the 3 cm cut-off to distinguish between LSBE and SSBE. While this is somewhat arbitrary, it has been noted that inter-observer agreement is poor for SSBE [47]. Besides segment length, the presence of mucosal nodularity, ulceration and strictures have been associated with risk of EAC; however, these may indicate prevalent neoplasia, rather than risk of future cancer, and should be assessed carefully with targeted biopsies or diagnostic endoscopic resection, if appropriate [48]. Presence of hiatus hernia and esophagitis are also associated with increased risk of progression to HGD and cancer, likely as a result of esophageal inflammation driving this process through increased risk of mutations.

Ideally, a future risk prediction model should take into account all these factors. However, such a model has not yet been developed and validated so, at the present time, segment length appears to be the only factor which can be used confidently to decide surveillance intervals in patients with NDBE.

9.3.2.2 Histological and molecular risk factors

The presence of glandular mucosa with intestinal metaplasia denotes higher cancer risk in BE. The grade of dysplasia is currently the most widely used biomarker of cancer progression risk in daily practice. There was a significantly increased incidence of EAC in patients with focal and diffuse HGD (14% and 56%, respectively) during a three-year follow-up [49]. The risk for LGD was five times higher than that of NDBE [37, 40]. Poor interobserver agreement and sampling error are the two major limitations in the use of dysplasia as a biomarker. Significant differences in progression rates have been

reported in patients with LGD confirmed by expert histopathologists (13.4% per year), compared with cases which were down-staged (0.49) [50] The impact of the consensus diagnosis on the progression rate was confirmed in a UK study [51]. Currently, the presence of dysplasia confirmed by two expert histopathologists is the best tissue biomarker available for assessment of cancer risk in patients with BE [22].

A number of molecular abnormalities occur during carcinogenesis, and some of these may become suitable to supplement or replace the current use of dysplasia, but first they will need to undergo rigorous validation process. Moreover, the technology has to be relatively automated and widely applicable for routine use in histopathology labs. Immunohistochemistry for nuclear p53 is currently the most promising out of all other potential biomarkers for risk stratification in clinical practice. It is easily applicable, reproducible, and serves as a good predictor of malignant progression [51]. Randomized controlled trial evidence needs to be available before these markers can be recommended for use in clinical practice.

9.3.3 Practical aspects and challenges in endoscopic surveillance

Prior to starting surveillance, patients should be carefully counseled regarding the benefits and risks of this approach, including the fact that there is no definite evidence that it will reduce risk of death. Moreover, the physical and psychological risks of endoscopy should be emphasized. It is not uncommon that patients will miss their follow-up endoscopy, and not all are willing to adhere to surveillance [52]. Another challenge is that surveillance does not guarantee to detect every early neoplasia, due to a variety of factors, including operator experience and sampling error.

Modern high-resolution and high-definition endoscopy systems allow the recognition of subtle mucosal abnormalities, so are therefore recommended for use in BE surveillance to detect early lesions. Other more advanced imaging techniques (narrow band imaging, auto fluorescence imaging, dye spray, etc) also exist, and this topic will be explored in later chapters. Nevertheless, the evidence is currently not sufficient to recommend their use in routine practice, so random four quadrant biopsies every 2 cm (Seattle protocol) remain part of the standard of care in BE surveillance [22]. The use of this protocol results in maximum yield for dysplasia, compared with other approaches [53].

However, it is well known that adherence to this protocol is poor among endoscopists (range 10–79%), with worse adherence for longer segments, which can result in a significant miss rate for dysplasia [54]. Another disadvantage of the Seattle protocol is that it is time-consuming and costly. Therefore, studies are needed to compare the cost-effectiveness of this practice with alternative techniques, such as image-enhanced endoscopy and targeted biopsies. The decision on frequency of surveillance can also be challenging.

Traditionally, previous guidelines recommend surveillance every 2–3 years for all patients. However, in light of recent data suggesting lower cancer progression rates, the more recent guidelines (Table 9.1) propose flexible surveillance intervals of up to five years, allowing clinicians to adjust the frequency according to the perceived individual cancer risk. One major dilemma in surveillance is that the vast majority of BE patients die of causes not related to EAC, and 95% of patients with EAC do not have previous diagnosis of BE [45]. This implies that surveillance is unlikely to have a major impact on mortality from EAC, which raises doubts about its cost-effectiveness.

Evidence from economic evaluations of surveillance is conflicting. Hirst *et al.* performed a systematic review of seven economic modeling studies, evaluating costs and outcomes of surveillance versus no surveillance, using Markov models. Surveillance was not cost-effective in few of the studies. One study from the USA found surveillance to be favorable at a cost of $16, 640 per quality-adjusted life-year. On the other hand, another study from the UK concluded that surveillance is more costly and less beneficial, compared with no surveillance, irrespective of the surveillance interval used and

despite using the 0.5% figure as the annual risk of cancer [55].

It is worth noting that these studies are subject to many limitations, not least because the evidence supporting parameter estimates is poor, and model assumptions are inconsistent – in particular, cancer recurrence rates, dysplasia progression and regression rates, and quality of life data [6]. A very recent study by Gordon *et al.* [56] incorporated the use of new technologies and modern endoscopic therapies for HGD and intra-mucosal cancer. Despite using the best available evidence for malignant progression, surveillance of NDBE was unlikely to be cost-effective for the majority of patients, and it varied largely, depending on progression rates between different grades of dysplasia. Authors reported that more targeted strategies that can identify and prioritize high-risk patients for surveillance may become cost-effective.

9.4 Conclusion

Significant progress has been made in the attempt to reduce mortality from EAC through early detection and treatment. Nevertheless, this area remains in need for research, particularly focusing on the comprehensive evaluation of emerging minimally invasive and novel screening tools, as well as deriving and validating BE risk prediction models. The current practice of surveillance is unlikely to be cost-effective, and methods to predict cancer progression risk are highly desirable. A proposed future screening and surveillance pathway is shown in Figure 9.1 below. This represents a future vision of how this process could potentially be cost-effective.

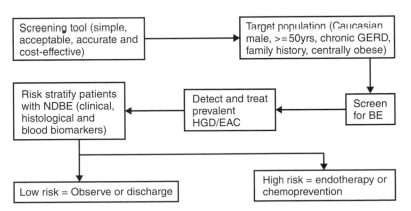

Figure 9.1 Suggested future pathway for screening and surveillance of BE with the aim of reducing mortality from EAC.

References

1 Pohl H, Sirovich B, Welch HG (2010). Esophageal adenocarcinoma incidence: are we reaching the peak? *Cancer Epidemiology Biomarkers and Prevention* **19**(6), 1468–70.

2 Pohl H, Welch HG (2005). The role of overdiagnosis and reclassification in the marked increase of esophageal adenocarcinoma incidence. *Journal of the National Cancer Institute* **97**(2), 142–6.

3 Auvinen MI, Sihvo EI, Ruohtula T, *et al.* (2002). Incipient angiogenesis in Barrett's epithelium and lymphangiogenesis in Barrett's adenocarcinoma. *Journal of Clinical Oncology* **20**(13), 2971–9.

4 Lao-Sirieix P, Fitzgerald RC (2012). Screening for oesophageal cancer. *Nature Reviews Clinical Oncology* **9**(5), 278–87.

5 Corley DA, Levin TR, Habel LA, *et al.* (2002). Surveillance and survival in Barrett's adenocarcinomas: A population-based study. *Gastroenterology* **122**(3), 633–40.

6 Hirst NG, Gordon LG, Whiteman DC, *et al.* (2011). Is endoscopic surveillance for non-dysplastic Barrett's esophagus cost-effective? Review of economic evaluations. *Journal of Gastroenterology and Hepatology* **26**(2), 247–54.

7 Dulai GS, Guha S, Kahn KL, *et al.* (2002). Preoperative prevalence of Barrett's esophagus in esophageal adenocarcinoma: A systematic review. *Gastroenterology* **122**(1), 26–33.

8 Jung KW, Talley NJ, Romero Y, *et al.* (2011). Epidemiology and natural history of intestinal metaplasia of the gastroesophageal junction and Barrett's esophagus: a population-based study. *American Journal of Gastroenterology* **106**(8), 1447–55; quiz 56.

9 Sikkema M, de Jonge PJ, Steyerberg EW, *et al.* (2010). Risk of esophageal adenocarcinoma and mortality in patients with Barrett's esophagus: a systematic review and meta-analysis. *Clinical Gastroenterology and Hepatology* **8**(3), 235–44; quiz e32.

10 Cooper GS, Kou TD, Chak A. (2009). Receipt of previous diagnoses and endoscopy and outcome from esophageal adenocarcinoma: a population-based study with temporal trends. *American Journal of Gastroenterology* **104**(6), 1356–62.

11 Lagergren J, Bergstrom R, Lindgren A, *et al.* (1999). Symptomatic gastroesophageal reflux as a risk factor for esophageal adenocarcinoma. *The New England Journal of Medicine* **340**(11), 825–31.

12 Ward EM, Wolfsen HC, Achem SR, *et al.* (2006). Barrett's esophagus is common in older men and women undergoing screening colonoscopy regardless of reflux symptoms. *American Journal of Gastroenterology* **101**(1), 12–7.

13 Ronkainen J, Aro P, Storskrubb T, *et al.* (2005). Prevalence of Barrett's esophagus in the general population: an endoscopic study. *Gastroenterology* **129**(6), 1825–31.

14 Balasubramanian G, Singh M, Gupta N, *et al.* (2012). Prevalence and predictors of columnar lined esophagus in gastroesophageal reflux disease (GERD) patients undergoing upper endoscopy. *American Journal of Gastroenterology* **107**(11), 1655–61.

15 Eloubeidi MA, Provenzale D. (2001). Clinical and demographic predictors of Barrett's esophagus among patients with gastroesophageal reflux disease: a multivariable analysis in veterans. *Journal of Clinical Gastroenterology* **33**(4), 306–9.

16 Wong A, Fitzgerald RC. (2005). Epidemiologic risk factors for Barrett's esophagus and associated adenocarcinoma. *Clinical Gastroenterology and Hepatology* **3**(1), 1–10.

17 Juhasz A, Mittal SK, Lee TH, *et al.* (2011). Prevalence of Barrett esophagus in first-degree relatives of patients with esophageal adenocarcinoma. *Journal of Clinical Gastroenterology* **45**(10), 867–71.

18 Su Z, Gay LJ, Strange A, *et al.* (2012). Common variants at the MHC locus and at chromosome 16q24.1 predispose to Barrett's esophagus. *Nature Genetics* **44**(10), 1131–6.

19 Orloff M, Peterson C, He X, *et al.* (2011). GErmline mutations in msr1, ascc1, and cthrc1 in patients with barrett esophagus and esophageal adenocarcinoma. *JAMA* **306**(4), 410–9.

20 Rubenstein JH, Mattek N, Eisen G (2010). Age- and sex-specific yield of Barrett's esophagus by endoscopy indication. *Gastrointestinal Endoscopy* **71**(1), 21–7.

21 Rubenstein JH, Scheiman JM, Sadeghi S, *et al.* (2011). Esophageal adenocarcinoma incidence in individuals with gastroesophageal reflux: synthesis and estimates from population studies. *American Journal of Gastroenterology* **106**(2), 254–60.

22 Fitzgerald RC, di Pietro M, Ragunath K, *et al.* (2013). British Society of Gastroenterology guidelines on the diagnosis and management of Barrett's oesophagus. *Gut* **63**(1), 7–42.

23 Spechler SJ, Sharma P, Souza RF, *et al.* (2011). American gastroenterological association technical review on the management of Barrett's esophagus. *Gastroenterology* **140**(3), e18–e52.

24 Hirota WK, Zuckerman MJ, Adler DG, *et al.* (2006). ASGE guideline: the role of endoscopy in the surveillance of premalignant conditions of the upper GI tract. *Gastrointestinal Endoscopy* **63**(4), 570–80.

25 Wang KK, Sampliner RE (2008). Updated guidelines 2008 for the diagnosis, surveillance and therapy of Barrett's esophagus. *American Journal of Gastroenterology* **103**(3), 788–97.

26 Gerson LB, Edson R, Lavori PW, *et al.* (2001). Use of a simple symptom questionnaire to predict Barrett's esophagus in patients with symptoms of gastroesophageal reflux. *American Journal of Gastroenterology* **96**(7), 2005–2012.

27 Locke GR, Zinsmeister AR, Talley NJ (2003). Can symptoms predict endoscopic findings in GERD? *Gastrointestinal Endoscopy* **58**(5), 661–70.

28 Falk GW, Chittajallu R, Goldblum JR, *et al.* (1997). Surveillance of patients with Barrett's esophagus for dysplasia

and cancer with balloon cytology. *Gastroenterology* **112**(6), 1787–97.

29 Rader AE, Faigel DO, Ditomasso J, *et al.* (2001). Cytological screening for Barrett's esophagus using a prototype flexible mesh catheter. *Digestive Diseases and Sciences* **46**(12), 2681–2686.

30 Kadri SR, Lao-Sirieix P, O'Donovan M, *et al.* (2010). Acceptability and accuracy of a non-endoscopic screening test for Barrett's oesophagus in primary care: cohort study. *BMJ* **341**, c4372.

31 Benaglia T, Sharples LD, Fitzgerald RC, *et al.* (2013). Health benefits and cost effectiveness of endoscopic and nonendoscopic cytosponge screening for Barrett's esophagus. *Gastroenterology* **144**(1), 62–73 e6.

32 Bhardwaj A, Hollenbeak CS, Pooran N, *et al.* (2009). A meta-analysis of the diagnostic accuracy of esophageal capsule endoscopy for Barrett's esophagus in patients with gastroesophageal reflux disease. *American Journal of Gastroenterology* **104**(6), 1533–9.

33 Rubenstein JH, Inadomi JM, Brill JV, *et al.* (2007). Cost utility of screening for Barrett's esophagus with esophageal capsule endoscopy versus conventional upper endoscopy. *Clinical Gastroenterology & Hepatology* **5**(3), 312–8.

34 Ramirez FC, Akins R, Shaukat M (2008). Screening of Barrett's esophagus with string-capsule endoscopy: a prospective blinded study of 100 consecutive patients using histology as the criterion standard. *Gastrointestinal Endoscopy* **68**(1), 25–31.

35 Sami SS, Subramanian V, Ortiz-Fernández-Sordó J, *et al.* (2013). *The utility of ultrathin endoscopy as a diagnostic tool for barrett's oesophagus (BO).* Systematic review and meta-analysis United European Gastroenterology Week; Berlin.

36 Zagari RM, Fuccio L, Wallander MA, *et al.* (2008). Gastro-oesophageal reflux symptoms, oesophagitis and barrett's oesophagus in the general population: The Loiano-Monghidoro study. *Gut* **57**(10), 1354–9.

37 Hvid-Jensen F, Pedersen L, Drewes AM, *et al.* (2011). Incidence of adenocarcinoma among patients with Barrett's esophagus. *New England Journal of Medicine* **365**(15), 1375–83.

38 Dent J, El-Serag HB, Wallander MA, *et al.* (2005). Epidemiology of gastro-oesophageal reflux disease: a systematic review. *Gut* **54**(5), 710–7.

39 Dunbar KB, Spechler SJ (2012). The risk of lymph-node metastases in patients with high-grade dysplasia or intramucosal carcinoma in Barrett's esophagus: a systematic review. *American Journal of Gastroenterology* **107**(6), 850–62.

40 Bhat S, Coleman HG, Yousef F, *et al.* (2011). Risk of malignant progression in Barrett's esophagus patients: results from a large population-based study. *Journal of the National Cancer Institute* **103**(13), 1049–57.

41 Desai TK, Krishnan K, Samala N, *et al.* (2012). The incidence of oesophageal adenocarcinoma in non-dysplastic Barrett's oesophagus: a meta-analysis. *Gut* **61**(7), 970–6.

42 Jess T, Rungoe C, Peyrin-Biroulet L (2012). Risk of colorectal cancer in patients with ulcerative colitis: a meta-analysis of population-based cohort studies. *Clinical Gastroenterology and Hepatology* **10**(6), 639–45.

43 de Valle MB, Bjornsson E, Lindkvist B (2012). Mortality and cancer risk related to primary sclerosing cholangitis in a Swedish population-based cohort. *Liver International* **32**(3), 441–8.

44 Rebbeck TR, Domchek SM (2008). Variation in breast cancer risk in BRCA1 and BRCA2 mutation carriers. *Breast Cancer Research* **10**(4), 108.

45 de Jonge PJ, van Blankenstein M, Grady WM, *et al.* (2014). Barrett's oesophagus: epidemiology, cancer risk and implications for management. *Gut* **63**(1), 191–202.

46 Coleman HG, Bhat S, Johnston BT, *et al.* (2012). Tobacco smoking increases the risk of high-grade dysplasia and cancer among patients with Barrett's esophagus. *Gastroenterology* **142**(2), 233–40.

47 Sharma P, Dent J, Armstrong D, *et al.* (2006). The development and validation of an endoscopic grading system for Barrett's esophagus: the Prague C & M criteria. *Gastroenterology* **131**(5), 1392–9.

48 Switzer-Taylor V, Schlup M, Lubcke R, *et al.* (2008). Barrett's esophagus: a retrospective analysis of 13 years surveillance. *Journal of Gastroenterology and Hepatology* **23**(9), 1362–7.

49 Buttar NS, Wang KK, Sebo TJ, *et al.* (2001). Extent of high-grade dysplasia in Barrett's esophagus correlates with risk of adenocarcinoma. *Gastroenterology* **120**(7), 1630–9.

50 Curvers WL, ten Kate FJ, Krishnadath KK, *et al.* (2010). Low-grade dysplasia in Barrett's esophagus: overdiagnosed and underestimated. *American Journal of Gastroenterology* **105**(7), 1523–30.

51 Kaye PV, Haider SA, Ilyas M, *et al.* (2009). Barrett's dysplasia and the Vienna classification: reproducibility, prediction of progression and impact of consensus reporting and p53 immunohistochemistry. *Histopathology* **54**(6), 699–712.

52 Ajumobi A, Bahjri K, Jackson C, *et al.* (2010). Surveillance in Barrett's esophagus: an audit of practice. *Digestive Diseases and Sciences* **55**(6), 1615–21.

53 Fitzgerald RC, Saeed IT, Khoo D, *et al.* (2001). Rigorous surveillance protocol increases detection of curable cancers associated with Barrett's esophagus. *Digestive Diseases and Sciences* **46**(9), 1892–8.

54 Abrams JA, Kapel RC, Lindberg GM, *et al.* (2009). Adherence to biopsy guidelines for Barrett's esophagus surveillance in the community setting in the United States. *Clinical Gastroenterology and Hepatology* **7**(7), 736–42.

55 Garside R, Pitt M, Somerville M, *et al.* (2006). Surveillance of Barrett's oesophagus: Exploring the uncertainty through systematic review, expert workshop and economic modelling. *Health Technology Assessment* **10**(8), iii–92.

56 Gordon LG, Mayne GC, Hirst NG, *et al.* (2014). Cost-effectiveness of endoscopic surveillance of non-dysplastic Barrett's esophagus. *Gastrointestinal Endoscopy* **79**(2), 242–56.

CHAPTER 10

New surface imaging technologies for dysplasia and cancer detection

David F. Boerwinkel, Wouter L. Curvers & Jacques J.G.H.M. Bergman

Department of Gastroenterology and Hepatology, Academic Medical Center, University of Amsterdam, Amsterdam, Netherlands

10.1 Introduction

Esophageal carcinoma has a dismal prognosis when detected at a symptomatic stage. Unfortunately, this is still the case for most patients diagnosed with squamous cell carcinoma or adenocarcinoma of the esophagus. However, when detected at an early stage, when the lesions are still confined to the superficial mucosal layers of the esophagus, this disease can be adequately treated with endoscopic therapy. Endoscopic resection or ablative techniques have a limited morbidity and mortality compared to esophagectomy and, due to the virtually absent risk of lymph node metastasis of intramucosal neoplasia, the five-year survival is excellent. Timely detection of esophageal neoplasia is, therefore, of crucial clinical importance.

For long, Barrett's esophagus (BE) has been recognized as the main precursor lesion for esophageal adenocarcinoma. Therefore, patients with BE are recommended to undergo regular surveillance endoscopy, in order to detect neoplastic progression of BE at an early stage.

In contrast to BE, no precursor lesion has been identified for esophageal squamous cell carcinoma (ESCC), which is the most prevalent subtype (90%) of esophageal carcinoma. ESCC is associated with smoking and alcohol consumption, and patients with a prior history of oropharyngeal or lung carcinoma are thought to have an increased risk of developing ESCC. ESCC has a particular geographic distribution and is especially prevalent in parts of China, Iran, India, France and Japan. In certain densely populated areas, such as northwest China, comprising over 100 million

people, incidence can reach a remarkable one in 1000. Therefore, regular screening endoscopy may be of use in these areas.

Premalignant stages of neoplasia, including low- and high-grade dysplasia and intramucosal cancer (IMC), are the targets of surveillance endoscopy. These lesions are usually flat and subtle, can be very focal and small, and in case of BE lesions may be found in an abnormal and inflamed looking esophagus.

In order to improve the yield of surveillance endoscopy in BE, a random biopsy protocol has been implemented; every visible abnormality is sampled for histology and, in addition, random quadrantic biopsies are obtained at every 2 cm of the BE segment. However, this process is laborious, and many endoscopists do not adhere to the protocol [1]. Due to the expenses associated with surveillance endoscopy, the labor-intensive process of obtaining and evaluating the large number of biopsies, and the burden on patients, the (cost-)effectiveness of screening has to be improved, both for BE-associated neoplasia and for ESCC.

Advanced endoscopic imaging techniques may improve the cost-effectiveness of diagnostic endoscopy, through increased targeted detection that may reduce, or even dismiss, the current practice of obtaining random biopsies. Moreover, advanced imaging may guide therapeutic decisions during ongoing endoscopy.

Advanced endoscopic imaging can be divided into wide-field detection and small-field differentiation techniques. Wide-field detection aims to draw attention to suspicious areas, while small-field differentiation techniques zoom in on those suspicious areas to discriminate between truly neoplastic or non-suspicious

---

Esophageal Cancer and Barrett's Esophagus, Third Edition. Edited by Prateek Sharma, Richard Sampliner and David Ilson.
© 2015 John Wiley & Sons, Ltd. Published 2015 by John Wiley & Sons, Ltd.

mucosa. Wide-field "red-flag" techniques generally image the mucosal surface, while differentiation may be achieved by detailed inspection of the mucosa, sub-surface imaging or functional imaging of the mucosal components.

This chapter will focus on new surface imaging technologies for the detection of early neoplasia in the esophagus, from exogenous dyes to complex optical filters and functional techniques.

10.2 Surface imaging in Barrett's esophagus

10.2.1 White light endoscopy

The cornerstone of endoscopic imaging for the detection of neoplasia in the esophagus is white light endoscopy (WLE). In recent years, the quality of WLE has increased markedly, mainly due to the pivotal switch from fiber optic endoscopes to electronic video endoscopy. Charge-coupled devices (CCD) in standard video endoscopes have a total number of pixels of 100,000–300,000 to generate a spatial resolution of about 100 μm. High-resolution – or high-definition – endoscopes have CCDs containing over 1,000,000 pixels. With a resolution of about 10 μm, these endoscopes enable imaging at near cellular levels.

No large comparative studies have been conducted to evaluate the performance of high-resolution white light endoscopy (HR-WLE), but secondary outcomes have suggested a gain in sensitivity for early neoplastic lesions, when compared to standard video endoscopy (Figure 10.1: see also Plate 10.1). High-quality monitors and cables complement HR-WLE, to increase image quality or to allow projection onto a larger screen while retaining image quality.

Gastrointestinal endoscopes usually have a focal distance with a fixed range (e.g. 1–9 cm), thus limiting detailed inspection of mucosal and vascular patterns. HR-WLE can be combined with magnification endoscopy (ME). Optical magnification is achieved by a movable lens that allows a variable focal distance without losing image quality. Some endoscopes use a lever on the endoscope handle for a continuous variation of focal distance, while others have a fixed zoom modus. Such a near focus mode allows quick switching between a focal distance of 5–100 mm to 2–6 mm.

Electronic magnification is a post-processing technique, which enlarges the central area of the image. Since only a part of the pixels is used, this may result in the loss of image quality, due to a loss of spatial resolution.

Detailed scanning of large surface areas is inefficient and laborious with ME. However, as an adjunct to HR-WLE, magnification may be a useful tool for detailed inspection, guiding targeted biopsies or delineation of lesions before resection.

Detection and differentiation of lesions ultimately relies on the endoscopists' ability to recognize the characteristics of early neoplasia. This process can benefit from image processors with image enhancement techniques to increase contrast. The main targets of image enhancement are surface enhancement, contrast enhancement and tone enhancement, which increases the contrast between dark and light, deep and superficial, vascular and mucosal structures, respectively. More complex image enhancement may be achieved by adding an exogenous dye to achieve a better visualization of the surface details, called chromoendoscopy. *Optical* chromoendoscopy, without the use of a dye, is performed by changing optical filters pre- or post-illumination, to highlight various components of the tissue with the switch of a button. Both types of chromoendoscopy – with dyes or optical filters – are discussed below.

10.2.2 Chromoendoscopy

There are two types of chromoendoscopy agents used in the esophagus in combination with HR-WLE and ME: vital stains and contrast stains. Vital stains (such as methylene blue and Lugol's solution) are actively absorbed by the epithelium. Contrast stains (e.g. indigo carmine) are not absorbed by the mucosal cells, but accumulate in pits and grooves along the epithelial surface, highlighting the superficial mucosal architecture. The materials required for chromoendoscopy (e.g. spraying catheters and dye) are inexpensive. However, variations in technique and interpretation of the staining patterns limit the application of chromoendoscopy in routine clinical practice.

10.2.2.1 Methylene blue

Methylene blue (MB) is a vital stain that is actively absorbed by the epithelial cells of the small bowel and

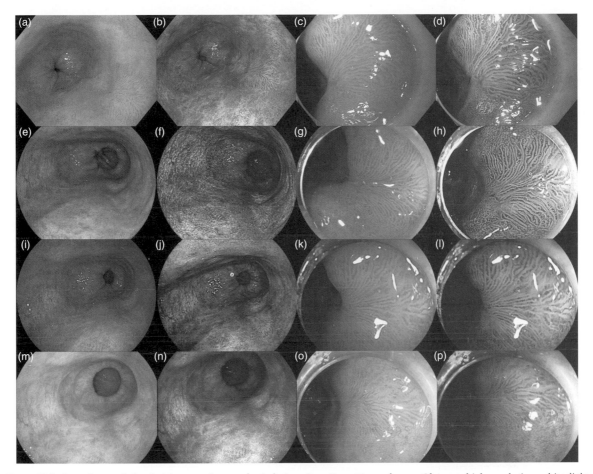

Figure 10.1 Overview and detailed images of a neoplastic lesions in a Barrett's esophagus: Olympus high resolution white light endoscopy (a, c); and narrow band imaging (b, d); Fujinon white light endoscopy (e.g.) and blue light imaging (f, h); Fujinon white light endoscopy (i,k); and Fujinon intelligent chromoendoscopy (j, l); Pentax white light endoscopy (m, o) and iSCAN (n, p). *(See insert for color representation of this figure.)*

the colon. With characteristics resembling small bowel epithelium, intestinal metaplasia of BE also absorbs MB, whereas gastric epithelium and squamous epithelium remain unstained. These features may be helpful in detecting esophageal intestinal metaplasia.

Several studies have demonstrated an increased detection and delineation of specialized intestinal metaplasia with MB chromoendoscopy [2]. Other studies have shown a benefit of MB endoscopy, in combination with magnification endoscopy, for the detection of early neoplasia [3]. However, a recent meta-analysis of nine studies for the assessment of the diagnostic yield of MB chromoendoscopy versus WLE, with random biopsies, showed that there was no incremental yield for MB

for the detection of IM and dysplasia [4]. Moreover, the technique is operator-dependent, time-consuming, and laborious [5]. In addition, it has been suggested that MB in combination with white light illumination might increase DNA damage in Barrett's mucosa [6]. Therefore, in our opinion, there is no relevant clinical utility of MB chromoendoscopy in imaging of BE.

10.2.2.2 Indigo carmine

Indigo carmine (IC) is a blue contrast stain that is not absorbed by epithelial cells. It enhances patterns in the mucosa by pooling in the mucosal ridges, thus increasing the contrast. Intestinal metaplasia was shown to correlate with villiform surface patterns, while dysplastic areas were observed to have distorted and irregular surfaces [7]. IC chromoendoscopy, like MB, is a laborious process. In combination with magnification endoscopy, the whole Barrett's segment has to be inspected at full magnification, with the possibility of missing certain areas. This technique may, therefore, be more suited for detailed inspection of suspicious areas than as a primary detection technique [8].

10.2.2.3   Acetic acid

When applied to Barrett's mucosa, acetic acid (1.5–3%) induces swelling of the mucosal surface, with enhancement of the architecture and congestion of the capillaries. In multiple prospective studies, pit patterns in BE were better visualized with acetic acid in combination with magnification endoscopy, compared to standard endoscopy with random biopsies [9]. For the detection of early BE neoplasia, recent publications have suggested that acetic acid may be beneficial [10], yet other studies have not demonstrated an additional value over HR-WLE [11]. A relative drawback of acetic acid is that it makes the mucosa more vulnerable to damage and bleeding by the tip of the endoscope or suctioning through the working channel. Although acetic acid increases the contrast of the mucosal pattern, the whitening caused by acetic acid decreases the visualization of the superficial patterns.

Given the low complexity and costs, acetic acid may be an easy applicable technique during routine BE surveillance, but its additional value has not been established irrefutably.

10.2.2.4   Other chromoendoscopic stains

Apart from methylene blue, indigo carmine and acetic acid, which have all been extensively studied in BE, various other stains have been subject of research:

• Toluidine blue (TB) is a vital stain mainly used for the detection of esophageal squamous cell carcinoma. It has been suggested that TB enhances the villous appearance of BE, yet this has not been formally assessed, nor has its value for the detection of BE neoplasia been studied [12].

• Crystal violet (CV) also is a vital stain, and positive staining was found to be associated with intestinal metaplasia while using a simple classification protocol and no magnification endoscopy [13]. However, CV has not been shown to improve the yield of neoplasia

detection in BE, and there have been some reports indicating that crystal violet may be carcinogenic [14].

• Lugol's staining (LS) is the main chromoendoscopic vital stain used for the detection and delineation of esophageal *squamous cell* carcinoma (see below) [15]. Lugol's is an iodine stain that has a high binding affinity for glycogen. It stains non-keratinized squamous epithelium brown. In areas with an increased metabolism and a high turnover of glycogen, such as inflammation or neoplasia, the mucosa remains unstained. This is also the case for columnar epithelium in BE. Lugol's may therefore be used to delineate the squamocolumnar junction, or to identify residual Barrett's islands after therapy. However, for the enhanced detection of BE associated neoplasia, LS has no role.

In summary, chromoendoscopy with exogenous applied dyes, in combination with high-resolution and/or magnification white-light endoscopy, has been studied extensively. Despite the availability of the dyes and required equipment, none of the techniques have been established in routine surveillance for non-dysplastic Barrett's esophagus, nor for the detection or work-up of early BE neoplasia. Among the many limitations that hamper widespread implementation of chromoendoscopy are large controversies within the literature, cumbersome procedures, operator dependency and, sometimes, even suggested carcinogenic effects of the involved dyes. Currently, therefore, chromoendoscopy as an adjunctive tool to (HR-)WLE assessment is not included in guidelines for BE surveillance [16].

10.2.3   Optical chromoendoscopy

In recent years, several endoscope manufacturers have developed electronic or optical chromoendoscopy modalities. Optical chromoendoscopy essentially acts in a comparable fashion to chromoendoscopy with topically applied dyes, by increasing the contrast of the surface epithelium. However, without the expenses and tedious process of dyes, optical chromoendoscopy may offer many advantages.

10.2.3.1   Narrow band imaging

Narrow band imaging (NBI) was introduced by Olympus (Tokyo, Japan) and makes use of the optical phenomenon that depth of light penetration into tissue is dependent on wavelength – the shorter the wavelength, the more superficial the penetration. In NBI, the band-pass ranges of the green and blue components of white light have been narrowed to 530–550 nm (green) and 390–445 nm (blue). The relative intensity of blue light has been increased while reducing the intensity of the red component, thereby enhancing the superficial mucosal architecture. Moreover, the blue band-pass filter corresponds to the absorption maximum of hemoglobin, which results in a better visualization of superficial vascular structures [17]. In combination with magnification endoscopy, NBI allows for inspection of the mucosal and vascular characteristics in great detail. Regular mucosal and vascular patterns upon NBI have been shown to correlate with non-dysplastic BE, while irregular features were associated with early neoplasia [18].

NBI has been investigated for the primary detection of early neoplasia. In the first study, no additional value in the diagnosis of neoplasia was shown when compared to HR-WLE in combination with indico carmine chromoendoscopy [8]. In a subsequent study, NBI demonstrated increased detection of patients with early neoplasia when compared to standard resolution WLE [20]. This effect was largely eliminated when NBI was compared to high-resolution WLE [19]. This study did show that, despite similar detection rates of neoplasia for NBI and HR-WLE, the number of random biopsies required may be reduced by NBI-targeted biopsies [19]. This may potentially impact on the cost-effectiveness of BE surveillance protocols.

NBI offers detailed inspection of mucosal and vascular structures and may, therefore, be better suited as a differentiation tool, rather than for primary detection [21]. NBI has thus been used as a differentiation tool in combination with autofluorescence imaging (see below). In this setting, NBI was able to reduce the high false-positive rates of autofluorescence imaging substantially, although a portion of true neoplastic areas were considered unsuspicious by NBI [22, 23]. Subsequent inter-observer studies, however, showed only moderate agreement [24]. In addition, NBI did not improve sensitivity or inter-observer agreement over HR-WLE.

Most studies have used still images obtained from a population enriched with patients with early neoplasia. A selection bias may thus have been introduced, and the results may not be translated easily to daily practice. Currently, therefore, standardized classification systems for the interpretation of NBI patterns are being developed

and validated, but have not yet reached clinical implementation.

Apart from neoplasia detection or differentiation, NBI may aid the careful delineation of lesions prior to endoscopic resection, and the detection of residual Barrett's epithelium after radio-frequency ablation. This has yet to be formally assessed.

NBI is relatively easy to use, since no additional stains have to be administered and the modality can be switched on and off by the push of a button. NBI can be incorporated in various kinds of endoscopes, and has recently become widely available. However, despite being the most rigorously studied optical chromoendoscopy modality to date, its value during BE surveillance for the detection or differentiation of early neoplasia has still not been fully established.

10.2.3.2 Fujinon Intelligent Chromoendoscopy and I-scan

Fujinon (Saitama, Japan) has developed Fujinon Intelligent ChromoEndoscopy (FICE), and Pentax (Tokyo, Japan) has developed I-scan.

FICE uses a post-processing algorithm to increase the intensity of blue light in the standard endoscopic image electronically, while decreasing the contribution of red and green [25]. With FICE, multiple settings can be integrated in the algorithm, thus allowing for variable spectral priorities, according to the mucosa under investigation. The adjunctive value of FICE has so far been adequately investigated only in one study, suggesting that FICE may be applied for the detection of esophageal abnormalities, with results comparable to conventional chromoendoscopy [26]. No data are currently available that demonstrate the additional value of FICE over standard or HR-WLE.

I-scan uses post-processing software to allow for analysis and modification of the 1.25 megapixel images. By adjusting the surface enhancement, contrast enhancement and tone enhancement, the surface characteristics can be highlighted [27]. I-scan has mainly been tested in the colon for the detection and differentiation of colonic polyps but, up to the present date, no studies on the detection of neoplasia in the esophagus have been published.

10.2.4 Fluorescence imaging

Autofluorescence imaging is based on the principle that certain endogenous substances, such as NADH (nicotinamide adenine dinucleotide), FAD (flavin adenine dinucleotide) and collagen emit light of longer wavelengths when excited with short-wavelength light (i.e. blue light). Each fluorophore has a characteristic emission range of wavelengths as a function of a given excitation wavelength, called the fluorescence spectrum. The emitted fluorescence spectra are highly dependent on the concentration, distribution and biochemical status of the fluorophores. In addition, structural alterations due to changed tissue architecture – thickening of the mucosa, increased number of blood vessels, enlarged nuclei – influence the optical characteristics. Spectroscopy studies using this autofluorescence principle have shown that neoplastic tissue in BE demonstrates decreased autofluorescence intensity in the green spectrum and increased intensity in the red spectrum, compared to non-neoplastic BE tissue [28, 29].

10.2.4.1 Endoscopic autofluorescence imaging

Autofluorescence (AF), as an endoscopic wide-field detection tool, was first introduced by Xillix Technologies Corp in a light-induced fluorescence endoscopy system (LIFE). The first feasibility studies with this system suggested that LIFE might improve the detection of early neoplasia in BE [30], but this was contradicted by a subsequent randomized crossover study [31]. The AF algorithm in LIFE had a high sensitivity for background inflammation, causing a high number of high false positives. No additional value for the detection of early neoplasia was, therefore, found for AF endoscopy. Moreover, early AF technology was incorporated in a fiber optic endoscopy system, which had inferior white light performance compared to video endoscopy.

These limitations were taken into account in the development of the video-autofluorescence imaging (AFI) system by Olympus. This system represented a major step forwards in image quality by combining autofluorescence endoscopy with high-resolution white light video-endoscopy (HR-WLE). Subtle mucosal abnormalities that were overlooked by fiber optic endoscopy could now possibly be detected with WLE. In the AFI mode of the endoscope, the image was composed of total emitted autofluorescence after blue light excitation (390–470 nm) and green reflectance (540–560 nm).

The first report on AFI showed promising results, with an increased detection of HGIN/IMC by AFI over WLE32. AFI was subsequently combined with narrow band imaging (NBI) into one "endoscopic trimodal imaging" (ETMI) system, to decrease the high false positive rate (Figure 10.2: see also Plate 10.2). In this system, high resolution WLE, AFI and NBI can be rapidly alternated, with a simple switch on the endoscope handle.

Autofluorescence imaging in the ETMI system was, at first, demonstrated to increase the detection of early neoplasia significantly, while NBI could decrease the false positive rate [22]. However, subsequent randomized crossover trials, comparing ETMI to standard video endoscopy (SVE) with random biopsies, could not confirm the previous positive results. Although AFI significantly increased the targeted detection of early neoplasia, SVE with random biopsies gave a superior performance on a patient basis [23, 33].

An adjusted AFI system was subsequently introduced, with a dual, small-band excitation autofluorescence algorithm. While the earlier generations of AFI were mainly based on architectural changes in the mucosal

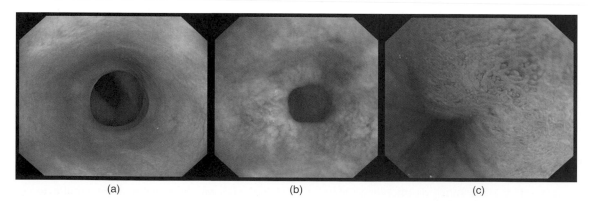

(a)   (b)   (c)

Figure 10.2 Early neoplastic lesion in Barrett's esophagus, imaged with a) high-resolution white light endoscopy; b) autofluorescence imaging; and c) narrow band imaging. *(See insert for color representation of this figure.)*

layer and submucosal collagen, the third generation was intended specifically to target fluorescent changes in the malignant cells themselves. However, when compared to the second generation AFI, this system did not show increased performance [34].

In line with previous observations with NBI, AFI may also be helpful in detecting additional lesions in BE, delineating lesions prior to resection or impact on the endoscopic therapy by detecting relevant lesions. A recent review of most AFI studies, however, concluded that the clinical impact on diagnosis and treatment of early BE neoplasia was rather limited (unpublished data).

Recent studies showed that AFI-false positive areas were associated with an increased content of molecular biomarkers for dysplasia. The use of a biomarker panel on a limited number of AFI targeted biopsies may thus potentially improve risk-stratification in Barrett's esophagus, avoiding laborious random sampling [35, 36].

In conclusion, endoscopic autofluorescence imaging for early neoplasia in BE aids in the targeted detection of early lesions, yet the subsequent impact on the total diagnostic and therapeutic process of BE patients is too small to justify routine application.

10.2.4.2 Fluorescent contrast agents

A recently emerged concept is the administration of fluorescently labeled exogenous substances that bind to specific molecular targets for malignant progression. Peptides, as a molecular probe, have shown tissue-specific binding in *ex vivo* studies using screening experiments and fluorescence microscopy [37]. Peptides are similar to antibodies in terms of binding affinity, but can be produced relatively cheaply and in large quantities. Another promising approach is fluorescently labeled lectins, which have a low toxicity, a high stability, and are inexpensive to produce. Lectins bind with high affinity to glycan targets in intestinal metaplasia, compared with low binding to HGIN/IMC, which results in good sensitivity for detecting early neoplasia [38].

These two approaches have different strengths and weaknesses. The peptide probes are more specific, but require a narrow field of view and may be costly to produce. Lectin probes are very cheap and, for agents such as wheat germ agglutinin, safety is not likely to be an issue, since it is a consumable product. However, lectins lack specificity, and it would be preferable if the fluorescent contrast agents would fluoresce outside the

autofluorescence emission wavelengths. Fluorescent contrast agents are still in an experimental phase and are not expected to be implemented in clinical practice in the upcoming years.

10.3 Surface imaging for esophageal squamous cell carcinoma

10.3.1 Lugol's solution

The most common method of enhanced imaging of early esophageal squamous cell carcinoma (ESCC) is the application of Lugol's solution (LS). LS is an iodine-based vital stain that is widely available, inexpensive and is easily sprayed on the esophageal mucosa, using a regular spraying catheter. In esophageal endoscopy, a 1–3% solution is generally used. Areas with a high glycogen metabolism, such as inflammation or neoplasia, have a low uptake of iodine and appear as unstained areas in a brown-stained esophagus.

Several studies, most of which have been conducted in Asian populations, have shown that unstained lesions after LS spraying are associated with early squamous neoplasia [15, 39]. Therefore, Lugol's has been used to investigate patients at risk for developing ESCC, such as patients with head and neck cancer, and subjects with heavy smoking and/or alcohol habits [40]. In Western populations, where ESCC has a low incidence rate, the additional value of LS for the detection of neoplastic lesions has been shown to be limited. However, in high-incidence, non-Western patient populations, the application of Lugol's is of high clinical value. In addition, spraying Lugol's solution improves the delineation of early ESCC, which is helpful in the endoscopic treatment of these lesions [41].

The application of LS has some limitations, one of which is the discomfort caused by esophageal spasms and retrosternal pain. Therefore, LS should not be applied in the proximal esophagus. In addition, LS has a caustic effect on the esophageal mucosa, which causes an inflammatory reaction and requires an interval period of four weeks to heal before endoscopic therapy can be performed. Moreover, LS cannot be administered in patients with iodine allergy or hyperthyroidism.

10.3.2 Narrow band imaging

The most promising optical contrast technique investigated for the detection of ESCC is narrow band imaging (NBI). NBI, especially when combined with zooming capabilities, is able to image the mucosal architecture in great detail [42]. Most studies on the use of NBI for ESCC have focused on the detection of synchronous or metachronous esophageal neoplasia in patients with primary head and neck cancers, where NBI showed a high accuracy in detecting early squamous lesions [43]. Investigations on intrapapillary capillary loops (IPCLs) in ESCC have demonstrated that changes in the mucosal microvasculature due to malignant progression can be visualized with NBI magnification endoscopy (e.g. dilated IPCLs, tortuous IPCLs, elongated IPCLs, caliber change and variety in IPCL shapes). These changes in IPCLs have been shown to follow a gradual process, associated with progressive transition to high-grade dysplasia and invasive carcinoma [44]. Moreover, IPCL patterns may be used to discriminate between intramucosal and submucosal invasive carcinoma [45].

To date, no large prospective randomized crossover trials comparing Lugol's staining to NBI for ESCC in the esophagus have been published, yet small comparative studies suggest that NBI performs equally as well as LS [46]. Since the application of LS is laborious and is associated with burdensome side-effects, NBI is an attractive alternative (Figure 10.3: see also Plate 10.3).

NBI appears to offer comparable performance to LS, but it is safer and lacks the abovementioned side effects. Moreover, NBI is currently widely available, since most standard diagnostic endoscopes are equipped with NBI. The use of NBI has no implications on therapeutic planning, which is the case with LS due to the inflammatory response. NBI can therefore be applied as a primary screening modality, followed by staging assessment of depth invasion using IPCL patterns. LS may subsequently be sprayed directly prior to the endoscopic therapy, to aid in the delineation of the lesion, or when NBI characteristics are indecisive.

10.4 Summary

In this chapter, we have focused on advanced surface imaging techniques for the detection and differentiation of early neoplastic lesions in the esophagus.

The main objective in endoscopic imaging for the diagnosis of early esophageal neoplasia is the primary detection of lesions. Subsequent differentiation of these lesions is of importance for further clinical management decisions, yet it is a secondary objective.

The main body of literature on advanced surface imaging has been published for early Barrett's neoplasia. In the last decade, despite the development of many novel sub-surface and functional differentiation techniques, the largest step forwards in wide-field surface imaging has been achieved by the increase of white light quality. The advent of HR-WLE has decreased the need for dye-assisted or optical chromoendoscopy. Narrow band imaging (NBI) and autofluorescence imaging (AFI) have been developed, studied, adjusted and commercialized in the last decade, yet the literature on the use of either of these modalities has reported limited additional value. Novel wide-field optical techniques have yet to emerge.

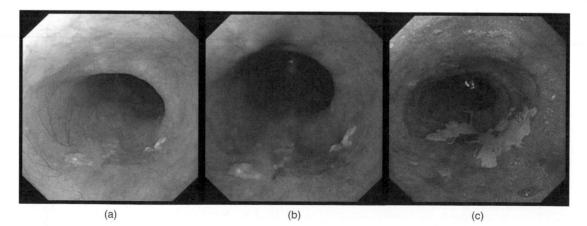

(a)   (b)   (c)

Figure 10.3 Early esophageal squamous cell carcinoma, imaged with a) white light endoscopy; b) narrow band imaging; and c) after Lugol's staining. *(See insert for color representation of this figure.)*

Advanced surface imaging for the detection of early squamous cell carcinoma (ESCC) in the esophagus has for a long time been based on WLE with Lugol's solution. Despite recent advances of HR-WLE and preliminary data on NBI as a wide-field optical chromoendoscopy tool, Lugol's remains the predominant adjunct in surface imaging for ESCC, especially in high-incidence areas with limited resources and endoscopic expertise.

With the current quality of high-resolution WLE, it is the endoscopist's ability to recognize and identify early neoplasia that will make the difference. Without proper training, all advanced imaging tools will merely be an intriguing piece of technology, rather than an aid in the diagnosis of patients with esophageal cancer. Future studies should be based on such comprehensive themes, with technology just being a part of the whole.

References

1 Peters FP, Curvers WL, Rosmolen WD, *et al.* (2008). Surveillance history of endoscopically treated patients with early Barrett's neoplasia: nonadherence to the Seattle biopsy protocol leads to sampling error. *Diseases of the Esophagus* **21**, 475–479.

2 Endo T, Awakawa T, Takahashi H, *et al.* (2002). Classification of Barrett's epithelium by magnifying endoscopy. *Gastrointestinal Endoscopy* **55**, 641–647.

3 Canto MI, Setrakian S, Willis J, *et al.* (2000). Methylene blue-directed biopsies improve detection of intestinal metaplasia and dysplasia in Barrett's esophagus. *Gastrointestinal Endoscopy* **51**, 560–568.

4 Ngamruengphong S, Sharma VK, Das A (2009). Diagnostic yield of methylene blue chromoendoscopy for detecting specialized intestinal metaplasia and dysplasia in Barrett's esophagus: a meta-analysis. *Gastrointestinal Endoscopy* **69**, 1021–1028.

5 Canto MI, Kalloo A (2006). Chromoendoscopy for Barrett's esophagus in the twenty-first century: to stain or not to stain? *Gastrointestinal Endoscopy* **64**, 200–205.

6 Olliver JR, Wild CP, Sahay P, *et al.* (2003). Chromoendoscopy with methylene blue and associated DNA damage in Barrett's esophagus. *Lancet* **362**, 373–374.

7 Sharma P, Weston AP, Topalovski M, *et al.* (2003). Magnification chromoendoscopy for the detection of intestinal metaplasia and dysplasia in Barrett's esophagus. *Gut* **52**, 24–27.

8 Kara MA, Peters FP, Rosmolen WD, *et al.* (2005). High-resolution endoscopy plus chromoendoscopy or narrow-band imaging in Barrett's esophagus: a prospective randomized crossover study. *Endoscopy* **37**, 929–936.

9 Hoffman A, Kiesslich R, Bender A, *et al.* (2006). Acetic acid-guided biopsies after magnifying endoscopy compared with random biopsies in the detection of Barrett's esophagus: a prospective randomized trial with crossover design. *Gastrointestinal Endoscopy* **64**, 1–8.

10 Longcroft-Wheaton G, Duku M, Mead R, *et al.* (2010). Acetic acid spray is an effective tool for the endoscopic detection of neoplasia in patients with Barrett's esophagus. *Clinical Gastroenterology and Hepatology* **8**, 843–847.

11 Curvers W, Baak L, Kiesslich R, *et al.* (2008). Chromoendoscopy and narrow-band imaging compared with high-resolution magnification endoscopy in Barrett's esophagus. *Gastroenterology* **134**, 670–679.

12 Eisen GM, Montgomery EA, Azumi N, *et al.* (1999). Qualitative mapping of Barrett's metaplasia: a prerequisite for intervention trials. *Gastrointestinal Endoscopy* **50**, 814–818.

13 Yuki T, Amano Y, Kushiyama Y, *et al.* (2006). Evaluation of modified crystal violet chromoendoscopy procedure using new mucosal pit pattern classification for detection of Barrett's dysplastic lesions. *Digestive and Liver Disease* **38**, 296–300.

14 Aidoo A, Gao N, Neft RE, *et al.* (1990). Evaluation of the genotoxicity of gentian violet in bacterial and mammalian cell systems. Teratog., Carcinog. *Mutagen* **10**, 449–462.

15 Dawsey SM, Fleischer DE, Wang GQ, *et al.* (1998). Mucosal iodine staining improves endoscopic visualization of squamous dysplasia and squamous cell carcinoma of the esophagus in Linxian, China. *Cancer* **83**, 220–231.

16 Wang KK, Sampliner RE (2008). Updated guidelines 2008 for the diagnosis, surveillance and therapy of Barrett's esophagus. *American Journal of Gastroenterology* **103**, 788–797.

17 Gono K, Obi T, Yamaguchi M, *et al.* (2004). Appearance of enhanced tissue features in narrow-band endoscopic imaging. *Journal of Biomedical Optics* **9**, 568–577.

18 Kara MA, Ennahachi M, Fockens P, *et al.* (2006). Detection and classification of the mucosal and vascular patterns (mucosal morphology) in Barrett's esophagus by using narrow band imaging. *Gastrointestinal Endoscopy* **64**, 155–166.

19 Sharma P, Hawes RH, Bansal A, *et al.* (2013). Standard endoscopy with random biopsies versus narrow band imaging targeted biopsies in Barrett's esophagus: a prospective, international, randomised controlled trial. *Gut* **62**, 15–21.

20 Wolfsen HC, Crook JE, Krishna M, *et al.* (2008). Prospective, controlled tandem endoscopy study of narrow band imaging for dysplasia detection in Barrett's Esophagus. *Gastroenterology* **135**, 24–31.

21 Curvers WL, Broek FJC van den, Reitsma JB, *et al.* (2009). Systematic review of narrow-band imaging for the detection and differentiation of abnormalities in the esophagus and stomach (with video). *Gastrointestinal Endoscopy* **69**, 307–317.

22 Curvers WL, Singh R, Song L-MW-K, *et al.* (2008). Endoscopic tri-modal imaging for detection of early neoplasia in Barrett's esophagus: a multi-centre feasibility study using high-resolution endoscopy, autofluorescence imaging and narrow band imaging incorporated in one endoscopy system. *Gut* **57**, 167–172.

23 Curvers WL, Vilsteren FG van, Baak LC, *et al.* (2011). Endoscopic trimodal imaging versus standard video endoscopy for detection of early Barrett's neoplasia: a multicenter, randomized, crossover study in general practice. *Gastrointestinal Endoscopy* **73**, 195–203.

24 Herrero LA, Curvers WL, Bansal A, *et al.* (2009). Zooming in on Barrett esophagus using narrow-band imaging: an international observer agreement study. *European Journal of Gastroenterology & Hepatology* **21**, 1068–1075.

25 Pohl J, May A, Rabenstein T, *et al.* (2007). Computed virtual chromoendoscopy: a new tool for enhancing tissue surface structures. *Endoscopy* **39**, 80–83.

26 Pohl J, May A, Rabenstein T, *et al.* (2007). Comparison of computed virtual chromoendoscopy and conventional chromoendoscopy with acetic acid for detection of neoplasia in Barrett's esophagus. *Endoscopy* **39**, 594–598.

27 Hancock S, Bowman E, Prabakaran J, *et al.* (2012). Use of i-scan Endoscopic Image Enhancement Technology in Clinical Practice to Assist in Diagnostic and Therapeutic Endoscopy: A Case Series and Review of the Literature. *Diagnostic and Therapeutic Endoscopy* **2012**, 193570.

28 Georgakoudi I, Jacobson BC, Dam J Van, *et al.* (2001). Fluorescence, reflectance, and light-scattering spectroscopy for evaluating dysplasia in patients with Barrett's esophagus. *Gastroenterology* **120**, 1620–1629.

29 Panjehpour M, Overholt BF, Vo-Dinh T, *et al.* (1996). Endoscopic fluorescence detection of high-grade dysplasia in Barrett's esophagus. *Gastroenterology* **111**, 93–101.

30 Haringsma J, Tytgat GN, Yano H, *et al.* (2001). Autofluorescence endoscopy: feasibility of detection of GI neoplasms unapparent to white light endoscopy with an evolving technology. *Gastrointestinal Endoscopy* **53**, 642–650.

31 Kara MA, Smits ME, Rosmolen WD, *et al.* (2005). A randomized crossover study comparing light-induced fluorescence endoscopy with standard videoendoscopy for the detection of early neoplasia in Barrett's esophagus. *Gastrointestinal Endoscopy* **61**, 671–678.

32 Kara MA, Peters FP, Ten Kate FJW, *et al.* (2005). Endoscopic video autofluorescence imaging may improve the detection of early neoplasia in patients with Barrett's esophagus. *Gastrointestinal Endoscopy* **61**, 679–685.

33 Curvers WL, Herrero LA, Wallace MB, *et al.* (2010). Endoscopic tri-modal imaging is more effective than standard endoscopy in identifying early-stage neoplasia in Barrett's esophagus. *Gastroenterology* **139**, 1106–1114.

34 Boerwinkel DF, Holz JA, Aalders MCG, *et al.* (2013). Third-generation autofluorescence endoscopy for the detection of early neoplasia in Barrett's esophagus: a pilot study. *Diseases of the Esophagus* **27**(3), 276–84.

35 Boerwinkel DF, Pietro M Di, Liu X, *et al.* (2012). Endoscopic TriModal imaging and biomarkers for neoplasia conjoined: a feasibility study in Barrett's esophagus. *Diseases of the Esophagus* **27**(5), 435–43.

36 Shariff KM, Pietro M di, Boerwinkel DF, *et al.* (2012). Time: A Prospective Study Combining Endoscopic Trimodal Imaging and Molecular Endpoints to Improve Risk Stratification in Barrett's Esophagus. *Gastroenterology* **142**, S165–S165.

37 Li M, Anastassiades CP, Joshi B, *et al.* (2010). Affinity peptide for targeted detection of dysplasia in Barrett's esophagus. *Gastroenterology* **139**, 1472–1480.

38 Bird-Lieberman EL, Neves AA, Lao-Sirieix P, *et al.* (2012). Molecular imaging using fluorescent lectins permits rapid endoscopic identification of dysplasia in Barrett's esophagus. *Nature Medicine* **18**, 315–321.

39 Dubuc J, Legoux J-L, Winnock M, *et al.* (2006). Endoscopic screening for esophageal squamous-cell carcinoma in high-risk patients: a prospective study conducted in 62 French endoscopy centers. *Endoscopy* **38**, 690–695.

40 Hashimoto CL, Iriya K, Baba ER, *et al.* (2005). Lugol's dye spray chromoendoscopy establishes early diagnosis of esophageal cancer in patients with primary head and neck cancer. *American Journal of Gastroenterology* **100**, 275–282.

41 Pech O, May A, Gossner L, *et al.* (2007). Curative endoscopic therapy in patients with early esophageal squamous-cell carcinoma or high-grade intraepithelial neoplasia. *Endoscopy* **39**, 30–35.

42 Ishihara R, Iishi H, Takeuchi Y, *et al.* (2008). Local recurrence of large squamous-cell carcinoma of the esophagus after endoscopic resection. *Gastrointestinal Endoscopy* **67**, 799–804.

43 Lee CT, Chang CY, Lee YC, *et al.* (2010). Narrow-band imaging with magnifying endoscopy for the screening of esophageal cancer in patients with primary head and neck cancers. *Endoscopy* **42**, 613–619.

44 Kumagai Y, Toi M, Inoue H. (2002). Dynamism of tumour vasculature in the early phase of cancer progression: outcomes from oesophageal *Cancer Research. The Lancet Oncology* **3**, 604–610.

45 Yoshida T, Inoue H, Usui S, *et al.* (2004). Narrow-band imaging system with magnifying endoscopy for superficial esophageal lesions. *Gastrointestinal Endoscopy* **59**, 288–295.

46 Lecleire S, Antonietti M, Iwanicki-Caron I, *et al.* (2011). Lugol chromo-endoscopy versus narrow band imaging for endoscopic screening of esophageal squamous-cell carcinoma in patients with a history of cured esophageal cancer: a feasibility study. *Diseases of the Esophagus* **24**, 418–422.

CHAPTER 11

New cellular imaging technologies for dysplasia and cancer detection

Helmut Neumann[1] & Ralf Kiesslich[2]

[1] Department of Medicine I, University of Erlangen-Nuremberg, Germany
[2] Department of Medicine II, Dr. Horst Schmidt Kliniken, Wiesbaden, Germany

11.1 Introduction

Barrett's esophagus (BE) represents a pre-cancerous condition in the distal esophagus, caused by gastroesophageal reflux disease [1]. Today, the most common definition of BE in Europe and the United States is that of columnar metaplasia containing goblet cells. However, in countries like Japan and the United Kingdom, any kind of columnar metaplasia in the distal esophagus is considered to be BE. It has been estimated that patients with BE have an up to 30-fold increased risk for the development of esophageal adenocarcinoma (EAC), compared with the general population, with an annual risk to develop cancer of approximately 0.5–1.0% [2, 3].

Within the past 30 years, a dramatic increase in the incidence of EAC has been noted. It is noteworthy that EAC has a poor prognosis, with an overall five-year survival rate of less than 15% when diagnosed at late stages [4]. Therefore, early diagnosis of EAC and its precursor lesions (i.e. BE) is of paramount importance to improve the outcome for affected patients. This is also highlighted by the fact that early esophageal cancer, which is still restricted to the mucosa without lymph node metastasis, can be treated endoscopically [5]. In the attempt to improve diagnosis of esophageal lesions, numerous advanced endoscopic imaging techniques have been introduced. These include wide field imaging techniques (e.g. high-definition imaging, dye-based and dye-less chromoendoscopy techniques) and small-field imaging techniques [6, 7]. The latter includes confocal laser endomicroscopy, endocytoscopy, optical coherence tomography, and molecular imaging techniques. Small-field imaging techniques allow detailed examination of cellular and sub-cellular features and are therefore also named "cellular imaging technologies".

In this review we will focus on these cellular imaging technologies for detection of esophageal lesions, including Barrett's esophagus and esophageal cancer.

11.2 Confocal laser endomicroscopy

Confocal laser endomicroscopy (CLE) was introduced in 2003, enabling the endoscopist to obtain real time *in vivo* histology during endoscopy [8]. CLE is based on tissue illumination with a low-power laser light of 488 nm wavelength, after application of fluorescence agents. These fluorescence agents can either be applied systemically or topically [9].

The most common used contrast agent for CLE is fluorescein sodium in a dilution of 10%. Dosages between 3–8 ml are administered intravenously, and the dye highlights the extracellular matrix within 5–10 seconds after injection. Potential adverse events include transient hypotension without shock (0.5%), nausea (0.39%), injection site erythema (0.35%), self-limited diffuse rash (0.04%), and mild epigastric pain (0.09%) [10]. Notably, fluorescein sodium does not allow for analysis of intercellular structures.

In order to visualize intercellular structures, one has to apply topical fluorescence agents. The most common used topically applied dye-agents are acriflavine hydrochloride and cresyl violet. While acriflavine highlights the nucleus, cresyl violet stains the cytoplasm, thereby enabling indirect visualization of the nucleus by measuring the nucleus-to-cytoplasm ratio. Recently, concerns have been raised regarding the use of acriflavine. As the dye accumulates in the nuclei of cells, potential mutagenic effects cannot be excluded. No concerns have been raised for cresyl violet.

Two types of endomicroscopy systems are available. One is integrated into the tip of a standard, high-resolution endoscope (iCLE; Pentax, Tokyo, Japan – see Figure 11.1: see also Plate 11.1), while the other is probe-based (pCLE; Cellvizio, Mauna Kea Technologies, Paris, France) and capable of passage through the working channel of a standard endoscope.

iCLE collects images at a manually adjustable scan rate of 1.6 frames per second, with a maximum resolution of 1024×1024 pixels (1 megapixel). By pushing a button on the handle of the endoscope, one can dynamically adjust the scanning depth (ranging from 0–250 μm) and also the laser power (ranging from 0–1000 μW).

For pCLE, different probes for various indications are available. pCLE devices use a dynamic laser power and a fixed imaging plane depth. Confocal images are streamed at a frame rate of 12 frames per second, thereby obtaining real-time videos of the intestinal mucosa. A special computer algorithm ("mosaicing") allows reconstruction of single video frames, either in real time or post-processed, with an increased field of view of up to 4×2 mm.

The most common used confocal probe for evaluation of esophageal disorders is the GastroFlex UHD probe. Lateral resolution of this probe is 1 μm, with a field of view of 240 μm and an imaging plane depth of 55–65 μm. For pCLE, the use of a clear distal cap to the endoscope before confocal imaging is recommended, as motion artifacts substantially impede confocal imaging at the squamocolumnar junction. Even administration of antispasmodic agents (e.g. Buscopan) may help to stabilize the confocal probe for subsequent high-magnification imaging of the mucosa.

Since the first study on CLE in BE, which was published by Kiesslich in 2006, various studies have shown the impact of CLE for *in vivo* diagnosis of BE and esophageal cancer. The initial study included 63 patients, and CLE was proven to readily identify

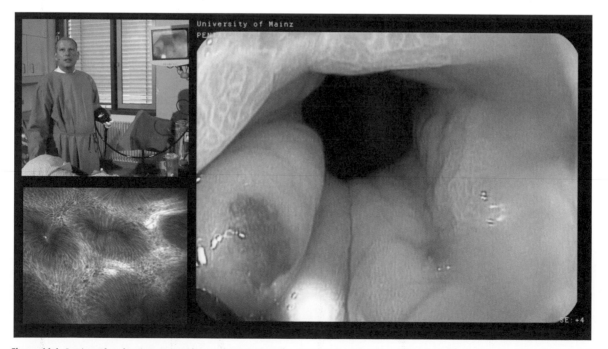

Figure 11.1 Setting of endomicroscopy. The confocal endoscope (iCLE) is handled like a conventional endoscope. The microscope is embedded in the distal tip and emits blue laser light onto the mucosa (right picture). Endomicroscopic images are displayed (lower left picture) by placing the microscope gently onto the mucosa. *(See insert for color representation of this figure.)*

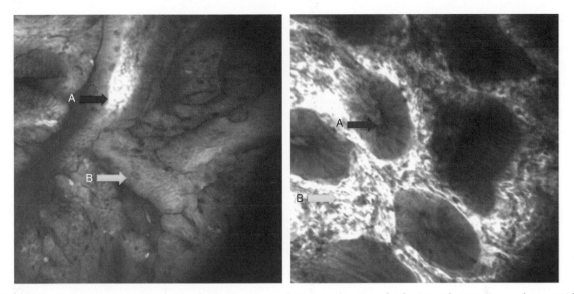

Figure 11.2 Endomicroscopy of non-dysplastic Barrett Esophagus. (Left): Superficial view of Barrett's esophagus with fluorescein-aided endomicroscopy. The villous architecture is readily seen. Single goblet cells (arrow B – defining intestinal metaplasia) and the basement membrane (arrow A) can be identified. (Right): Deeper layers of the mucosa are seen. Here, the lamina propria with the vascular network is seen (arrow A). Single Barrett glands can be identified.

specialized intestinal epithelium-containing goblet cells [8]. Goblet cells could easily be identified, as CLE displayed the mucin of goblet cells as very dark oval- to round-appearing structures within the columnar-lined epithelium (see Figures 11.2 and 11.3). Overall, confocal imaging could predict BE and associated neoplasia with a sensitivity of 98% and 93%, a specificity of 94% and 98% and an accuracy of 97%, respectively. These data have been confirmed by two prospective randomized controlled trials.

One study by Dunbar *et al.* determined whether CLE with optical biopsies and targeted mucosal biopsy has the potential to improve the diagnostic yield of endoscopically unapparent, BE-associated neoplasia, compared with standard endoscopy with a four-quadrant, random biopsy protocol [11]. It was shown that CLE with targeted biopsy almost doubled the diagnostic yield for neoplasia, and was equivalent to the standard protocol for the final diagnosis of neoplasia. Moreover, two-thirds of patients in the surveillance group did not need any mucosal biopsies at all.

Another, international multicenter study examined patients with high-definition white light endoscopy (HD-WLE), narrow-band imaging (NBI), and pCLE [12]. All suspicious lesions on HD-WLE or NBI and

four-quadrant random locations were documented. These locations were examined with pCLE, and a presumptive diagnosis of benign or neoplastic (defined as high-grade intraepithelial neoplasia or cancer) tissue was performed in real time. Finally, biopsies were taken from all locations and were reviewed blinded to endoscopic and endomicroscopic data. The study reported a sensitivity and specificity for HD-WLE of 34% and 93%, respectively, compared with 68% and 88%, respectively, for HD-WLE or pCLE, which was statistically significantly different. The sensitivity and specificity for HD-WLE or NBI were 45% and 88%, respectively, compared with 76% and 84%, respectively, for HD-WLE, NBI, or pCLE. It was concluded that pCLE combined with HD-WLE significantly improved the ability to detect neoplasia in BE patients compared with HD-WLE.

Wallace and co-workers aimed to determine the preliminary evaluation accuracy and inter-observer agreement of pCLE in BE [13]. Overall, eleven experts in advanced imaging from four different endoscopy centers from the United States and Europe evaluated the images. The sensitivity for the diagnosis of neoplasia was 88% and the specificity was 96%. Moreover, a substantial agreement on the pCLE diagnosis (86%) was noted, with a kappa value of 0.72. Endomicroscopists

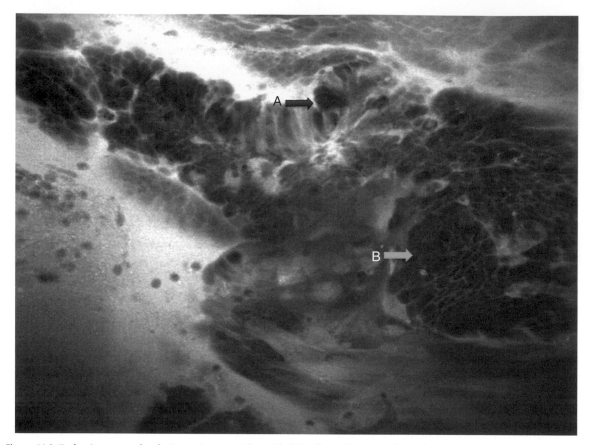

Figure 11.3 Endomicroscopy of early Barrett's cancer. The epithelial cells are disorganized and the color turns into black, which is an endomicroscopic sign of neoplasia (arrow A). Furthermore, malignant infiltration into the lamina propria is readily visible (arrow B).

with prior pCLE experience had an overall sensitivity of 91%, a specificity of 100%, and almost perfect agreement of 92%. These study results suggest that pCLE for the diagnosis of neoplasia in BE has a very high accuracy and reliability.

Various endoscopic modalities are currently available for treatment of BE, including endoscopic mucosal resection (EMR), argon plasma coagulation and radiofrequency ablation (RFA) [14]. Notably, eradication of all glandular mucosa in the distal esophagus cannot be reliably determined at endoscopy. Very recently, Wallace *et al.* assessed if use of pCLE in addition to HD-WLE could aid in determination of residual BE after mucosal ablation or resection of neoplasia in BE [15]. The study was halted at the planned interim analysis, based on *a priori* criteria. Among the 119 patients with follow-up, there was no difference in the proportion of patients achieving optimal outcomes in

the two groups (26% for HD-WLE, 27% with HD-WLE plus pCLE). Accordingly, this study does not yield any evidence that the addition of pCLE to HD-WLE for detection of residual BE or neoplasia can provide improved treatment.

11.3 Endocytoscopy

Endocytoscopy (EC; Olympus, Tokyo, Japan) is based on the principle of contact light microscopy. Endocytoscopy enables high-magnification imaging of the superficial mucosal layer up to 1390-fold. The images are displayed on a monitor at 30 frames per second. Two different types of endocytoscopy systems exist. One is integrated into the distal tip of an endoscope (iEC), while the other is probe-based (pEC) and is advanced through the accessory channel of a standard endoscope [16].

Before endocytoscopic imaging, extensive washing of the mucosa and mucolysis, which can be achieved with topical application of N-acetylcysteine, is recommended. Following these washing steps, pre-staining of the mucosa with absorptive staining agents has to be accomplished. Typically used dye agents for EC are methylene blue, toluidine blue or cresyl violet at high concentrations. The dyes are topically applied to the mucosa by using standard spraying catheters, and endocytoscopic imaging can be performed after an appropriate time of exposure of the dye (approximately 60 seconds).

One recent study from Japan allocated patients in a 1 : 1 : 1 ratio to three distinct staining methods: 0.05% cresyl violet alone, 1% methylene blue alone, or cresyl violet plus methylene blue (double staining) [17]. Normal rectal mucosa was stained with each dye, and videos of EC images were recorded. Methylene blue alone and the double staining resulted in recognizable nuclei within comparable periods of time, whereas cresyl violet alone was unable to identify nuclei. Gland formation became recognizable earlier after double staining with cresyl violet and methylene blue. Accordingly, the "double stain" approach is currently recommended for endocytoscopic imaging.

Notably, repeat staining of the mucosa is mostly necessary while using absorptive contrast agents. A clear, 4 mm hood attached to the scope, and mild suction, may help to stabilize the endoscope while obtaining high-magnification imaging of the mucosa. Interpretation of endocytoscopic images is based on architectural details (e.g. epithelial structure), cellular features (e.g. size, arrangement of cells) and vascular pattern morphology (e.g. size, leakage, and tortuosity). Most importantly endocytoscopy also allows assessment of cytological features such as the density of cells, the size and shape of nuclei, and the nucleus-to-cytoplasm ratio [18].

Currently, endocytoscopy is not commercially available in Europe or the United States, and has been mostly evaluated by Japanese colleagues for colorectal polyps and early cancer. Accordingly, only limited data are available for its use in BE and associated cancer. One early pilot study described an overall accuracy of endocytoscopy for differentiating between nonmalignant and malignant tissue of 82% [19].

Pohl *et al.* assessed the accuracy of endocytoscopy in correlation with histology at 166 biopsy sites from 16 patients [20]. Two different magnification settings were used (×1125 and ×450). Notably, adequate assessment of endocytoscopy images was impossible in 49% of the pre-marked areas with magnification ×450, and in 22% with magnification ×1125. 23% of images with lower magnification were interpretable to identify characteristics of neoplasia, and 41% with higher magnification. Inter-observer agreement was only fair at best (κ up to 0.45). Positive and negative predictive values for high grade intraepithelial neoplasia or cancer were 0.29 and 0.87, respectively, for magnification ×450 (0.44 and 0.83, for magnification ×1125). Therefore, it was concluded that endoscopic histology using endocytoscopy lacks sufficient image quality to be of assistance in identifying neoplastic areas.

Very recently, Eleftheriadis and co-workers from Kudo's group in Tokyo studied the endocytoscopic visualization of squamous cell islands within Barrett's epithelium [21]. *In vivo* high-magnification imaging using endocytoscopy visualized, after double staining, regular Barrett's epithelium, while higher magnification (×480) additionally revealed the orifices of glandular structures. Furthermore, typical squamous cell papillary protrusions were identified within regular glandular Barrett's mucosa.

11.4 Optical coherence tomography

The technique of optical coherence tomography (OCT) has recently been reviewed by the American Society for Gastrointestinal Endoscopy (ASGE) Technology Committee [22]. OCT obtains cross-sectional images of the tissue on the order of a low-power microscope. The technique is comparable to ultrasound. Instead of an acoustic signal, light is used to provide high-resolution imaging. Newer developments have yielded in frequency-domain OCT that provides faster real-time imaging. Currently, one frequency-domain OCT system is approved by the FDA. Volumetric laser endomicroscopy (VLE; Ninepoint Medical, Cambridge, MA) performs a cross-sectional scan through a 6 cm length, 3 mm deep, over a period of 90 seconds. Within this time, over 4000 longitudinal images and 1200 cross-sectional images are created. Accordingly, VLE enables visualization of the esophageal mucosa, submucosa and lamina propria at a 7 μm resolution in real time. Compared to CLE, with a field of view of approximately 0.25 mm², VLE offers a field of view of approximately 10,000 mm².

One early study demonstrated the efficacy of OCT to distinguish squamous mucosa, gastric cardia, Barrett's esophagus, and cancer [23]. In addition, OCT was proven to be reliable for identifying sub-squamous BE [24]. Evans and co-workers aimed to establish OCT image characteristics of intramucosal cancer and high-grade intraepithelial neoplasia in BE [25]. Biopsy-correlated OCT images were acquired from patients with BE, and a blinded investigator reviewed the biopsy-correlated OCT images and scored each for surface maturation and gland architecture. Sensitivity and specificity for diagnosing intramucosal cancer and high-grade intraepithelial neoplasia in BE were 83% and 75%, respectively.

Another, prospective, double-blinded study evaluated the accuracy of OCT for the diagnosis and the exclusion of dysplasia in patients with BE [26]. A total of 314 OCT images were obtained and analyzed by using histology as the reference standard. OCT showed a sensitivity, specificity, and accuracy of 68%, 82%, and 78%, respectively. Positive and negative predictive values were measured to be 53% and 89%, respectively.

Very recently, Sauk *et al.* evaluated inter- and intra-observer agreements for differentiating squamous mucosa, gastric cardia mucosa, and BE among ten readers [27]. Notably, the study showed an excellent agreement for the differentiation of BE versus non-BE mucosa ($\kappa = 0.811$) and for differentiating BE versus gastric cardia versus squamous mucosa ($\kappa = 0.866$). Most recently, OCT has also been studied after radiofrequency ablation (RFA) of BE [28, 29]. In this context, it was shown that OCT-visible glands, immediately after RFA, correlated with the presence of residual BE at follow-up (83% sensitivity, 95% specificity, 91% accuracy).

11.5 Molecular imaging in Barrett's

Endoscopic molecular imaging is based on *in vivo* visualization and characterization of disease-specific molecular alterations representing *in vivo* immunohistochemistry [30]. As molecular targets are too small for direct visualization, optically active probes, which are usually labeled with fluorescein derivatives, are used to highlight subtle changes. After application of these probes, confocal laser endomicroscopy is performed for subsequent visualization and characterization of the probe binding to a specific molecular target. Animal studies have already shown that molecular imaging of single cells is feasible. In this context, molecular targeting of somatostatin receptor-positive tumor cells *in vivo* was demonstrated in a nude mouse xenograft model after injection of a carboxyfluorescein-labeled ligand [31]. In addition, differentiation of tumor cells, based on their epithelial growth factor receptor and vascular epithelial growth factor expression patterns, was achieved *in vivo* in a rodent model with human colorectal cancer xenografts [32, 33].

Gorospe *et al.* from the Minnesota group recently analyzed the potential of CLE in detecting BE by using a novel bioprobe in *ex vivo* tissue [34]. The fluorescent glucose analog showed preferential uptake in dysplastic mucosa to supply contrast. Overall accuracy in detecting dysplasia was 79%. Very recently, a new fluorescently labeled synthetic peptide, termed ASY-FITC, that specifically targets esophageal adenocarcinoma, has been tested in humans for the first time [35]. The molecular probe enabled visualization of neoplasia in the esophagus using *in vivo* endomicroscopy, and might therefore prove useful in the early detection of esophageal adenocarcinoma. Additionally, recent data also indicated the potential of *in vivo* molecular imaging in humans for diagnosis of inflammatory bowel diseases and colonic polyps [36, 37].

11.6 Conclusion

New endoscopic cellular imaging technologies have improved our possibilities for dysplasia and cancer detection in Barrett's and esophageal cancer. Endocytoscopy enables high-magnification imaging of the very superficial mucosal layer, and has the advantage of direct nucleus visualization, thereby potentially allowing *in vivo* diagnosis of low-grade and high-grade intraepithelial neoplasia and cancer. Confocal laser endomicroscopy enables cellular imaging of architectural and cellular features up to an imaging plane depth of 250 μm.

The recently introduced frequency-domain optical coherence tomography allows visualization of the esophageal mucosa, submucosa and lamina propria at a high resolution in real time. Molecular imaging now allows *in vivo* imaging and characterization of molecular alterations in real time. It is anticipated that, within the next few years, cellular imaging techniques will open new avenues for an individualized diagnosis and therapy of patients with Barrett's esophagus and esophageal cancer.

References

1 Vieth M, Langner C, Neumann H, *et al.* (2012). Barrett's esophagus. Practical issues for daily routine diagnosis. *Pathology – Research and Practice* **208**, 261–8.

2 Tytgat GN (1995). Does endoscopic surveillance in esophageal columnar metaplasia (Barrett's esophagus) have any real value? *Endoscopy* **27**, 19–26.

3 Haggitt RC (1994). Barrett's esophagus, dysplasia and adenocarcinoma. *Human Pathology* **25**, 982–93.

4 Edge SB Byrd D Compton CC Fritz AG Greene FL, Trotti A (American joint committee of cancer) (2010). *Cancer Staging Manual* **7**, 103–115.

5 Pech O, Manner H, Ell C (2011). Endoscopic resection. *Gastrointestinal Endoscopy Clinics of North America* **21**, 81–94.

6 Neumann H, Neurath MF, Vieth M, *et al.* (2013). Innovative techniques in evaluating the esophagus; imaging of esophageal morphology and function; and drugs for esophageal disease. *Annals of the New York Academy of Sciences* **1300**, 11–28.

7 Sharma P, Savides TJ, Canto MI, *et al.* (2012). The American Society for Gastrointestinal Endoscopy PIVI (Preservation and Incorporation of Valuable Endoscopic Innovations) on imaging in Barrett's Esophagus. *Gastrointestinal Endoscopy* **76**, 252–4.

8 Kiesslich R, Gossner L, Goetz M, *et al.* (2006). *In vivo* histology of Barrett's esophagus and associated neoplasia by confocal laser endomicroscopy. *Clinical Gastroenterology and Hepatology* **4**, 979–87.

9 Neumann H, Kiesslich R, Wallace MB, *et al.* (2010). Confocal laser endomicroscopy: technical advances and clinical applications. *Gastroenterology* **139**, 388–92.

10 Wallace MB, Meining A, Canto MI, *et al* (2010). The safety of intravenous fluorescein for confocal laser endomicroscopy in the gastrointestinal tract. *Alimentary Pharmacology & Therapeutics* **31**, 548–52.

11 Dunbar KB, Okolo P 3rd, Montgomery E, *et al.* (2009). Confocal laser endomicroscopy in Barrett's esophagus and endoscopically inapparent Barrett's neoplasia: a prospective, randomized, double-blind, controlled, crossover trial. *Gastrointestinal Endoscopy* **70**, 645–54.

12 Sharma P, Meining AR, Coron E, *et al.* (2011). Real-time increased detection of neoplastic tissue in Barrett's esophagus with probe-based confocal laser endomicroscopy: final results of an international multicenter, prospective, randomized, controlled trial. *Gastrointestinal Endoscopy* **74**, 465–72.

13 Wallace MB, Sharma P, Lightdale C, *et al.* (2010). Preliminary accuracy and interobserver agreement for the detection of intraepithelial neoplasia in Barrett's esophagus with probe-based confocal laser endomicroscopy. *Gastrointestinal Endoscopy* **72**, 19–24.

14 Vieth M, Neumann H (2013). Barrett oesophagus: Is RFA the overall answer to all Barrett oesophagus issues? *Nature Reviews Gastroenterology & Hepatology* **10**, 388–9.

15 Wallace MB, Crook JE, Saunders M, *et al.* (2012). Multicenter, randomized, controlled trial of confocal laser endomicroscopy assessment of residual metaplasia after mucosal ablation or resection of GI neoplasia in Barrett's esophagus. *Gastrointestinal Endoscopy* **76**, 539–47.

16 Neumann H, Fuchs FS, Vieth M, *et al.* (2011). Review article: *in vivo* imaging by endocytoscopy. *Alimentary Pharmacology & Therapeutics* **33**, 1183–93.

17 Ichimasa K, Kudo SE, Mori Y, *et al.* (2013). Double staining with crystal violet and methylene blue is appropriate for colonic endocytoscopy: An *in vivo* prospective pilot study. *Journal of Digestive Endoscopy* **26**(3), 403–8.

18 Neumann H, Vieth M, Neurath MF, *et al.* (2013). Endocytoscopy allows accurate *in vivo* differentiation of mucosal inflammatory cells in IBD: a pilot study. *Inflammatory Bowel Diseases* **19**, 356–62.

19 Inoue H, Sasajima K, Kaga M, *et al.* (2006). Endoscopic *in vivo* evaluation of tissue atypia in the esophagus using a newly designed integrated endocytoscope: a pilot trial. *Endoscopy* **38**, 891–5.

20 Pohl H, Koch M, Khalifa A, *et al.* (2007). Evaluation of endocytoscopy in the surveillance of patients with Barrett's esophagus. *Endoscopy* **39**, 492–6.

21 Eleftheriadis N, Inoue H, Ikeda H, *et al.* (2013). Endocytoscopic visualization of squamous cell islands within Barrett's epithelium. *World Journal of Gastrointestinal Endoscopy* **5**, 174–9.

22 ASGE Technology Committee (2013). Enhanced imaging in the GI tract: spectroscopy and optical coherence tomography. *Gastrointestinal Endoscopy* **78**, 568–73.

23 Zuccaro G, Gladkova N, Vargo J, *et al.* (2001). Optical coherence tomography of the esophagus and proximal stomach in health and disease. *American Journal of Gastroenterology* **96**, 2633–9.

24 Cobb MJ, Hwang JH, Upton MP, *et al.* (2010). Imaging of subsquamous Barrett's epithelium with ultrahigh-resolution optical coherence tomography: a histologic correlation study. *Gastrointestinal Endoscopy* **71**, 223–30.

25 Evans JA, Poneros JM, Bouma BE, *et al.* (2006). Optical coherence tomography to identify intramucosal carcinoma and high-grade dysplasia in Barrett's esophagus. *Clinical Gastroenterology and Hepatology* **4**, 38–43.

26 Isenberg G, Sivak MV Jr, Chak A, *et al.* (2005). Accuracy of endoscopic optical coherence tomography in the detection of dysplasia in Barrett's esophagus: a prospective, double-blinded study. *Gastrointestinal Endoscopy* **62**, 825–31.

27 Sauk J, Coron E, Kava L, *et al.* (2013). Interobserver agreement for the detection of Barrett's esophagus with optical frequency domain imaging. *Digestive Diseases and Sciences* **58**, 2261–5.

28 Zhou C, Tsai TH, Lee HC, *et al.* (2012). Characterization of buried glands before and after radiofrequency ablation by using 3-dimensional optical coherence tomography (with videos). *Gastrointestinal Endoscopy* **76**, 32–40.

29 Tsai TH, Zhou C, Tao YK, *et al.* (2012). Structural markers observed with endoscopic 3-dimensional optical coherence tomography correlating with Barrett's esophagus radiofrequency ablation treatment response (with videos). *Gastrointestinal Endoscopy* **76**, 1104–12.

30 Kiesslich R, Goetz M, Hoffman A, *et al.* (2011). New imaging techniques and opportunities in endoscopy. *Nature Reviews Gastroenterology & Hepatology* **8**, 547–53.

31 Fottner C, Mettler E, Goetz M, *et al.* (2010). *In vivo* molecular imaging of somatostatin receptors in pancreatic islet cells and neuroendocrine tumors by miniaturized confocal laser-scanning fluorescence microscopy. *Endocrinology* **151**, 2179–88.

32 Goetz M, Ziebart A, Foersch S, *et al.* (2010). *In vivo* molecular imaging of colorectal cancer with confocal endomicroscopy by targeting epidermal growth factor receptor. *Gastroenterology* **138**, 435–46.

33 Foersch S, Kiesslich R, Waldner MJ, *et al.* (2010). Molecular imaging of VEGF in gastrointestinal cancer *in vivo* using confocal laser endomicroscopy. *Gut* **59**, 1046–55.

34 Gorospe EC, Leggett CL, Sun G, *et al.* (2012). Diagnostic performance of two confocal endomicroscopy systems in detecting Barrett's dysplasia: a pilot study using a novel bioprobe in ex vivo tissue. *Gastrointestinal Endoscopy* **76**, 933–8.

35 Sturm MB, Joshi BP, Lu S, *et al.* (2013). Targeted imaging of esophageal neoplasia with a fluorescently labeled peptide: first-in-human results. *Science Translational Medicine* **5**, 184–61.

36 Atreya R, Neumann H, Neufert C, *et al.* (2014). *In vivo* molecular imaging using fluorescent anti-TNF antibodies and confocal laser endomicroscopy predicts response to biological therapy in Crohn's. *Nature Medicine* **20**, 313–318.

37 Hsiung PL, Hardy J, Friedland S, *et al.* (2008). Detection of colonic dysplasia *in vivo* using a targeted heptapeptide and confocal microendoscopy. *Nature Medicine* **14**, 454–458.

CHAPTER 12

The role of endoscopic ultrasound in esophageal cancer

Samad Soudagar & Neil Gupta

Division of Gastroenterology and Nutrition, Loyola University Medical Center, Maywood, IL, USA

12.1 Background

Endoscopic ultrasound (EUS) has been a revolutionary tool in aiding diagnosis and management for gastrointestinal (GI) disease processes, including esophageal, gastric, rectal, and pancreato-biliary malignancies. With regards to esophageal cancer, the high-resolution images that EUS provides of the GI tract, along with associated extraluminal organs, including the mediastinum and nearby lymph nodes, has allowed a stark improvement in disease staging over prior "gold standards", including computed tomography (CT) scans and positron emission tomography (PET) imaging. As a consequence, the addition of EUS to esophageal cancer staging has allowed for a more accurate pre-treatment staging. This, in turn, has resulted in better treatment stratification as to which patients should be managed endoscopically, surgically, or with neoadjuvant chemotherapy and/or radiotherapy.

12.2 Equipment

Initial EUS equipment developed in the 1980s consisted of radial scanning echoendoscopes, which combined regular viewing GI luminal endoscopes with ultrasonography. These endoscopes have an ultrasound transducer attached at the tip, which has the capability of being rotated 360° and provides a cross-sectional view of the surrounding GI tract and associated extraluminal structures, perpendicular to the long axis or direction of insertion of the endoscope. The transducer is surrounded by a balloon, which is insufflated with water

and allows for the creation of a water interface between the ultrasound probe and GI lumen, eliminating artifact and allowing for high quality and accurate images. Proximal to the ultrasound is the endoscopic viewing optic, which provides an oblique view of the GI lumen and intended lesion.

In addition, the development of the curvilinear echoendoscope has been used to provide targeted, non-oblique (in contrast to the radial echoendoscope) ultrasound images for the intention of fine needle aspiration (FNA). Specifically, the linear scope provides images at an angle of 80–105° from its long axis or from the angle of insertion. FNA can be performed by varying sizes of needles (i.e. 19, 22, 25 gauge), introduced through the tip of the endoscope, with concurrent ultrasound guided visualization of the intended lesion.

These standard echoendoscopes usually use ultrasound frequencies between 5–12 MHz and allow penetration of depths 5–6 cm from the transducer. The images obtained are, however, often limited, due to their lower resolution. Higher-clarity images have thus been pursued through the use of high-frequency ultrasound probes or miniprobes, which are typically inserted through the working channel of a standard endoscope. By using ultrasound frequencies between 12–20 MHz (and even up to 30 MHz), higher-resolution images can be obtained, although limited in depth of penetration to 1–2 cm [1].

12.3 Visualized EUS anatomy

When examining the esophageal lumen, the five normal-appearing alternating hyper- and hypo-echoic layers of the esophagus can be seen, in order to assess any overt esophageal wall abnormalities. From closest to the ultrasound, the layers identified by a typical echoendoscope operating at frequencies between 5–12 MHz are as follows: superficial mucosa; deep mucosa; submucosa; muscularis propria; and serosa or adventitia. A high-frequency US probe operating at higher frequencies can provide a more detailed view of lumen through visualization of nine esophageal wall layers. Proper identification of these layers is of extreme importance in the process of accurately staging disease.

EUS also provides visualization of several lymph node chains often relevant in the staging of esophageal cancer. These include nodes in the posterior and inferior mediastinum, consisting of paraesophageal and pulmonary ligament chains, along with posteriorly located subcarinal nodes. Additionally, the left lower paratracheal nodes are accessible by EUS, with variable evaluation possible of the upper paratracheal, right lower paratracheal, and aortopulmonary nodal chains (depending on size, proximity to esophagus, and distance from trachea). Chains located in the anterior upper mediastinum usually cannot be visualized by EUS, due to air interference within the trachea [2]. Other visualized lymph nodes include celiac and cervical chains, with celiac nodal identification appearing to have the highest endosonographic accuracy.

Distant organ metastases can also be evaluated using EUS. These include the left adrenal gland, which is most effectively visualized by EUS, providing a 98% accuracy versus 69% for transabdominal ultrasound [3]. Liver metastases can also be seen using EUS, as there is a role for liver surveillance using EUS in patients in whom traditional imaging modalities are non-diagnostic [4]. Using EUS to evaluate the esophageal lumen, associated nearby lymph nodes, and distant organs that may have metastases, is essential in definitively staging esophageal disease.

12.4 Obstacles to accurate EUS staging

Approximately 20–40% of patients with esophageal adenocarcinoma present with high-grade malignant stenosis, precluding endosonographic visualization using the standard echoendoscopes that are routinely available [5–7]. Appropriate staging of tumors requires pre-EUS dilation of these strictures, utilizing Savary or balloon dilation of the lumen to facilitate echoendoscope passage. Utilizing this method, one study noted advanced disease (stage III/IV) in 90% of patients with malignant strictures [8], while others noted T3/T4 disease in 29–78% of patients, with nodal involvement in 75% and distal metastases in 10% [9, 10]. An additional study noted upstaging of disease in 19% of patients following stricture dilation and subsequent echoendoscope staging [11].

As seen with these studies, the presence of malignant strictures is usually indicative of higher-stage, more locally advanced disease, which is typically not amenable to surgical resection. Therefore, although associated with an increased risk of perforation (reported to be as high as 24%) [5], dilation of malignant strictures is frequently necessary to stage and dictate initial therapy. However, the presence of a malignant stricture that prevents complete EUS examination may be a predictive marker for individuals who may not be surgical candidates. As a result, it remains uncertain whether routine pre-dilation of these strictures to complete EUS examination actually changes the clinical management of the patient's cancer.

Alternative means to stage these patients in lieu of esophageal dilation include the use of ultrasound probes (including high-frequency and wire-guided) which, with their small-caliber diameter, can often be advanced through partially obstructing tumors. Although this often allows for complete endosonographic visualization of the tumor and peri-tumoral area with similar accuracy to standard echoendoscopes, its yield, as noted above, is limited due to greater depths of invasion and its lack of ability to perform FNA.

Apart from such mechanical/structural limitations to EUS functionality, variability in operator findings can also compromise the accuracy of EUS findings. Data has shown that the extent of disease, and the experience of echoendosonographers in interpreting EUS, can influence whether agreement can be reached during T staging. For example, inexperienced endosonographers have been shown to disagree with regards to all stages of T disease (particularly T4), while even those categorized as experienced have shown disagreement when dealing with T2 staging [12–14]. One study found over-staging of T disease by all operators 14% of the time, with under-staging being more common (28%) by inexperienced operators, compared to 3% with experienced ones [15]. These findings suggest that experienced operators are less likely to miss the extent of tumor invasion, avoiding costly errors when staging patients and determining subsequent management.

Inexperienced operator errors are thought to contribute to the relative lack of agreement with their peers and can occur for a range of reasons, including a lack of understanding of echo-anatomy (precluding appropriate visualization of target lesion), to inappropriate delineation between esophageal layers due to improper ultrasound technique. To reach a suitable number of EUS examinations that would minimize these errors and variability in findings, studies have concluded that reliable results can be obtained after more than 75–100 EUS examinations have been performed by the operator. This has been shown to have a dramatic increase in diagnostic accuracy of T staging from as low as 60% to as high as 90%, attributed to a learning effect gained with experience from additional examinations [15, 16].

However, a more recent study dealing with experienced endosonographers defined by even greater EUS examinations (>100–300) showed that even high EUS examination experience may still not prevent high inter-observer variability [17]. These findings suggest that, although increasing operator experience is likely to yield an improvement in diagnostic yields, EUS findings remain subjective and operator-dependent.

12.5 Esophageal cancer staging and impact on treatment intervention

EUS has provided an important means of appropriately staging esophageal cancer (Table 12.1), and is recommended by multiple societies, including the National Comprehensive Cancer Network (NCCN) and several American and European gastroenterology and oncologic societies [18–20].

The role of EUS is even more pronounced when noting that the prognosis of esophageal disease has been shown to depend on the extent of primary tumor invasion and the presence of lymph node or organ metastases, all of which can be routinely determined by EUS [21]. By accurately determining tumor depth using EUS, the extent of metastases can be predicted, noting correlations between the two factors. For instance, localized disease for T1a has only a 5–9% chance of lymph node metastasis compared with T1b disease, which has a markedly higher 19–44% chance of metastasis [22–24]. As a result, T1b disease has a lower five-year survival rate ($\approx$58%) versus T1a disease

Table 12.1 Esophageal cancer TNM staging.

Primary tumor (T stage)	
TX	Primary tumor cannot be assessed.
T0	No evidence of primary tumor.
Tis	High-grade dysplasia.
T1	Tumor invades lamina propria, muscularis mucosae, or submucosa.
T1a	Tumor invades lamina propria or muscularis mucosae.
T1b	Tumor invades submucosa.
T2	Tumor invades muscularis propria.
T3	Tumor invades adventitia.
T4	Tumor invades adjacent structures.
T4a	Resectable tumor invading pleura, pericardium, or diaphragm.
T4b	Unresectable tumor invading other adjacent structures, such as aorta, vertebral body, trachea, etc.
Regional lymph nodes (N stage)	
NX	Regional lymph nodes cannot be assessed.
N0	No regional lymph node metastasis.
N1	Metastases in 1–2 regional lymph nodes.
N2	Metastases in 3–6 regional lymph nodes.
N3	Metastases in $\geq$ 7 regional lymph nodes.
Distant metastasis (M stage)	
M0	No distant metastasis.
M1	Distant metastasis.

($\approx$91%) [25]. Consequently, accurate pre-treatment staging is important in risk stratifying these patients to determine the appropriate initial therapy, while avoiding invasive treatments in those patients who would not benefit from such therapy.

12.6 T staging

Prior standards of treatment for esophageal cancer consisted solely of surgical resection, with the possible addition of neoadjuvant or definitive chemotherapy. The introduction of advanced endoscopic methods, including endoscopic mucosal resection (EMR), has provided another means of treating less invasive, localized cancer. Determining which of these treatments is pursued depends primarily on the extent of esophageal wall disease involvement, as determined by EUS, which has become the "gold standard" method for T staging of pre-treatment esophageal disease.

12.6.1 Staging for endoscopic versus surgical resection candidates

The role for endoscopic resection (EMR) largely depends on the extent to which EUS provides accurate superficial disease staging. Specifically, T1a disease (limited to the lamina propria with or without muscularis mucosa involvement) can often be treated with endoscopic resection, while T1b (invading the submucosa) is referred for surgical intervention. This differentiation is all the more important when considering that EMR provides a markedly lower morbidity (1–3%) and mortality rate (0%), along with quality of life, when compared to esophageal surgery [26, 27].

Data regarding EUS accuracy for submucosal invasion has varied, with rates found to be as low as 33% to as high as 85%, with some concern for under-diagnosis in up to two-thirds of patients. Citing such conflicting findings over the past decades, a comprehensive meta-analysis, focusing solely on superficial esophageal cancer (T1a and T1b) disease, utilized 19 studies and over 1000 patients, and reported a sensitivity and specificity of 85% and 87%, respectively, for T1a staging and 86% for both with T1b staging [28]. These high rates of superficial T staging indicate that EUS has a strong role in dictating possible endoscopic versus surgical therapy in these patients. However, the performance of EUS still remains sub-optimal when compared to staging EMR and, therefore, EUS should not replace a staging EMR in patients without clear tumor invasion into the muscularis propria, who may be candidates for endoscopic therapy.

To further expand on this differentiation and guide management, these superficial esophageal lesions are being evaluated increasingly by high-frequency ultrasound probes, which often allow better differentiation of tumor invasion through layers of the esophageal wall (80–90% diagnostic accuracy rate for mucosal and submucosal invasion versus 70–80% for standard, radial EUS) [29]. The potential drawback for this improved superficial T staging is the lower depth of penetration that the higher-frequency ultrasound probes provide. This often prevents appropriate nodal metastatic evaluation, as seen with two studies noting lower nodal diagnostic accuracy rates with probe-based EUS versus those provided by traditional radial EUS (48% versus 90% and 56% to 67%, respectively) [29, 30]. High-frequency probes may also compromise evaluation of the thickness of tumor as it extends through the esophageal wall and beyond. To prevent such a possible compromise in staging, it may be prudent to use high-frequency probes in patients in whom there is a high degree of suspicion of superficial cancer burden that may be amenable to EMR.

12.6.2 Staging for surgical resection versus neoadjuvant chemoradiotherapy candidates

Individuals with T1b and T2 disease without lymph node metastases are candidates for esophagectomy as the initial therapeutic approach. Greater tumor invasion (T3/T4, Figure 12.1), with or without nodal involvement, is generally treated with neoadjuvant chemoradiotherapy. Therefore, as the extent of disease burden, as determined by T staging, determines which of these treatments to proceed with, it is essential that accurate T staging be obtained.

EUS has become the diagnostic tool of choice for local staging, as seen through several studies noting high diagnostic yields for T staging. For example, two comprehensive meta-analyses, which included 13 and 43 studies, respectively, found sensitivities for EUS mediated T staging ranging from 70% to greater than 80% for T1 and T2 staging and > 90% for T3 and T4 staging [31, 32]. Specificities for disease staging were also high (>90%) and trending to 96% and 97% for T2 and T4 staging respectively [19].

An additional study, when evaluating for more extensive disease, showed that EUS can detect T4 lesions at rates as high as 86% [33]. To further aid overall disease staging, extra-esophageal tumor extension was predicted in one study with high accuracy (>90%) for T3/T4 lesions that were at least 16 mm in thickness by EUS, with lesions less than 8 mm predicted to be T1/T2 lesions [34]. By providing data that can, therefore, predict disease burden, while also yielding highly accurate T staging, EUS is a necessary and integral component of determining treatment (surgery versus neoadjuvant radiotherapy) for esophageal tumors, whose management is often predicated on the extent of their local T stage of disease.

12.6.3 Staging using EUS versus other imaging modalities

When comparing diagnostic yields for T staging, EUS has been noted to have a higher accuracy compared to previously used "gold standard" staging modalities.

One study comparing patients with esophageal cancer noted a higher accuracy for EUS (71%) versus that of CT

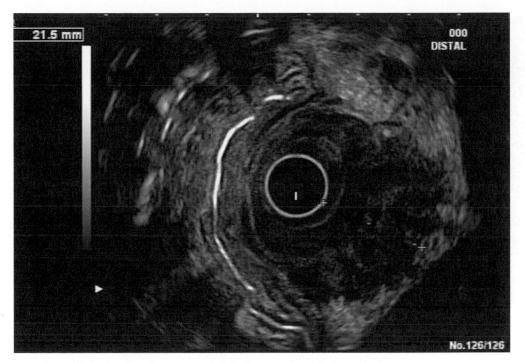

Figure 12.1 Esophageal lesion invading the esophageal wall adventitia, designated as T3 tumor.

and PET imaging (42%) [35], while an additional study noted an accuracy of 90% for EUS versus 50% with CT [36]. Additional studies comparing non-EUS imaging modalities (CT and PET) showed sensitivity and specificity rates ranging from 40–65% and 35–85% for T staging, which are less than the EUS rates in comparable studies (70–90%) [35–37].

12.7   N staging

Nodal disease involvement is of great importance when determining whether surgical (T1b or T2 disease in absence of nodal metastases) or neoadjuvant chemoradiotherapy (nodal involvement) interventions are to be pursued.

12.7.1   Staging for neoadjuvant chemoradiotherapy candidates (nodal disease)

The presence of malignant lymph nodes portends a worse survival rate for patients, with one study noting median survival rates of 66, 14.5, and 6.5 months for 0, 1–2, and greater than 2 malignant appearing lymph

nodes on EUS, respectively [38]. EUS is able to evaluate nodal involvement in the mediastinal, paraesophageal, celiac, peri-gastric, gastrohepatic ligament, and cervical regions, which can be routinely involved in more extensive esophageal cancer.

Of these, EUS appears to provide the greatest diagnostic accuracy for celiac nodes. One study noted a sensitivity and specificity of malignancy diagnosis of 83% and 98% for celiac nodes, versus 79% and 63% for mediastinal lymph nodes [39]. Typical EUS findings suggestive of lymph node involvement include size greater than 1 cm, round shape, well defined/smooth border, and hypoechoic pattern (Figure 12.2). The presence of all four features predicts malignancy in 80–100% of lymph nodes [40, 41].

The diagnostic yield of detecting malignancy in suspicious lymph nodes is aided by the use of FNA to confirm malignancy. One study noted an accuracy of 90% for EUS with FNA, compared to 70% for EUS alone [42], when evaluating for malignant lymph nodes. This finding was further verified by a meta-analysis of 44 studies that found an improvement in diagnostic accuracy from 85% with EUS to 97% when EUS was combined with FNA [32]. An additional study noted upgrading of tumor staging following lymph node sampling in 80% of

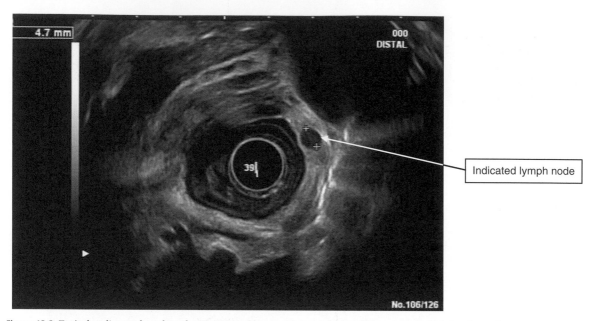

Figure 12.2 Typical malignant lymph node, represented by round shape, hypoechoic nature, well defined margins.

patients with a change in management indicated, based on the adjusted loco-regional staging in 20% [43].

12.7.2   Staging using EUS versus other modalities

EUS has been noted to have a significantly higher diagnostic accuracy for nodal staging over alternative modalities. A meta-analysis showed that EUS and EUS with FNA had higher sensitivity for detecting regional lymph node metastases (80%), compared with CT (50%) and PET-CT (57%) [44]. Two studies evaluating patients with esophageal cancer undergoing perioperative staging noted that EUS and EUS with FNA had higher diagnostic accuracies (60–90%) when identifying regional lymph nodes versus CT (27–60%) [45, 46]. Remarkably, both studies showed that EUS findings of lymph node involvement directly changed patient management (avoiding direct surgery) in 34% [45] and 77% [46] of these patients, respectively.

12.8   M staging

The role of EUS in evaluating for metastatic lesions remains limited, and is usually deferred to alternative diagnostic modalities. However, EUS is able to effectively visualize distant lymph node involvement, primarily of celiac lymph nodes, which had previously been constituted as metastatic disease (now regional). Additional EUS yield arises from visualization of liver metastases (if non-diagnostic using other modalities), the left adrenal gland (higher diagnostic accuracy than abdominal ultrasound), and through FNA aspiration of ascites fluid to confirm malignant cytology.

Alternative imaging modalities, such as PET/CT imaging, however, remain the standard for evaluating metastatic disease. Of these, PET CT appears to be superior to CT, with higher sensitivities, specificities and accuracy for detecting metastatic lesions, most often through detection of distant involved lymph nodes [47].

12.9   Restaging after chemoradiotherapy and surveillance for disease recurrence

EUS is often used for restaging purposes, following neoadjuvant chemoradiotherapy, to dictate whether a potentially resectable tumor exists. Its role for restaging has been a source of controversy, due to variable rates of diagnostic accuracy after neoadjuvant therapy.

One study, evaluating patients post-neoadjuvant chemotherapy, noted a relatively low EUS mediated diagnostic yield of 60% for T and N staging, as verified on post-surgical resection pathological staging [48]. Other, similar studies have noted lower accuracy rates for tumor burden post-treatment, ranging from 17% to 50% for T staging and 38–71% for N staging in varying post-chemoradiotherapy populations [49–51]. This decreased accuracy is thought to be from operator over-staging of disease, resulting from post-treatment fibrosis being mistaken for residual tumor. Similarly, treatment non-responders in these populations had a significantly higher diagnostic accuracy for staging than responders (95% to 26%), likely due to lack of tumor response to treatment, and corresponding minimal tumor distortion and higher architecture preservation [48].

Other methods of restaging disease have also been pursued, including assessing response to treatment by evaluating for a decrease in tumor size. Studies have shown that a greater than 50% reduction in maximal cross-sectional area of the mass post-treatment predicts tumor regression, with an EUS mediated positive predictive value of 80% via this assessment [52]. Although this method is yet to be uniformly applied for restaging purposes, it provides an additional means of stratifying patients who would likely be downstaged at post-treatment surgical resection (responders).

In addition to restaging disease following treatment, EUS has a role in evaluating for recurrence in those who have received definitive treatment. Often, these patients present without overt signs of malignancy (negative endoscopic and radiographic evaluation), but may still have localized findings that can be endosono-graphically identified. Higher diagnostic accuracies have been noted for cancer recurrence with EUS in asymp-tomatic patients post-surgical resection, compared with endoscopy or radiographic evaluation. One study evalu-ating asymptomatic patients post esophagectomy noted a sensitivity and specificity of 100% and 96%, respec-tively, for EUS-mediated diagnosis of disease recurrence [53]. Several additional studies have appreciated simi-larly high sensitivities and specificities of greater than 90% for loco-regional disease recurrence [54, 55].

Although evidence exists to suggest that up to two-thirds of patients who have disease recurrence are asymptomatic, and that EUS may provide an effective means for diagnosing early loco-regional recurrence in them (thus allowing early, timely intervention) [56], it is unclear whether there is a survival benefit from such routine surveillance. Thus, the role of EUS in post-treatment management is unclear, and more data are required to definitively institute such a surveillance protocol. The decision to pursue EUS should, therefore, be made based on a patient's symptomatic presentation or, if suspicion of disease recurrence remains high in an asymptomatic patient, especially in the setting of a negative endoscopic or radiographic examination.

12.10 Conclusion/summary

EUS has been an evolving clinical tool in the care of esophageal cancer since its inception in practice two decades ago. It is critical to the appropriate staging of loco-regional disease. In conjunction with additional imaging modalities, including PET and CT imaging, EUS allows for prognosis of the course of the disease and dictates corresponding treatment interventions. Its accuracy for detecting tumor depth to assess T staging and lymph node involvement is high, with sensitivities and specificities greater than 80–90%. This allows treat-ing physicians to adjust and alter treatment regimens confidently, allowing for timely neoadjuvant chemora-diotherapy if indicated, while preventing unnecessary comorbid surgical resections when inappropriate.

Although limitations to EUS remain, the clinical data added to a patient's case is invaluable, and EUS is now routinely recommended for pre-treatment staging in esophageal cancer. Additionally, there appears to be a role, although somewhat limited, in restaging patients following treatment and, possibly, in surveillance for disease recurrence. As the incidence of esophageal cancer continues to rise worldwide, the use of EUS continues to expand and evolve, and will remain a cornerstone of management.

References

1 Byrne M, Jowell PS (2002). Gastrointestinal imaging: endo-scopic ultrasound. *Gastro* **122**, 1631–1648.
2 Jue TL, Sharaf RN, Appalaneni V, *et al.* (2011). Role of EUS for the evaluation of mediastinal adenopathy. *Gastrointestinal Endoscopy* **74**(2), 239–45.
3 Dietrich CF, Wehrmann T, Hoffmann C *et al.* (1997). Detec-tion of the adrenal glands by endoscopic or transabdominal ultrasound. *Endoscopy* **29**(9), 859–64.

4 Prasad P, Schmulewitz N, Patel A *et al.* (2004). Detection of occult liver metastases during EUS for staging of malignancies. *Gastrointestinal Endoscopy* **59**(1), 49–53.

5 Van Dam J, Rice TW, Catalano MF, Kirby T, Sivak MV, Jr. (1993). High-grade malignant stricture is predictive of esophageal tumor stage. Risks of endosonographic evaluation. *Cancer* **71**(10), 2910–7.

6 Hancock SM, Gopal DV, Frick TJ, Pfau PR (2011). Dilation of malignant strictures in endoscopic ultrasound staging of esophageal cancer and metastatic spread of disease. *Diagnostic and Therapeutic Endoscopy* 356538.

7 Jacobson BC, Shami VM, Faigel DO, Larghi A, Kahaleh M, Dye C, *et al.* (2007). Through-the-scope balloon dilation for endoscopic ultrasound staging of stenosing esophageal cancer. *Digestive Diseases and Sciences* **52**(3), 817–22.

8 Catalano MF, Van Dam J, Sivak MV, Jr. (1995). Malignant esophageal strictures: staging accuracy of endoscopic ultrasonography. *Gastrointestinal Endoscopy* **41**(6), 535–9.

9 Kallimanis GE, Gupta PK, al-Kawas FH, Tio LT, Benjamin SB, Bertagnolli ME, *et al.* (1995). Endoscopic ultrasound for staging esophageal cancer, with or without dilation, is clinically important and safe. *Gastrointestinal Endoscopy* **41**(6), 540–6.

10 Pfau PR, Ginsberg GG, Lew RJ, Faigel DO, Smith DB, Kochman ML (2000). Esophageal dilation for endosonographic evaluation of malignant esophageal strictures is safe and effective. *American Journal of Gastroenterology* **95**(10), 2813–5.

11 Wallace MB, Hawes RH, Sahai AV, Van Velse A, Hoffman BJ (2000). Dilation of malignant esophageal stenosis to allow EUS guided fine-needle aspiration: safety and effect on patient management. *Gastrointestinal Endoscopy* **51**(3), 309–13.

12 Catalano MF, Sivak MV Jr, Bedford RA, *et al.* (1995). Observer variation and reproducibility of endoscopic ultrasonography. *Gastrointestinal Endoscopy* **41**, 115.

13 Burtin P, Napoleon B, Palazzo L *et al.* (1996). Interob server agreement in endoscopic ultrasonography staging of esophageal and cardia cancer. *Gastrointestinal Endoscopy* **43**(1), 20–4.

14 Burtin P, Berg P, Bour B, *et al.* (1995). Evaluation of the teaching of echo-endoscopy. Application to the assessment of invasiveness of cancer of the esophagus and the cardia. *Gastroentérologie Clinique et Biologiqu* **19**, 15.

15 Fockens P, Van den Brande JH, van Dullemen HM, *et al.* (1996). Endosonographic T-staging of esophageal carcinoma: a learning curve. *Gastrointestinal Endoscopy* **44**, 58.

16 Schlick T, Heintz A, Junginger T (1999). The examiner's learning effect and its influence on the quality of endoscopic ultrasonography in carcinoma of the esophagus and gastric cardia. *Surgical Endoscopy* **13**, 894.

17 Meining A, Rösch T, Wolf A, *et al.* (2003). High inter-observer variability in endosonographic staging of upper gastrointestinal cancers. *Zeitschrift für Gastroenterologie* **41**(5), 391–4.

18 Ajani JA, Barthel JS, Bentrem DJ, D'Amico TA, Das P, Denlinger CS, *et al.* (2011). Esophageal and esophagogastric junction cancers. *Journal of the National Comprehensive Cancer Network* **9**(8), 830–87.

19 Allum WH, Blazeby JM, Griffin SM, Cunningham D, Jankowski JA, Wong R (2011). Guidelines for the management of oesophageal and gastric cancer. *Gut* **60**(11), 1449–72.

20 Stahl M, Budach W, Meyer HJ, Cervantes A (2010). Esophageal cancer: Clinical Practice Guidelines for diagnosis, treatment and follow-up. *Annals of Oncology* **21**(Suppl 5), v46–9.

21 Daly JM, Karnell LH, Menck HR (1996). National Cancer Data Base report on esophageal carcinoma. *Cancer* **78**, 1820–1828.

22 Ide H, Nakamura T, Hayashi K, *et al.* (1994). Esophageal squamous cell carcinoma: pathology and prognosis. *World Journal of Surgery* **18**, 321–330

23 [No authors listed] (2003). The Paris endoscopic classification of superficial neoplastic lesions: esophagus, stomach, and colon: November 30 to December 1, 2002. *Gastrointestinal Endoscopy* **58**(6 Suppl), S3–S43.

24 Kodama M, Kakegawa T (1998). Treatment of superficial cancer of the esophagus: a summary of responses to a questionnaire on superficial cancer of the esophagus in Japan . *Surgery* **123**, 432–439.

25 Liu L, Hofstetter WL, Rashid A, *et al.* (2005). Significance of the depth of tumor invasion and lymph node metastasis in superficially invasive (T1) esophageal adenocarcinoma. *American Journal of Surgical Pathology* **29**(8), 1079–85.

26 Crumley AB, Going JJ, Mcewan K, *et al.* (2011). Endoscopic mucosal resection for gastroesophageal cancer in a U.K. population (Long-term follow-up of a consecutive series). *Surgical Endoscopy* **25**, 543–548.

27 Pech O, Behrens A, May A, *et al.* (2008). Long-term results and risk factor analysis for recurrence after curative endoscopic therapy in 349 patients with high-grade intraepithelial neoplasia and mucosal adenocarcinoma in Barrett's oesophagus. *Gut* **57**, 1200–1206.

28 Thosani N, Singh H, Kapadia A, *et al.* (2012). Diagnostic accuracy of EUS in differentiating mucosal versus submucosal invasion of superficial esophageal cancers: a systematic review and meta-analysis. *Gastrointestinal Endoscopy* **75**, 242.

29 Hasegawa N, Niwa Y, Arisawa T, *et al.* (1996). Preoperative staging of superficial esophageal carcinoma: comparison of an ultrasound probe and standard endoscopic ultrasonography. *Gastrointestinal Endoscopy* **44**, 388.

30 Nesje LB, Svanes K, Viste A, *et al.* (2000). Comparison of a linear miniature ultrasound probe and a radial-scanning echoendoscope in TN staging of esophageal cancer. *Scandinavian Journal of Gastroenterology* **35**, 997.

31 Kelly S, Harris KM, Berry E, *et al.* (2001). A systematic review of the staging performance of endoscopic

ultrasound in gastro-oesophageal carcinoma. *Gut* **49**, 534–539.

32 Puli SR, Reddy JB, Bechtold ML, *et al.* (2008). Staging accuracy of esophageal cancer by endoscopic ultrasound: a meta-analysis and systematic review. *World Journal of Gastroenterology* **14**(10), 1479–90.

33 Rösch T (1995). Endosonographic staging of esophageal cancer: a review of literature results. *Gastrointestinal Endoscopy Clinics of North America* **5**, 537.

34 Brugge WR, Lee MJ, Carey RW, Mathisen DJ (1997). Endoscopic ultrasound staging criteria for esophageal cancer. *Gastrointestinal Endoscopy* **45**, 147.

35 Lowe VJ, Booya F, Fletcher JG, *et al.* (2005). Comparison of positron emission tomography, computed tomography, and endoscopic ultrasound in the initial staging of patients with esophageal cancer. *Molecular Imaging and Biology* **7**, 422.

36 Massari M, Cioffi U, De Simone M, *et al.* (1997). Endoscopic ultrasonography by preoperative staging of esophageal carcinoma. *Surgical Laparoscopy, Endoscopy & Percutaneous Techniques* **7**, 162.

37 Meltzer CC, Luketich JD, Friedman D, *et al.* (2000). Whole-body FDG positron emission tomographic imaging for staging esophageal cancer comparison with computed tomography. *Clinical Nuclear Medicine* **25**(11), 882–7.

38 Chen J, Xu R, .Hunt GC, *et al.* (2006). Influence of the number of malignant regional lymph nodes detected by endoscopic ultrasonography on survival stratification in esophageal adenocarcinoma. *Clinical Gastroenterology and Hepatology* **4**(5), 573–9.

39 Catalano MF, Alcocer E, Chak A, *et al.* (1999). Evaluation of metastatic celiac axis lymph nodes in patients with esophageal carcinoma: accuracy of EUS. *Gastrointestinal Endoscopy* **50**, 352.

40 Catalano MF, Sivak MV Jr, Rice T, *et al.* (1994). Endosonographic features predictive of lymph node metastasis. *Gastrointestinal Endoscopy* **40**, 442.

41 Bhutani MS, Hawes RH, Hoffman BJ (1997). A comparison of the accuracy of echo features during endoscopic ultrasound (EUS) and EUS-guided fine-needle aspiration for diagnosis of malignant lymph node invasion. *Gastrointestinal Endoscopy* **45**, 474.

42 Vazquez-Sequeiros E, Norton ID, Clain JE, *et al.* (2001). Impact of EUS-guided fine-needle aspiration on lymph node staging in patients with esophageal carcinoma. *Gastrointestinal Endoscopy* **53**, 751.

43 Giovannini M, Monges G, Seitz JF, *et al.* (1999). Distant lymph node metastases in esophageal cancer: impact of endoscopic ultrasound-guided biopsy. *Endoscopy* **31**, 536.

44 van Vliet EP, Heijenbrok-Kal MH, Hunink MG, *et al.* (2008). Staging investigations for oesophageal cancer: a meta-analysis. *British Journal of Cancer* **98**, 547.

45 Pfau PR, Perlman SB, Stanko P, *et al.* (2007). The role and clinical value of EUS in a multimodality esophageal carcinoma staging program with CT and positron emission tomography. *Gastrointestinal Endoscopy* **65**(3), 377–84.

46 Vazquez-Sequeiros E, Wiersema MJ, Clain JE, *et al.* (2003). Impact of lymph node staging on therapy of esophageal carcinoma. *Gastroenterology* **125**, 1626.

47 Yoon YC, Lee KS, Shim YM, *et al.* (2003). Metastasis to regional lymph nodes in patients with esophageal squamous cell carcinoma: CT versus FDG PET for presurgical detection prospective study. *Radiology* **227**(3), 764–70.

48 Ribeiro A, Franceschi D, Parra J, *et al.* (2006). Endoscopic ultrasound restaging after neoadjuvant chemotherapy in esophageal cancer. *American Journal of Gastroenterology* **101**(6), 1216–21.

49 Zuccaro G Jr, Rice TW, Goldblum J, *et al.* (1999). Endoscopic ultrasound cannot determine suitability for esophagectomy after aggressive chemoradiotherapy for esophageal cancer. *American Journal of Gastroenterology* **94**, 906.

50 Schneider PM, Metzger R, Schaefer H, *et al.* (2008)Response evaluation by endoscopy, rebiopsy, and endoscopic ultrasound does not accurately predict histopathologic regression after neoadjuvant chemoradiation for esophageal cancer. *Annals of Surgery* **248**, 902.

51 Laterza E, de Manzoni G, Guglielmi A, *et al.* (1999). Endoscopic ultrasonography in the staging of esophageal carcinoma after preoperative radiotherapy and chemotherapy. *Annals of Thoracic Surgery* **67**, 1466.

52 Willis J, Cooper GS, Isenberg G, *et al.* (2002). Correlation of EUS measurement with pathologic assessment of neoadjuvant therapy response in esophageal carcinoma. *Gastrointestinal Endoscopy* **55**, 655.

53 Catalano MF, Sivak MV Jr, Rice TW, Van Dam J (1995). Postoperative screening for anastomotic recurrence of esophageal carcinoma by endoscopic ultrasonography. *Gastrointestinal Endoscopy* **42**, 540.

54 Müller C, Kähler G, Scheele J (2000). Endosonographic examination of gastrointestinal anastomoses with suspected locoregional tumor recurrence. *Surgical Endoscopy* **14**, 45.

55 Lightdale CJ, Botet JF, Kelsen DP, *et al.* (1989). Diagnosis of recurrent upper gastrointestinal cancer at the surgical anastomosis by endoscopic ultrasound. *Gastrointestinal Endoscopy* **35**(5), 407–12.

56 Fockens P, Manshanden CG, van Lanschot JJ, *et al.* (1997). Prospective study on the value of endosonographic follow-up after surgery for esophageal carcinoma. *Gastrointestinal Endoscopy* **46**, 487.

CHAPTER 13

Staging of esophageal adenocarcinoma by CT, PET, and other modalities

Florian Lordick[1], Katja Ott[2], Matthias Ebert[3], Lars Grenacher[4], Bernd-Joachim Krause[5] & Christian Wittekind[6]

[1] University Cancer Center Leipzig (UCCL), University Medicine Leipzig, Germany

[2] Department of Surgery, University of Heidelberg, Germany

[3] Department of Medicine II, Gastroenterology, University of Mannheim, Germany

[4] Department of Diagnostic and Interventional Radiology, University of Heidelberg, Germany

[5] Department of Nuclear Medicine, University of Rostock, Germany

[6] Institute of Pathology, University Medicine Leipzig, Germany

13.1 Introduction

According to contemporary guidelines, the treatment of esophageal adenocarcinoma is stage-dependent (Figure 13.1) [1].

In the 7th edition of the T (tumor) N (node) M (metastases) classification, all adenocarcinomas of the esophago-gastric junction (AEG) which, for clinical purposes, have been classified as AEG type I, II and III by Siewert and coworkers (Figure 13.2) [2], are now classified as to the anatomical extent, according to the TNM of esophageal tumors.

The TNM staging of esophageal tumors is delineated in Table 13.1 [3]. It must be emphasized that this clarification in the TNM system has been implemented without the intention to simplify the various different treatment strategies that may exist between the different Siewert type tumors.

It is important to realize that most strategic treatment decisions in esophageal cancer are based on the results of clinical staging. This is true for choosing an endoscopic or surgical approach for local treatment of early tumors [4–6], and even more so for the indication for preoperative (neoadjuvant) treatment, which has become an evidence-based and recommended standard of care in clinical stages II and III [1, 7, 8]. To avoid "overtreatment" or "undertreatment", which both may harm patients, sophisticated staging procedures are of utmost importance in the contemporary management of esophageal cancer.

13.2 Endoscopic staging

Upper gastrointestinal endoscopy and endoscopic biopsy are the investigations of choice for the primary diagnosis of esophageal cancer. Endoscopy should determine the exact anatomical localization of the tumor. Based on endoscopic assessment, and in conjunction with other imaging modalities, tumors should be grouped according to Siewert's classification (Figure 13.2), which is essential for the selection of further treatment planning.

Precise local staging is required to determine the depth of tumor spread in early tumors which may be amenable to endoscopic resection. Endoscopic mucosal resection (EMR) and endoscopic submucosal dissection (ESD) can eradicate mucosal cancer. Endoscopic resection is an essential method to stage early tumors. It is indicated for the assessment of areas of Barrett's epithelium with dysplasia and nodularity where invasive disease is suspected. The depth of resection is usually into the submucosa. In a comparative study, Wani et al. found submucosa in 88% of EMR samples, compared with 1% of biopsy samples. The overall interobserver agreement for the diagnosis of neoplasia was significantly greater for EMR than biopsy specimens [9].

Esophageal Cancer and Barrett's Esophagus, Third Edition. Edited by Prateek Sharma, Richard Sampliner and David Ilson.
© 2015 John Wiley & Sons, Ltd. Published 2015 by John Wiley & Sons, Ltd.

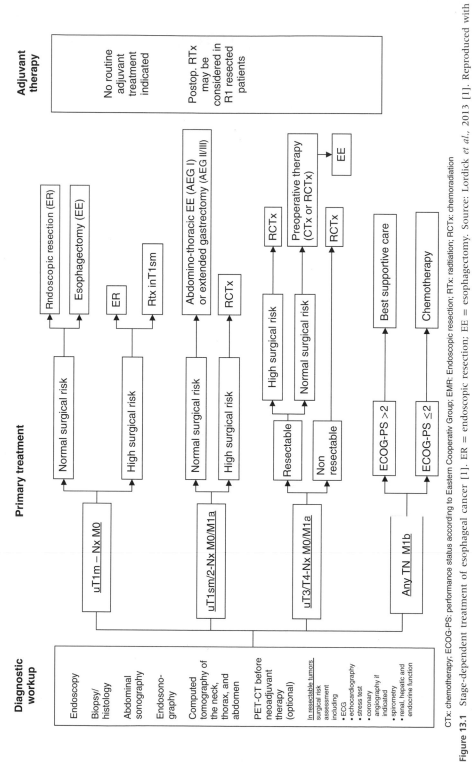

Figure 13.1 Stage-dependent treatment of esophageal cancer [1]. ER = endoscopic resection; EE = esophagectomy. Source: Lordick *et al.*, 2013 [1]. Reproduced with permission from Springer-Verlag.

CTx: chemotherapy; ECOG-PS: performance status according to Eastern Cooperativ Group; EMR: Endoscopic resection; RTx: radiation; RCTx: chemoradiation

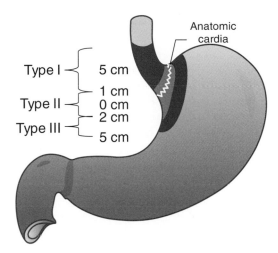

Figure 13.2   Classification of adenocarcinoma of the esophago-gastric junction (AEG). Adapted from Siewert *et al.*, 1987 [2].

It allows assessment not only of depth of penetration, but also of degree of differentiation and vascular and lymphatic involvement. EMR is superior to endoscopic ultrasound (EUS) in staging T1 cancers [10–12].

A differentiation must be made between mucosal (T1m = T1a/pT1a) and submucosal (T1sm = T1b/pT1b)) cancer. The sub-categorization of submucosal infiltration in thirds, according to the Japanese classification for gastric cancers (sm1, sm2, sm3), has also gained importance [10]. While esophageal adenocarcinomas very rarely have lymph node metastases as long as they are limited to the mucosal layer, the frequency of lymph node metastases ranges from 10–20% in sm1 cancers to 50–60% in sm3 cancers [14, 15].

The role of EUS in the assessment of the T and N categories are delineated in detail in the previous chapter. Most importantly, EUS has to be performed in a high-volume center and by an experienced investigator. Otherwise the results are not reliable [16].

In a systematic review, the authors Kwee and Kwee included 23 studies investigating the diagnostic accuracy of EUS for the T staging. Due to the heterogeneity of the included studies, they did not perform a pooled analysis. The diagnostic accuracy of T staging varied between 65% and 92% [17]. In a meta-analysis of 22 studies, Puli *et al.* [18] found a pooled sensitivity and specificity for the EUS-based T staging of 88% and 100% (T1), 82% and 96% (T2), 90% and 95% (T3) and 99% and 97% (T4), respectively. Clear limitations in the

Table 13.1 TNM classification of esophageal tumors.

Primary tumor (T)	
TX	Primary tumor cannot be assessed
T0	No evidence of primary tumor
Tis	Carcinoma *in situ*/high-grade dysplasia
T1	Tumor invades the lamina propria, muscularis mucosae or submucosa
T1a	Tumor invades lamina propria or muscularis mucosae
T1b	Tumor invades the submucosa
T2	Tumor invades the muscularis propria
T3	Tumor invades the adventitia
T4	Tumor invades adjacent structures
T4a	Tumor invades the pleura, pericardium, or diaphragm
T4b	Tumor invades other adjacent structures, e.g. aorta, vertebral body, or trachea

Regional lymph nodes (N)	
NX	Regional lymph nodes cannot be assessed
N0	No regional lymph node metastases
N1	Metastases in 1 or 2 regional lymph nodes
N2	Metastases in 3 to 6 regional lymph nodes
N3	Metastases in 7 or more regional lymph nodes

Distant metastases (M)	
M0	No distant metastases
M1	Distant metastases

Stage grouping

Stage 0	Tis	N0	M0
Stage IA	T1	N0	M0
Stage IB	T2	N0	M0
Stage IIA	T3	N0	M0
Stage IIB	T1, T2	N1	M0
Stage IIIA	T4a	N0	M0
Stage IIIB	T3	N1	M0
Stage IIIC	T1, T2	N2	M0
Stage IV	T3	N2	M0
	T4a	N1, N2	M0
	T4b	Any N	M0
	Any T	N3	M0
	Any T	Any N	M1

Source: Sobin *et al.*, 2010 [3]. Reproduced with permission of Wiley.

accuracy of EUS T staging were found for the definition of serosal involvement in Siewert-type-III-tumors, in case of tumor stenosis, as well as in ulcerating lesions and in diffuse type tumors according to Laurén [17–20].

In contrast to the acceptable accuracy for defining the depth of tumor infiltration, the accuracy of EUS-based N staging is not sufficient. The reason for this is that, in smaller lymph nodes, microscopic metastasis are not detected reliably. Furthermore, in enlarged lymph nodes, a clear distinction between inflammation and malignancy is often not possible [18, 21]. In the meta-analysis of Puli *et al.*, the correct EUS-based diagnosis of a pN1 category was reported with a pooled sensitivity of 58% and a specificity of 87%. For the correct endosonographic diagnosis of a pN2 category, the corresponding values were 65% and 92%, respectively [18]. In case of suspected malignancy, a fine-needle aspiration (FNA) can be done if the decision for or against pre-operative treatment is based on this criterion (which is not the case in the centers of the authors of this article). The EUS-guided FNA seems to have a high sensitivity and specificity, according to the experience from selected centers [22, 23].

The role for EUS in detecting distant metastases is limited. In some cases, liver metastases or ascites which are not detected by CT or abdominal ultrasound can be visualized by EUS.

13.3   Staging by external ultrasonography

B-mode-ultrasonography (US) has a broad availability in clinical practice. The sensitivity to detect liver metastases in tumor patients is 53–81% and the specificity is 59–98% [24]. Studies in patients with gastrointestinal cancers report a sensitivity of 77% [25] and 81% [26] in detecting liver metastases. When contrast-enhanced US is performed, the accuracy for the detection of liver metastases is in the range of multi-detector computed tomography (MDCT) and magnetic resonance tomography (MRT) [27]. For the detection of cervical lymph node metastases, B-mode-US has an accuracy at least similar to that of MDCT [28]. External US is also an important and useful confirmatory investigation for lesions that appeared suspicious on MDCT or PET-CT [29]. A US-guided FNA can be done to validate metastatic lymph node infiltration [30]. However, we prefer the complete removal and histopathological assessment of a suspicious lesion to have more precise diagnostic information and – in case of lymph node metastases – more material for additional molecular investigations, which may be needed for selecting the most appropriate systemic treatment [31, 32].

13.4   Staging by radiological examinations

13.4.1   Computed tomography (CT)

Patients with esophageal cancer who have a curative treatment option should be investigated with a MDCT. Studies should be performed after intravenous contrast enhancement. The slice thickness should be < 3 mm. The minimal requirement is a biphasic protocol including a native and a portal-venous phase, while a clear recommendation to examine the arterial phase cannot be made. Oral contrast should also be used. We recommend distension of the wall of the stomach and esophagus with negative contrast, for example, water in conjunction with spasmolytic treatment of the smooth muscle cells (e.g. by butylscopolamine). This technique is called a hydro-CT [33]. The use of multiplanar reformat images in addition to axial images improves the topographic visualization and the accuracy in discriminating T3 versus T4 disease, due to the possibility of evaluating invasion of the tumor into its surrounding structures in multiple planes [34, 35].

If these requirements are respected, the accuracy of T staging is estimated to be 77–89 % [17]. As with EUS, the accuracy of MDCT for the identification of metastatic lymph node invasion is sub-optimal [17]. The size of lymph nodes alone is not an appropriate parameter for defining metastatic infiltration.

The sensitivity and specificity for detecting distant metastases by CT are 70% and 72%, respectively. For lung lesions, even those smaller than 3 mm, modern CT technology allows for a very high sensitivity, while the specificity is lower. Due to its good sensitivity, a CT of the chest is recommended, and conventional X-ray of the thorax should not be performed.

13.4.2   Magnetic resonance imaging (MRI)

If a CT cannot be performed, MRI is the preferred alternative method. Slice thickness should be < 3 mm. 1.5 Tesla field strength, T1-/T2-standard registration and contrast-enhanced sequences should be applied. The literature does not unanimously recommend one specific examination protocol. There is also no clear recommendation for one of the available contrast media for improving the detection rate of distant metastases [36, 37].

MRI is also useful in the characterization of indeterminate liver lesions detected on CT and is an alternative if the dignity of liver lesions cannot be clarified with contrast-enhanced ultrasound [38, 39].

New functional imaging techniques, such as diffusion-weighted MRI, show promising results [40], and should be under consideration as complementary, future techniques.

13.4.3 Barium swallows

In the time before high-quality CT became available, barium swallows were used to define the localization of esophageal tumors. Nowadays, this information is obtained by multiplanar CT reconstruction techniques and video endoscopy. Therefore, barium swallows are no longer routinely indicated for preoperative staging [41, 42]. However, barium swallows or alternatively orally ingested aqueous low-osmolality agents can be useful to detect esophago-tracheal fistulas, or to document complete tumor obstructions.

13.5 Staging by positron emission tomography (PET)

13.5.1 Technique

The combination of metabolic assessment by PET and integrated CT provides both functional and anatomical data. The major advantage of the combined investigation is that the patient position is unchanged between each procedure which allows for reliable co-registration of the PET and the CT data. Several technical issues remain to be evaluated such as the use of iodinated contrast media for CT and optimal PET tracer doses and uptake periods. The low-dose CTs that are often done in conjunction with PET are not sufficient for making an appropriate anatomical staging. Contrast-enhanced MDCTs are indispensable and have to be done either simultaneously with PET or in addition to PET-CT.

The most widely used PET tracer for the assessment of esophageal cancer is 18F-fluorodeoxyglucose (FDG), which is a glucose analogue [43]. 83–95% esophageal cancers are FDG avid and therefore can be detected accurately [44, 45]. Experiences with other tracers, such as the "proliferation marker" 3'-deoxy-3'-(18)F-fluorothimidine (FLT) or the "angiogenesis marker" 18F-Galacto-RGD, are limited [46–48]. A disadvantage of FLT is its high accumulation in the liver, which limits the detection of liver metastases [47].

A study undertaken in esophageal cancer revealed the tumor uptake of 18F-FDG to be significantly higher, compared with the 18F-FLT uptake. Consequently, 18F-FLT scans showed more false-negative findings, but fewer false-positive findings, than 18F-FDG scans. Disappointingly, neither uptake of 18F-FDG nor 18F-FLT did correlate with proliferation measured by Ki-67 expression on histopathology [46]. Observations like this underline the recent statement made by Anthony F. Shields: "PET Imaging of Tumor Growth: Not as Easy as it Looks." [49].

13.5.2 FDG-PET for staging

Due to its physically determined limitations in spatial resolution, PET is not *per se* the optimal tool for defining the T category in esophageal cancer. In contrast, PET may add important information for defining the N- and M categories. In a systematic review, it was shown that the sensitivity and specificity for FDG-PET in nodal staging are 51% and 84%, respectively. For the detection of distant metastases, the corresponding numbers are 67% and 91% [46]. In a recent meta-analysis, the authors draw the conclusion that EUS, CT, and FDG-PET each play a distinctive role in the detection of nodal and distant metastases in esophageal cancer. For N staging, EUS is the most sensitive investigation, while CT and FDG-PET are more specific. For M staging, FDG-PET has probably a higher sensitivity than CT. Its combined use could, however, be of clinical value, with FDG-PET detecting possible metastases and CT confirming or excluding their presence and precisely determining their location [50]. Expert panels and guideline commissions recently recommended the use of FDG-PET for the detection of distant metastases in esophageal cancer [51, 52].

The specificity of PET is still limited, and false-positive findings are reported in up to 20% of cases. Therefore, treatment decisions should not be based on PET results alone. Positive findings which would lead to relevant treatment limitations need to be confirmed by other methods, especially by histopathology.

13.5.3 FDG-PET and stage-independent prognostic information

The Standardized Uptake Value (SUV) is often used for (semi-)quantitative analysis of PET-acquired data [53].

The SUV is calculated either pixel-wise, or over a region of interest (ROI), for each image of a dynamic series at specific time points (t). The SUV is the ratio of tissue radioactivity concentration (e.g. in MBq/kg = kBq/g) at time t – called $c(t)$ – and the injected dose of a tracer (e.g. in MBq) at the time of injection ($t = 0$). This value is corrected for the body weight (e.g. in kg) or lean body weight or the body surface area. For $c(t)$, either the maximum or mean value of a ROI is taken. In the newer literature, a change from region of interest-based SUV calculation to volume of interest-based SUV calculation can be observed [54].

An experienced group from the Memorial Sloan Kettering Cancer Center analyzed 40 patients with esophageal cancer who had been assessed with FDG-PET prior to esophagectomy. The median SUV in their patients was 4.5. Patients with a higher SUV had a significantly worse prognosis than patients with a SUV of less than 4.5 [55]. The survival advantage associated with a SUVmax of 4.5 or less was also seen in early stage patients (defined as no enlarged lymph nodes on CT and PET, and cT1-2 cN0 categories by EUS), as well as in patients with histopathologically confirmed early-stage disease (pT1-2pN0). However, the initial SUV as a prognostic marker is still a matter of debate.

13.6   The value of FDG-PET to predict response to pre-operative treatment

Pre-operative therapy has become a standard approach in stage II and III esophageal cancer and AEG [1]. Histopathologic remission and clinical response following neoadjuvant treatment are important surrogate markers for relapse-free and overall survival [56–58]. CT and endoscopy are of limited value in assessing response to preoperative treatment in esophageal cancer, as morphological changes occur relatively late, and the discrimination of vital tumor from scar is difficult. Clinical evaluation of dysphagia scores has been shown to be inaccurate [59]. Even post-treatment cytology and biopsies failed to accurately assess response to preoperative treatment, because residual tumor is often located at the radial margins and, therefore, is not endoscopically accessible [60, 61].

Recently, PET Response Criteria in solid Tumors (PERCIST 1.0) have been advocated [62]. The authors argued that anatomic imaging alone using standard World Health Organization (WHO) criteria, and Response Criteria in Solid Tumors (RECIST), have important limitations, particularly in assessing the activity of newer cancer therapies that stabilize disease rather than shrink it. FDG-PET appears particularly valuable in such cases. Validation studies are ongoing in several diseases and during different forms of treatment.

13.6.1   Post-therapeutic staging

Numerous studies have investigated post-therapeutic PET scanning in order to define its predictive and prognostic value (Table 13.2). Unfortunately, many studies investigated mixed populations of patients with adenocarcinoma and with squamous cell carcinoma, which limits the conclusions that can be drawn. In summary, most studies show a correlation of metabolic response as assessed by FDG-PET with response and survival. However, clear cut-offs do not exist, or have not yet been validated in prospective multicentre studies. Finally, the positive predictive value of PET to predict complete histopathologic response does not seem to be high enough to justify treatment decisions against surgical resection of the tumor.

13.6.2   Pre-therapeutic response prediction

Several groups examined the correlation of pre-therapeutic FDG uptake and treatment response (Table 13.3). In summary, the results are conflicting. While some investigators found a correlation between higher SUVs and response to chemotherapy or chemo-radiation, others did not. Prospective validation studies confirming specific techniques and cut-offs are lacking.

13.6.3   Early metabolic response assessment

Early sequential PET assessment during neoadjuvant chemotherapy of esophageal adenocarcinoma and AEG has been intensively studied. Cut-offs have been prospectively validated, and have been used prospectively in the interventional MUNICON studies [74, 77]. As a first step, changes of the metabolic tumor activity were quantified in consecutive phase II studies. After two weeks of induction chemotherapy, significant decreases of the SUVs were measured. A drop of $\geq 35\%$ was the most accurate cut-off value to predict later clinical and histopathological response [75, 76].

Table 13.2 Predictive and prognostic impact of SUVs from FDG-PET following preoperative chemoradiotherapy in patients with esophageal cancer.

Author	Year	Tumor	n	Correlation with response p value	Correlation with prognosis p value
Monjazeb et al. [63]	2010	AC/SCC	163	0.18	0.01
Javeri et al. [64]	2009	AC	151	0.06	0.01
Vallböhmer et al. [65]	2009	AC/SCC	119	0.056	n.s.
Kim et al. [66]	2007	SCC	62	n.d.	0.033
Levine et al. [67]	2006	AC/SCC	64	0.004	n.d.
Wieder et al. [68]	2004	SCC	38	0.011	n.d.
Swisher et al. [69]	2004	AC/SCC	83	0.03	0.01
Downey et al. [70]	2003	AC/SCC	39	n.d.	0.088
Flamen et al. [71]	2002	AC/SCC	36	0.001	0.002
Brucher et al. [72]	2001	SCC	27	0.001	0.001

AC = adenocarcinoma; n = number; n.d. = not determined; n.s. = not significant; SCC = squamous cell cancer.

Table 13.3 Predictive impact of SUVs from FDG-PET prior to preoperative chemo- or chemoradiotherapy in patients with esophageal cancer.

Author	Year	Tumor	n	SUV	Correlation with response
Rizk et al. [73]	2009	AC	189	absolute	$P = 0.02$
Javeri et al. [64]	2009	AC	161	absolute	$P = 0.06$
Lordick et al. [74]	2007	AC	110	median	$P = 0.018$
Levine et al. [67]	2006	AC/SCC	64	absolute	$P = 0.005$
Ott et al. [76]	2006	AC	65	median	$P = 0.16$
Swisher et al. [69]	2004	AC/SCC	56	absolute	$P = 0.56$
Wieder et al. [68]	2004	SCC	33	absolute	$P = 0.23$

AC = adenocarcinoma; n = number; SCC = squamous cell cancer; SUV = standard uptake value.

Metabolic response to neoadjuvant chemotherapy was also shown to be an independent prognostic factor [76]. Furthermore, early metabolic changes measured by FDG-PET revealed to be more sensitive for response prediction than early morphologic changes measured by MDCT [68]. This suggested that interim PET could be used to tailor treatment according to the chemo-sensitivity of the disease. This concept was realized in the MUNICON trials [74, 77]. Investigators from New York re-assessed the findings from the Munich investigators and validated the –35% SUV cut-off for patients receiving neoadjuvant chemotherapy [78]. In contrast to the Munich team, they did an interim staging PET after six, not two, weeks of neoadjuvant chemotherapy. Based on this finding, they meanwhile started an interventional clinical trial within the CALGB network.

Of note, the concept of interim staging and early response assessment is particularly valid in patients receiving chemotherapy without simultaneous radiation. In contrast, when radiation is added, the interim PET shows less compelling results [79–83]. This indicates that cell death induced by radiation therapy may follow different mechanisms and timelines than chemotherapy-induced apoptosis. Radiation induces more inflammatory reactions and scar formation, which may lead to false-positive and false-negative features.

13.7 Conclusion: summary of recommended staging procedures

Optimal staging is an indispensable prerequisite for adequate treatment planning. It is the basis of optimal treatment outcome and also for a rational allocation of economic resources. Current international guidelines come to the following recommendations for the staging of esophageal adenocarcinoma and AEG [1, 52, 84]:

13.7.1 T staging

Endoscopic resection is the preferred approach for assessing depth of infiltration in early cancers (T1). EUS is more accurate for T staging in more advanced lesions, because of the precise visualization of the separate layers of the esophageal wall. The value of MDCT is limited for early stage disease, but has a good accuracy to define the T category in larger tumors when done with optimal technique. Studies with PET-CT have reported failure to detect early T categories (T1 and T2) and mucinous or diffuse type tumors. In addition, smooth muscle activity and inflammation due to reflux disease may produce false-positive results. Therefore, PET-CT is not indicated for the definition of the T category, but it has its value for N and M staging.

13.7.2 N staging

The assessment of nodal disease by each technique is variable according to the anatomical relationship of lymph nodes to the primary tumor. EUS, in combination with MDCT, has the highest sensitivity for detecting involved lymph nodes, although accuracy varies considerably between different investigators and studies. While PET-CT can identify local nodes, FDG uptake by the adjacent tumor often obscures the uptake by metastatic nodes. For regional and distant nodal disease, PET-CT has a similar or better accuracy than conventional EUS and CT. Thus, a combined approach including CT, EUS and PET-CT has the highest possible yield for accurately assessing local, regional and distal nodal status [50, 52, 85].

13.7.3 M staging

Conventional imaging with EUS and CT has a wide range of accuracy for detecting metastatic disease. The addition of PET has significantly improved detection rates, and this is particularly advantageous for identification of unsuspected metastatic disease, which is present in up to 30% of patients at presentation. Therefore, PET-CT is recommended to exclude metastatic spread before the curative treatment of esophageal cancer and AEG. The American College of Surgical Oncology Group trial of PET to identify unsuspected metastatic disease has demonstrated some limitations, with 3.7% false-positive and 5% false-negative rates [86]. Therefore, further evaluation (including surgical excision or biopsy) of PET/CT-positive nodes or single "hot spots" is recommended when these would lead to a change in the treatment concept. PET has similar limitations to CT in detecting peritoneal disease and very small metastatic lesions.

References

1 Lordick F, Hölscher AH, Haustermans K, Wittekind C (2013). Multimodal treatment of esophageal cancer. *Langenbeck's Archives of Surgery* **398**, 177–87.

2 Siewert JR, Hölscher AH, Becker K, Gössner W (1987). Kardiacarcinom: Versuch einer therapeutisch relevanten Klassifikation. *Der Chirurg* **58**, 25–32.

3 Sobin LH, Gospodarowicz MK, Wittekind C (2010). *TNM classification of malignant tumours*, 7th edition. JohnWiley & Sons, Chichester, UK.

4 Pech O, Bollschweiler E, Manner H *et al*. (2011). Comparison between endoscopic and surgical resection of mucosal esophageal adenocarcinoma in Barrett's esophagus at two high-volume centers. *Annals of Surgery* **254**, 67–72.

5 Mariette C, Piessen G. (2012) Oesophageal cancer: how radical should surgery be? *European Journal of Surgical Oncology* **38**, 210–213.

6 Siewert JR, Feith M, Werner M, Stein HJ (2000). Adenocarcinoma of the esophago-gastric junction; results of surgical therapy based on anatomical/topographic classification in 1,002 consecutive patients. *Annals of Surgery* **232**, 353–61.

7 Sjoquist KM, Burmeister BH, Smithers BM *et al*. (2011). Survival after neoadjuvant chemotherapy or chemoradiotherapy for resectable oesophageal carcinoma: an updated meta-analysis. *The Lancet Oncology* **12**, 681–692.

8 van Hagen P, Hulshof MC, van Lanschot JJ *et al*. (2012). Preoperative chemoradiotherapy for esophageal or junctional cancer. *New England Journal of Medicine* **366**, 2074–2084.

9 Wani S, Mathur SC, Curvers WL, *et al*. (2010). Greater interobserver agreement by endoscopic mucosal resection than biopsy samples in Barrett's dysplasia. *Clinical Gastroenterology and Hepatology* **8**, 783–8.

10 Curvers WL, Bansal A, Sharma P, *et al*. (2008). Endoscopic work-up of early Barrett's neoplasia. *Endoscopy* **40**, 1000–7.

11 Mino-Kenudson M, Hull MJ, Brown I, *et al*. (2007). EMR for Barrett's esophagus-related superficial neoplasms offers better diagnostic reproducibility than mucosal biopsy. *Gastrointestinal Endoscopy* **66**, 660–6.

12 Peters FP, Brakenhoff KP, Curvers WL, *et al.* (2008). Histologic evaluation of resection specimens obtained at 293 endoscopic resections in Barrett's esophagus. *Gastrointestinal Endoscopy* **67**, 604–9.

13 Curvers WL, Bansal A, Sharma P, Bergman JJ (2008). Endoscopic workup of early Barrett's neoplasia. *Endoscopy* **40**, 1000–7.

14 Bollschweiler E, Baldus SE, Schröder W, Prenzel K, Gutschow Ch, Schneider PM, Hölscher AH (2006). High rate of lymph node metastasis in submucosal esophageal squamous-cell carcinomas and adenocarcinomas. *Endoscopy* **38**, 144–51.

15 Hölscher AH, Bollschweiler E, Schröder W, *et al.* (2011). Prognostic impact of upper, middle, and lower third mucosal or submucosal infiltration in early esophageal cancer. *Annals of Surgery* **254**, 802–7.

16 van Vliet EP, Eijkemans MJ, Poley JW *et al.* (2006). Staging of esophageal carcinoma in a low-volume EUS center compared with reported results from high-volume centers. *Gastrointestinal Endoscopy* **63**, 938–947.

17 Kwee RM, Kwee TC (2007). Imaging in local staging of gastric cancer: a systematic review. *Journal of Clinical Oncology* **25**, 2107–16.

18 Puli SR, Batapati Krishna Reddy J, *et al.* (2008). How good is endoscopic ultrasound for TNM staging of gastric cancers? A meta-analysis and systematic review. *World Journal of Gastroenterology* **14**, 4011–4019.

19 Blackshaw G, Lewis WG, Hopper AN *et al.* (2008). Prospective comparison of endosonography, computed tomography, and histopathological stage of junctional oesophagogastric cancer. *Clinical Radiology* **63**, 1092–98.

20 Heeren PA, van Westreenen HL, Geersing GJ *et al.* (2004). Influence of tumor characteristics on the accuracy of endoscopic ultrasonography in staging cancer of the esophagus and esophagogastric junction. *Endoscopy* **36**, 966–71.

21 Kwee RM, Kwee TC (2009). Imaging in assessing lymph node status in gastric cancer. *Gastric Cancer* **12**, 6–22.

22 Chen VK, Eloubeidi MA (2004). Endoscopic ultrasound-guided fine needle aspiration is superior to lymph node echofeatures: a prospective evaluation of mediastinal and peri-intestinal lymphadenopathy. *American Journal of Gastroenterology* **99**, 28–633.

23 Yasuda I, Tsurumi H, Omar S *et al.* (2006). Endoscopic ultrasound-guided fine-needle aspiration biopsy for lymphadenopathy of unknown origin. *Endoscopy* **38**, 919–24.

24 Oldenburg A, Albrecht T (2008). Baseline and contrast-enhanced ultrasound of the liver in tumor patients. *Ultraschall in der Medizin* **29**, 488–98.

25 Piscaglia F, Corradi F, Mancini M *et al.* (2007). Real time contrast enhanced ultrasonography in detection of liver metastases from gastrointestinal cancer. *BMC Cancer* **7**, 171–9.

26 Dietrich CF, Kratzer W, Strobe D *et al.* (2006). Assessment of metastatic liver disease in patients with primary extrahepatic tumors by contrast-enhanced sonography versus CT and MRI. *World Journal of Gastroenterology* **12**, 1699–1705.

27 Claudon M, Cosgrove D, Albrecht T *et al.* (2008). Guidelines and good clinical practice recommendations for contrast enhanced ultrasound (CEUS) – update (2008). *Ultraschall in der Medizin* **29**, 28–44.

28 Schreurs LM, Verhoef CC, van der Jagt EJ *et al.* (2008). Current relevance of cervical ultrasonography in staging cancer of the esophagus and gastroesophageal junction. *European Journal of Radiology* **67**, 105–11.

29 Omloo JM, van Heijl M, Smits NJ *et al.* (2009). Additional value of external ultrasonography of the neck after CT and PET scanning in the preoperative assessment of patients with esophageal cancer. *Digestive Surgery* **26**, 43–49.

30 van Overhagen H, Lameris JS, Berger MY *et al.* (1992). Assessment of distant metastases with ultrasound-guided fine-needle aspiration biopsy and cytologic study in carcinoma of the esophagus and gastroesophageal junction. *Gastrointestinal Radiology* **17**, 305–310.

31 Lordick F, Röcken C (2013). The identification of predictive factors for perioperative chemotherapy in esophago-gastric cancer. *Annals of Oncology* **24**, 1135–8.

32 Warneke VS, Behrens HM, Haag J, *et al.* (2013) Prognostic and Putative Predictive Biomarkers of Gastric Cancer for Personalized Medicine. *Diagnostic Molecular Pathology* **22**(3), 127–37.

33 Grenacher L, Schwarz M, Lordick F, *et al.* (2012). S3-Guideline: Diagnosis and Treatment of Gastric Carcinoma. *Fortschritte auf dem Gebiete der Röntgenstrahlen und der Nuklearmedizin* **184**, 706–12.

34 Bhandari S, Shim CS, Kim JH, *et al.* (2004). Usefulness of three-dimensional, multidetector row CT (virtual gastroscopy and multiplanar reconstruction) in the evaluation of gastric cancer: a comparison with conventional endoscopy, EUS, and histopathology. *Gastrointestinal Endoscopy* **59**, 619–26.

35 Fukuya T, Honda H, Kaneko K, *et al.* (1997). Efficacy of helical CT in T-staging of gastric cancer. *Journal of Computer Assisted Tomography* **21**, 73–81.

36 Anzidei M, Napoli A, Zaccagna F, *et al.* (2009). Diagnostic performance of 64-MDCT and 1.5-T MRI with high-resolution sequences in the T staging of gastric cancer: a comparative analysis with histopathology. *La Radiologia Medica* **114**, 1065–79.

37 Hammerstingl R, Huppertz A, Breuer J, *et al.* (2008). Diagnostic efficacy of gadoxetic acid (Primovist)-enhanced MRI and spiral CT for a therapeutic strategy: comparison with intraoperative and histopathologic findings in focal liver lesions. *European Radiology* **18**, 457–67.

38 Halavaara J, Breuer J, Ayuso C, *et al.* (2006). Liver tumor characterization: comparison between liver-specific gadoxetic acid disodium-enhanced MRI and biphasic CT – multicenter trial. *Journal of Computer Assisted Tomography* **30**, 345–54.

39 Semelka RC, Martin DR, Balci C, *et al.* (2001). Focal liver lesions: comparison of dual-phase CT and multisequence multiplanar MR imaging including dynamic gadolinium enhancement. *Journal of Magnetic Resonance Imaging* **13**, 397–401.

40 Weber MA, Bender K, von Gall CC, *et al.* (2013). Assessment of diffusion-weighted MRI and 18F-fluoro-deoxyglucose PET/CT in monitoring early response to neoadjuvant chemotherapy in adenocarcinoma of the esophagogastric junction. *Journal of Gastrointestinal and Liver Diseases* **22**, 45–52.

41 SIGN (2006). *Management of oesophageal and gastric cancer.* NHS.

42 Peeters M, Lerut T, Vlayen J. *et al.* (2008). *Wetenschappelijke ondersteuning van het College voor Oncologie: een nationale praktijkrichtlijn voor de aanpak van slokdarm – en maagkanker.* Brussel: Federaal Kenniscentrum voor de Gezondheidszorg (KCE), **75**.

43 Lordick F, Ott K, Krause BJ (2010). New trends for staging and therapy for localized gastroesophageal cancer: the role of PET. *Annals of Oncology* **21**(Suppl 7), vii294–vii299.

44 Flamen P, Lerut A, Van Cutsem E, *et al.* (2000). Utility of positron emission tomography for the staging of patients with potentially operable esophageal carcinoma. *Journal of Clinical Oncology* **18**, 3202–10.

45 Räsänen JV, Sihvo EI, Knuuti MJ, *et al.* (2003). Prospective analysis of accuracy of positron emission tomography, computed tomography, and endoscopic ultrasonography in staging of adenocarcinoma of the esophagus and the esophagogastric junction. *Annals of Surgical Oncology* **10**, 954–60.

46 van Westreenen HL, Cobben DCP, Jager PL, *et al.* (2005). Comparison of 18F-FLT PET and 18F-FDG PET in Esophageal Cancer. *Journal of Nuclear Medicine* **46**, 400–4.

47 Herrmann K, Ott K, Buck AK, *et al.* (2007). Imaging gastric cancer with positron emission tomography (PET) and the radiotracers 3′-deoxy-3′-[18F]fluorothymidine (FLT) and FDG – a comparative analysis. *Journal of Nuclear Medicine* **48**, 1945–50.

48 Beer AJ, Lorenzen S, Metz S, *et al.* (2008). Comparison of Integrin {alpha}v{beta}3 Expression and Glucose Metabolism in Primary and Metastatic Lesions in Cancer Patients: A PET Study Using 18F-Galacto-RGD and 18F-FDG. *Journal of Nuclear Medicine* **49**, 22–9.

49 Shields AF (2012). PET Imaging of Tumor Growth: Not as Easy as it Looks. *Clinical Cancer Research* **18**, 1189–91.

50 van Vliet EP, Heijenbrok-Kal MH, Hunink MG, *et al.* (2008). Staging investigations for oesophageal cancer: a meta-analysis. *British Journal of Cancer* **98**, 547–57.

51 Fletcher JW, Djulbegovic B, Soares HP, *et al.* (2008). Recommendations on the use of 18F-FDG PET in oncology. *Journal of Nuclear Medicine* **49**, 480–508.

52 Allum WH, Blazeby JM, Griffin SM, *et al.* (2011). Guidelines for the management of oesophageal and gastric cancer. *Gut* **60**, 1449–72.

53 Schomburg A, Bender H, Reichel C, *et al.* (1996). Standardized uptake values of fluorine-18 fluorodeoxyglucose: the value of different normalization procedures. *European Journal of Nuclear Medicine* **23**, 571–4.

54 Boellaard R, O-Doherty MJ, Weber WA, *et al.* (2010). FDG PET and PET/CT: EANM procedure guidelines for tumour PET imaging: version 1.0. *European Journal of Nuclear Medicine and Molecular Imaging* **37**, 181–200.

55 Rizk N, Downey RJ, Akhurst T, *et al.* (2006). Preoperative 18[F]-fluorodeoxyglucose positron emission tomography standardized uptake values predict survival after esophageal adenocarcinoma resection. *Annals of Thoracic Surgery* **81**, 1076–81.

56 Ott K, Blank S, Becker K, *et al.* (2013). Factors predicting prognosis and recurrence in patients with esophago-gastric adenocarcinoma and histopathological response with less than 10 % residual tumor. *Langenbeck's Archives of Surgery* **398**, 239–49.

57 Lorenzen S, Blank S, Lordick F, *et al.* (2012). Prediction of Response and Prognosis by a Score Including Only Pretherapeutic Parameters in 410 Neoadjuvant Treated Gastric Cancer Patients. *Annals of Surgical Oncology* **19**, 2119–27.

58 Langer R, Ott K, Feith M, *et al.* (2009). Prognostic significance of histopathological tumor regression after neoadjuvant chemotherapy in esophageal adenocarcinomas. *Modern Pathology* **22**, 1555–63.

59 Ribi K, Koeberle D, Schuller JC, *et al.* (2009). Is a change in patient-reported dysphagia after induction chemotherapy in locally advanced esophageal cancer a predictive factor for pathological response to neoadjuvant chemoradiation? *Support Care Cancer* **17**, 1109–16.

60 Peng HQ, Halsey K, Sun CC, *et al.* (2009). Clinical utility of postchemoradiation endoscopic brush cytology and biopsy in predicting residual esophageal adenocarcinoma. *Cancer Cytopathology* **117**, 463–72.

61 Sarkaria IS, Rizk NP, Bains MS, *et al.* (2009). Post-treatment endoscopic biopsy is a poor-predictor of pathologic response in patients undergoing chemoradiation therapy for esophageal cancer. *Annals of Surgery* **249**, 764–7.

62 Wahl RL, Jacene H, Kasamon Y, Lodge MA (2009). From RECIST to PERCIST: Evolving Considerations for PET response criteria in solid tumors. *Journal of Nuclear Medicine* **50**(Suppl 1), 122S–150S.

63 Monjazeb AM, Riedlinger G, Aklilu M, *et al.* (2010). Outcomes of patients with esophageal cancer staged with [18F] fluorodeoxyglucose positron emission tomography (FDG-PET): can postchemoradiotherapy FDG-PET predict the utility of resection? *Journal of Clinical Oncology* **28**, 4714–21.

64 Javeri H, Xiao L, Rohren E, *et al.* (2009).The higher the decrease in the standardized uptake value of positron emission tomography after chemoradiation, the better the survival of patients with gastroesophageal adenocarcinoma. *Cancer* **115**, 5184–92.

65 Vallböhmer D, Hölscher AH, Dietlein M, *et al.* (2009). [^{18}F]-Fluorodeoxyglucose-positron emission tomography for the assessment of histopathologic response and prognosis after completion of neoadjuvant chemoradiation in esophageal cancer. *Annals of Surgery* **250**, 888–94.

66 Kim MK, Ryu JS, Kim SB, *et al.* (2007). Value of complete metabolic response by [^{18}F]-fluorodeoxyglucose-positron emission tomography in oesophageal cancer for prediction of pathologic response and survival after preoperative chemoradiotherapy. *European Journal of Cancer* **43**, 1385–91.

67 Levine EA, Farmer MR, Clark P, *et al.* (2006). Predictive value of 18-fluoro-deoxy-glucose-positron emission tomography (^{18}F-FDG-PET) in the identification of responders to chemoradiation therapy for the treatment of locally advanced esophageal cancer. *Annals of Surgery* **243**, 472–8.

68 Wieder HA, Beer AJ, Lordick F, *et al.* (2005). Comparison of changes in tumor metabolic activity and tumor size during chemotherapy of adenocarcinomas of the esophagogastric junction. *Journal of Nuclear Medicine* **46**, 2029–34.

69 Swisher SG, Erasmus J, Maish M, *et al.* (2004). 2-Fluoro-2-deoxy-D-glucose positron emission tomography imaging is predictive of pathologic response and survival after preoperative chemoradiation in patients with esophageal carcinoma. *Cancer* **101**, 1776–85.

70 Downey RJ, Akhurst T, Ilson D, *et al.* (2003). Whole body ^{18}FDG-PET and the response of esophageal cancer to induction therapy: results of a prospective trial. *Journal of Clinical Oncology* **21**, 428–32.

71 Flamen P, Van Cutsem E, Lerut A, *et al.* (2002). Positron emission tomography for assessment of the response to induction radiochemotherapy in locally advanced oesophageal cancer. *Annals of Oncology* **13**, 361–8.

72 Brücher BL, Weber W, Bauer M, *et al.* (2001). Neoadjuvant therapy of esophageal squamous cell carcinoma: response evaluation by positron emission tomography. *Annals of Surgery* **233**, 300–9.

73 Rizk NP, Tang L, Adusumilli PS, *et al.* (2009). Predictive value of initial PET-SUVmax in patients with locally advanced esophageal and gastroesophageal junction adenocarcinoma. *Journal of Thoracic Oncology* **4**, 875–9.

74 Lordick F, Ott K, Krause BJ, *et al.* (2007). PET to assess early metabolic response and to guide treatment of adenocarcinoma of the oesophagogastric junction: the MUNICON phase II trial. *The Lancet Oncology* **8**, 797–805.

75 Weber WA, Ott K, Becker K, *et al.* (2001). Prediction of response to preoperative chemotherapy in adenocarcinomas of the esophagogastric junction by metabolic imaging. *Journal of Clinical Oncology* **19**, 3058–65.

76 Ott K, Weber WA, Lordick F, *et al.* (2006). Metabolic imaging predicts response, survival, and recurrence in adenocarcinomas of the esophagogastric junction. *Journal of Clinical Oncology* **24**, 4692–8.

77 Lordick F, Meyer zum Büschenfelde C, Hermann K, *et al.* (2011). *PET-guided treatment in locally advanced adenocarcinoma of the esophagogastric junction (AEG): the MUNICON II study* (best abstract oral presentation). 2011 ASCO Gastrointestinal Cancer Symposium, San Francisco, CA, USA, abstract 3.

78 Ilson DH, Minsky BD, Ku GY, *et al.* (2012). Phase 2 trial of induction and concurrent chemoradiotherapy with weekly irinotecan and cisplatin followed by surgery for esophageal cancer. *Cancer* **118**, 2820–7.

79 Gillham CM, Lucey JA, Keogan M, *et al.* (2006). (^{18})FDG uptake during induction chemoradiation for oesophageal cancer fails to predict histomorphological tumour response. *British Journal of Cancer* **95**, 1174–9.

80 Klaeser B, Nitzsche E, Schuller JC, *et al.* (2009). Limited predictive value of FDG-PET for response assessment in the preoperative treatment of esophageal cancer: results of a prospective multi-center trial (SAKK 75/02). *Onkologie* **32**, 724–30.

81 Malik V, Lucey JA, Duffy GJ, *et al.* (2010). Early Repeated 18F-FDG PET Scans During Neoadjuvant Chemoradiation Fail to Predict Histopathologic Response or Survival Benefit in Adenocarcinoma of the Esophagus. *Journal of Nuclear Medicine* **51**, 1863–9.

82 van Heijl M, Omloo JM, van Berge Henegouwen MI (2011). Fluorodeoxyglucose positron emission tomography for evaluating early response during neoadjuvant chemoradiotherapy in patients with potentially curable esophageal cancer. *Annals of Surgery* **253**, 56–63.

83 Cuenca X, Hennequin C, Hindié E, *et al.* (2013). Evaluation of early response to concomitant chemoradiotherapy by interim 18F-FDG PET/CT imaging in patients with locally advanced oesophageal carcinomas. *European Journal of Nuclear Medicine and Molecular Imaging* **40**, 477–85.

84 National Comprehensive Cancer Network Practical Treatment Guidelines (2013). *Esophageal and Esophagogastric Junction Cancers*, Version 2. nccn.org.

85 Chowdhury FU, Bradley KM, Gleeson FV (2008). The role of 18F-FDG PET/CT in the evaluation of oesophageal carcinoma. *Clinical Radiology* **63**, 1297–309.

86 Meyers BF, Downey RJ, Decker PA, *et al.* (2007). The utility of positron emission tomography in staging of potentially operable carcinoma of the thoracic esophagus: results of the American College of Surgeons Oncology Group Z0060 trial. *Journal of Thoracic and Cardiovascular Surgery* **133**, 738–45.

CHAPTER 14

Medical management of Barrett's esophagus

Sachin Wani[1,2]

[1]Division of Gastroenterology and Hepatology, University of Colorado Anschutz Medical Center, Aurora, CO, USA
[2]Division of Gastroenterology and Hepatology, Veterans Affairs Medical Center, Denver, CO, USA

14.1 Introduction

Barrett's esophagus is a metaplastic change in the esophageal lining from the usual squamous mucosa to columnar epithelium and is the most important risk factor for development of esophageal adenocarcinoma [1]. Over the past few decades, the incidence of esophageal adenocarcinoma and incidence-based mortality has increased rapidly in the United States and other Western countries, albeit at a slower rate since the 1990s [2]. The most recent estimates suggest that 17,460 people will be diagnosed with esophageal cancer, and 15,070 people will die from this disease annually [3]. Given the dearth of population-based studies, the true prevalence of Barrett's esophagus in the United States is not known, but estimates based on other population-based studies suggest that more than three million adults may harbor Barrett's esophagus [4].

Medical management of this premalignant condition, once diagnosed, includes: assessment and management of symptoms of gastroesophageal reflux; healing of erosive esophagitis; enrolment in surveillance programs for early detection of dysplasia and esophageal adenocarcinoma; acid suppression and healing of mucosa during and post endoscopic eradication therapies; and, finally, prevention of progression to Barrett's related neoplasia (chemoprevention). This chapter focuses on all of the above aspects, with the exception of surveillance and chemoprevention, which has been addressed in separate chapters.

14.2 Assessment of symptoms

It is estimated that approximately 5% of patients with chronic heartburn symptoms have Barrett's esophagus on a population basis [1, 5–7]. A recent systematic review and meta-analysis showed that symptoms of gastroesophageal reflux disease are not associated with short segments of Barrett's esophagus, but increased the odds of long segment Barrett's esophagus (fixed effects odds ratio (OR): 4.92 (95% CI 2.01–12)) [8]. The vast majority of patients with Barrett's esophagus experience chronic symptoms of gastroesophageal reflux (heartburn and regurgitation). However, the exact proportion of individuals with asymptomatic Barrett's esophagus is not known.

The prevalence of Barrett's esophagus was 65 of 961 (6.8%) among patients who underwent upper endoscopy along with scheduled colonoscopy. The prevalence of Barrett's esophagus in patients with no prior history of heartburn was 5.6% [9]. Another study reported a Barrett's prevalence of 25% among asymptomatic male veterans older than 50 years of age undergoing screening sigmoidoscopy for colorectal cancer screening [10]. In a similarly designed study, Ward *et al* reported a 15% prevalence of Barrett's esophagus in asymptomatic individuals [11].

Assessment of symptoms should include assessment of frequency and duration of heartburn and regurgitation, and presence of nocturnal heartburn and regurgitation. The presence of dysphagia or odynophagia, and onset of these symptoms, should

Supported by the American Gastroenterological Association Takeda Research Scholar Award in GERD and Barrett's esophagus.

be assessed. The most common causes of dysphagia in patients with chronic gastroesophageal reflux disease and Barrett's esophagus include severe grades of erosive esophagitis, peptic stricture, Schatzki ring or esophageal adenocarcinoma. Similar to patients with chronic reflux symptoms [5], patients with Barrett's esophagus, and alarm symptoms of dysphagia, bleeding, anemia, weight loss and recurrent vomiting, should be referred for an upper endoscopy.

14.3   Acid suppressive therapies in management of reflux symptoms

Patients with Barrett's esophagus experience more reflux than patients with severe erosive esophagitis and peptic strictures, and this is true regardless of concomitant symptoms of reflux [12, 13]. Recently, Savarino *et al.* compared characteristics of reflux episodes in consecutive patients with Barrett's esophagus ($n = 100$), erosive esophagitis ($n = 50$), and healthy volunteers ($n = 48$), using multichannel intraluminal impedance-pH off proton pump inhibitor (PPI) therapy. Patients with Barrett's esophagus had significantly greater acid and weakly acidic reflux episodes, compared with patients with erosive esophagitis and controls [14]. Proton pump inhibitors (PPIs) are routinely prescribed as first-line and maintenance therapy for patients with Barrett's esophagus. The primary goal of PPI therapy is symptom control, and several studies have demonstrated the effectiveness of PPI therapy in eliminating gastroesophageal reflux disease symptoms [15–19].

14.4   Normalization of intraesophageal acid exposure

Several studies have reported that normalization of intraesophageal pH cannot be achieved in a significant proportion of patients with Barrett's esophagus even on high-dose PPI therapy and in patients with complete resolution of symptoms (Table 14.1) [15–23].

In a randomized, double-blind, three-way crossover study, Spechler *et al.* compared intraesophageal acidity and intragastric acidity in 31 patients with long-segment Barrett's esophagus treated with three different dosing regimens of esomeprazole (40 mg TID, 40 mg BID and 20 mg TID). Although all three regimens

Table 14.1 Summary of studies reporting proportion of Barrett's esophagus patients on high dose PPI therapy with abnormal intraesophageal acid exposure.

Author and year	Number of patients	PPI regimen	Proportion with abnormal pH studies
Katzka *et al.*, 1994	5	Omeprazole 20–60 mg/day	80%
Ouatu-Lascar *et al.*, 1998	30	Lansoprazole 15–30 mg/day	40%
Fass *et al.*, 2000	25	Omeprazole 40 mg BID	16%
Basu *et al.*, 2002	45	Omeprazole 20 mg BID	22%
Yeh *et al.*, 2003	13	Esomeprazole 40–80 mg/day	62%
Gerson *et al.*, 2004	48	Variable PPI regimen	50%
Sarela *et al.*, 2004	32	BID PPI regimen	47%
Wani *et al.*, 2005	46	Rabeprazole 20 mg BID	26%
Spechler *et al.*, 2006	31	Esomeprazole 40 mg TID	16%
		40 mg BID	23%
		20 mg TID	19%
Krishnan *et al.*, 2012	37	BID PPI regimen	20%

achieved intragastric pH of > 4.0 in 80–88% of patients, pathologic esophageal pH exposure (defined as pH < 4.0 for > 5% of time) was seen in 16–23% of patients [15].

Wani *et al.* evaluated esophageal acid exposure in 46 patients with Barrett's esophagus on BID PPI therapy and determined clinical factors predicting normalization of intraesophageal pH. Twelve patients (26.1%) had an abnormal result (median total percentage time pH < 4: 9.3%), and factors such as age, length of Barrett's esophagus and hiatal hernia size could not predict persistent abnormal intraesophageal pH on high-dose PPI therapy [20]. Similarly, in another study, Krishnan *et al.* showed that 20% of BE patients referred for endoscopic eradication therapy had abnormal distal esophageal acid exposure, despite twice-daily PPI therapy [21].

Pathophysiologic mechanisms that may explain pathologic esophageal pH exposure in patients with Barrett's esophagus, despite achieving adequate symptom control, include: marked hypotension of the lower esophageal sphincter; delayed esophageal acid clearance; increase in frequency and duration of esophageal acid exposure; hiatal hernias; and associated poor esophageal contractility and ineffective peristalsis, leading to defective clearance of the refluxed gastric contents [15, 20, 24, 25]. It is unlikely that gastric acid hypersecretion or abnormal gastric resistance to PPIs contribute to the above described phenomenon [15]. The clinical implication of continued esophageal acid exposure in patients with Barrett's esophagus is not clear, and needs to be defined in future studies. At the present time, 24-hour pH monitoring to document normalization of esophageal acid exposure is not routinely recommended.

14.5 Management of erosive esophagitis

The goals of PPI therapy in patients with Barrett's esophagus and erosive esophagitis are symptom relief and healing of erosive esophagitis. There are limited data evaluating the effectiveness of PPI therapy with regards to symptom relief and healing of erosive esophagitis. The available literature includes small studies that focus on end points other than those listed above, such as regression of columnar lined esophagus [26–30]. An expert panel, based on indirect evidence, concluded that the rate of symptom relief and healing of esophagitis using PPI therapy in patients with Barrett's esophagus is similar to patients with Los Angeles grades C and D esophagitis, but inferior to patients with grades A and B esophagitis, and it was unanimously agreed that long-term PPI therapy is effective in patients with Barrett's esophagus [26].

In a prospective study that included 172 patients with erosive esophagitis with reflux symptoms without a prior diagnosis of Barrett's esophagus, Barrett's esophagus was detected in 12% of patients after repeat endoscopy after treatment with standard doses of PPI therapy [31]. Similarly, another retrospective study showed that Barrett's esophagus was detected in 9% of 102 patients with erosive esophagitis undergoing endoscopy for any indication. The presence of severe esophagitis (grade 4 erosive esophagitis, $p = 0.01$) and presentation of GI bleeding ($p = 0.01$) were associated with the detection of Barrett's esophagus

at follow-up endoscopy [32]. Thus, the presence of denuded esophageal epithelium related to erosive esophagitis may obscure the accurate detection of columnar lined distal esophagus. Therefore, follow-up upper endoscopy is recommended after eight weeks of twice daily high-dose PPI therapy in patients with severe esophagitis, to ensure healing and to rule out the presence of Barrett's esophagus [5].

14.6 Maintenance of healed mucosa after endoscopic eradication therapies

The basic premise of endoscopic eradication therapies in patients with Barrett's related neoplasia is that removal of the neoplastic mucosa by endoscopic mucosal resection, and/or mucosal ablation followed by acid suppression, will result in re-epithelialization with squamous mucosa [33]. Mucosal healing during endoscopic eradication therapies, and maintenance of healing, is routinely achieved with high dose PPI therapy administered twice a day. Successful ablation cannot be achieved in all patients, and a recent study from UK showed that complete eradication of intestinal metaplasia could be achieved in only 62% of patients (198 out of a total of 335 patients with Barrett's esophagus achieved complete eradication) [34].

It has been proposed that inadequate reflux control may play a role in the persistence of intestinal metaplasia in patients undergoing ablative therapies. In a recent study, Krishnan et al. enrolled 37 patients referred for ablation, who underwent high resolution manometry and 24-hour impedance-pH testing followed by radiofrequency ablation. Comparison of complete responders (patients who achieved complete eradication of intestinal metaplasia in < 3 sessions, $n = 22$) with incomplete responders (residual intestinal metaplasia or dysplasia at third endoscopy, $n = 15$) showed that complete responders had fewer weakly acidic events (29.5 vs. 52, $p = 0.03$) and total reflux events (33.5 vs. 60, $p = 0.03$) compared with incomplete responders. Length of Barrett's segment and size of hiatal hernia were other predictors of persistent intestinal metaplasia after radiofrequency ablation [21].

Although several ablation methods exist, radiofrequency ablation is currently the most widely used, given the level 1 evidence demonstrating a decrease in the risk of neoplastic progression among patients with dysplastic Barrett's esophagus and wide availability of devices for its application [35]. A follow-up study to the randomized controlled trial found, after two years, that 95% and 93% of patients achieved remission of dysplasia and intestinal metaplasia, respectively. However, a significant proportion of patients (55%) required repeat ablation treatments after the first year to achieve these endpoints [36].

Recent reports have described variable rates of recurrence of intestinal metaplasia and dysplasia post-ablation in patients who achieve the endpoint of complete eradication of intestinal metaplasia, ranging from 6–33% [34, 37, 38]. While some of the variability may be accounted for by differences in the definition of recurrence and techniques for ablation, differences in acid suppression regimens have been proposed as an explanation for *recurrent* intestinal metaplasia. The Netherlands group prescribed not only twice-daily dosing of a PPI, post-ablation and during follow-up, but also included a H2RA at bedtime, along with sucralfate suspension after each ablation [37, 39]. Long-term acid suppression with twice-daily dosing with PPI therapy has been recommended to maintain remission. Future studies should evaluate the impact of differences in acid suppression regimens on rates of recurrent intestinal metaplasia and dysplasia, and identifying individuals in whom a step-down approach of once-daily PPI or on-demand PPI therapy can be adopted.

14.7 Conclusions

Medical management of Barrett's esophagus, once diagnosed, includes assessment and management of symptoms of gastroesophageal reflux, healing of erosive esophagitis, and acid suppression and healing of mucosa during and post endoscopic eradication therapies. The vast majority of patients with Barrett's esophagus experience chronic symptoms of gastroesophageal reflux (heartburn and regurgitation). However, the exact proportion of individuals with asymptomatic Barrett's esophagus is not known. Assessment of symptoms should include assessment of frequency and duration of heartburn and regurgitation, and presence of nocturnal heartburn and regurgitation. Patients with Barrett's esophagus and alarm symptoms such as dysphagia should be referred for an upper endoscopy.

PPIs are routinely prescribed as first-line and maintenance therapy for patients with Barrett's esophagus, with the primary goal of symptom control. Several studies have reported that normalization of intraesophageal pH cannot be achieved in a significant proportion of patients with Barrett's esophagus, even on high-dose PPI therapy and in patients with complete resolution of symptoms. Although 24-hour pH monitoring to document normalization of esophageal acid exposure is not routinely recommended, the clinical implication of continued esophageal acid exposure in patients with Barrett's esophagus needs to be explored in future studies.

The presence of denuded esophageal epithelium related to erosive esophagitis may obscure the accurate detection of columnar-lined distal esophagus. Hence, follow-up upper endoscopy is recommended after eight weeks of twice daily high-dose PPI therapy in patients with severe esophagitis, to ensure healing and to rule out the presence of Barrett's esophagus. Finally, acid suppression with high-dose PPI therapy is recommended to induce and maintain remission in Barrett's esophagus patients undergoing endoscopic eradication therapies.

References

1 Sharma P (2009). Clinical practice. Barrett's esophagus. *New England Journal of Medicine* **361**, 2548–56.

2 Hur C, Miller M, Kong CY, *et al.* (2013). Trends in esophageal adenocarcinoma incidence and mortality. *Cancer* **119**, 1149–58.

3 Siegel R, Naishadham D, Jemal A (2012). Cancer statistics, 2012. *CA: A Cancer Journal for Clinicians* **62**, 10–29.

4 Ronkainen J, Aro P, Storskrubb T, *et al.* (2005). Prevalence of Barrett's esophagus in the general population: an endoscopic study. *Gastroenterology* **129**, 1825–31.

5 Shaheen NJ, Weinberg DS, Denberg TD, *et al.* (2012). Upper endoscopy for gastroesophageal reflux disease: best practice advice from the clinical guidelines committee of the American College of Physicians. *Annals of Internal Medicine* **157**, 808–16.

6 Westhoff B, Brotze S, Weston A, *et al.* (2005). The frequency of Barrett's esophagus in high-risk patients with chronic GERD. *Gastrointestinal Endoscopy* **61**, 226–31.

7 Csendes A, Smok G, Burdiles P, *et al.* (2000). Prevalence of Barrett's esophagus by endoscopy and histologic studies: a prospective evaluation of 306 control subjects and 376 patients with symptoms of gastroesophageal reflux. *Diseases of the Esophagus* **13**, 5–11.

8 Taylor JB, Rubenstein JH (2010). Meta-analyses of the effect of symptoms of gastroesophageal reflux on the risk of Barrett's esophagus. *American Journal of Gastroenterology* **105**, 1729, 1730–7; quiz 1738.

9 Rex DK, Cummings OW, Shaw M, *et al.* (2003). Screening for Barrett's esophagus in colonoscopy patients with and without heartburn. *Gastroenterology* **125**, 1670–7.

10 Gerson LB, Shetler K, Triadafilopoulos G (2002). Prevalence of Barrett's esophagus in asymptomatic individuals. *Gastroenterology* **123**, 461–7.

11 Ward EM, Wolfsen HC, Achem SR, *et al.* (2006). Barrett's esophagus is common in older men and women undergoing screening colonoscopy regardless of reflux symptoms. *American Journal of Gastroenterology* **101**, 12–7.

12 Stein HJ, Barlow AP, DeMeester TR, *et al.* (1992). Complications of gastroesophageal reflux disease. Role of the lower esophageal sphincter, esophageal acid and acid/alkaline exposure, and duodenogastric reflux. *Annals of Surgery* **216**, 35–43.

13 Niemantsverdriet EC, Timmer R, Breumelhof R, *et al.* (1997). The roles of excessive gastro-oesophageal reflux, disordered oesophageal motility and decreased mucosal sensitivity in the pathogenesis of Barrett's oesophagus. *European Journal of Gastroenterology & Hepatology* **9**, 515–9.

14 Savarino E, Zentilin P, Frazzoni M, *et al.* (2010). Characteristics of gastro-esophageal reflux episodes in Barrett's esophagus, erosive esophagitis and healthy volunteers. *Neurogastroenterology & Motility* **22**, 1061–e280.

15 Spechler SJ, Sharma P, Traxler B, *et al.* (2006). Gastric and esophageal pH in patients with Barrett's esophagus treated with three esomeprazole dosages: a randomized, double-blind, crossover trial. *American Journal of Gastroenterology* **101**, 1964–71.

16 Ouatu-Lascar R, Triadafilopoulos G (1998). Complete elimination of reflux symptoms does not guarantee normalization of intraesophageal acid reflux in patients with Barrett's esophagus. *American Journal of Gastroenterology* **93**, 711–6.

17 Katzka DA, Castell DO (1994). Successful elimination of reflux symptoms does not insure adequate control of acid reflux in patients with Barrett's esophagus. *American Journal of Gastroenterology* **89**, 989–91.

18 Yeh RW, Gerson LB, Triadafilopoulos G (2003). Efficacy of esomeprazole in controlling reflux symptoms, intraesophageal, and intragastric pH in patients with Barrett's esophagus. *Diseases of the Esophagus* **16**, 193–8.

19 Gerson LB, Boparai V, Ullah N, *et al.* (2004). Oesophageal and gastric pH profiles in patients with gastro-oesophageal reflux disease and Barrett's oesophagus treated with proton pump inhibitors. *Alimentary Pharmacology & Therapeutics* **20**, 637–43.

20 Wani S, Sampliner RE, Weston AP, *et al.* (2005). Lack of predictors of normalization of oesophageal acid exposure in Barrett's oesophagus. *Alimentary Pharmacology & Therapeutics* **22**, 627–33.

21 Krishnan K, Pandolfino JE, Kahrilas PJ, *et al.* (2012). Increased risk for persistent intestinal metaplasia in patients with Barrett's esophagus and uncontrolled reflux exposure before radiofrequency ablation. *Gastroenterology* **143**, 576–81.

22 Fass R, Sampliner RE, Malagon IB, *et al.* (2000). Failure of oesophageal acid control in candidates for Barrett's oesophagus reversal on a very high dose of proton pump inhibitor. *Alimentary Pharmacology & Therapeutics* **14**, 597–602.

23 Basu KK, Bale R, West KP, *et al.* (2002). Persistent acid reflux and symptoms in patients with Barrett's oesophagus on proton-pump inhibitor therapy. *European Journal of Gastroenterology & Hepatology* **14**, 1187–92.

24 Bremner RM, Crookes PF, DeMeester TR, *et al.* (1992). Concentration of refluxed acid and esophageal mucosal injury. *American Journal of Surgery* **164**, 522–6; discussion 526–7.

25 Parrilla P, Ortiz A, Martinez de Haro LF, *et al.* (1990). Evaluation of the magnitude of gastro-oesophageal reflux in Barrett's oesophagus. *Gut* **31**, 964–7.

26 Sharma P, McQuaid K, Dent J, *et al.* (2004). A critical review of the diagnosis and management of Barrett's esophagus: the AGA Chicago Workshop. *Gastroenterology* **127**, 310–30.

27 Sharma P, Sampliner RE, Camargo E (1997). Normalization of esophageal pH with high-dose proton pump inhibitor therapy does not result in regression of Barrett's esophagus. *American Journal of Gastroenterology* **92**, 582–5.

28 Sampliner RE (1994). Effect of up to 3 years of high-dose lansoprazole on Barrett's esophagus. *American Journal of Gastroenterology* **89**, 1844–8.

29 Peters FT, Ganesh S, Kuipers EJ, *et al.* Endoscopic regression of Barrett's oesophagus during omeprazole treatment; a randomised double blind study. *Gut* (1999) **45**, 489–94.

30 Wilkinson SP, Biddlestone L, Gore S, *et al.* (1999). Regression of columnar-lined (Barrett's) oesophagus with omeprazole 40 mg daily: results of 5 years of continuous therapy. *Alimentary Pharmacology & Therapeutics* **13**, 1205–9.

31 Hanna S, Rastogi A, Weston AP, *et al.* (2006). Detection of Barrett's esophagus after endoscopic healing of erosive esophagitis. *American Journal of Gastroenterology* **101**, 1416–20.

32 Modiano N, Gerson LB (2009). Risk factors for the detection of Barrett's esophagus in patients with erosive esophagitis. *Gastrointestinal Endoscopy* **69**, 1014–20.

33 Wani S, Early D, Edmundowicz S, *et al.* (2012). Management of high-grade dysplasia and intramucosal adenocarcinoma in Barrett's esophagus. *Clinical Gastroenterology and Hepatology* **10**, 704–11.

34 Haidry RJ, Dunn JM, Butt MA, *et al.* (2013). Radiofrequency ablation and endoscopic mucosal resection for dysplastic Barrett's esophagus and early esophageal adenocarcinoma: outcomes of the UK National Halo RFA Registry. *Gastroenterology* **145**, 87–95.

35 Shaheen NJ, Sharma P, Overholt BF, *et al.* (2009). Radiofrequency ablation in Barrett's esophagus with dysplasia. *New England Journal of Medicine* **360**, 2277–88.

36 Shaheen NJ, Overholt BF, Sampliner RE, *et al.* (2011). Durability of radiofrequency ablation in Barrett's esophagus with dysplasia. *Gastroenterology* **141**, 460–8.

37 Phoa KN, Pouw RE, van Vilsteren FG, *et al.* (2013). Remission of Barrett's esophagus with early neoplasia 5 years after radiofrequency ablation with endoscopic resection: a Netherlands cohort study. *Gastroenterology* **145**, 96–104.

38 Gupta M, Iyer PG, Lutzke L, *et al.* (2013). Recurrence of esophageal intestinal metaplasia after endoscopic mucosal resection and radiofrequency ablation of Barrett's esophagus: results from a US Multicenter Consortium. *Gastroenterology* **145**, 79–86 e1.

39 Pouw RE, Wirths K, Eisendrath P, *et al.* (2010). Efficacy of radiofrequency ablation combined with endoscopic resection for barrett's esophagus with early neoplasia. *Clinical Gastroenterology and Hepatology* **8**, 23–9.

CHAPTER 15

Thermal therapies and photodynamic therapy for early esophageal neoplasia

Jacques Deviere

Department of Gastroenterology, Hepatopancreatology and Digestive Oncology, Erasme University Hospital, Université Libre de Bruxelles, Brussels, Belgium

15.1 Introduction

Barrett's esophagus (BE), defined as the replacement of squamous esophageal epithelium by intestinal metaplasia in the distal esophagus, is a premalignant lesion that may further develop into dysplasia and lead to adenocarcinoma of the esophagus. A better knowledge of this disease, and the developments of endoscopic therapies over the last 30 years, have profoundly changed our approach to early esophageal neoplasia associated with BE.

Progress has been made in endoscopic work-up, thanks to dramatic improvements in endoscopic imaging, which have allowed better identification, recognition and characterization of the suspected lesions, as well as in pathological definitions and interpretation, thus limiting the risk of understaging (by lack of recognition) and/or overstaging (by unappropriated interpretation) [1].

Once only performed in referral centers, endoscopic resection (ER) of focal early tumors is now performed in many centers, while referral centers now have programs that include endoscopic mucosal resection, endoscopic submucosal dissection in selected cases and ablation of residual Barrett's, to prevent the development of metachronous lesions after focal ablation. After removal of a focal lesion or, in case of high-grade intestinal neoplasia (HGIN) without visible lesion, radiofrequency ablation (RFA) has gained credibility and proved efficacy over the last five years [2, 3]. It is now considered by many as the reference technique for ablation of residual Barrett after resection of a focal lesion, or for selected treatments of dysplasia in the absence of visible lesions, as developed in another chapter.

However, already in the nineties, other thermal ablation techniques have been used in the setting of BE and early esophageal adenocarcinoma. Some have disappeared such as multipolar electrocoagulation (MPEC), others have seen their utility changing or have not yet gained acceptance. They include photodynamic therapy (PDT), argon plasma coagulation (APC) and cryotherapy (CT). This chapter summarizes the knowledge acquired with these techniques and tries to define the potential residual niches of application as well as possible further progresses which could be made in thermal ablation.

One of the rationales behind thermal and PDT ablation was that, in an anacid environment, the destruction of BE mucosa leads to a squamous reepithelialization, with a possible impact on the risk of tumor development by reversing the pathophysiological sequence that leads to adenocarcinoma [4–6].

Thermal endoscopic therapies and PDT are technically easier than mucosal resection, and their indications have been directed towards :

1 The destruction of non-dysplastic intestinal metaplasia (IM), leading to its replacement by squamous epithelium in the hope of having a direct impact on the risk of tumor development.

2 The destruction of BE associated with low grade intestinal neoplasia (LGIN), with the same purpose.

3 The destruction of remaining BE after ER of a focal lesion, with the hope of reducing the risk of metachronous tumor development.

4 The treatment of HGIN or intramucosal adenocarcinoma.

Esophageal Cancer and Barrett's Esophagus, Third Edition. Edited by Prateek Sharma, Richard Sampliner and David Ilson.
© 2015 John Wiley & Sons, Ltd. Published 2015 by John Wiley & Sons, Ltd.

15.2 Photodynamic therapy

Throughout the 1990s and early 2000s, PDT has been the most widely used ablation technique for treatment of early neoplasia in BE [7–9]. Although often classified as thermal therapy, it uses the interaction between drug, light and oxygen. After accumulation of the drug (a photosensitizer) in the targeted tissue, it is illuminated at an appropriate wavelength. Energy is absorbed by the photosensitizer and results in the creation of free oxygen radicals, leading to cell death and apoptosis. Tissue damage is delayed, and usually becomes visible 12–24 hours after the procedure.

Two photosensitizers which were mainly used for PDT of early Barrett's neoplasia. The only one approved by FDA, and therefore used in the USA, is sodium porfimer (or Photofrim 2). It is also, unfortunately, the one associated with the highest rate of complications [8–10]. 5-aminolevulinic acid (5-ALA) was mainly used in Europe [7], and differs by its much more limited accumulation at the mucosal layer into the esophagus (which probably explains its much lower risk of stenosis after treatment).

PDT has been used for the treatment of HGIN or early cancer in high-risk patients, and offered a 50–96% eradication rate of neoplasia, as well as regression of BE in approximately 50% of the cases, with follow up ranging from 12–60 months. The recurrence rate, at more than two years was, however, significant, ranging from 10–75%. Recurrence risk was associated with advanced age, smoking and the presence of residual non-dysplastic BE, a feature unfortunately observed frequently [11].

Although of potential interest in the absence of other alternative treatment to surgery, these results have become insufficient to justify routine use, and made the technique obsolete in this indication when ER became more widespread. This is also due to the complications associated with PDT, which include :

1 Cutaneous photosensitivity, mainly observed with sodium porfimer, requiring strict sun-blocking protection during at least two weeks and resulting in significant skin complications in up to 20% of cases.

2 Retrosternal pain and odynophagia also present for up to two weeks.

3 Symptomatic stenosis formation in approximately one-third of the patients treated with sodium porfimer. This is not or rarely observed after 5-ALA treatment. The rate of symptomatic strictures even increased after previous EMR [10], which further reduces applicability (at least when Photofrim is used as photosensitizer), when EMR of visible lesions has become standard.

Although the number of publications has dramatically dropped over the last five years, a recently published randomized controlled trial comparing 5-ALA and photofrim PDT confirmed the relatively low rate of complete remission of HGIN obtained with both techniques at five years (less than 50% for both sensitizers), and the better risk profile of 5-ALA in terms of complications. Both techniques were followed by squamous reepithelialization, but with a high incidence of buried glands (48 and 20% after photofrin and 5-ALA, respectively), and 14% of new cancer incidence [12].

The issue of buried glands exists with most ablation techniques [6, 13], and was recently also described in association with subsquamous adenocarcinoma and HGIN after RFA [14]. It was, however, first described after PDT. Interestingly, not only are the genetic abnormalities present before PDT, and potentially responsible for the malignant potential, still present in residual or subsquamousmetaplastic glands after treatment [15], but PDT itself, through production of reactive oxygen species, might induce new genetic abnormalities involved in BE progression towards cancer [16].

For all these reasons, considering the primary indications of PDT, namely treatment of neoplasia and prevention of recurrences, the technique has not reached the level of reasonable expectations, and has been largely abandoned, even in referral enthusiastic centers.

15.3 Argon plasma coagulation

APC is a modality that requires an argon gas source, high-frequency electric current and a dedicated catheter that delivers the gas and the current to the tissue. When coming out of the catheter, the gas is ionized by the electrode and delivers high-frequency current to the tissue. Ideally, the probe should not be in contact with the tissue, allowing the current to travel through the gas. The coagulation depth is reported to be controlled to 1–3 mm, due to the physical properties of the electrically insulating zone of tissue desiccation, which confers increased electrical resistance and contributes to limit depth of coagulation. Depth of injury is, however, dependent on generator power setting (30–90 watts), argon gas flow rate (1–2 liters/min), probe-tissue distance (2–5 mm) and duration of application [27]. When applied in BE, APC generates a white coagulum, either circumferentially, point by point for a short segment, or by achieving longitudinal strips in a backward direction during withdrawal of the endoscope.

The first wave of enthusiasm with APC treatment came from clinical series and trials exploring its use in ablation of non-dysplastic BE or low grade intestinal neoplasia LGIN [17–25]. It was fascinating to see that, in a anacid environment, destroying the mucosa using non-expensive equipment enabled an endoscopic squamous reepithelialization to be obtained in 70–100% of cases (Table 15.1), with the hope that it could reverse the sequence which leads to the development of adenocarcinoma and avoid the need for surveillance. In terms of squamous reepithelialization, APC achieved results similar or superior to PDT [25] with much lower complications, which consisted of pain and odynophagia, with very rare perforations or stenoses.

It is interesting to note that it is almost ten years since the first reports on clinical application of APC in non-dysplastic BE, that level 1 evidence of its ability to induce partial or complete replacement of intestinal metaplasia by squamous mucosa has become available [28]. This was done in an interesting group of patients undergoing APC or surveillance after surgery. Overall, at one year, complete "ablation" was achieved in 63% of the treated group and 15% of the surveillance

group ($p < 0.01$). No patient had dysplasia at the end of follow-up and, interestingly, in a subgroup of patients with buried glands, they noticed a reduction of their frequency between one month and one year of follow-up. This is the opposite of what was observed after APC application without surgical fundoplication.

Indeed, the enthusiasm went down when longer follow-up became available, showing a high incidence (up to 68%) of recurrence at mid-term follow-up, especially in patients with initial long-segment BE and those who reduced their PPI dose [24] (Table 15.2).

Buried glands, which were observed in median 15% of the cases, even when complete squamous reepithelialization was obtained, have rapidly become a matter of concern. This was confirmed when cases of carcinoma arising in these buried glands were reported [12, 26], which was obviously contradicting the first purpose of such treatment, namely to avoid progression to cancer. With such observations, it was doubtful that this goal was achieved and ablation surely was not allowed to avoid surveillance. On the contrary, reepithelialization might render this surveillance less effective, due to the fact that early lesions arising under the neosquamous epithelium would become more difficult to detect.

We recently reviewed a cohort of 32 patients with non-dysplastic BE treated by APC in the 1990s, and for whom a 16-years follow-up was available [29]. Even if a complete endoscopic eradication was still present at the end of follow-up in 50% of the cases, we observed (over

Table 15.1 Studies on argon plasma coagulation (APC) in non-dysplastic Barrett's esophagus: short-term result.

Authors	Patients	APC/MPEC sessions (median, range)	APC power setting (W)	Length of Barrett (cms) (range)	PPI doses during treatment (mg/day)	Endoscopic ablation (%)	Residual intestinal metaplasia (%)
Mork et al. (1998)	15	4 (1–8)	60	median 4 (2–8)	60	86.7	0
Van Laethem et al. (1998)	31	2.4 (1–4)	60	mean 4.5 (3–11)	40	81	24
Byrne et al. (1998)	30	4 (2–7)	60	median 5 (3–17)	20–40	100	30
Grade et al. (1999)	9	mean 1.7	60	mean 3.5 (UK)	60–90	100	22
Pereira -Lima et al. (2000)	33	mean 1.9	65–70	median 4 (0.5–7)	60	100	0
Schultz et al. (2000)	73	2 (1–4)	90	median 4 (1–12)	120	98.6	0
Morris et al. (2001)	53	mean 3	UK	mean 6 (3–15)	20–60	UK	30
Basu et al. (2002)	50	4 (1–8)	30	mean 5.9 (3–19)	20	68	44
Kahaleh et al. (2002)	39	3 (1–4)	60	mean 4.7 (2–11)	40	70	18
Dulai et al. (2005)	24	mean 3.6	60	≥2 < 7	80	81	35

Table 15.2 Studies on argon plasma coagulation (APC) in non-dysplastic Barrett's esophagus: long-term results.

Authors	Patients	APC power setting (W)	PPI doses maintenance (mg/day)	Median follow-up (months)	Intestinal metaplasia on follow-up (%)
Mork *et al.* (1998)	15	60	20–60	6–13	7.6
Van Laethem *et al.* (1998)	31	60	10 or 40	12	47
Byrne *et al.* (1998)	30	60	20	9	30
Pereira-Lima *et al.* (2000)	33	65–70	30	10.6	3
Schultz *et al.* (2000)	73	90	20 or 40	12	0%
Morris *et al.* (2001)	53	UK	20–60	38.5	UK
Basu *et al.* (2002)	50	30	20–60	14	68
Kahaleh *et al.* (2002)	39	60	20 or 40	36	62
Madisch *et al.* (2005)	66	90	120	51	12

a total of 376 patients years of follow-up) three cancers, including two appearing underneath the neosquamous epithelium. Overall, we had an incidence of cancer of 0.8%/patient-year, which is clearly not different from the incidence reported in surveillance series.

Given all these data, it may be concluded that APC ablation (and currently any ablation technique probably) is not recommended in management of non-dysplastic BE, and there are insufficient data to justify its use in LGIN. Combined with the need for life-long high doses of PPI therapy, available data showed that thermal ablation increases the cost of management/ surveillance of non-dysplastic BE, and is associated with potential complications without any demonstrated clinical benefit.

Another indication where APC was evaluated in some series is the ablation of BE with high-grade intestinal neoplasia or cancer. Apart from some cases reported in series including non-dysplastic BE, two studies focused on APC treatment in patients unfit for surgery [30, 31]. They reported a complete response to treatment in 80% and 86% of the cases, while progression to cancer was observed in 11% and 10% over a mean follow-up of 37 and 12 months, respectively. The absence of mucosal resection in these series did not allow evaluation of the depth of penetration of initial tumors, and authors never claimed to use APC in other groups than patients unfit for surgery. The development of ER in these indications rendered the application of APC, as a single treatment, obsolete in this indication.

Up to recently, the use of APC in BE was limited to a minimum. It was sometimes useful for ablation of small

residual bridges after piecemeal endoscopic resection, although avoidance of such bridges is the cornerstone of adequate ER.

However, with the spread of ER for treatment of early Barrett's neoplasia, the problem of metachronous neoplasia occurring in any remaining segment has become prominent. These metachronous lesions are observed in up to 20% of patients [32]. It has become widely accepted that, after resection of a visible lesion, the remaining non-neoplastic Barrett segment should either be resected (which allows precise pathological staging concerning multifocal neoplasia) or ablated.

RFA has become popular for ablation of residual Barrett's, and is an accepted technique in this indication [33]. However, it is a technique significantly more expensive than APC, which is still not covered by health insurance in several countries, particularly in Europe, and has never been shown to be better than APC in face-to-face randomized controlled trials (RCT). Although series from referral centers report a low incidence of residual buried glands, a complete reepithelialization is not observed in every case [34].

The group of Wiesbaden [35] recently reported on an long-term randomized follow-up study comparing APC (*n* = 33 patients) of residual Barrett's with surveillance (*n* = 30 patients) in patients in whom complete remission from early Barrett's cancer or HGIN had been achieved following endoscopic resection. All patients were on high-dose, 24-hour pHmetry-adjusted, PPIs. Recurrence of neoplasia after a mean follow-up of 27 months was observed in one in 33 (1%) and 11 in 30

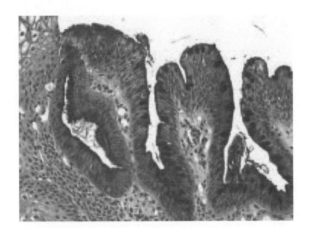

Figure 7.1 Periodic acid-Schiff (PAS)/Alcian blue at pH 2.5 demonstrates incomplete intestinal metaplasia. Goblet cells containing acid mucin stain intensely blue with Alcian blue (right), while the adjacent columnar cells containing neutral mucin stain with PAS (left).

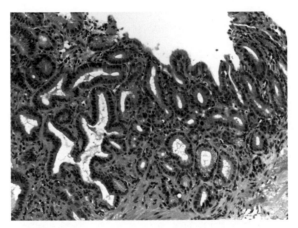

Figure 7.4 Barrett's gastric foveolar-type dysplasia, low-grade. H&E-stained section of Barrett's esophageal biopsy showing full-thickness mucosal replacement by crowded glands and non-villiform architecture. The cells demonstrate basally oriented monolayered and uniform nuclei, with abundant pale eosinophilic to mucinous cytoplasm.

Esophageal Cancer and Barrett's Esophagus, Third Edition. Edited by Prateek Sharma, Richard Sampliner and David Ilson.
© 2015 John Wiley & Sons, Ltd. Published 2015 by John Wiley & Sons, Ltd.

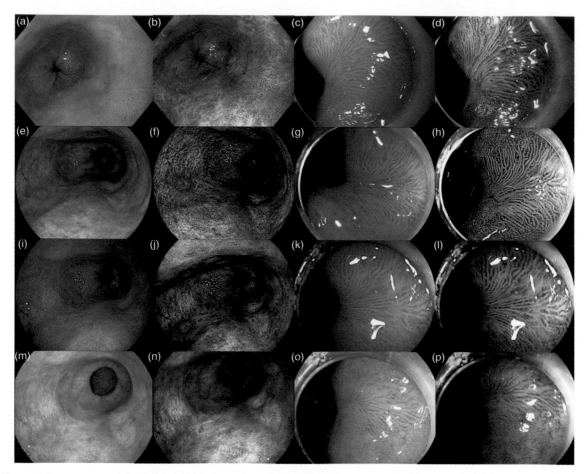

Figure 10.1 Overview and detailed images of a neoplastic lesions in a Barrett's esophagus: Olympus high resolution white light endoscopy (a, c); and narrow band imaging (b, d); Fujinon white light endoscopy (e.g.) and blue light imaging (f, h); Fujinon white light endoscopy (i, k); and Fujinon intelligent chromoendoscopy (j, l); Pentax white light endoscopy (m, o) and iSCAN (n, p).

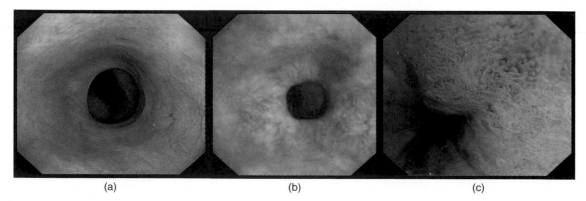

Figure 10.2 Early neoplastic lesion in Barrett's esophagus, imaged with a) high-resolution white light endoscopy; b) autofluorescence imaging; and c) narrow band imaging.

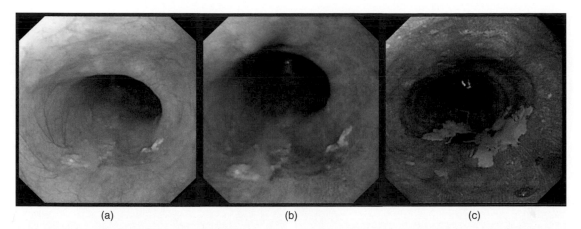

(a)   (b)   (c)

Figure 10.3 Early esophageal squamous cell carcinoma, imaged with a) white light endoscopy; b) narrow band imaging; and c) after Lugol's staining.

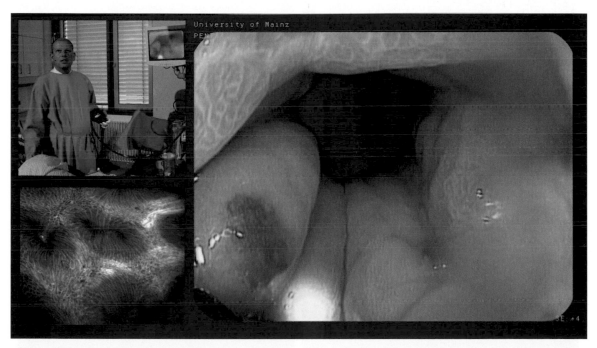

Figure 11.1 Setting of endomicroscopy. The confocal endoscope (iCLE) is handled like a conventional endoscope. The microscope is embedded in the distal tip and emits blue laser light onto the mucosa (right picture). Endomicroscopic images are displayed (lower left picture) by placing the microscope gently onto the mucosa.

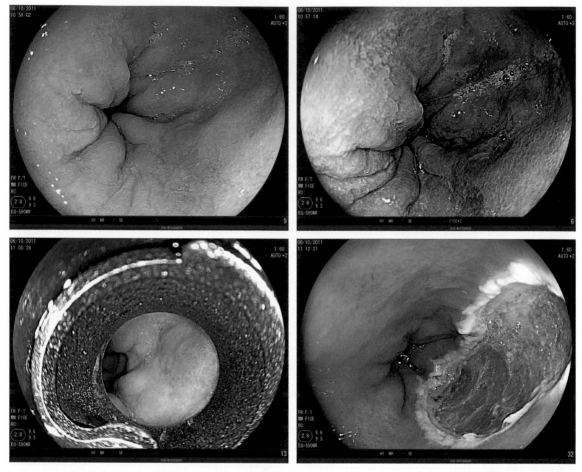

Figure 18.1 **a-d** ER-L of a subtle type IIb Barrett's neoplasia.

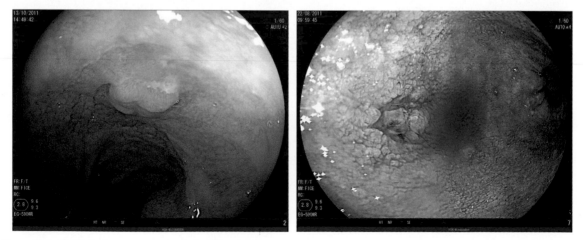

Figure 18.2 a-b ER-C of a recurrent neoplasia with scaring.

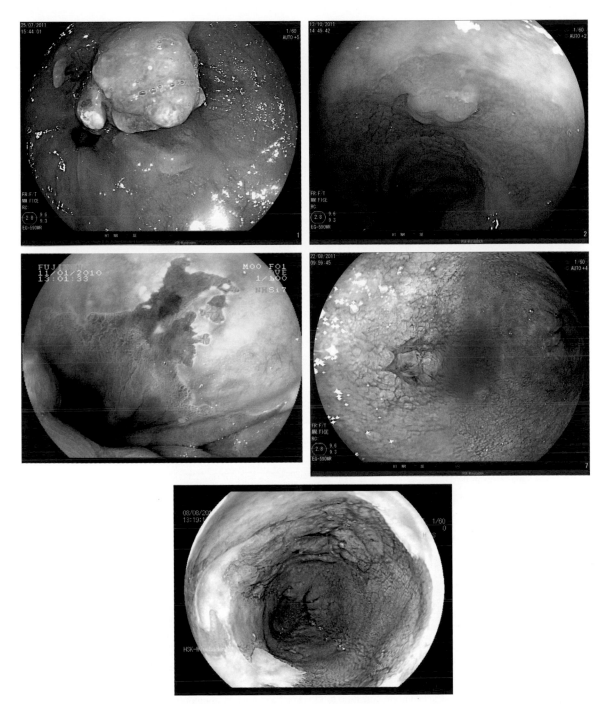

Figure 18.4 Endoscopic examples of different macroscopic types of early Barrett's neoplasia: (a) Type I–polypoid lesion. (b) Type IIa–slightly elevated lesion. (c) Type IIb–flat lesion in mucosal level. (d) Type IIc–depressed lesion. (e) Type IIa + c–mixed type lesion.

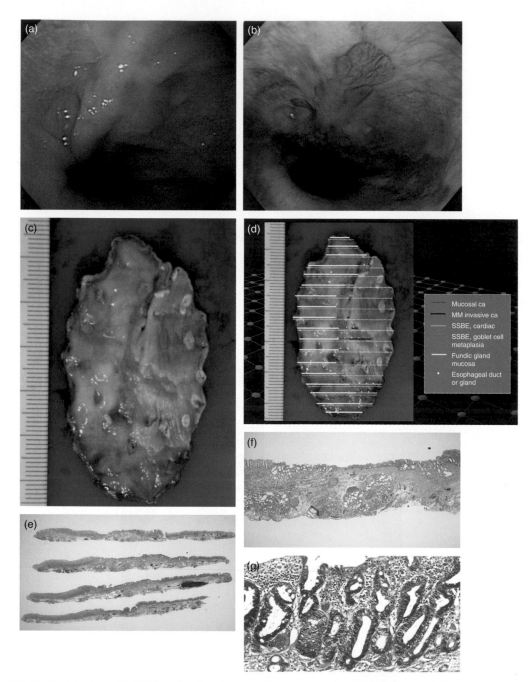

Figure 19.2 *En bloc* resection with ESD for a junctional cancer arisen from short-segment Barrett epithelium. **a**. Avascular edematous mucosa on the end of the gastric fold in the junction. **b**. Elongated columnar epithelium with dysplasia (or well-differentiated adenocarcinoma) in squamous epithelium. **c**. *En bloc* material resected by ESD. **d**. Histological assessment (well-differentiated adenocarcinoma developed from short-segment Barrett epithelium–size of tumor: 19 × 15 mm; depth of invasion: MM). **e**. Low power views of serial section. **f**. Esophageal glands in submucosal layer and columnar epithelium in mucosal layer. **g**. Well-differentiated adenocarcinoma (high power view).

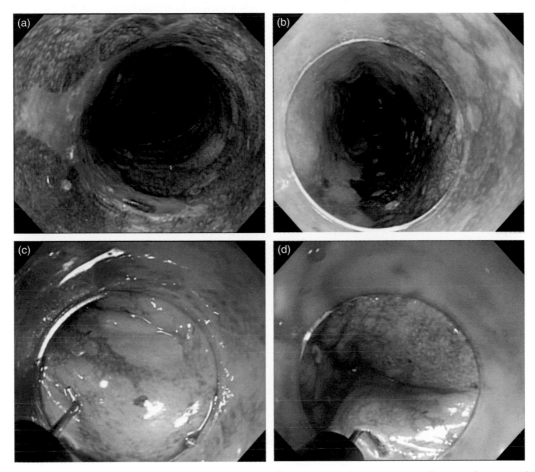

Figure 19.3 *En bloc* resection with ESD for a superficial squamous cell carcinoma in the esophagus. **a**. Chromoendoscopy with Iodine staining. The unstained area with a clear border through iodine staining represents widespread squamous cell carcinoma of the middle thoracic esophagus. The lesion extends from the anterior wall to the posterior wall, and is subtotal. Excision of such a lesion with conventional EMR leads to multiple piecemeal resection and makes accurate postoperative pathological evaluation impossible. Since the remaining non-neoplastic mucosa may also be excised, the risk of stricture due to circumferential excision is greater. **b**. While the mucosa is touched slightly with the hook knife stored in the sheath, marking is made by applying current for a moment with forced coagulation at 40 W. Non-neoplastic epithelial mucosa is a small portion, due to the subtotal lesion. For prevention of stricture, however, it is important to leave this portion. **c**. The mucosal incision is initiated after a submucosal local injection. With the use of a hook knife, when the back of the knife is pressed lightly on the mucosa to apply current for a moment with a dry cut effect 5, 60 W, a small hole is bored into the mucosa for insertion of the point of the knife into the submucosal layer. **d**. The muscularis mucosae are hooked with the knife inserted into the submucosal layer and elevated to the luminal side for the incision by applying a current. A sufficient local injection is needed to prevent perforation. Also, it is important to control the direction of the knife to the luminal side. **e**. Endoscopic view during incision of the mucosa. The translucent submucosal layer and a vessel are observed on the right side. The muscularis propria is invisible because of the sufficient local injection. A mucosal incision with hooking in this state causes no perforation. **f**. Endoscopic view during dissection of the submucosal layer. The view of the submucosal layer is obtained by opening the layer with a transparent hood attached at the tip of the endoscope. The submucosal layer is dissected while hooking the fibers and the vessels with the tip of the hook knife. To prevent perforation and bleeding, it is important to perform dissection while directly observing the submucosal layer. **g**. Endoscopic view immediately after ESD completed. Sub-circumferential excision was performed, leaving the ≈5 mm wide non-neoplastic mucosa. Fibers of the submucosal layer are left on the ulcer floor, and no muscularis propria is exposed. Because the esophagus lacks serosa, the exposure of the muscularis propria may cause mediastinal emphysema. Consequently, it is important to dissect at the inferior third of the submucosal layer. **h**. Iodine stained view of excised specimen. The clear and irregular iodine unstained border and existence of the non-neoplastic mucosa stained by iodine at the excised margins reveal negative surgical margins. The lesion was pathologically diagnosed as squamous cell carcinoma of 53 × 40 mm with LPM in invasion depth, and complete excision was confirmed.

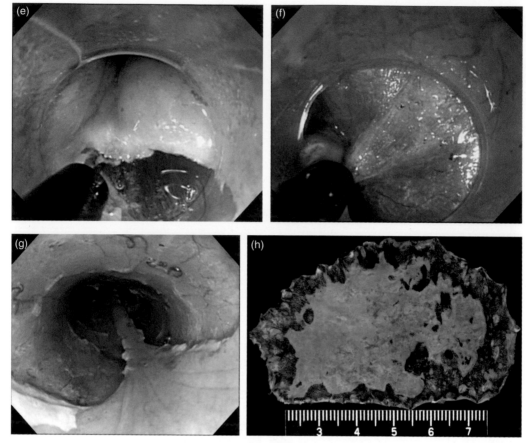

Figure 19.3 (*Continued*)

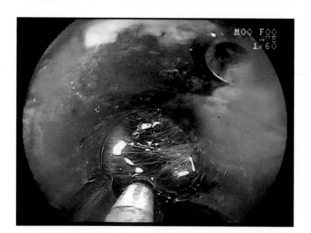

Figure 19.5 Endoscopic view of submucosal dissection using a needle knife through an ST hood. The submucosal fibers are hooked by the tip of a needle knife, while opening the incised mucosa with the tip of the ST hood.

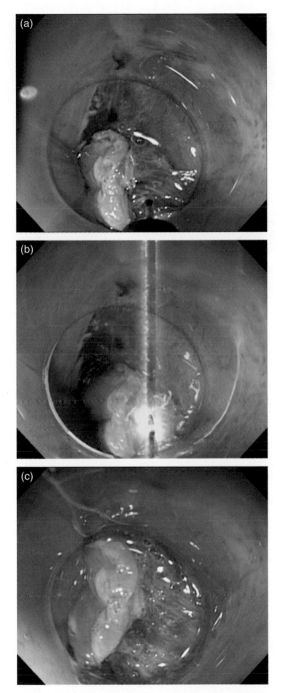

Figure 19.6 Bleeding prevention during dissection. For a small vessel about 0.5 mm in diameter, the slow excision of the vessel by applying current, with the spray mode effect 2, 60 W, allows dissection without bleeding. It is important for prevention of bleeding to slowly incise the vessel.

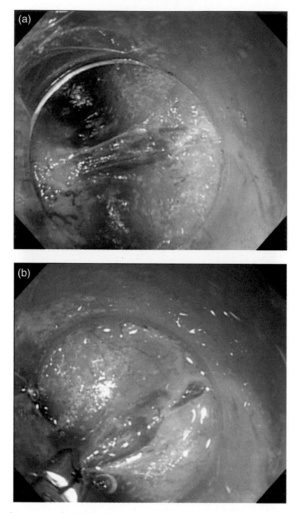

Figure 19.7 Pre-coagulation. **a**. When a vessel thicker than 1 mm or an artery is observed, pre-coagulation becomes a very useful method for prevention of bleeding. Fibers around the vessel are sufficiently dissected to expose the vessel. **b**. The vessel is grasped with a rotatable coagulation forceps. At this time, the direction of the forceps is adjusted to an angle perpendicular to the vessel. Electrification is performed with soft coagulation, effect 5, 40 W. Since damage to the muscularis propria due to electrification may cause delayed perforation, it is important to apply current while slowly pulling the site away from the muscularis propria grasped by the forceps.

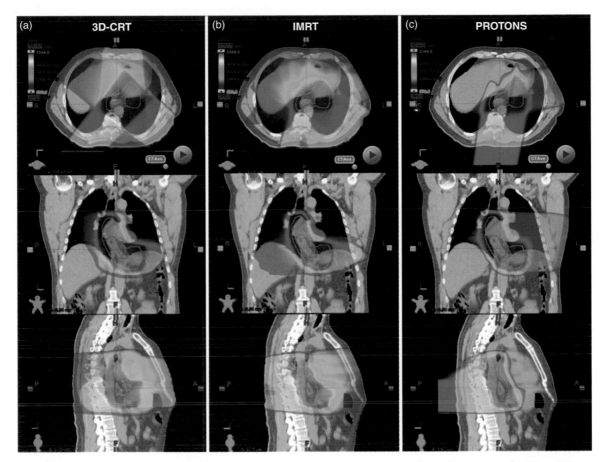

Figure 25.1 Comparative radiation treatment plans. a) 3D-CRT; b) IMRT; c) Proton beam; d) DVH comparison between treatment modalities. In this case, both IMRT and protons provide improved lung and cardiac sparing compared with 3D-CRT. Proton beam decreases liver dose compared to other modalities.

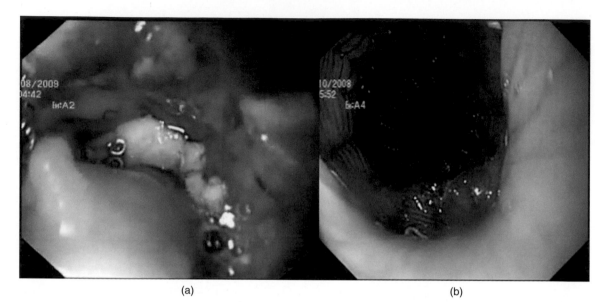

Figure 27.1 (a) Stenosis from esophageal cancer. (b) Reconstruction of luminal perviety with placement of an esophageal stent.

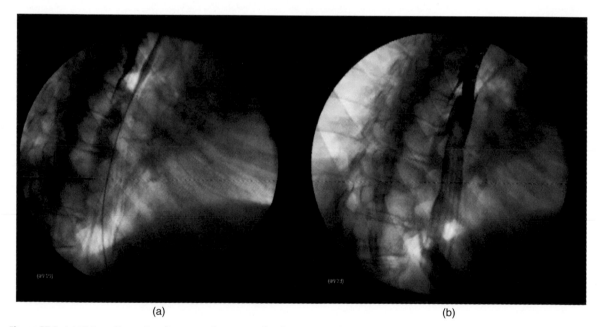

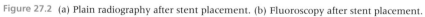

Figure 27.2 (a) Plain radiography after stent placement. (b) Fluoroscopy after stent placement.

(36%) patients in the ablation and the surveillance group, respectively. Given these results, APC ablation of residual non-neoplastic BE combined with PPI therapy became standard in their center. The major complications consisted of stricture formation, requiring bougie dilation, in three patients. These results compare favorably with ablation using RFA, and a trial comparing both ablation techniques in this indication would be desirable to evaluate both their efficacy and their cost-effectiveness.

Although, with various frequencies, all thermal methods of ablation carry a significant risk of stenosis and, as far as APC is concerned, the fear of creating deep wall injury may limit the completeness of ablation. Initially described on isolated organs [36, 37], submucosal injection of saline may prevent muscular damage and, possibly, facilitate mucosal destruction. This coagulation/injection technique has been recently described to assist complete resection of recurrent fibrotic colon polyps [38]. In line with that, Erbe (Tuebingen, Germany) has recently developed a system which combines their "Erbejet" submucosal injection system with an APC probe. Clinical trials are ongoing, and will probably focus not only on the potential decrease of complications but also on a potentially more complete and homogeneous ablation, resulting in a lower incidence of buried glands.

15.4 Cryotherapy

Another thermal method uses liquid nitrogen as cryogen (delivered at a temperature of $-196°C$) to destroy the esophageal mucosa. Three studies using this system have been published so far. The first one [39] included inoperable patients with HGIN and early cancer, and demonstrated elimination or downgrading of HGIN or intramucosal cancer in 68% and 80% of patients, respectively, at a median follow-up of 12 months. Two other studies demonstrated complete eradication of HGIN in more than 95% of the cases, and complete eradication of intestinal metaplasia (IM) in 57% and 84%, over a relatively short follow-up period of 10 and 24 months, [40, 41].

Although of potential interest, the role of this technique in the armamentarium of early Barrett's cancer management has still to be defined, and it is currently under investigation.

15.5 Conclusion

Thermal therapies or PDT are clearly not indicated in non-dysplastic Barrett's, like any other current ablation technique. PDT has shown effectiveness in managing HGIN but, due to its high rate of recurrence and incidence of severe complications, it has become obsolete with the advent of endoscopic resection and more effective ablation techniques. The same is true for APC in primary management of HGIN and intramucosal neoplasia. However, APC still has a potential role for ablation of residual Barrett's after ER of HGIN or early cancer. New techniques combining submucosal injection and APC might further improve the results of this technique in this indication.

References

1 Boerwinkel DF, Swager AF, Curvers WL, Bergman JJ (2014). The clinical consequences of advanced imaging techniques in Barrett's esophagus. *Gastroenterology* **146**, 622–9.

2 Shaheen NJ, Sharma P, Overholt BF, Wolfsen HC, *et al.* (2009). Radiofrequency ablation in Barrett's esophagus with dysplasia. *New England Journal of Medicine* **360**, 2277–88.

3 Phoa KN, Pouw RE, van Vilsteren FG, Sondermeijer CM, *et al.* (2013). Remission of Barrett's esophagus with early neoplasia 5 years after radiofrequency ablation with endoscopic resection: a Netherlands cohort study. *Gastroenterology* **145**, 96–104.

4 Barham CP, Jones RL, Biddlestone LR, Hardwick RH, *et al.* (1997). Photothermal laser ablation of Barrett's oesophagus: endoscopic and histological evidence of squamous re-epithelialisation. *Gut* **41**, 281–4.

5 Byrne JP, Armstrong GR, Attwood SE (1998). Restoration of the normal squamous lining in Barrett's esophagus by argon beam plasma coagulation. *American Journal of Gastroenterology* **93**, 1810–5.

6 Van Laethem JL, Cremer M, Peny MO, Delhaye M, Devière (1998). Eradication of Barrett's mucosa with argon plasma coagulation and acid suppression: immediate and mid term results. *Gut* **43**, 747–51.

7 Pech O, Gossner L, May A, Rabenstein T *et al.* (2005). Long-term results of photodynamic therapy with 5-aminolevulinic acid for superficial Barrett's cancer and high-grade intraepithelial neoplasia. *Gastrointestinal Endoscopy* **62**, 24–30.

8 Overholt BF, Wang KK, Burdick JS, Lightdale CJ, *et al.* (2007). Five-year efficacy and safety of photodynamic therapy with Photofrin in Barrett's high-grade dysplasia. *Gastrointestinal Endoscopy* **66**, 460–8.

9 P Overholt BF, Lightdale CJ, Wang KK, Canto MI, *et al.* (2005). hotodynamic therapy with porfimer sodium for ablation of high-grade dysplasia in Barrett's esophagus: international, partially blinded, randomized phase III trial. *Gastrointestinal Endoscopy* **62**, 488–98.

10 Prasad GA, Wang KK, Buttar NS, Wongkeesong LM, *et al.* (2007). Predictors of stricture formation after photodynamic therapy for high-grade dysplasia in Barrett's esophagus. *Gastrointestinal Endoscopy* **65**, 60–6.

11 Badreddine RJ, Prasad GA, Wang KK, Song LM, *et al.* (2010). Prevalence and predictors of recurrent neoplasia after ablation of Barrett's esophagus. *Gastrointestinal Endoscopy* **71**, 697–703.

12 Dunn JM, Mackenzie GD, Banks MR, Mosse CA, *et al.* (2013). A randomized controlled trial of ALA vs photofrin photodynamic therapy for high-grade dysplasia arising in Barrett's esophagus. *Lasers in Medical Science* **28**, 707–15.

13 Van Laethem JL, Peny MO, Salmon I, Cremer M, Devière (2000). Intramucosal adenocarcinoma arising under squamous re-epithelialisation of Barrett's oesophagus. *Gut* **46**, 574–7.

14 Titi M, Overhiser A, Ulusarac O, Falk GW, *et al.* (2012). Development of subsquamous high-grade dysplasia and adenocarcinoma after successful radiofrequency ablation of Barrett's esophagus. *Gastroenterology* **143**, 564–6.

15 Barr H, Schepherd NA, Dix A, Roberts DJ, *et al.* (1996). Eradication of high-grade dysplasia in columnar-lined (Barrett's) oesophagus by photodynamic therapy with endogenously generated protoporhyrin IX. *Lancet* **348**, 584–5.

16 Farhadi A, Fields J, Banan A, Keshavarzian A (2002). Reactive oxygen species: are they involved in the pathogenesis of GERD, Barrett's esophagus, and the latter's progression toward esophageal cancer ? *American Journal of Gastroenterology* **97**, 22–6.

17 Madisch A, Michlke S, Bayerdorffer E, Wiedemann B, *et al.* (2005). Long term follow up after ablation of Barrett's esophagus with argon plasma coagulation. *World Journal of Gastroenterology* **11**, 1182–6.

18 Kahaleh M, Van Laethem JL, Nagy N, Cremer M, *et al.* (2002). Long term follow-up and factors predictive of recurrence in Barrett's esophagus treated by argon plasma therapy and acid suppression. *Endoscopy* **12**, 950–5.

19 Schulz H, Michlke S, Antos D, Schentke KU, *et al.* (2000). Ablation of Barrett's epithelium by endoscopic argon plasma coagulation in combination with high-dose omeprazole. *Gastrointestinal Endoscopy* **51**, 659–63.

20 Pereira-Lima JC, Busnello JV, Saul C, Toneloto EB *et al.* (2000). High power setting argon plasma coagulation for the eradication of Barrett's esophagus. *American Journal of Gastroenterology* **95**, 1661–8.

21 Morris CD, Byrne JP, Armstrong GR, Attwood SE (2001). Prevention of the neoplastic progression of Barrett's oesophagus by endoscopic argon beam plasma ablation. *British Journal of Surgery* **88**, 1357–62.

22 Mork H, Barth T, Kreipe HH, Kraus M, *et al.* (1998). Reconstitution of squamous epithelium in Barrett's oesophagus with endoscopic argon plasma coagulation: a prospective study. *Scandinavian Journal of Gastroenterology* **33**, 1130–4.

23 Byrne JP, Armstrong GR, Attwood SE (1998). Restoration of the normal squamous lining in Barrett's esophagus by argon beam plasma coagulation. *American Journal of Gastroenterology* **93**, 1810–5.

24 Basu KK, Pick B, Bale R, West KP, *et al.* (2002). Efficacy and one year follow up of argon plasma coagulation therapy for ablation for Barrett's oesophagus: factors determining persistence and recurrence of Barrett's epithelium. *Gut* **51**, 776–80.

25 Kelty CJ, Ackroyd R, Brown NJ, Stephenson TJ, *et al.* (2004). Endoscopic ablation of Barrett's oesophagus: a randomized-controlled trial of photodynamic therapy vs argon plasma coagulation. *Alimentary Pharmacology & Therapeutics* **20**, 1289–96.

26 Shand A, Dallal H, Palmer K, Ghosh S, *et al.* (2001). Adenocarcinoma arising in columnar lined oesophagus following treatment with argon plasma coagulation. *Gut* **48**, 580–1.

27 Ginsberg GG, Barkun AN, Bosco JJ, Burdick JS, *et al.* (2002). The argon plasma coagulator. *Gastrointestinal Endoscopy* **55**, 807–10.

28 Ackroyd R, Tam W, Schoeman M, Devitt PG, *et al.* (2004) Prospective randomized controlled trial of argon plasma coagulation ablation vs endoscopic surveillance of patients with Barrett's esophagus after antireflux surgery. *Gastrointestinal Endoscopy* **59**, 1–7.

29 Milashka M, Calomme A, Van Laethem J-L, Blero D, Eisendrath P, Le Moine O, Deviere J (2014). Sixteen-year follow-up of Barrett's esophagus endoscopically treated with argon plasma coagulation. *United European Gastroenterology Journal* **2**, 367–373

30 Attwood SE, Lewis CJ, Caplin S, Hemming K, *et al.* (2003). Argon beam plasma coagulation as therapy for high-grade dysplasia in Barrett's esophagus. *Clinical Gastroenterology and Hepatology* **1**, 258–63.

31 Van Laethem JL, Jagodzinski R, Peny MO, Cremer M, *et al.* (2001). Argon plasma coagulation in the treatment of Barrett's high-grade dysplasia and *in situ* adenocarcinoma. *Endoscopy* **33**, 257–61.

32 Pech O, May A, Manner H, Behrens A, *et al.* (2014). Long-term efficacy and safety of endoscopic resection for patients with mucosal adenocarcinoma of the esophagus. *Gastroenterology* **146**, 652–60.

33 Pouw RE, Wirths K, Eisendrath P, Sondermeijer CM, *et al.* (2010). Efficacy of radiofrequency ablation combined with endoscopic resection for Barrett's esophagus with early neoplasia. *Clinical Gastroenterology and Hepatology* **8**, 23–9.

34 Van Vilsteren FG, Alvarez Herrero L, Pouw RE, Schrijnders D, *et al.* (2013). Predictive factors for initial treatment response after circumferential radiofrequency ablation for Barrett's esophagus with early neoplasia: a prospective multicenter study. *Endoscopy* **45**, 516–25.

35 Manner H, Rabenstein T, Pech O, Braun K, *et al.* (2014). Ablation of residual Barrett's epithelium after endoscopic resection: a randomized long-term follow-up study of argon plasma coagulation vs surveillance (APE study). *Endoscopy* **46**, 6–12.

36 Fujishiro M, Yahagi N, Nakamura M, *et al.* (2006). Submucosal injection of normal saline may prevent damage from argon plasma coagulation. An experimental study using resected procine esophagus, stomach and colon. *Surgical Laparoscopy, Endoscopy & Percutaneous Techniques* **16**, 307–11.

37 Norton ID, Wang L, Levine SA, *et al.* (2002). Efficacy of colonic submucosal saline solution injection for the reduction of iatrogenic thermal injury. *Gastrointestinal Endoscopy* **56**, 95–9.

38 Tsiamoulos ZP, Bourikas LA, Saunders BP (2012). Endoscopic mucosal ablation: a new argon plasma coagulation/injection technique to assist complete resection of recurrent, fibrotic colon polyps (with video). *Gastrointestinal Endoscopy* **75**, 400–4.

39 Dumot JA, Vargo JJ, Falk GW, *et al.* (2009). An open-label, prospective trial of cryospray ablation for Barrett's esophagus high-grade dysplasia and early esophageal cancer in high-risk patients. *Gastrointestinal Endoscopy* **70**, 635–44.

40 Shaheen NJ, Greenwald BD, Beery AF, *et al.* (2010). Safety and efficacy of endoscopic spray cryotherapy for Barrett's esophagus with high-grade dysplasia. *Gastrointestinal Endoscopy* **71**, 680–5.

41 Gosain S, Mercer K, Twaddell WS, *et al.* (2013). Liquid nitrogen spray cryotherapy in Barrett's esophagus with high-grade dysplasia: long-term results. *Gastrointestinal Endoscopy* **78**, 260–5.

CHAPTER 16

RFA for early esophageal neoplasia

Daniel K. Chan, Cadman L. Leggett & Kenneth K. Wang

Barrett's Esophagus Unit, Division of Gastroenterology and Hepatology, Mayo Clinic, Rochester, MN, USA

16.1 Background

Barrett's esophagus (BE) is a pre-neoplastic condition where normal stratified squamous esophageal mucosa is replaced by specialized columnar epithelium in the setting of chronic gastroesophageal reflux [1]. BE can progress to BE with low-grade dysplasia (LGD), high-grade dysplasia (HGD) and, eventually, to esophageal adenocarcinoma. HGD dysplasia has the highest risk of developing into esophageal adenocarcinoma, with a 30% risk over five years [2].

Endoscopic therapy is recommended over esophagectomy for individuals with BE complicated by HGD or intramucosal adenocarcinoma (IMC), as this treatment modality is associated with less morbidity and mortality, and early esophageal cancer is associated with a low rate of lymphatic metastasis [3, 4]. The primary goal of endoscopic therapy for BE with early esophageal neoplasia is to achieve complete eradication of the cancer and, for best long-term results, complete remission of the intestinal metaplasia (CR-IM). Endoscopic therapy for early cancer in BE involves initial endoscopic mucosal resection (EMR) or endoscopic submucosal dissection of any visible neoplastic mucosal abnormalities, followed by mucosal ablation of the remaining columnar mucosa [5, 6]. Resection is required, as it is the best method by which the cancer can be assessed in terms of depth of invasion.

Initially, photodynamic therapy was the preferred mucosal ablation technique, using intravenously administered porfimer sodium that was activated 48 hours after infusion by red light to induce tissue damage. However, complications such as photosensitivity and a high esophageal stricture rate limited its use. Although initial strictures rates were only 16%, it is clear that the therapy was fibrogenic. In addition, patients had more chest pain, as well as cutaneous photosensitivity that often spanned several months. More recently, radio frequency ablation (RFA) has become the mucosal ablation technique of choice, because of its improved side-effect profile and improvement in treatment efficiency [7].

16.2 Device and procedural technique

RFA is a thermal ablative modality that uses alternating electrical current to generate an electromagnetic field, which causes charged ions to rapidly oscillate and release thermal energy. Cauterized tissue acquires a higher resistance and serves as an insulator against further damage and, as such, limits injury to a superficial depth. RFA requires a seamless contact between the interface and the esophagus [8].

The first commercially available RFA device was the ablation balloon (formerly HALO^{360+}, now Barrx™ 360 RFA Balloon Catheter), which was followed by the creation of a focal ablation device (formerly HALO^{90}, now Barrx™ 90 RFA Focal Catheter) (Covidien GI Solutions). The Barrx™ 360 RFA Balloon Catheter is used for circumferential ablation. This system comprises of tightly spaced (<250 μm) radiofrequency electrodes that deliver high power (≈300 W) from the Barrx™ Flex Energy Generator to three separate sequential segments along a three-centimeter balloon.

Treatment must be started by first clearing mucous from the mucosal surface using a mucolytic agent such as N-acetyl-cysteine. This is sprayed on the surface and then removed using endoscopic suctioning. A wire is left in the antrum of the stomach. The treatment

Esophageal Cancer and Barrett's Esophagus, Third Edition. Edited by Prateek Sharma, Richard Sampliner and David Ilson.
© 2015 John Wiley & Sons, Ltd. Published 2015 by John Wiley & Sons, Ltd.

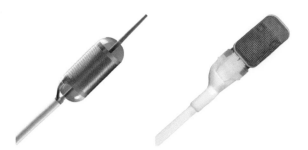

Figure 16.1 Barrx™ 360 RFA Balloon Catheter and Barrx™ 90 RFA Focal Catheter. Source: Barrx.com. Reproduced with permission of Barrx.

balloons vary in size from 18–34 mm in diameter, with the treatment coil length always remaining static at 3 cm. The depth of penetration extends to 500–1000 μm. The ablation catheter size is selected by first using a sizing balloon that is initially placed over a wire into the proximal esophagus. The balloon is calibrated outside of the esophagus, as the diameter is measured by the amount of air infused. For this reason, the air pump that automatically inflates the balloons must be kept free of debris. An air filter is provided with both the treatment and sizing balloons that should be used.

The Barrx™ 90 RFA Focal Catheter also contains an array of radio frequency electrodes and is mechanistically similar to the Barrx™ 360 RFA Balloon Catheter. However, it is not circumferential and, thus, it is used to treat focal areas of BE and cauterizes a region approximately 2 cm^2 in area. The Barrx™ Flex Energy Generator also powers the Barrx™ 90 RFA Focal Catheter (Figure 16.1).

Circumferential ablation of BE with the Barrx™ 360 RFA Balloon Catheter comprises the following steps:

1 *Size*: Esophageal landmarks are endoscopically identified by measuring between the top of intestinal metaplasia to the top of the gastric folds. The Barrx™ 360 Soft Sizing Balloon is positioned over a guidewire 1 cm above the measured distance to the Barrett's mucosa and is automatically inflated to select for an appropriately sized ablation catheter. The guidewire is left in place (Figure 16.2a).

2 *Ablate*: The selected ablation catheter is introduced over the guidewire and positioned side-by-side to the endoscope so that it is under direct visualization. The proximal edge of the ablation catheter is aligned slightly above the proximal border of metaplasia. The balloon is automatically inflated, delivering 300 W of

energy at 12–15 J/cm^2 when treating patients with early cancer. Generally, 12 Joules has been used in the United States, although European groups tend to favor 15 Joules. The catheter is advanced distally 2.5–3.0 cm, and ablation is repeated until the top of the gastric folds are reached. Overlap between treatment segments is minimal, to prevent stricture formation (Figure 16.2b-d).

3 *Clean and repeat*: Coagulum from the ablation zone is removed using a Barrx™ RFA Cleaning Cap on the endoscope, and the Barrx™ 360 RFA Balloon Catheter electrode is cleaned externally. Over the same guidewire, the Barrx™ 360 RFA Balloon Catheter is reintroduced and the ablation steps repeated. Once completed, the ablation catheter is removed and the area inspected under endoscopy (Figure 16.2e).

Focal ablation of BE with the Barrx™ 90 RFA Focal Catheter consists of the following similar steps:

1 *Mount and identify*: The Barrx™ 90 RFA Balloon Catheter is mounted to the distal end of the endoscope using a catheter strap. Esophageal landmarks are then endoscopically identified with the catheter in place. The mucosa should also be prior cleaned with N-acetyl-cysteine (Figure 16.3a).

2 *Ablate*: The endoscope is deflected, to allow for contact of the attached Barrx™ 90 RFA Balloon Catheter to the mucosal surface. The Barrx™ Flex Energy Generator delivers 300 W of energy at 10–12 J/cm^2. For focal therapy, this amount of energy is repeated for a total of two treatments (Figure 16.3b).

3 *Clean and repeat*: The coagulum is removed endoscopically, and the Barrx™ 90 RFA Balloon Catheter is cleaned externally and then reintroduced. The ablation steps are repeated and the area is immediately inspected endoscopically (Figure 16.3c).

The focal device now comes in three successively larger sizes, including the Barrx™ 60 RFA Focal Catheter, which is the smallest of the friction-fitted focal devices, the Barrx™ 90 RFA Focal Catheter, and finally the Barrx™ Ultra Long RFA Focal Catheter, which is 4 cm in length and the same width as the Barrx™ 90 RFA Focal Catheter. These are the most commonly used focal ablation devices. The most recent development of RFA ablation catheter technology allows for passage through the working channel of

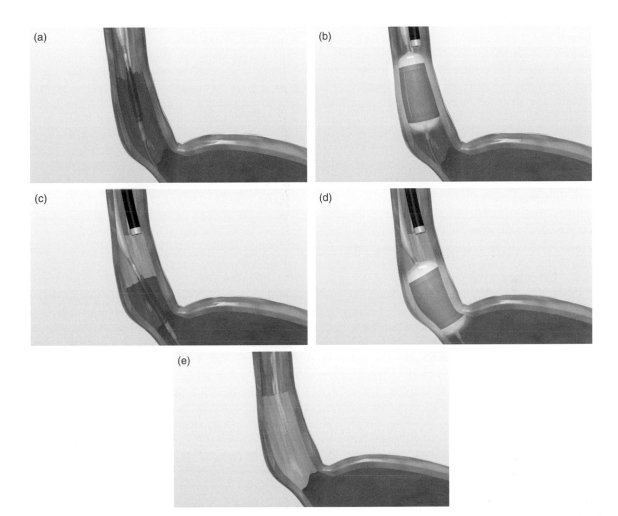

Figure 16.2 Circumferential ablation of BE with the The Barrx™ 360 RFA Balloon Catheter. Source: Barrx.com. Reproduced with permission of Barrx.

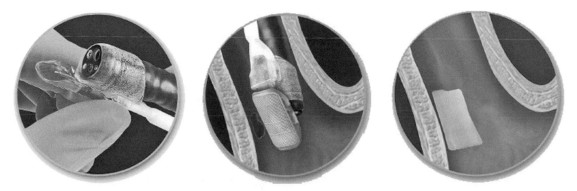

Figure 16.3 Focal ablation of BE with the Barrx™ 90 RFA Focal Catheter. Source: Barrx.com. Reproduced with permission of Barrx.

a flexible endoscope. The recently released Barrx™ Channel RFA Endoscopic Catheter allows for passage in a folded manner with direct visualization through a semi-translucent electrode. It promises to simplify the RFA workflow by eliminating some endoscopy introductions. It is designed to have the same procedural steps as the Barrx™ 90 RFA Focal Catheter (http://barrx. com/channel/wp-content/themes/barrx-channel/files/ printable-brochure.pdf).

Recent operational improvements include using the Barrx™ 90 RFA Focal Catheter system with omission of the cleaning step between two ablation passes as this has been demonstrated to have similar efficiency to the standard procedure with cleaning [10].

16.3 Efficacy and durability of radiofrequency ablation

The AIM Dysplasia Trial demonstrated the efficacy and safety of RFA in the treatment of BE in comparison to a sham-control group without ablative therapy. In a 19-site multicenter trial with 12-month follow-up, it was found that those in the control group without RFA were more likely to have disease progression (16.3%), to develop esophageal cancer (9.3% vs. 1.2%), and those with HGD progress to esophageal cancer at a rate of 19.0% compared to 2.4%. CR-IM was achieved at a relative rate of 33.3 (95% CI, 4.8–231.7) for RFA versus sham, and complete remission of dysplasia (CR-D) for HGD at a relative rate of 4.2 (95% CI, 1.7–10.4) [11].

The durability of the AIM Dysplasia Trial was evaluated by measuring two- and three-year outcomes, which showed that after two years 93% of patients achieved CR-IM, and 95% CR-D. In those with initial HGD, 89% achieved CR-IM, and 93% CR-D. After three years, 91% had achieved CR-IM and 98% CR-D though, of note, only 56 of 106 patients remained in analysis at two years [12].

With five years of longitudinal follow-up after RFA for early neoplasia, Phoa et al. found that, in a cohort of 46 patients with five-year follow-up, 93% (95% CI, 82.5-97.8%) achieved CR-IM, as evaluated by endoscopic ultrasound and endoscopic resection of neosquamous epithelium. Three of 54 patients of the total cohort had recurrence of dysplasia. Of these patients, LGD was discovered at five years in one individual, HGD was seen at 52 months in another

and, finally, carcinoma was found in the third. Each was treated successfully with endoscopic resection and ablation [5].

Lyday et al. demonstrated that the efficacy of RFA seen in initial studies in tertiary centers was generalizable to the community-based practice. Retrospectively studying 429 patients in a multicenter registry of four community-based gastroenterology practices over a four-year interval, they found 72–77% achievement of CR-IM and 89–100% achievement of CR-D [13].

RFA is also effective and durable in patients with long-segment BE (LSBE) (≥3 to < 8 cm) and ultra-long segment BE (ULSBE) (≥8 cm). Dulai et al. studied 38 patients with LSBE and 34 patients with ULSBE. A total of 79% achieved CR-IM and 87% CR-D. On multivariate regression analysis, increasing BE length was associated with a decreased likelihood for eradicating IM (OR 0.87, 95% CI, 0.75–1.00), but this was not observed for dysplasia (OR 1.13, 95% CI, 0.95–1.35) [14].

Since 2009, numerous studies have further examined the efficacy and durability of RFA in the treatment of BE (Figure 16.4). In 2013, Orman et al. summarized and analyzed many of these studies by performing a meta-analysis of 13 peer-reviewed publications and five abstracts [6]. In pooled meta-analysis, the overall percentage of patient achieving CR-IM was 78% (95% CI, 70–86%) and CR-D 91% (95% CI, 87–95%). Stratification by pretreatment histology revealed a decreased relative risk reduction with increasing dysplasia.

For HGD amongst six studies, the relative risk was 0.92 (95% CI, 0.87–0.98) and, for IMC among three studies, the relative risk was 0.99 (95% CI, 0.92–1.18). Individually, the studies had conflicting observations of this finding. It has been postulated that perhaps higher grade dysplasia could be a surrogate marker for increased BE length, with associated decrease in CR-IM rates [14]. Another hypothesis is that higher grade dysplasia is associated with more invasive neoplasia penetrating deeper into the submucosa. This explanation, however, is less likely, as the rates of esophageal adenocarcinoma would be expected to increase, and the incidence of cancer was 0.1% per year, which is lower than the 1.7% per year cancer rate in non-RFA post-ablation patients with HGD [15].

Regarding durability, Orman et al. observed that BE recurred in 13% (95% CI, 9–18%), based on the reported recurrence rates of six studies (Figure 16.5). The rate of recurrence was similar in larger and smaller

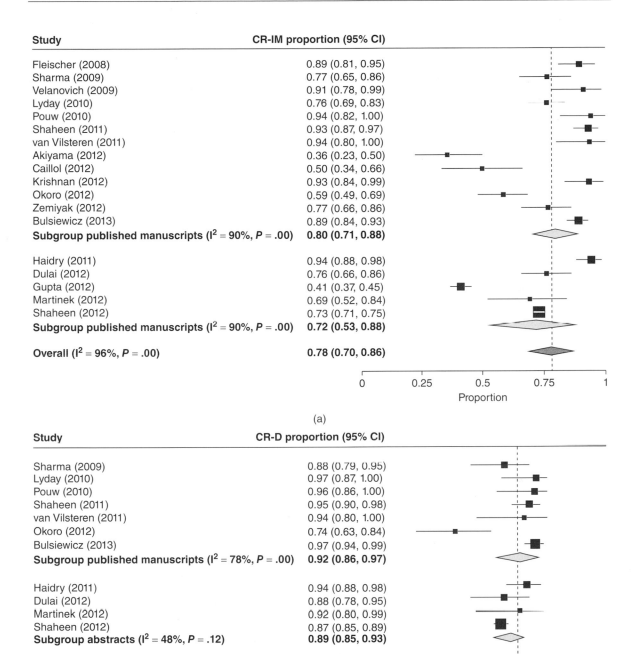

Figure 16.4 Forest plots of the proportion of patients achieving (A) CR-IM and (B) CR-D after treatment of BE with RFA, stratified according to publication as a peer-reviewed article vs abstract. Source: Orman *et al.*, 2013 [6]. Reproduced with permission from Elsevier.

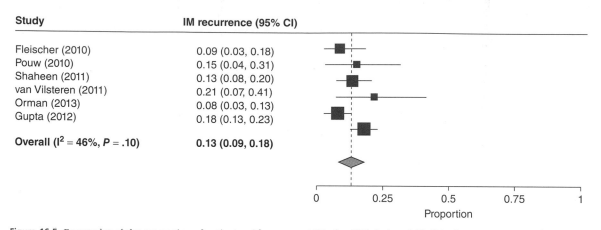

Figure 16.5 Forest plot of the proportion of patients with recurrent IM after RFA-induced CR-IM. Source: Orman *et al.*, 2013 [6]. Reproduced with permission from Elsevier.

studies. Over 1.5 years, there were five patients from one study with dysplasia at time of recurrence [16], and four patients from two studies with EAC [16, 12]. The overall risk for progression to dysplasia was 0.9%, and 0.7% for EAC [6]. Factors associated with recurrence include long-segment BE, piecemeal resection, multifocal neoplasia, and time until CR-IM [17].

16.4   Initial treatment response to RFA and risk factors for failed ablation

Approximately 80–90% of patients with BE treated with RFA reach CR-IM after an average of 2–3 sessions [6]. A subset of patients only reach CR-D, and some simply fail to respond to RFA. There is currently no consensus regarding the definition of RFA failure in the literature. Some studies describe RFA failure as less than 50% regression in the surface area of the BE segment three months after initial circumferential RFA (c-RFA) [18]. This definition, however, is limited in that it does not account for the response in treatment of dysplasia. Although surveillance biopsies are not included in the treatment protocol for RFA, we propose that failure to respond to RFA be defined by lack of improvement in the BE segment area and grade of dysplasia after two RFA sessions.

Several studies have looked at patient demographic and endoscopic factors for persistent intestinal metaplasia and dysplasia with RFA. A multi-center trial that treated 278 patients with c-RFA found that 36 patients had poor initial response (defined as < 50% regression of BE at three months following c-RFA). Four independent predictors of poor response in this cohort were active reflux esophagitis (OR 37.4; 95% CI 3.2–433.2); endoscopic resection scar regeneration with Barrett's epithelium (OR 4.7; 95% CI 1.1–20.0); esophageal narrowing pre-RFA (OR 3.9; 95% CI 1.0–15.1); and number of years of neoplasia pre-RFA (OR 1.2; 95% CI 1.0–1.4) [9, 10].

A retrospective study of 244 patients treated with RFA for BE with dysplasia showed that 20% of patients did not achieve CR-IM (defined as endoscopic and histological resolution of IM). In this cohort, incomplete eradication of intestinal metaplasia was associated with a longer BE segment (5.5 vs. 4.0 cm, *p* = 0.03); incomplete healing between treatment sessions (45% vs. 15%; p=0.004); and a greater number of treatment sessions (4 vs. 3, *p* = 0.007) [18].

Several retrospective studies have looked at the role of gastroesophageal reflux and acid suppression in regard to response to RFA. A retrospective study of 45 patients who underwent 24-hour pH monitoring while on acid suppression therapy showed that patients who had normal-to-mild esophageal acid exposure (pH < 4 for < 8% of study duration), and who had small hiatal hernias, were more likely to achieve CR-IM, compared with patients who had moderate-to-severe esophageal acid exposure and large hiatal hernias [19]. Thus far, prospective studies that have demonstrated the benefit of improved acid control are lacking.

16.5 Endoscopic mucosal resection in combination with radiofrequency ablation

Early esophageal neoplasia often presents with endoscopically visible mucosal irregularities (nodules) that can be targeted with endoscopic mucosal resection (EMR). Several studies have addressed the safety and efficacy of RFA following EMR [20–23]. In these studies, RFA was performed at least 4–6 weeks following EMR, to allow for adequate mucosal healing. It is postulated that scar tissue associated with EMR healing may hamper treatment with RFA. These studies retrospectively compared patients who underwent RFA for non-nodular BE with patients who underwent EMR followed by RFA for nodular BE.

In general, RFA following EMR is well-tolerated and does not necessarily increase the risk of complications including stricture formation. The efficacy of treatment was also similar between groups, with one study showing CR-D and CR-IM rates of 94% and 88% respectively in the EMR followed by RFA group, compared to 83% and 78% respectively in the RFA-only group [24]. A study assessing the feasibility of EMR immediately following c-RFA concluded that, although feasible, this approach is associated with a higher rate of complications, including perforation, bleeding and stenosis [25].

16.6 Safety and tolerability of radiofrequency ablation

A large multicenter trial on photodynamic therapy for ablation of high-grade dysplasia in BE showed that 94% of the treated group had treatment-related adverse events [26]. The most common adverse events included photosensitivity reactions (69%), esophageal strictures (36%), vomiting (32%) and non-cardiac chest pain (20%). Compared to photodynamic therapy, RFA is associated with less adverse events. Most strictures were managed endoscopically, with few dilation procedures compared with multiple dilation sessions with photodynamic therapy-associated strictures.

Other treatment-related adverse events associated with RFA included non-cardiac chest pain (3%, CI 1–6%) and bleeding (1%, CI 1–5%). Despite heterogeneity in the definition of adverse events between studies, RFA appears to be well-tolerated, and most adverse events can be managed endoscopically. Increasing BE length was associated with an increased risk of complications (OR 1.10, 95% CI 1.01–1.21) and a trend toward increased risk of strictures (OR 1.08, 95% CI, 0.97–1.20) in one study [27]. A large single-center study showed that patients who developed a stricture were more likely to use NSAIDs (70% vs 45%), to have antireflux surgery before treatment (15% vs 3%), and to have a history of prior erosive esophagitis (35% vs 12%), compared with patients who did not develop a stricture [6].

16.7 Subsquamous Intestinal metaplasia after radiofrequency ablation

Subsquamous intestinal metaplasia (SSIM) refers to Barrett's glands that are found buried under squamous epithelium. RFA is thought to lead to SSIM through a process of re-epithelization with neosquamous epithelium over partially treated BE. However, buried intestinal metaplasia is not unique to post-ablation mucosa and is, in fact, observed in up to 28% of pre-ablation biopsy samples [28]. Although the risk of neoplastic progression of SSIM is thought to be low, there are several reports of SSIM evolving into esophageal adenocarcinoma, raising concern for surveillance following ablation [29].

The diagnosis of SSIM is challenging in multiple regards. SSIM is indistinguishable from squamous epithelium under high resolution white light endoscopy and narrow band imaging, and it is usually only identified on surveillance biopsies. The histological diagnosis can also be challenging. Biopsy size, depth (down to the lamina propria) and orientation are key components in the assessment for SSIM. It is also often difficult to determine whether glands are truly buried or if they connect to the adjacent mucosal surface.

A systematic review of 31 studies involving 953 RFA patients concluded that the prevalence of SSIM was only 0.9% in post-RFA patients [28]. A notable limitation is the number of studies with adequate biopsy depth to evaluate for SSIM. Surveillance biopsies also represent a small fraction of the esophageal mucosa, and may underestimate the true prevalence of SSIM in this population. Cross-sectional imaging with three-dimensional optical coherence tomography was used in 18 patients undergoing RFA, and found SSIM in 63% of patients who achieved CR-IM [30]. Further advances in imaging technology, including the use of volumetric laser endomicroscopy, will help to further define the prevalence SSIM.

16.8 Surveillance following radiofrequency ablation

Current guidelines recommend that surveillance be continued after ablation, at similar intervals to that used before ablation, for the first year. If no recurrence is identified, the intervals between surveillance can be lengthened. Common practice is to perform surveillance biopsies at the squamocolumnar junction and at the normal appearing esophagus over the area of previous BE. Biopsies are also performed on any columnar appearing islands within the tubular esophagus. Surveillance intervals in patients with early esophageal neoplasia are initially every three months. Once CR-IM is achieved, intervals can be extended to six months for a year, then continued annually.

16.9 Conclusions

RFA has become the ablation modality of choice to treat non-nodular BE complicated by early neoplasia. Randomized controlled studies have shown that RFA is safe, well tolerated and effective in achieving CR-D and CR-IM with durable results. Although most patients respond to RFA, several factors are associated with poor initial response, including uncontrolled gastroesophageal reflux. Poor contact of the ablation catheter with the mucosa, as in a narrow esophagus, or in the presence of a hiatal hernia, can also lead to poor response.

Recurrence is observed in a small subset of patients and is associated with longer BE segments, the presence of multifocal neoplasia, and time until CR-IM. Ongoing surveillance over regenerated squamous epithelium is important to detect subsquamous BE and recurrent dysplasia. Recurrent disease can be managed with repeat ablation in the absence of mucosal irregularities. New RFA devices are being developed, including most recently a catheter that can be passed through the working channel of an endoscope to treat focal BE.

References

1 Dent J (2011). Barrett's Esophagus: A Historical Perspective, an Update on Core Practicalities and Predictions on Future Evolutions of Management. *Journal of Gastroenterology and Hepatology* **26**(Suppl 1), 11–30.

2 Rastogi A, Puli S, El-Serag HB, Bansal A, Wani S, Sharma P (2008). Incidence of Esophageal Adenocarcinoma in Patients with Barrett's Esophagus and High-Grade Dysplasia: a Meta-Analysis. *Gastrointestinal Endoscopy* **67**(3), 394–8.

3 Prasad, GA, Wang KK, Buttar NS, Wongkeesong L-M, Krishnadath KK, Nichols FC, Lutzke LS, Borkenhagen LS (2007). Long-Term Survival Following Endoscopic and Surgical Treatment of High-Grade Dysplasia in Barrett's Esophagus. *Gastroenterology* **132**(4), 1226–33.

4 Stein HJ, Feith M, Bruecher BLDM, Naehrig J, Sarbia M, Siewert JR (2005). Early Esophageal Cancer. *Transactions of the … Meeting of the American Surgical Association* **123** (&NA;), 260–269.

5 Phoa KN, Pouw RE, van Vilsteren FGI, Sondermeijer CMT, Ten Kate FJW, Visser M, Meijer SL *et al.* (2013). Remission of Barrett's Esophagus With Early Neoplasia 5 Years After Radiofrequency Ablation With Endoscopic Resection: A Netherlands Cohort Study. *Gastroenterology* **145**(1), 96–104.

6 Orman ES, Li N, Shaheen NJ (2013). Efficacy and Durability of Radiofrequency Ablation for Barrett's Esophagus: Systematic Review and Meta-Analysis. *Clinical Gastroenterology and Hepatology: the Official Clinical Practice Journal of the American Gastroenterological Association* **11**(10), 1245–55.

7 Inadomi JM, Somsouk M, Madanick RD, Thomas JP, Shaheen NJ (2009). A Cost-Utility Analysis of Ablative Therapy for Barrett's Esophagus. *Gastroenterology* **136**(7), 2101–2114.

8 Bulsiewicz WJ, Shaheen NJ (2011). The Role of Radiofrequency Ablation in the Management of Barrett's Esophagus. *Gastrointestinal Endoscopy Clinics of North America* **21**(1), 95–109.

9 Van Vilsteren FGI, Herrero LA, Pouw RE, Schrijnders D, Sondermeijer CMT, Bisschops R, Esteban JM *et al.* (2013). Predictive Factors for Initial Treatment Response after Circumferential Radiofrequency Ablation for Barrett's Esophagus with Early Neoplasia: a Prospective Multicenter Study. *Endoscopy* **45**(7), 516–25.

10 Van Vilsteren, FGI, Phoa KN, Herrero LA, Pouw RE, Sondermeijer CMT, Visser M, Ten Kate FJW *et al.* (2013). A Simplified Regimen for Focal Radiofrequency Ablation of Barrett's Mucosa: a Randomized Multicenter Trial Comparing Two Ablation Regimens. *Gastrointestinal Endoscopy* **78**(1), 30–8.

11 Shaheen NJ, Sharma P, Overholt BF, Wolfsen HC, Sampliner RE, Wang KK, Galanko JA, *et al.* (2009). Radiofrequency Ablation in Barrett's Esophagus with Dysplasia. *The New England Journal of Medicine* **360**(22), 2277–88.

12 Shaheen, NJ, Overholt BF, Sampliner RE, Wolfsen HC, Wang KK, Fleischer DE, Sharma VK, *et al.* (2011). Durability

of Radiofrequency Ablation in Barrett's Esophagus with Dysplasia. *Gastroenterology* **141**(2), 460–8.

13 Lyday, WD, Corbett FS, Kuperman DA, Kalvaria I, Mavrelis PG, Shughoury AB, Pruitt RE (2010). Radiofrequency Ablation of Barrett's Esophagus: Outcomes of 429 Patients from a Multicenter Community Practice Registry. *Endoscopy* **42**(4), 272–8.

14 Dulai, PS, Pohl H, Levenick JM, Gordon SR, MacKenzie TA, Rothstein RI (2013). Radiofrequency Ablation for Long- and Ultralong-Segment Barrett's Esophagus: a Comparative Long-Term Follow-up Study. *Gastrointestinal Endoscopy* **77**(4), 534–41.

15 Wani, S, Puli SR, Shaheen NJ, Westhoff B, Slehria S, Bansal A, Rastogi A, Sayana H, Sharma P (2009). Esophageal Adenocarcinoma in Barrett's Esophagus after Endoscopic Ablative Therapy: a Meta-Analysis and Systematic Review. *The American Journal of Gastroenterology* **104**(2), 502–13.

16 Orman, ES, Kim HP, Bulsiewicz WJ, Cotton CC, Dellon ES, Spacek MB, Chen X, Madanick RD, Pasricha S, Shaheen NJ (2013). Intestinal Metaplasia Recurs Infrequently in Patients Successfully Treated for Barrett's Esophagus with Radiofrequency Ablation. *The American Journal of Gastroenterology* **108**(2), 187–95; quiz 196.

17 Pech, O, Behrens A, May A, Nachbar L, Gossner L, Rabenstein T, Manner H, *et al.* (2008). Long-Term Results and Risk Factor Analysis for Recurrence after Curative Endoscopic Therapy in 349 Patients with High-Grade Intraepithelial Neoplasia and Mucosal Adenocarcinoma in Barrett's Oesophagus. *Gut* **57**(9), 1200–6.

18 Bulsiewicz WJ, Kim HP, Dellon ES, Cotton CC, Pasricha S, Madanick RD, Spacek MB, *et al.* (2013). Safety and Efficacy of Endoscopic Mucosal Therapy With Radiofrequency Ablation for Patients With Neoplastic Barrett's Esophagus. *Clinical Gastroenterology and Hepatology: the Official Clinical Practice Journal of the American Gastroenterological Association* **11**(6), 636–42.

19 Akiyama, J, Marcus SN, Triadafilopoulos G (2012). Effective Intra-Esophageal Acid Control Is Associated with Improved Radiofrequency Ablation Outcomes in Barrett's Esophagus. *Digestive Diseases and Sciences* **57**(10), 2625–32.

20 Okoro, NI, Tomizawa Y, Dunagan KT, Lutzke LS, Wang KK, Prasad GA (2012). Safety of Prior Endoscopic Mucosal Resection in Patients Receiving Radiofrequency Ablation of Barrett's Esophagus. *Clinical Gastroenterology and Hepatology: the Official Clinical Practice Journal of the American Gastroenterological Association* **10**(2), 150–4.

21 Herrero, LA, van Vilsteren FGI, Pouw RE, ten Kate FJW, Visser M, Seldenrijk CA, Henegouwen MIvB, Fockens P, Weusten BLaM, Bergman JJGHM (2011). Endoscopic Radiofrequency Ablation Combined with Endoscopic Resection for Early Neoplasia in Barrett's Esophagus Longer Than 10 cm. *Gastrointestinal Endoscopy* **73**(4), 682–90.

22 Goers, TA, Leão P, Cassera MA, Dunst CM, Swanström LL (2011). Concomitant Endoscopic Radiofrequency Ablation and Laparoscopic Reflux Operative Results in More Effective and Efficient Treatment of Barrett Esophagus. *Journal of the American College of Surgeons* **213**(4), 486–92.

23 Pouw, RE, Wirths K, Eisendrath P, Sondermeijer CM, Ten Kate FJ, Fockens P, Devière J, Neuhaus H, Bergman JJ (2010). Efficacy of Radiofrequency Ablation Combined with Endoscopic Resection for Barrett's Esophagus with Early Neoplasia. *Clinical Gastroenterology and Hepatology: the Official Clinical Practice Journal of the American Gastroenterological Association* **8**(1), 23–9.

24 Kim HP, Bulsiewicz WJ, Cotton CC, Dellon ES, Spacek MB, Chen X, Madanick RD, Pasricha S, Shaheen NJ (2012). Focal Endoscopic Mucosal Resection before Radiofrequency Ablation Is Equally Effective and Safe Compared with Radiofrequency Ablation Alone for the Eradication of Barrett's Esophagus with Advanced Neoplasia. *Gastrointestinal Endoscopy* **76**(4), 733–9.

25 Van Vilsteren FGI, Herrero LA, Pouw RE, Visser M, Ten Kate FJW, van Berge Henegouwen MI, Schoon EJ, Weusten BL, Bergman JJ (2012). Radiofrequency Ablation and Endoscopic Resection in a Single Session for Barrett's Esophagus Containing Early Neoplasia: a Feasibility Study. *Endoscopy* **44**(12), 1096–104.

26 Overholt, BF, Wang KK, Burdick JS, Lightdale CJ, Kimmey M, Nava HR, Sivak MV, *et al.* (2007). Five-Year Efficacy and Safety of Photodynamic Therapy with Photofrin in Barrett's High-Grade Dysplasia. *Gastrointestinal Endoscopy* **66**(3), 460–8.

27 Gupta, M, Iyer PG, Lutzke L, Gorospe EC, Abrams JA, Falk GW, Ginsberg GG, *et al.* (2013). Recurrence of Esophageal Intestinal Metaplasia After Endoscopic Mucosal Resection and Radiofrequency Ablation of Barrett's Esophagus: Results From a US Multicenter Consortium. *Gastroenterology* **145**(1), 79–86.

28 Gray, NA, Odze RD, Spechler SJ (2011). Buried Metaplasia after Endoscopic Ablation of Barrett's Esophagus: a Systematic Review. *The American Journal of Gastroenterology* **106**(11), 1899–908; quiz 1909.

29 Titi, M, Overhiser A, Ulusarac O, Falk GW, Chak A, Wang K, Sharma P (2012). Development of Subsquamous High-Grade Dysplasia and Adenocarcinoma after Successful Radiofrequency Ablation of Barrett's Esophagus. *Gastroenterology* **143**(3), 564–6.

30 Zhou, C, Tsai T-H, Lee H-C, Kirtane T, Figueiredo M, Tao YK, Ahsen OO, *et al.* (2012). Characterization of Buried Glands before and after Radiofrequency Ablation by Using 3-Dimensional Optical Coherence Tomography (with Videos). *Gastrointestinal Endoscopy* **76**(1), 32–40.

31 Krishnan, K, Pandolfino JE, Kahrilas PJ, Keefer L, Boris L, Komanduri S (2012). Increased Risk for Persistent Intestinal Metaplasia in Patients with Barrett's Esophagus and Uncontrolled Reflux Exposure before Radiofrequency Ablation. *Gastroenterology* **143**(3), 576–81.

CHAPTER 17

The role of endoscopic cryotherapy for treatment and palliation

Kristle Lee Lynch, Eun Ji Shin & Marcia Irene Canto

Division of Gastroenterology and Hepatology, Johns Hopkins University, Baltimore, MD, USA

17.1 Introduction

The incidence of Barrett's esophagus (BE) and esophageal adenocarcinoma (EAC) has risen significantly in the last decade. More importantly, EAC is a deadly disease. The overall mortality of EAC has increased seven-fold in the past three decades, and the five-year survival rate ranges between 10% and 20% [1]. In the past esophagectomy was recommended for the management of high grade dysplasia (HGD) given the risk of progression to or presence of EAC [2]. However, surgery is associated with significant morbidity (20–50%) and mortality (2–5%) [3, 4]. In addition, there are a multitude of patients who cannot undergo esophagectomy due to poor surgical candidacy, metastatic disease, or personal preference.

Thus, alternative endoscopic treatments have been aggressively developed over the past decade. Options for endoluminal therapy include cryotherapy, radiofrequency ablation (RFA), argon plasma coagulation (APC), electrocoagulation, photodynamic therapy (PDT), endoscopic mucosal resection (EMR), and endoscopic submucosal resection (ESR). This chapter will focus on cryotherapy for the management of BE and EAC.

17.2 Cryotherapy mechanisms of tissue injury

"Cryotherapy" originates from the Greek *cryo*, meaning *cold*, and *therapy*, meaning *cure*. It is used widely in the medical field as the therapeutic application of extreme cold to human tissue. Cryoablative therapies rely on controlled, local freezing, caused by the removal of thermal energy (heat) from the tissues – hence, it is an energy-deprivation strategy [5]. Cryotherapy has been employed for treating various conditions, including various skins lesions and malignancies, liver tumors, lung tumors, retinoblastoma, cervical intraepithelial neoplasm, Kaposi's sarcoma, prostate cancer, hemorrhoids, joint pain, nerve entrapment syndromes, and cardiac arrhythmias [6].

There are several proposed mechanisms of tissue injury resulting from freezing tissue. When extreme cold is applied to tissue, rapid intracellular and extracellular freezing occurs, resulting in cell necrosis via several mechanisms. Direct freezing of the cell results in diffuse ice formation, cell membrane interruption, and protein denaturation [7]. Vascular flow is compromised as lower temperatures lead to the complete cessation of blood flow. In addition to necrosis, studies in animal models have revealed that freezing tissue leads to self-induced apoptosis [8].

The act of thawing also produces significant damage to cells via various pathways. First, as the ice crystals melt shearing forces disrupt the cell membranes. Next, the increase in fluid culminates in a hypotonic environment, causing the diffusion of water into the cells and resulting in the bursting of cell membranes. Finally, thawing results in vasodilation and increased vascular permeability, leading to platelet aggregation, microthrombi production and ultimately, circulatory failure [9].

Given the unique processes of cell damage during freezing and thawing, freeze-thaw cycles are typically performed on target lesions during each

Esophageal Cancer and Barrett's Esophagus, Third Edition. Edited by Prateek Sharma, Richard Sampliner and David Ilson.
© 2015 John Wiley & Sons, Ltd. Published 2015 by John Wiley & Sons, Ltd.

treatment session. The duration of the application of cryotherapy, in combination with the number of freeze-thaw cycles, controls the depth of injury. Like other gastrointestinal mucosal ablative techniques, such as radiofrequency ablation, healing of the cryoablative-induced injury and tissue regeneration are potentially enhanced by an acidic environment. Hence, acid suppression is generally recommended to promote replacement of Barrett's esophagus with neosquamous epithelium.

17.3 Types of cryotherapy: devices, dosing, and endoscopic application

Cryotherapy is delivered via an endoscopic spray catheter, resulting in tissue destruction without direct contact. The first endoscopic application of cryotherapy was described by Pasricha *et al.* (Johns Hopkins University, Baltimore, Maryland), using nitrous oxide and carbon dioxide as cryogens in an animal model and a patient with an obstructing gastric cancer [10]. Since then, there have been three unique cryotherapy delivery systems developed in the United States using liquid nitrogen, carbon dioxide, and nitrogen gas (Table 17.1). All three systems are approved by the Food and Drug Administration (FDA) and are commercially available for clinical use.

17.3.1 Liquid nitrogen cryotherapy

Liquid nitrogen cryotherapy was first developed in Maryland, USA and described by Johnston *et al.* in 2003 [11]. It involves delivery of liquid nitrogen through a heated catheter passed through the biopsy channel in the endoscope. The liquid nitrogen spray results in very cold tissue freeze, with an estimated temperature of −196° Celsius. This treatment modality was previously described as a "low pressure" cryotherapy system because the flow rate from the tip of the catheter is low (2–4 psi) but in reality the immediate expansion of liquid nitrogen into a gaseous state can generate up to 24 liters of nitrogen gas. Hence, a decompression large-bore orogastric tube is required to decrease the resultant gastric distension.

The current second generation liquid nitrogen spray cryotherapy device introduced in 2007 (truFreeze, CSA Medical, Maryland) replaced the first generation system (CryoSpray) to improve flexibility of the catheter and provide improved laminar flow and decreased intraluminal pressures. Although gaseous distention is less, orogastric tube suction is still required. The system consists of a console that contains a liquid nitrogen holding tank and a disposable multi-layered stainless steel reinforced 7 French catheter which is coated with a polymer that can be electrically heated (Figure 17.1). The release of liquid nitrogen and heating of the catheter are controlled by a dual foot pedal.

The technique of liquid nitrogen cryospray involves passing the catheter through the endoscope channel and placing the tip approximately 1–2 cm from the mucosal surface. A plastic cap on the tip of the endoscope has been used to focus the ice and maintain a distance from the mucosa. After visible ice forms, the catheter tip is moved with the endoscope to "spray" the other areas of BE, typically from distal to proximal. With a side-firing

Table 17.1 Types of endoscopic cryotherapy.

Cryogen	Device	Method of application	Contact with mucosa	Estimated tissue temperature	Dosing in clinical studies
Liquid nitrogen	CryoSpray	Heated catheter (through-the-scope), forward and side firing "spray"	Non-contact	−196° Celsius	20 seconds freeze, 45 second thaw, 3 cycles
Carbon dioxide gas	Polar wand	Polyethylene catheter (through-the-scope), forward firing "spray"	Non-contact	−78° Celsius	15 seconds freeze, thaw until ice melts, × 6–8 cycles
Nitrous oxide gas	CryoBalloon ablation system	Balloon catheter (through-the-scope), circumferential and focal side firing	Contact	−80° Celsius	Research in progress

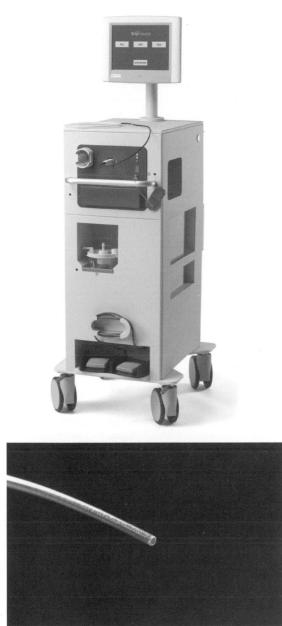

Figure 17.1 The liquid nitrogen device for cryotherapy consists of a console with a holding tank (1A) and a flexible multilayered no. 7 French catheter (1B). Source: CSA Medical, Maryland. Reproduced with permission of CSA Medical.

catheter, a hemi-circumferential zone of ice is created and the cryospray is sustained until all target areas of the BE have frozen for the predetermined time (cryogen dose). The ice then thaws, usually for the same number of seconds.

The dosing of liquid nitrogen cryogen has varied. Studies have reported 15–20 seconds of ice, followed by a minimum 45 seconds of thaw (typically timed), repeated for three cycles [12]. Repeat treatments are typically performed after 4–6 weeks, depending upon the indication and extent of the BE. Replacement of BE mucosa with neo-squamous epithelium can be seen.

17.3.2 Carbon dioxide cryotherapy

The second type of cryotherapy device (Polar Wand, GI Supply, Camp Hill, Pennsylvania), which was developed at the Johns Hopkins Hospital in Baltimore, Maryland, originally employed nitrogen gas, but second-generation devices apply compressed carbon dioxide gas. The first clinical use of this device in 2003 [13], was as a salvage therapy for refractory gastrointestinal bleeding due to gastric antral vascular ectasia, watermelon stomach, and radiation proctitis. It was subsequently used for Barrett's esophagus [14].

The current device consists of a portable console which houses the carbon dioxide tank and suction canister. It has a tunable control of suction strength (Figure 17.2A). The carbon dioxide is released from a 0.005 inch hole at the tip of a flexible plastic catheter (Figure 17.2B), which rapidly cools tissue to −78 degrees Celsius through the Joules-Thompson effect. The compressed carbon dioxide gas expands rapidly at a flow rate of approximately 6–8 liters/minute but, unlike the liquid nitrogen, there is no need for an orogastric tube for decompression. Excess carbon dioxide gas is removed simultaneously during cryogen delivery, with a slim plastic suction catheter attached to the tip of the endoscope (Figure 17.2B).

Several cycles of freezing and thawing per treatment session are typically administered. In a porcine animal model, increasing duration and number of freeze cycles are associated with increased depth of cryotherapy injury in the esophagus and stomach [15]. The average depth of tissue injury (measured from mucosal surface) due to a single application of 15 seconds of carbon dioxide cryotherapy in porcine esophagus ranged from 1.2–2.5 mm, depending upon the number of freeze-thaw applications. With the cryogen dose commonly used in patients (15 seconds × 6–8 cycles), injury could be seen in the submucosa but this did not lead to transmural necrosis. At two weeks, there was complete regeneration of the tissue. In patients

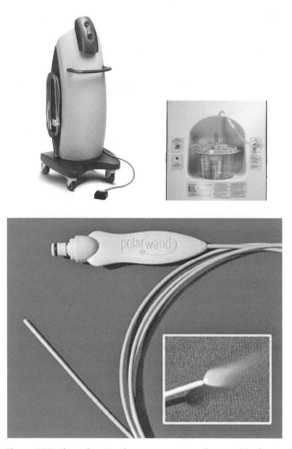

Figure 17.2 The Polar Wand system consists of a portable device on wheels (A), containing the suction canister with carbon dioxide gas in a tank stored at the back, a suction catheter attached to the endoscope, and a through-the-scope plastic delivery catheter (B). Source: GI Supply, Camp Hill, PA. Reproduced with permission of GI Supply.

cryotherapy treatments are typically repeated every 4–8 weeks until eradication is achieved [14].

17.3.3 Nitrous oxide cryotherapy

The third and the newest type of endoscopic cryotherapy system, the CryoBalloon Ablation System (C2 Therapeutics, Redwood, California), was first reported in 2011 [16]. The initial paper reported laboratory and animal model use of the balloon-based system using one application of 6–12 seconds of ice, a relatively lower dose of cryogen compared to other systems [16].

CryoBalloon therapy involves delivery of liquid nitrous oxide through a balloon catheter passed through the endoscope channel (Figure 17.3). The cryogen is contained in a small portable cartridge containing liquid nitrous oxide, placed in a battery-powered "gun-like" handle, which contains the cartridge heater and delivery valve controlled by a trigger (Figure 17.3A). The balloon at the end of the catheter is inflated and simultaneously cooled by the gas expansion (Figure 17.3B). It makes contact with the mucosa and causes the thermal injury (Figure 17.3C), unlike the other two types of delivery systems (Table 17.1). Furthermore, in contrast to the other two types of cryotherapy, the gas is contained within the balloon and exits through the proximal end of the catheter. Hence, the gas does not escape into the gastrointestinal tract and there is no need for a suction catheter.

The CryoBalloon system has an appealing small size, light weight, and portability. It is still under development, but preliminary data provide encouraging results. A circumferential balloon and focal balloon device are in clinical trials for ablation of BE. The latter provides a focused ablation area of about $2 \, cm^2$ (Figure 17.3C).

17.4 Efficacy and safety in Barrett's esophagus

In the past decade, the majority of published studies have involved liquid nitrogen cryotherapy for treatment of Barrett's esophagus with all grades of dysplasia, as well as esophageal adenocarcinoma for curative and palliative intent. A pilot study by Johnston in 2005 described 11 patients with BE, ranging from non-dysplastic to multifocal HGD, who were reviewed prospectively. Complete eradication of intestinal metaplasia (CE-IM) was achieved initially in 100% of patients and after six months, in 78% of patients [17].

Subsequent studies on the outcomes and safety of liquid nitrogen cryotherapy have also reported encouraging treatment outcomes in BE patients with HGD. A single center cohort study by Dumot in 2009 investigated 30 patients with either HGD or IMCA who were ineligible for or refused esophagectomy. After treatment, 68% of the patients with HGD and 80% of the patients with intramucosal adenocarcinoma had downgrading of their worst pathologic dysplasia grade at a median follow-up of 12 months. The safety profile for the liquid nitrogen cryotherapy is very good; a total of ten patients reported mild to moderate chest pain, lasting up to seven days.

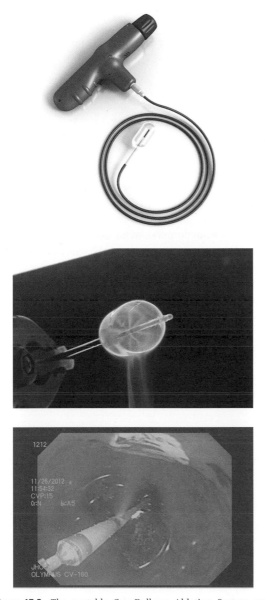

Figure 17.3 The portable CryoBalloon Ablation System consists of liquid nitrous oxide in a small cartridge placed in a battery-powered handle (A), which contains the cartridge heater and delivery valve. The nitrous oxide gas passes through a balloon catheter (B) that is passed through the endoscopic channel. The CryoBalloon is inflated when the trigger is pulled. The nitrous oxide liquid converts to gas, which expands the balloon and provides mucosal contact for freezing. The focal CryoBalloon allows directional application of cryogen from a tiny opening in the central catheter to areas of Barrett's esophagus (C). Source: C2 Therapeutics, Redwood City, CA. Reproduced with permission of C2 Therapeutics.

Three patients had mild to moderate strictures that were all dilated. One patient developed a lip ulcer [18].

Greenwald *et al.* expanded on this study and reported a multicenter retrospective cohort study of patients, some of which overlapped with the previous study. There were 45 BE patients with HGD who were to undergo treatment with liquid nitrogen cryotherapy, but only 17 patients completed the treatment and follow-up. Out of these 17 patients, 53% achieved CE-IM. Adverse events reported in this study included the one patient with Marfan's syndrome with a gastric perforation, and three patients who developed esophageal strictures [12].

These early results were not especially promising. However, a subsequent larger retrospective cohort study of 60 BE patients with HGD followed patients post-procedurally to a mean of 10.5 months. Almost all of the patients (97%) achieved complete eradication of high-grade dysplasia (CE-HGD), and 34 patients (57%) achieved CE-IM. There were no perforations post-procedurally while three patients (5%) developed strictures [19].

The most recent albeit small study of liquid nitrogen cryotherapy published in 2013 reported excellent results with long-term follow-up. This was a prospective single-arm study of 32 BE patients with HGD who underwent treatment with cryotherapy, some of which overlapped with the previous study. At a two-year follow-up interval, 100% of patients had achieved CE-HGD and 84% had achieved CE-IM. At a median 37 months follow-up interval, 97% of patients had CE-HGD and 81% had CE-IM. There were no serious adverse events reported in this study, though three patients (9%) developed strictures [20]. The same group reported the incidence and patterns of recurrence of BE HGD after liquid nitrogen cryotherapy in a retrospective cohort of prospectively collected data from 36 patients [21]. Eleven patients (30%) developed recurrent BE, with or without dysplasia in a median of 6.5 months – usually in the "hot zone" below the gastroesophageal junction, similar to the location of RFA recurrences. After retreatment, 33 patients (92%) achieved a complete response.

For carbon dioxide cryotherapy, a small prospective single arm clinical trial of carbon dioxide cryotherapy suggests comparable high efficacy in BE patients. Xue *et al.* treated 22 patients with non-dysplastic BE, of which 20 completed treatment. A median of three sessions (range 1–3) were needed. No complications were noted. Over a median follow-up of ten months (range 6–18 months), 91% achieved complete ablation of BE. At six months, recurrence was seen in 13.6% of the entire cohort and 15% of the complete responders.

Preliminary data from a prospective, non-randomized single-center study suggest comparable efficacy of carbon dioxide cryotherapy for BE with high grade dysplasia or cancer. Researchers treated these patients with carbon dioxide cryogen, dosed at 4–8 cycles of 10–15 seconds of freeze, followed by thaw until the visible ice melted, while excess gas was suctioned from the stomach [22]. No special diet or pain medications were prescribed. At the time, 44 patients were treated; 25 of these had failed conventional treatments with RFA, PDT, or had EMR margin positive for neoplasia. The rest of the patients received cryotherapy as primary treatment for BE with HGD. Complete resolution of HGD was seen in 91% [22]. Only two patients experienced transient post-procedural pain and no serious adverse events were noted. This study suggests that carbon dioxide cryotherapy may be considered for the treatment of BE with HGD in patients who have failed RFA and/or EMR.

For CryoBalloon therapy, a human feasibility pilot study using a circumferential CryoBalloon reported safety and efficacy in BE patients treated prior to planned esophagectomy. Thirteen patients underwent 21 ablations with this, through the scope balloon-based cryotherapy device. Esophagectomy then occurred 0, 4, or 7 days post-procedure. Circumferential necrosis, extending into the superficial muscularis propria, was achieved in a majority of patients who underwent ablation for at least ten seconds. There were no significant adverse events. At three days post-procedure, 89% of patients were pain-free and 22% had dysphagia [23].

A preliminary prospective multicenter non-randomized international trial presented at the United European Gastroenterology Week (UEGW), 2013, reported successful focal ablation of BE using and eight seconds of ice, with minimal side effects. Twenty-six patients had 36 ablations using the CryoBalloon focal ablation system. Complete regression of BE in treated areas was noted in 60% of patients in the six-second group, and 81% of patients in the eight-second group. Pain scores were low (0–2) immediately post-procedure

and two days post-treatment. No strictures were noted at median follow-up of 49–54 months. Minor asymptomatic balloon mucosal lacerations not needing treatment were noted in four patients, resulting in device design changes.

17.5 Cryotherapy for the treatment of esophageal carcinoma

Cryotherapy induces cellular death via direct injury as well as indirect methods. The formation of ice crystals directly injures cells, disrupting organelles and mitochondria. Vascular stasis and intravascular thrombin formation leads to tissue ischemia. Apoptosis has been seen to occur in cells that are not directly destroyed by freezing. Additionally, in cancer cells immune-mediated toxicity may lead to cell death. This anti-inflammatory response occurs in areas with sub-lethal injury [24].

Cryotherapy has also been successfully used for the palliation of EAC. In a multicenter retrospective study, there were 49 patients from ten centers who were treated with liquid nitrogen cryotherapy (one or more sessions). Out of the 49 patients who completed treatment, 46 had EAC and three had squamous cell carcinoma. Patients with endoluminal disease were deemed inoperable due to comorbidities or refusal of esophagectomy. Patients with invasive cancer either failed or were ineligible for systemic therapy such as radiation and chemotherapy. Complete regression of luminal cancer occurred in 75% of patients at a median of ten months follow-up. There were no serious adverse events reported, and 16% of patients developed benign strictures [25]. Thus, these data on the use of cryotherapy for palliation in esophageal cancer are highly encouraging because of the relatively high efficacy and adequate safety profile in patients with limited therapeutic options.

Cryotherapy may be a viable outpatient endoscopic treatment option for patients with obstructing tumors and cancers that recur after chemotherapy and/or radiation therapy. It may also be considered for local treatment of high-risk inoperable patients with BE adenocarcinomas in non-lifting nodular lesions, depressed and ulcerated lesions (Paris IIc and III class), or deep margin-positive invasive EAC following endoscopic mucosal resection. Furthermore, compared to alternative endoscopic cancer palliative therapies for EAC such as photodynamic therapy (REF) that result in extreme photosensitivity, pain and esophageal strictures, cryotherapy is an attractive and viable treatment option.

More studies are needed to assess curative and palliative treatment outcomes, particularly longer-term complete response rate, remission rate, and potential for improved quality of life.

17.6   Summary and future directions

In summary, cryotherapy shows great capacity for therapeutic use in early studies, but more data are needed. The efficacy rate for CE-IM reported in long-term follow-up studies peaks at 84% and is potentially comparable to that of RFA [15]. The efficacy for eradication of dysplasia may be very high, peaking at 97%. Additionally, the safety profile of cryotherapy is acceptable with rare reports of serious adverse events such as perforation. The rate of stricture formation with liquid nitrogen cryotherapy is 9% and no stricture reported yet for carbon dioxide cryotherapy. Post-treatment chest pain also appears to be minimal in cryotherapy-treated patients, seemingly lower than in post-RFA patients. In addition to a potentially lower adverse event rate, cryotherapy provides dose-dependent injury and cell death. Hence, it can be applied to nodular BE and EAC, unlike the current RFA system, which delivers a fixed energy delivery and ablation depth of about 1.0 mm.

The future of cryotherapy is promising, given its low cost, straightforward technique of application, and utility in altered anatomy. With more widespread use, improved technique in cryotherapy will develop and may result in decreased frequency of treatment sessions and improved efficacy [20]. The next step in evaluating this treatment should include large randomized controlled trials to establish optimal dosimetry for successful ablation with maintenance of excellent safety profile. Eventually, head-to-head trials comparing cryotherapy with established treatment modalities such as RFA are needed. Lastly, further studies on the routine use of cryotherapy for cure and palliation of EAC are warranted, as an alternative treatment to esophagectomy or as an adjunctive or rescue therapy after chemoradiation therapy.

References

1 Pohl H, Welch HG (2005). The role of overdiagnosis and reclassification in the marked increase of esophageal adenocarcinoma incidence. *Journal of the National Cancer Institute* **97**(2), 142–6.

2 Montgomery E, Canto MI (2006). Management of high-grade dysplasia in patients with Barrett's esophagus. *Clinical Gastroenterology and Hepatology* **4**(12), 1434–9.

3 Enestvedt BK, Ginsberg GG (2013). Advances in endoluminal therapy for esophageal cancer. *Gastrointestinal Endoscopy Clinics of North America* **23**(1), 17–39.

4 Garman KS, Shaheen NJ (2011). Ablative therapies for Barrett's esophagus. *Current Gastroenterology Reports* **13**(3), 226–39.

5 Baust JG, Gage AA, Bjerklund Johansen TE, Baust JM (2013). Mechanisms of cryoablation: Clinical consequences on malignant tumors. *Cryobiology* **68**(1), 1–11.

6 Dumot JA, Greenwald BD (2011). Cryotherapy for Barrett's esophagus: does the gas really matter? *Endoscopy* **43**(5), 432–3.

7 Greenwald BD, Lightdale CJ, Abrams JA, Horwhat JD, Chuttani R, Komanduri S, *et al.* (2011). Barrett's esophagus: endoscopic treatments II. *Annals of the New York Academy of Sciences* **1232**, 156–74.

8 Forest V, Peoc'h M, Campos L, Guyotat D, Vergnon JM (2005). Effects of cryotherapy or chemotherapy on apoptosis in a non-small-cell lung cancer xenografted into SCID mice. *Cryobiology* **50**(1), 29–37.

9 Halsey KD, Greenwald BD (2010). Cryotherapy in the management of esophageal dysplasia and malignancy. *Gastrointestinal Endoscopy Clinics of North America* **20**(1), 75–87, vi–vii.

10 Pasricha PJ, Hill S, Wadwa KS, Gislason GT, Okolo PI, 3rd, Magee CA, *et al.* (1999). Endoscopic cryotherapy: experimental results and first clinical use. *Gastrointestinal Endoscopy* **49**(5), 627–31.

11 Johnston MH (2003). Cryotherapy and other newer techniques. *Gastrointestinal Endoscopy Clinics of North America* **13**(3), 491–504.

12 Greenwald BD, Dumot JA, Horwhat JD, Lightdale CJ, Abrams JA (2010). Safety, tolerability, and efficacy of endoscopic low-pressure liquid nitrogen spray cryotherapy in the esophagus. *Diseases of the Esophagus* **23**(1), 13–9.

13 Kantsevoy SV, Cruz-Correa MR, Vaughn CA, Jagannath SB, Pasricha PJ, Kalloo AN (2003). Endoscopic cryotherapy for the treatment of bleeding mucosal vascular lesions of the GI tract: a pilot study. *Gastrointestinal Endoscopy* **57**(3), 403–6.

14 Xue HB, Tan HH, Liu WZ, Chen XY, Feng N, Gao YJ, *et al.* (2011). A pilot study of endoscopic spray cryotherapy by pressurized carbon dioxide gas for Barrett's esophagus. *Endoscopy* **43**(5), 379–85.

15 Shin EJ, Amateau SK, Kim Y, Gabrielson KL, Montgomery EA, Khashab MA, *et al.* (2012). Dose-dependent depth of tissue injury with carbon dioxide cryotherapy in porcine GI tract. *Gastrointestinal Endoscopy* **75**(5), 1062–7.

16 Friedland S, Triadafilopoulos G (2011). A novel device for ablation of abnormal esophageal mucosa (with video). *Gastrointestinal Endoscopy* **74**(1), 182–8.

17 Johnston MH, Eastone JA, Horwhat JD, Cartledge J, Mathews JS, Foggy JR (2005). Cryoablation of Barrett's esophagus: a pilot study. *Gastrointestinal Endoscopy* **62**(6), 842–8.

18 Dumot JA, Vargo JJ, 2nd, Falk GW, Frey L, Lopez R, Rice TW (2009). An open-label, prospective trial of cryospray ablation for Barrett's esophagus high-grade dysplasia and early esophageal cancer in high-risk patients. *Gastrointestinal Endoscopy* **70**(4), 635–44.

19 Shaheen NJ, Greenwald BD, Peery AF, Dumot JA, Nishioka NS, Wolfsen HC, *et al.* (2010). Safety and efficacy of endoscopic spray cryotherapy for Barrett's esophagus with high-grade dysplasia. *Gastrointestinal Endoscopy* **71**(4), 680–5.

20 Gosain S, Mercer K, Twaddell WS, Uradomo L, Greenwald BD (2013). Liquid nitrogen spray cryotherapy in Barrett's esophagus with high-grade dysplasia: long-term results. *Gastrointestinal Endoscopy* **78**(2), 260–5.

21 Halsey KD, Chang JW, Waldt A, Greenwald BD (2011). Recurrent disease following endoscopic ablation of Barrett's high-grade dysplasia with spray cryotherapy. *Endoscopy* **43**(10), 844–8.

22 Canto MI GE, Shin EJ, Dunbar KB, Montgomery E, Kalloo, AN, Okolo P (2009). Carbon dioxide (CO_2) cryotherapy is a safe and effective treatment for Barrett's esophagus with HGD/intramucosal carcinoma. *Gastrointestinal Endoscopy* **69**(5), AB341.

23 DeMeester DR OA, Bergman JJ, Grant KS, Jobe BA, Niebish S, Peters JH, Schölvinck D, van Berge Henegouwen M, Weisten BL (2012). Initial Human Experience With a Novel Through-the-Scope Cryoballoon Device for Mucosal Ablation. *Gastroenterology* **145**(5, Supplement 1), S–1038.

24 Mohammed A, Miller S, Douglas-Moore J, Miller M (2013). Cryotherapy and its applications in the management of urologic malignancies: A review of its use in prostate and renal cancers. *Urologic Oncology* **32**(1), 39.e19–27.

25 Greenwald BD, Dumot JA, Abrams JA, Lightdale CJ, David DS, Nishioka NS, *et al.* (2010). Endoscopic spray cryotherapy for esophageal cancer: safety and efficacy. *Gastrointestinal Endoscopy* **71**(4), 686–93.

CHAPTER 18

Endoscopic resection

Oliver Pech

Department of Gastroenterology and interventional Endoscopy, St. John of God Hospital, Teaching Hospital of the University of Regensburg, Germany

18.1 Introduction

Endoscopic (mucosal) resection (ER or EMR) of localizable early Barrett's neoplasia has become the treatment of choice in recent years. On the one side, it serves as a diagnostic tool for the staging and also as a curative treatment method [1]. ER can be considered curative in low-grade dysplasia (LGD), high-grade dysplasia (HGD) and mucosal adenocarcinoma in Barrett's esophagus, and it is the preferred therapy over any ablative and surgical treatment.

ER of Barrett's neoplasia has been shown to be safe and effective in several studies from different centers with long follow-up. In a matched pair analysis comparing ER with radical esophageal resection, both methods were equal regarding rate of complete remission and long-term survival. ER had a significantly lower rate of major complications (0 vs 32%), but was associated with a higher rate of local recurrences (6.6% vs 0%) [2].

In contrast to ablative treatment methods such as photodynamic therapy, argon-plasma-coagulation, cryotherapy and radiofrequency ablation, ER allows histological assessment of the resected specimen in order to assess the exact infiltration depth of the tumor, and whether any risk factors for local or distant metastasis such as infiltration of lymph (L-status) or blood vessels (V-status) is present. Biopsy diagnosis is not always exact, and ER also serves as an important staging tool. A recently published Australian series demonstrated that diagnosis changed in 48% after ER, with downstaging in 28% and upstaging in 20%. Submucosal infiltration was detected in 9% after ER [3].

In addition to the assessment of the histological risk factors, the pathologist can also provide important information about freedom from neoplasia at the lateral and (more importantly) basal margins [1]. When the margin of the resected specimen shows neoplastic cells, there is a chance that dysplasia or cancer was not completely resected, requiring further treatment.

18.2 ER techniques

The goal of ER must always be a complete removal of the whole neoplastic lesion resecting the mucosa and major parts of the submucosal layer. This can be performed as a single resection for small lesions (<20 mm), or as a "piecemeal" resection in larger lesions.

ER is an advanced endoscopic procedure, requiring proper training in experienced high-volume centers. The perforation rate of six trainees during their first 120 ERs (20 ER/trainee) in anesthetized pigs was 5% [4].

18.2.1 Cap-ER (ER-C)

More than 20 years ago, the ER-C was introduced by Dr. Inoue and co-workers for ER of early esophageal cancer [5]. ER with the cap technique uses a specially developed transparent plastic cap that is attached to the distal tip of the endoscope. Sometimes, taping the cap to the endoscope is helpful to prevent slipping of the cap from the tip of the endoscope. The crucial part of every curative ER is high-quality imaging of the whole Barrett's segment and careful delineation of the lesion. The borders of the lesion should be marked with a distance of 5 mm, either with electrocautery, using the tip of the snare or an APC probe, since injecting underneath a discrete neoplastic lesion often makes it difficult to identify the borders of the target lesion afterwards. In addition, some peri-procedural bleeding might obscure the view.

Esophageal Cancer and Barrett's Esophagus, Third Edition. Edited by Prateek Sharma, Richard Sampliner and David Ilson.
© 2015 John Wiley & Sons, Ltd. Published 2015 by John Wiley & Sons, Ltd.

Submucosal injection with a saline-epinephrine solution under the target lesion prior resection should prevent perforation of the muscularis propria. After injection, the lesion is sucked into the cap. Then, the specially designed crescent snare, which has previously been loaded into a rim on the lower edge of the cap, is closed tightly, and the sucked-in tissue is resected with a blended cutting current. Pre-loading of the snare is usually done in distance to the target lesion (e.g. the gastric antrum) by applying slight suction to the mucosa and carefully advancing the snare until it is placed exactly in the rim at the distal margin of the cap.

The cap technique is ideal for piecemeal resection of larger lesions. For further resections, the margin of the cap should be placed exactly at the margin of the previous resection site, with only little overlap, in order to prevent perforation by sucking the muscle layer into the cap, but also to prevent leaving behind residual neoplastic islands and bridges (Figure 18.1: see also Plate 18.1).

18.2.2 ER with a ligation device (ER-L)

For treatment of early Barrett's neoplasia, a widely used method is ER with a ligation device. Those devices were originally used for ligation of esophageal varices. With this method, the target lesion is sucked into the cylinder of the ligation device, and a rubber band is then released over the lesion to create a pseudopolyp that has the rubber band at its base. Usually, prior submucosal injection is not necessary. Afterwards, the pseudopolyp with the target lesion is resected with a reusable snare. The snare is usually placed underneath the rubber band, in order to achieve larger resection specimens (Figure 18.2: see also Plate 18.2).

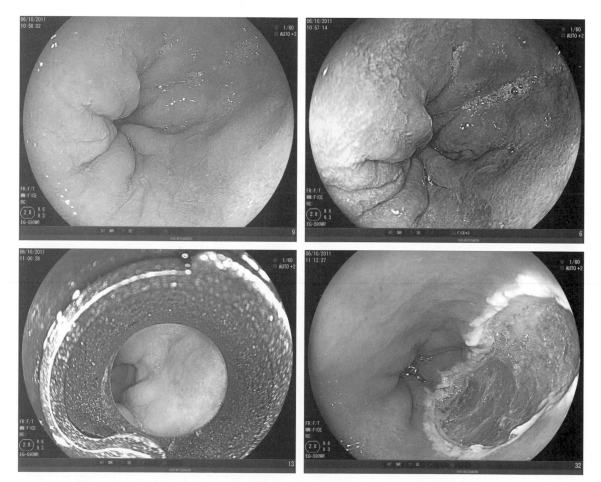

Figure 18.1 a-d ER-L of a subtle type IIb Barrett's neoplasia. *(See insert for color representation of this figure.)*

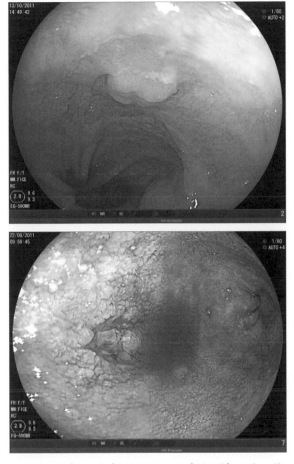

Figure 18.2 a-b ER-C of a recurrent neoplasia with scaring. *(See insert for color representation of this figure.)*

Nowadays, a ligation cylinder with six rubber bands, and the possibility to advance a snare through the working channel of a diagnostic endoscope, is the most frequently used ER technique, described as multiband mucosectomy (MBM). Using MBM enables the endoscopist to perform up to six resections without having to withdraw and reintroduce the endoscope. This device is widely used for piecemeal resections of larger neoplastic lesions.

Both ER with a ligation device and with the cap can be performed in the esophagus, with similar results and complication rates. A prospective randomized trial with 100 consecutive ER in 70 patients, comparing ER with a reusable ligation device with cap-ER, was able to demonstrate that there is no difference regarding size of the resection specimens, the resection area

and complication rate [6]. Complications were minor bleedings in each group, but no perforation or other severe complications were observed. However, another retrospective study from the Amsterdam group showed that ER with MBM was faster and safer than cap resection. Mild bleedings occurred significantly more often after cap-ER (20% vs 6%) [7]. Another prospective randomized trial by the same group demonstrated that ER with MBM was faster (34 vs 50 minutes) and cheaper (€240 vs €322) than with the cap [8]. There were more perforations observed with the cap (3 vs 1), but the difference was not statistically significant.

The major drawback of ER with the suck-and-cut technique appears to be that only small lesions with a diameter of less than 20 mm can be resected *en bloc* with tumor-free lateral margins. Ulcerated lesions often have fibrosis attaching the submucosa to the lamina muscularis propria, often resulting in failure of the lesion to lift. In these cases, ER is not advisable, or should only be performed with caution. Larger lesions can usually be resected completely with the "piecemeal" technique, but this method appears to be associated with a higher recurrence rate, probably due to small neoplastic residues resulting from insufficient overlapping of the resection areas.

For "piecemeal" ER, the ligation device or cap has to be placed at the margin of the prior resection area and careful suction has to be applied. The endoscopist has to be very careful to avoid small neoplastic remnants between the resection areas. Alternatively, there is a danger of sucking the proper muscle layer of the previous resection into the pseudopolyp, leading to a perforation. To minimize the risk of complications and of insufficient resection, only an experienced endoscopist in high-volume centers should perform this procedure. *En bloc* resection allows more accurate histological evaluation of the neoplastic lesion, especially of the lateral and basal margins. A new resection technique – endoscopic submucosal dissection (ESD) – was therefore developed.

18.3   ER in HGIN and early Barrett's cancer

ER is the treatment of choice in HGD and early mucosal cancer in Barrett's esophagus, since the risk for lymph node and distant metastasis is almost absent. Large series from several groups are demonstrating the safety and efficacy of this treatment approach, even after long-term follow-up. [3,9–13]. Risk stratification should be carried out in accordance with known risk factors, such as grade of differentiation, lymph vessel or venous infiltration and the infiltration depth of the carcinoma (m1 – m3/m4). Also, the macroscopic type of the lesion, according to the Paris classification, is helpful to predict the probability of submucosal invasion [14,15] (Figures 18.3 and 18.4: see also Plate 18.4); Table 18.1).

Several groups have published studies on ER of early Barrett's neopalsia, with excellent results. Ell *et al.* reported the first series on ER of early Barrett's adenocarcinoma, or HGIN, in 2000 [9]. 64 patients were included, and complete local remission could be achieved in 82.5%. The recurrence rate was 14% after a mean follow-up of 12 months. However, the rate of recurrence and metachronous neoplasia rises significantly with increased follow-up. A further study published by the same group reported a high complete remission rate of 98% in 115 patients but, after a follow-up of 34 months, the recurrence rate of rate of metachronous neoplasia was 31% [10].

The high recurrence rate remained a problem of endoscopic therapy for several years, and a close follow-up of all patients treated with ER was necessary in order to obtain an early diagnosis of recurrence. In almost all patients, endoscopic re-treatment was possible.

In a large series on endoscopic treatment of early Barrett's neoplasia in 349 patients, the risk factors for

recurrence of neoplasia were analyzed in a multivariate analysis [12] (Table 18.2). After treatment, 96.6% of all included patients achieved complete remission, and recurrent or metachronous neoplasia was observed in 21.5% after a median follow-up of 64 months. Most patients could be re-treated successfully, and long-term complete response was achieved in 94.5%.

These data clearly demonstrate that ablation of the remaining Barrett's metaplasia after removal of the neoplastic lesion by ER is an essential step in the successful treatment of HGD and mucosal Barrett's adenocarcinoma. For ablation, radio frequency ablation (RFA) and argon-plasma-coagulation (APC) are usually applied.

Another technique to remove the whole Barrett's mucosa at risk is complete radical ER in several steps. The Hamburg group was the first to describe radical complete ER, in 12 patients with early Barrett's neoplasia [16]. The complete Barrett's segment was resected in one to five sessions, with a median of five ERs per session (range 1–19). Complications occurred in six cases, with four bleedings and two strictures. All complications were managed endoscopically. The median follow-up in this small series was nine months, and no recurrences were observed.

The concept of complete ER was also investigated in an European multicenter trial which included 169 patients with early Barrett's neoplasia [17]. Stepwise radical ER was performed in four experienced centers in order to completely eradicate Barrett's esophagus with neoplasia. Complete eradication of neoplasia and Barrett's epithelium could be achieved in 97.6% and 85.2% of patients, respectively. One patient showed progression of cancer and died from metastatic disease, and four patients developed recurrence after a median follow-up of 32 months. Symptomatic esophageal stenosis was also a major problem in this series, and was observed in almost 50% of patients.

A prospective randomized trial compared complete radical ER with focal ER of all neoplastic lesions, followed by ablation of the remaining Barrett's epithelium with RFA [18]. 47 patients with HGIN and early Barrett's cancer and a Barrett's length of less than 5 cm were included. There was no significant difference between the radical ER arm and the ER + RFA arm regarding complete remission of neoplasia (100% vs 96%) and of intestinal metaplasia (92% vs 96%). However, there was a significant difference in complication

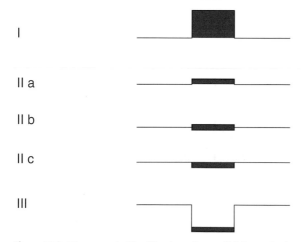

Figure 18.3 Macroscopic Classification of superficial neoplastic lesions.

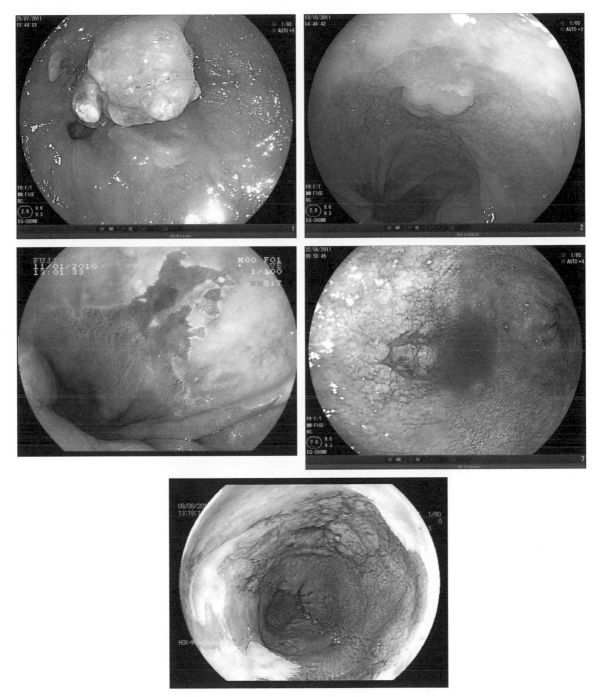

Figure 18.4 Endoscopic examples of different macroscopic types of early Barrett's neoplasia: (a) Type I – polypoid lesion. (b) Type IIa – slightly elevated lesion. (c) Type IIb – flat lesion in mucosal level. (d) Type IIc – depressed lesion. (e) Type IIa + c – mixed type lesion. *(See insert for color representation of this figure.)*

Table 18.1 Macroscopic appearance of early Barrett's neoplasia according to the Paris classification, and percentage of submucosal infiltration according to [14,15].

Macroscopic type	Number of lesions	Endoscopic appearance	% submucosal infiltration
Type I	70	Polypoid/ elevated	13%
Type IIa	181	Slightly elevated	13%
Type IIb	96	Mucosal level	3%
Type IIc	20	Slightly depressed	25%
Type IIa + c	125	Mixed elevated and depressed	14%
Type III	–	Ulcerated	–

Table 18.2 Risk factors for recurrence after endoscopic resection of early Barrett's neoplasia.

Variables	Relative risk (95% CI)	P
Long-segment Barrett's esophagus	1.9 (1.06 to 3.3)	0.03
Time until CR achieved >10 months	0.3 (0.12 to 0.75)	0.009
"Piecemeal" resection	2.44 (1.13 to 4.89)	0.02
Multifocal neoplasia	2.1 (1.16 to 3.99)	0.01
No ablative therapy of BE after CR	0.4 (0.26 to 0.66)	0.0003

Reproduced from Pech, 2008 [12], with permission of the BMJ.
BE – Barrett's esophagus; CR – complete remission.

rate. 88% of patients in the radical ER group developed strictures, compared with 14% in the combined treatment group. In addition, significantly less treatment sessions were needed with ER + RFA (6 vs 3).

One of the major advantages of radical ER of neoplastic Barrett's esophagus is the possibility that the whole Barrett's segment can be evaluated by the pathologist in order to detect and stage even endoscopically not visualized neoplasia. The downside of complete radical ER of the whole Barrett's segment is the high stricture rate associated with this method, requiring repeated dilatation. Therefore, a combination of ER of all visible neoplastic lesions, followed by thermal ablation of the remaining Barrett's epithelium, is the superior treatment strategy, combining the positive sides of tissue acquisition with a low complication rate associated with ablation [12,19,20].

18.4 ER of submucosal Barrett's adenocarcinoma

Submucosal infiltration is associated with an increased lymph node risk rising up to 41%, and it seems to be correlated with the depth of infiltration of the tumor into the submucosal layer. Cancer infiltrating the upper third of the submucosa (pT1sm1) has a risk varying between 0 and 21%. Cancer invading the mid and lower part of the submucosa (pT1sm2/3) goes along with metastatic lymph nodes in 36–54% [21–28]. These data are mainly from older retrospective surgical series, in a time period when exact determination of the tumor infiltration depth had little clinical relevance. In contrast to ER specimens, which are sliced every 1–2 millimeters, surgical resection specimens were routinely cut in 5 mm slices and, therefore, deeper infiltrating parts of the tumor were not detected. This explains that the actual infiltration depth was underestimated in those surgical series, resulting in an incorrect lymph node metastasis rate. In addition, further risk factors such as poor differentiation grade and lymphatic and vascular invasion were usually not reported, making it impossible to draw final conclusions from these series.

Some data are suggesting that ER can safely be performed in so-called "low-risk" submucosal cancer (sm1-cancer with invasion up to 500µm, G1/2, L0, V0) [21,27]. A recently published study by the Wiesbaden group included 67 patients, with submucosal Barrett's cancer invading only the upper layer of the submucosa without any risk factors [29]. Risk factors for lymph node metastasis were adopted from Japanese data on early gastric cancer and were poor differentiation grade, ulcerated lesion, lymph vessel infiltration and tumor size >20 mm. In this large series, all patients were treated by ER, but only one patient developed a lymph node metastasis. This was detected by EUS nine months after treatment, resulting in a lymph node risk of 1.5%, which is below the usual mortality rate of esophagectomy.

18.5 Conclusions

ER is the treatment of choice for HGD and mucosal Barrett's adenocarcinoma. It is not only an effective treatment method, but also serves as a diagnostic tool, enabling an exact assessment of the tumor infiltration depth and the presence of risk factors such as lymph vessel infiltration. To avoid tumor recurrence or metachronous neoplasia, ER should always be followed by careful ablation of the remaining Barrett's epithelium. Therefore, successful endoscopic treatment of early neoplastic lesions is always a two-step procedure.

- Step 1: ER of all HGD and adenocarcinomas.
- Step 2: Ablation of the remaining non-dysplastic Barrett's esophagus.

According to recent data, ER of early Barrett's adenocarcinoma with incipient infiltration of the submucosa up to 500 μm, without any further risk factors, seem to be also eligible for ER. This is because the risk of lymph node metastatis seems to be below the mortality rate of radical esophageal resection.

References

1 Pech O, May A, Rabenstein T, Ell C (2007). Endoscopic resection of early oesophageal cancer. *Gut* **56**, 1625–1634.

2 Pech O, Bollschweiler E, Manner H, Leers J, Ell C, Hölscher AH (2011). Comparison between Endoscopic and Surgical Resection of Mucosal Esophageal Adenocarcinoma in Barrett's Esophagus at Two High-Volume Centers. *Annals of Surgery* **254**(1), 67–72

3 Moss A, Bourke MJ, Hourigan LF, Gupta S, Williams SJ, Tran K, Swan MP, Hopper AD, Kwan V, Bailey AA (2010). Endoscopic resection for Barrett's high-grade dysplasia and early esophageal adenocarcinoma: an essential staging procedure with long-term therapeutic benefit. *American Journal of Gastroenterology* **105**(6), 1276–83.

4 van Vilsteren FG, Pouw RE, Herrero LA, Peters FP, Bisschops R, Houben M, Peters FT, Schenk BE, Weusten BL, Visser M, Ten Kate FJ, Fockens P, Schoon EJ, Bergman JJ (2012). Learning to perform endoscopic resection of esophageal neoplasia is associated with significant complications even within a structured training program. *Endoscopy* **44**(1), 4–12.

5 Inoue H, Endo M (1993). A new simplified technique of endoscopic esophageal mucosal resection using a cap-fitted panendoscope. *Surgical Endoscopy* **6**, 264–5.

6 May A, Gossner L, Behrens A, *et al.* (2003). A prospective randomized trial of two different suck-and-cut mucosectomy techniques in 100 consecutive resections in patients with early cancer of the esophagus. *Gastrointestinal Endoscopy* **58**, 167–75

7 Peters FP, Kara MA, Curvers WL, Rosmolen WD, Fockens P, Krishnadath KK, Ten Kate FJ, Bergman JJ (2007). Multiband mucosectomy for endoscopic resection of Barrett's esophagus: feasibility study with matched historical controls. *European Journal of Gastroenterology & Hepatology* **19**(4), 311–5.

8 Pouw RE, van Vilsteren FG, Peters FP, Herrero LA, Ten Kate FJ, Visser M, Schenk BE, Schoon EJ, Peters FT, Houben M, Bisschops R, Weusten BL, Bergman JJ (2011). Randomized trial on endoscopic resection-cap versus multiband mucosectomy for piecemeal endoscopic resection of early Barrett's neoplasia. *Gastrointestinal Endoscopy* **74**(1), 35–43

9 Ell C, May A, Gossner L, Pech O, Günter E, Mayer G, Henrich R, Vieth M, Müller H, Seitz G, Stolte M (2000). Endoscopic mucosal resection of early cancer and high-grade dysplasia in Barrett's esophagus. *Gastroenterology* **118**(4), 670–7.

10 May A, Gossner L, Pech O, Fritz A, Günter E, Mayer G, *et al.* (2002). Local endoscopic therapy for intraepithelial high-grade neoplasia and early adenocarcinoma in Barrett's oesophagus: acute-phase and intermediate results of a new treatment approach. *European Journal of Gastroenterology & Hepatology* **14**(10), 1085–91.

11 Ell C, May A, Pech O, *et al.* (2007). Curative endoscopic resection of early esophageal adenocarcinomas (Barrett's cancer). *Gastrointestinal Endoscopy* **65**, 3–10.

12 Pech O, Behrens A, May A, *et al.* (2008). Long-term results and risk factor analysis for recurrence after curative endoscopic therapy in 349 patients with high-grade intraepithelial neoplasia and mucosal adenocarcinoma in Barrett's oesophagus. *Gut* **57**, 1200–1206.

13 Chennat J, Konda VJA, Ross AS, Herreros de Tejada A, Noffsinger A, Hart J, Lin S, Ferguson MK, Posner MC, Waxman I (2009). Complete Barrett's Eradication Endoscopic Mucosal Resection (CBE-EMR): An Effective Treatment Modality for High Grade Dysplasia (HGD) and Intramucosal Carcinoma (IMC) – An American Single Center Experience. *American Journal of Gastroenterology* **104**(11), 2684–92

14 Pech O, Gossner L, Manner H, *et al.* (2007). Prospective evaluation of the macroscopic types and location of early Barrett's neoplasia in 380 lesions. *Endoscopy* **39**, 588–59

15 Peters FP, Brakenhoff KP, Curvers WL, *et al.* (2008). Histologic evaluation of resection specimens obtained at 293 endoscopic resections in Barrett!s esophagus. *Gastrointestinal Endoscopy* **67**, 604–609

16 Seewald S, Akaraviputh T, Seitz U, *et al.* (2003). Circumferential EMR and complete removal of Barrett's epithelium: a new approach to management of Barrett's esophagus containing high-grade intraepithelial neoplasia and intramucosal carcinoma. *Gastrointestinal Endoscopy* **57**, 854–9

17 Pouw RE, Seewald S, Gondrie JJ, Deprez PH, Piessevaux H, Pohl H, Rösch T, Soehendra N, Bergman JJ (2010). Stepwise radical endoscopic resection for eradication of Barrett's oesophagus with early neoplasia in a cohort of 169 patients. *Gut* **59**(9), 1169–77

18 van Vilsteren FG, Pouw RE, Seewald S, Alvarez Herrero L, Sondermeijer CM, Visser M, Ten Kate FJ, Yu Kim Teng KC, Soehendra N, Rösch T, Weusten BL, Bergman JJ (2011). Stepwise radical endoscopic resection versus radiofrequency ablation for Barrett's oesophagus with high-grade dysplasia

or early cancer: a multicentre randomised trial. *Gut* **60**(6), 765–73.

19 Pouw RE, Wirths K, Eisendrath P, Sondermeijer CM, Ten Kate FJ, Fockens P, Devière J, Neuhaus H, Bergman JJ (2010). Efficacy of radiofrequency ablation combined with endoscopic resection for Barrett's esophagus with early neoplasia. *Clinical Gastroenterology and Hepatology* **8**(1), 23–9.

20 Phoa KN, Pouw RE, van Vilsteren FG, Sondermeijer CM, Ten Kate FJ, Visser M, Meijer SL, van Berge Henegouwen MI, Weusten BL, Schoon EJ, Mallant-Hent RC, Bergman JJ (2013). Predictive factors for initial treatment response after circumferential radiofrequency ablation for Barrett's esophagus with early neoplasia: a prospective multicenter study. *Gastroenterology* **145**(1), 96–104.

21 Buskens CJ, Westerterp M, Lagarde SM, Bergman JJ, ten Kate FJ, van Lanschot JJ (2004). Prediction of appropriateness of local endoscopic treatment for high-grade dysplasia and early adenocarcinoma by EUS and histopathologic features. *Gastrointestinal Endoscopy* **60**, 703–710.

22 Stein HJ, Feith M, Bruecher BLDM, Nahrig J, Siewert JR (2005). Early esophageal squamous cell and adenocarcinoma: pattern of lymphatic spread and prognostic factors for long term survival after surgical resection. *Annals of Surgery* **242**, 566–573.

23 Rice TW, Blackstone EH, Goldblum JR, DeCamp MM, Murthy SC, Falk GW, Ormsby AH, Rybicki LA, Richter JE, Adelstein DJ (2001). Superficial adenocarcinoma of the esophagus. *Journal of Thoracic and Cardiovascular Surgery* **122**, 1077–1090.

24 Oh DS, Hagen JA, Chandrasoma PT, Dunst CM, Demeester SR, Alavi M, Bremner CG, Lipham J, Rizzetto C, Cote R, Demeester TR (2006). Clinical biology and surgical therapy of intramucosal adenocarcinoma of the esophagus. *Journal of the American College of Surgeons* **203**, 152–161.

25 Bollschweiler E, Baldus SE, Schröder W, Prenzel K, Gutschow C, Schneider PM, Hölscher AH (2006). High rate of lymph-node metastasis in submucosal esophageal squamous-cell carcinomas and adenocarcinomas. *Endoscopy* **38**, 149–156.

26 Ancona E, Rampado S, Cassaro M, Battaglia G, Ruol A, Castoro C, Portale G, Cavallin F, Rugge M (2008). Prediction of lymph node status in superficial esophageal carcinoma. *Annals of Surgical Oncology* **15**(11), 3278–88.

27 Manner H, May A, Pech O, Gossner L, Rabenstein T, Günter E, Vieth M, Stolte M, Ell C (2008). Early Barrett's carcinoma with "low-risk" submucosal invasion: long-term results of endoscopic resection with a curative intent. *American Journal of Gastroenterology* **103**(10), 2589–97

28 Badreddine RJ, Prasad GA, Lewis JT, Lutzke LS, Borkenhagen LS, Dunagan KT, Wang KK (2010). Depth of submucosal invasion does not predict lymph node metastasis and survival of patients with esophageal carcinoma. *Clinical Gastroenterology and Hepatology* **8**(3), 248–53.

29 Manner H, Pech O, Heldmann Y, May A, Pohl J, Behrens A, Gossner L, Stolte M, Vieth M, Ell C (2013). Efficacy, safety and long-term results of endoscopic treatment for early-stage adenocarcinoma oft he esophagus with low-risk sm1 invasion. *Clinical Gastroenterology and Hepatology* **11**(6), 630–5.

CHAPTER 19

Endoscopic submucosal dissection

Hironori Yamamoto[1], Tsuneo Oyama[2] & Takuji Gotoda[3]

[1] Department of Medicine, Division of Gastroenterology, Jichi Medical University, Shimotsuke, Tochigi, Japan
[2] Department of Endoscopy, Saku Central Hospital Advanced Care Center, Nagano, Japan
[3] Department of Gastroenterology and Hepatology, Tokyo Medical University, Tokyo, Japan

19.1 Introduction

Patients who are identified to have no risk, or a lower risk, for developing lymph node metastasis than the perioperative risks associated with surgery, are ideal candidates for endoscopic resection. Endoscopic resection allows complete pathological staging of the cancer, which is critical as it allows stratification and refinement of further treatment [1].

The major advantage of endoscopic resection is its ability to provide pathological staging without precluding future surgical therapy [2]. After endoscopic resection, pathological assessment of depth of cancer invasion, degree of differentiation of the cancer, and lympho-vascular invasion allow the risk of lymph node metastasis to be predicted using published data of patients with similar findings. The risk of developing lymph node metastasis or distant metastasis is then weighed against the risk of surgery. The final staging can only be done through formal histological analysis, which endoscopic excision can achieve [3].

Conventional esophageal EMR procedures include the EEMR-tube method described by Makuuchi et al. [4], the EMRC method described by Inoue et al. [5], and the EAM method described by Tanabe et al. [6]. In all of these procedures, a flat lesion is deformed into a polyp-like shape, to be snared using aspiration or a grasper as an extension of a polypectomy. All are simple, but the rate of en bloc resection was as low as 23–57%, because the resected area per resection was limited to 15.1–23.9 mm [6, 7]. Therefore, the local recurrence rate was reported to be as high as 7.8–20% [8, 9]. In addition, more fractionated resections tended to lead to a higher local recurrence rate [10].

Standard EMR techniques cannot be used to resect lesions larger than 15 mm in one piece [11]. Specimens obtained following piecemeal resections are difficult to analyze by the pathologist, and render pathological staging inadequate. This is a major factor leading to the high-risk of recurrence when this technique is used on larger lesions. Therefore, en bloc resection is essential to investigate the risk factors of lymph node metastasis fully and reduce the risk of recurrence. Endoscopic submucosal dissection (ESD) was developed for precise and large en bloc resections.

19.2 Indications of ESD for esophageal cancer

19.2.1 Squamous cell carcinoma

ESD is indicated for cancer with no or minimal risk of lymph node metastasis. When the lesions are classified, according to the depth of invasion, as intraepithelial carcinoma (EP), restricted within the proper mucosal layer (LPM), adjacent to or invading but not beyond the muscularis mucosa (MM), invading the submucosal layer to a depth of one-third (SM1), or more than one-third (SM2 and 3) of the layer thickness (Figure 19.1), then the incidence of lymph node metastasis was reported to be 0%, 0–5.6%, 8–18%, 11–53%, and 30–54%, respectively [12–14]. Therefore, under the 2007 Japan Esophageal Society guidelines for the treatment of esophageal cancer, the absolute indication for endoscopic mucosal resection (EMR) is defined as EP-LPM esophageal cancer as well as two-thirds or less extension of the circumference, while the relative

Esophageal Cancer and Barrett's Esophagus, Third Edition. Edited by Prateek Sharma, Richard Sampliner and David Ilson.
© 2015 John Wiley & Sons, Ltd. Published 2015 by John Wiley & Sons, Ltd.

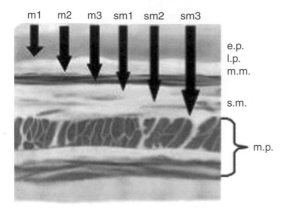

Figure 19.1 Sub-classification of esophageal mucosa and submucosal layer. The condition of cancer limited to the basement membrane is classified as EP, the condition of cancer to the lamina propria is LPM, and the condition of cancer reached or infiltrated the muscularis mucosae is MM. For the surgically excised specimen, the submucosal layer is divided equally into three layers, classified as SM1, SM2, and SM3. However, for the endoscopic excised specimen, the infiltration from the inferior end of the muscularis mucosae to 200 μm is classified as SM1, and the further infiltration as SM2. Source: Soetikno *et al.* (2003) [16]. Reproduced with permission of Elsevier.

indication is defined as MM-SM1 esophageal cancer with as well as three-quarters or more mucosal defect after EMR [15].

Oyama reported that an analysis of 749 patients with MM-SM1 cancer revealed that the incidence of lymph node metastasis of MM cancer was 9.3%, while that of SM1 was 19.3%. Risk factors for lymph node metastasis represented a 50 mm or more longitudinal extension, poorly differentiated carcinoma, and positive vascular invasion, and the incidence of lymph node metastasis was 4.6% in the absence of these risk factors [14].

19.2.2   Barrett's esophageal cancer

There are limited superficial cases among patients with Barrett's esophageal cancer, which is more prevalent in Western countries than Asian countries. The incidence of lymph node metastasis in the disease has not been well documented. Bollschweiler *et al.* reported that analysis of pT1 esophageal adenocarcinoma in 36 patients revealed that the incidence of lymph node metastasis of mucosal cancer was 0%, while SM1, SM2, and SM3 as well as all types of submucosal invasive cancer were 22%, 0%, 78%, and 41%, respectively [17].

In a more recently published systematic review, the rate of lymph node metastasis has been reported

in 1874 patients who had esophagectomy performed for high-grade dysplasia or intramucosal carcinoma in Barrett's esophagus. No metastases were found in the 524 patients who had a final pathology diagnosis of high-grade dysplasia, whereas 26 (1.93%, 95% CI 1.19–2.66%) of the 1350 patients with a final pathology diagnosis of intramucosal carcinoma had positive lymph nodes. However, considering that esophagectomy has a mortality rate that often exceeds 2%, with substantial morbidity and no guarantee of curing metastatic disease, the risk of lymph node metastases alone does not warrant the choice of esophagectomy over endoscopic therapy for high-grade dysplasia and intramucosal carcinoma in Barrett's esophagus [18]. Therefore, Barrett's esophageal cancer restricted within the mucosa, and high-grade dysplasia, can be considered as indication for the endoscopic treatment.

Using ESD, complete *en bloc* resection of a superficial Barrett's esophageal cancer and junctional cancer is also possible, which enables accurate histopathological examination to evaluate the curability of the resection (Figure 19.2a–g: see also Plate 19.2).

19.3   Preoperative examination

Endoscopy, endosonography, and computed tomography (CT) should be conducted to examine the depth of invasion, presence of lymph node metastasis, and metastasis to other organs.

Since squamous cell carcinoma does not stain with iodine staining, the range of lateral advancement can be easily determined. However, the range of lateral advancement of Barrett's esophageal adenocarcinoma may sometimes be difficult to determine. Therefore, lateral margin is diagnosed by using chromoendoscopy with indigo carmine spray or magnifying endoscopy, as well as biopsy of the peripheral tissue.

19.4   Techniques of ESD [19–22] for esophageal cancer

19.4.1   Marking

The thickness of the esophageal wall can vary, depending on the air content; it may become as thin as about 2–3 mm when the wall is extended. When a needle-type knife such as a needle knife (KD-1L-1, Olympus Co., Tokyo, Japan) or a Flush knife (Fujifilm,

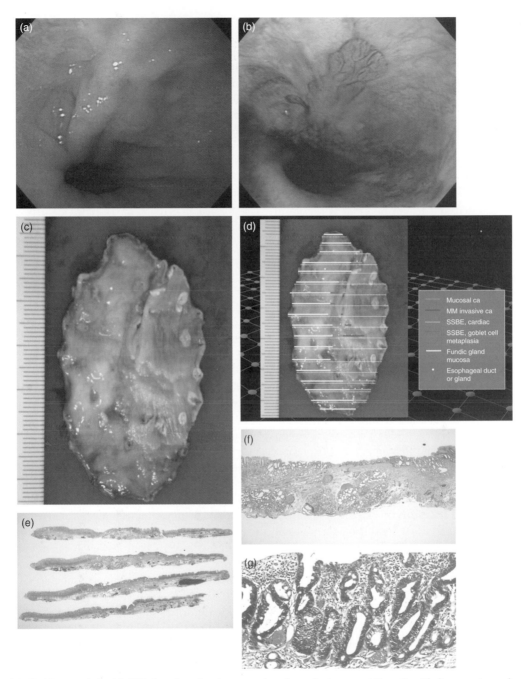

Figure 19.2 *En bloc* resection with ESD for a junctional cancer arisen from short-segment Barrett epithelium. **a**. Avascular edematous mucosa on the end of the gastric fold in the junction. **b**. Elongated columnar epithelium with dysplasia (or well-differentiated adenocarcinoma) in squamous epithelium. **c**. *En bloc* material resected by ESD. **d**. Histological assessment (well-differentiated adenocarcinoma developed from short-segment Barrett epithelium – size of tumor: 19 × 15 mm; depth of invasion: MM). **e**. Low power views of serial section. **f**. Esophageal glands in submucosal layer and columnar epithelium in mucosal layer. **g**. Well-differentiated adenocarcinoma (high power view). *(See insert for color representation of this figure.)*

Tokyo, Japan) is used for marking, it should be used with soft coagulation (Figure 19.3a, b: see also Plate 19.3) to avoid perforation. Using a ball-tipped Flush knife (Flush knife-BT: Fujifilm, Tokyo, Japan), clear marking can be made with the ball tip using soft coagulation. A Hook knife (KD-620LR, Olympus Co., Tokyo, Japan) and TT knife (KD-640L, Olympus Co., Tokyo, Japan) are attached to the mucosa, with a knife stored in the sheath, and energization for a moment using forced coagulation (60 W) (ICC200 or VIO300D, Erbe, Tübingen, Germany) can provide a mark safely. A Flex knife (KD- 630L, Olympus Co., Tokyo, Japan) should be adjusted to a length of 1 mm at the tip to prevent perforation.

19.4.2   Submucosal injection

Since the proper muscular layer of the esophageal wall is thinner than that of the gastric wall, and is always in motion due to the heart beating, sufficient space should be secured between the mucosa and proper muscular layer through submucosal injection. Therefore, it is ideal to use solutions with higher viscosity than that of physiological saline, such as 0.4% sodium hyaluronate solution (MucoUp; Seikagaku Corp, Tokyo, Japan) [23] and 10% glycerol (Glyceol; Chugai Pharmaceutical Co, Tokyo, Japan). Submucosal injection of sodium hyaluronate creates a long-lasting mucosal protrusion that usually lasts more than an hour [19, 24]. To prevent bleeding, epinephrine should be added at 5 µg/ml into the local administration solution.

19.4.3   Mucosal incision

ENDO CUT mode (Endocut I) is suitable for mucosal incisions because it can prevent over-incision with a single cut. The mucosa on the anal side is initially incised. In order to avoid the risk of perforation, a mucosal incision should be made after making a sufficient submucosal bulge using sodium hyaluronate solution. A 1.5 mm ball-tipped Flush knife is a suitable knife for esophageal ESD. When a needle-type knife, such as a Flush knife, is used for mucosal incision, the mucosa should be cut from the oral side to the anal side, or cut the lateral way by lifting up the mucosa toward the direction of the luminal side. When a Hook knife is used, perforation can be prevented by inserting the hook part into the submucosal layer and performing an electrization incision during elevation of the mucosa (Figure 19.3c–e: see also Plate 19.3). A deep incision

may damage vessels, leading to bleeding. It is important initially to incise the mucosa shallowly, and to incise deeper under observation of the submucosal layer.

The mucosa on the oral side is then incised in a similar manner. After the submucosal layer on the oral side is well visualized, a lateral mucosal incision is performed. If a needle-type knife is used, the mucosa should be hooked with the knife to elevate it toward the lumen for cutting. With a Hook knife, the hook is turned to the esophageal lumen, and inserted into the submucosal layer, sliding the back of the knife. The mucosa is elevated to the lumen and an electrization incision is performed. In general, the IT knife (KD-610L, Olympus Co., Tokyo, Japan) is not used for esophageal ESD, due to a high risk of perforation, but it may occasionally be useful for mucosal incision from the anal side to the oral side (ENDO CUT mode, 3 W, 60 W). The optimal device should be selected and used according to the site and conditions.

19.4.4   Submucosal dissection

For submucosal dissection, an electrosurgical mode with a high hemostatic capability, such as Swift coagulation and dry cut, should be selected, because it easily enables control of bleeding. There are two strategies for submucosal dissection. In one strategy, after a mucosal incision, dissection of the submucosal layer is performed sequentially from the oral side to the anal side. Circumferential incision may cause leakage of the locally administered solution, leading to an insufficient bulge in the submucosal layer. To prevent this, a partial mucosal incision is initially made, followed by submucosal dissection, which may sustain the bulge in the submucosal layer. Then dissection is performed from the oral to the anal side (Figure 19.3f: see also Plate 19.3), during which an additional submucosal injection is performed if appropriate.

To perform the submucosal dissection safely with a needle-type knife and a Hook knife, the submucosal layer should be maintained with a sufficient bulge, then the fibers of the submucosal tissue are hooked with the knife, directing it toward a safer space, followed by repeated brief energization. The knife can be used safely in the direction from the closed to the open space after the incised part is opened using an ST hood (DH-15GR, Fujinon Corp., Saitama, Japan; Figure 19.4) or transparent hood and the fibers are hooked (Figure 19.5: see also Plate 19.5) [25]. A needle knife is applied in

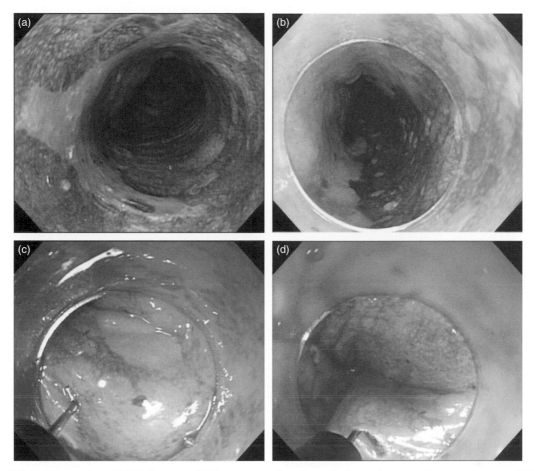

Figure 19.3 *En bloc* resection with ESD for a superficial squamous cell carcinoma in the esophagus. **a**. Chromoendoscopy with Iodine staining. The unstained area with a clear border through iodine staining represents widespread squamous cell carcinoma of the middle thoracic esophagus. The lesion extends from the anterior wall to the posterior wall, and is subtotal. Excision of such a lesion with conventional EMR leads to multiple piecemeal resection and makes accurate postoperative pathological evaluation impossible. Since the remaining non-neoplastic mucosa may also be excised, the risk of stricture due to circumferential excision is greater. **b**. While the mucosa is touched slightly with the hook knife stored in the sheath, marking is made by applying current for a moment with forced coagulation at 40 W. Non-neoplastic epithelial mucosa is a small portion, due to the subtotal lesion. For prevention of stricture, however, it is important to leave this portion. **c**. The mucosal incision is initiated after a submucosal local injection. With the use of a hook knife, when the back of the knife is pressed lightly on the mucosa to apply current for a moment with a dry cut effect 5, 60 W, a small hole is bored into the mucosa for insertion of the point of the knife into the submucosal layer. **d**. The muscularis mucosae are hooked with the knife inserted into the submucosal layer and elevated to the luminal side for the incision by applying a current. A sufficient local injection is needed to prevent perforation. Also, it is important to control the direction of the knife to the luminal side. **e**. Endoscopic view during incision of the mucosa. The translucent submucosal layer and a vessel are observed on the right side. The muscularis propria is invisible because of the sufficient local injection. A mucosal incision with hooking in this state causes no perforation. **f**. Endoscopic view during dissection of the submucosal layer. The view of the submucosal layer is obtained by opening the layer with a transparent hood attached at the tip of the endoscope. The submucosal layer is dissected while hooking the fibers and the vessels with the tip of the hook knife. To prevent perforation and bleeding, it is important to perform dissection while directly observing the submucosal layer. **g**. Endoscopic view immediately after ESD completed. Sub-circumferential excision was performed, leaving the ≈5 mm wide non-neoplastic mucosa. Fibers of the submucosal layer are left on the ulcer floor, and no muscularis propria is exposed. Because the esophagus lacks serosa, the exposure of the muscularis propria may cause mediastinal emphysema. Consequently, it is important to dissect at the inferior third of the submucosal layer. **h**. Iodine stained view of excised specimen. The clear and irregular iodine unstained border and existence of the non-neoplastic mucosa stained by iodine at the excised margins reveal negative surgical margins. The lesion was pathologically diagnosed as squamous cell carcinoma of 53 × 40 mm with LPM in invasion depth, and complete excision was confirmed. *(See insert for color representation of this figure.)*

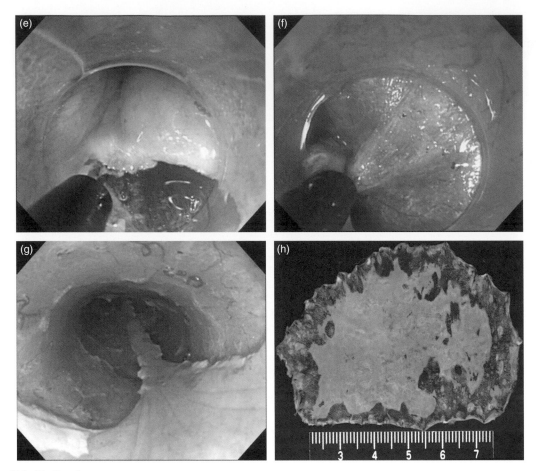

Figure 19.3 (*Continued*)

the direction from the center to the lateral sides of the lesion. A Hook knife is used to incise, by pulling after the fibers are hooked.

In the other strategy, a local injection is administered after a circumferential incision, followed by a tunnel-shaped dissection of the center of the lesion, and the fibers on both sides are dissected [26]. In the former strategy, dissection from the oral side may cause gradual inversion of the lesion, leading to insufficient traction of the submucosal layer, which can make residual dissection difficult. Tunnel-shaped dissection of the central part enables traction and countertraction using a transparent hood, providing more efficient dissection.

With either strategy, the entire lesion is resected in one piece using ESD (Figure 19.3g, h).

In patients with Barrett's esophageal cancer, the submucosal layer may be accompanied by severe fibrosis,

due to scarring after reflux esophagitis or esophageal ulcers. In this case, a submucosal topical injection of highly viscous sodium hyaluronate may be useful. If the lesion will not bulge sufficiently, then the operator should forego endoscopic dissection and choose another treatment.

19.4.5 Hemostasis using knife [27]

When bleeding occurs during mucosal incision or dissection, the area should be flushed using a water jet system as soon as possible, to find the origin of the bleeding. For oozing bleed, a knife tip is brought close to the origin, and electrical discharge is done with Spray mode to obtain hemostasis (effect 2 and 20 W with a needle-type knife, effect 2 and 60 W with a Hook knife). Since prolonged electrization may cause perforation, electrization should be performed momentarily.

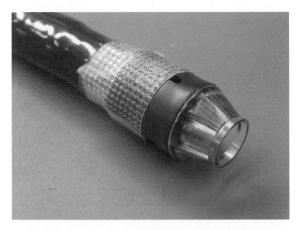

Figure 19.1 The ST hood attached at the tip of the endoscope (DH-15GR, Fujinon Corporation). The tip of the ST hood is tapered to 7 mm at the opening. The tip of the hood provides a 1 mm long nail hook to facilitate opening the incised wound.

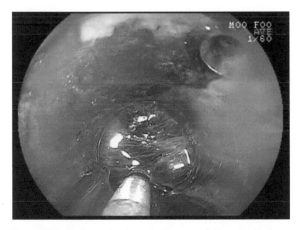

Figure 19.5 Endoscopic view of submucosal dissection using a needle knife through an ST hood. The submucosal fibers are hooked by the tip of a needle knife, while opening the incised mucosa with the tip of the ST hood. *(See insert for color representation of this figure.)*

Electrization by pushing the tip into the lesion may also cause perforation, so it is important to maintain optimal distance, using a transparent hood.

Coagulation with the origin of bleeding unclear may cause coagulation of the blood and blackening, leading to further impairment in the field of vision. A water jet system must be used to confirm the precise origin of the bleeding. A scope equipped with a water jet should be selected for esophageal ESD.

19.4.6 Hemostatic procedures using a hemostatic forceps

A hemostatic forceps (HemoStat-Y, Pentax Co., Tokyo, FD-410LR Olympus, Tokyo, Japan) is useful in cases of more active or spurting bleeding. After flushing with a water jet to clear the origin of bleeding, the origin is grasped accurately with the hemostatic forceps. After that, re-flushing with a water jet may enable us to determine whether the origin is grasped accurately. The forceps is then elevated a little, and soft coagulation is performed, with the forceps kept from the proper muscular layer, followed by electrization with effect 5 and 40 W momentarily to obtain hemostasis.

In the hemostatic procedures using a hemostatic forceps, an accurate grasp is the most important factor. An accurate grasp of the bleeding point may provide reliable hemostasis, while an inaccurate grasp will not provide hemostasis by electrization. Unnecessary electrization may cause delayed perforation, so an accurate grasp should be ensured. Since the wall of the esophagus is thinner than that of the stomach, to prevent delayed and other types of perforation, care should be taken not to widen the contact area excessively due to a wider grasp of the tissue and pushing of the forceps into the tissue, if a regular mono-polar hemostatic forceps is used during esophageal ESD. A bipolar hemostatic forceps (HemoStat-Y, PENTAX Co., Tokyo, Japan), which will not provide deep coagulation, is useful for preventing such perforation.

19.4.7 Prevention of bleeding

Bleeding may worsen the visual field, leading to a higher risk of accidents. Inadvertent coagulation may cause coagulation of the blood, which creates an impaired field of vision. Incision and dissection while preventing bleeding is more desirable than hastily attempting hemostasis after bleeding starts. Regular transparent hoods or ST hoods are available for full observation of the submucosal layer. If small vessels, with a diameter of 0.5 mm, are observed, bleeding can be prevented through a careful incision, using spray coagulation (effect 2 and 20 W with needle-type knife, effect 2 and 60 W with Hook knife) (Figure 19.6a–c: see also Plate 19.6). If vessels with a larger diameter are observed, bleeding can be prevented through pre-coagulation, which consists of grasping these vessels with a hemostatic forceps (Figure 19.7a and b: see also Plate 19.7), soft coagulation, and short-time electrization with effect 5 and 40 W, followed by an incision.

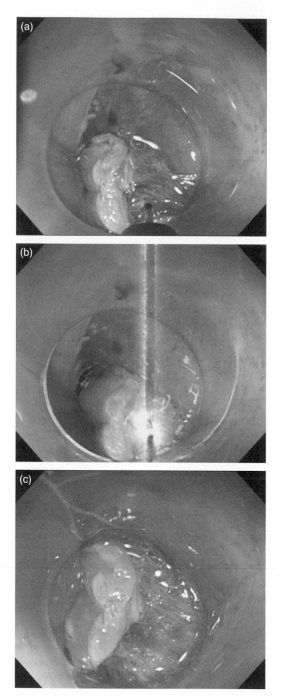

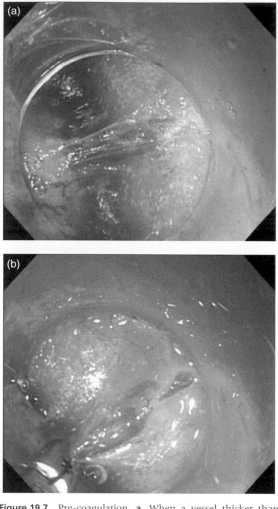

Figure 19.7 Pre-coagulation. **a**. When a vessel thicker than 1 mm or an artery is observed, pre-coagulation becomes a very useful method for prevention of bleeding. Fibers around the vessel are sufficiently dissected to expose the vessel. **b**. The vessel is grasped with a rotatable coagulation forceps. At this time, the direction of the forceps is adjusted to an angle perpendicular to the vessel. Electrification is performed with soft coagulation, effect 5, 40 W. Since damage to the muscularis propria due to electrification may cause delayed perforation, it is important to apply current while slowly pulling the site away from the muscularis propria grasped by the forceps. *(See insert for color representation of this figure.)*

Figure 19.6 Bleeding prevention during dissection. For a small vessel about 0.5 mm in diameter, the slow excision of the vessel by applying current, with the spray mode effect 2, 60 W, allows dissection without bleeding. It is important for prevention of bleeding to slowly incise the vessel. *(See insert for color representation of this figure.)*

19.5 Complications

Complications of esophageal ESD typically include perforations, mediastinal emphysema, subcutaneous emphysema, and aspiration pneumonia. Perforations may cause mediastinal emphysema, which increases the intramediastinal pressure, crushing the esophageal lumen and leading to difficulty in securing the visual field. Severe mediastinal emphysema may be complicated by pneumothorax, leading to shock, so electrocardiography, arterial oxygen saturation, and blood pressure (using automated sphygmomanometer) monitoring should be conducted during ESD, as well as periodic observation for subcutaneous emphysema through palpation.

Since the esophagus has no serous membrane, and the intramediastinal pressure is lower than that of the esophageal lumen, mediastinal emphysema may appear without perforation. Dissection immediately above the proper muscular layer may damage the proper muscular layer during electrization, which may often cause mediastinal emphysema. Therefore, it is important to dissect the submucosal layer, leaving the lowest one-third, without exposure of the proper muscular layer.

Under intubation general anesthesia, the mediastinal pressure is higher than the intraesophageal pressure, enabling prevention of mediastinal emphysema and/or subcutaneous emphysema. Therefore, intubation general anesthesia is preferable for a sub-circumferential or large lesion that is expected to take two or more hours to complete the resection of the lesion.

Recently, carbon dioxide (CO_2) has been used for insufflation during ESD. CO_2 is absorbed faster than air in the body, and it is rapidly expelled through respiration. Use of CO_2 insufflation in ESD procedures not only reduces patient discomfort, but also reduce the risk of severe mediastinal emphysema and pneumothorax in case of perforation.

19.6 Sedation and anesthesia

Commonly, sedation is performed using a combination of narcotic analgesics, including pentazocine, petidine, and butorphanol with benzodiazepine sedatives, including midazolam and diazepam. When the effect is insufficient, sedatives will be added if appropriate.

Propofol is administered to heavy drinkers or in the case of ineffective sedation. As induction of sedation, 1% propofol is slowly administered intravenously at 1–2 mg/kg (0.1–0.2 ml/kg). Since bolus intravenous administration always causes respiratory inhibition,

up to 2 ml is administered intravenously, followed by observation for 30 seconds, and then re-administered. As a maintenance dose, 1% propofol is administered intravenously at 3–5 mg/kg/h (0.3–0.5 mL/kg/h). Propofol has a narrow spectrum of safety and efficacy, so it is preferable for a trained anesthesiologist to administer the drug.

In addition, intubation general anesthesia is preferable for sub-circumferential resections or large lesions with a diameter of 5 cm or more, when the procedure is expected to take two or more hours.

19.7 Results

Oyama performed esophageal ESD in 102 patients, and reported that the rates of *en bloc* resection, local recurrence, perforation, and mediastinal emphysema were 95%, 0%, 0%, and 6%, respectively [28]. Fujishiro performed esophageal ESD in 58 patients and reported that the rates of *en bloc* resection, R0 resection (*en bloc* and negative resection margin), and perforation were 100%, 78%, and 6.9%, respectively. All cases of perforation were treated conservatively, and there were no serious adverse events [29].

19.8 Training

Because the esophagus has a thin proper muscular layer, electrization with a knife contacted to the proper muscular layer may easily cause perforation. Esophageal perforation may lead to mediastinal emphysema, subcutaneous emphysema, and pneumothorax, which may cause shock. Therefore, sufficient training is needed. [30, 31].

The first step in training is learning by observation. It is very important to learn the standard procedure of ESD by visiting a facility staffed by expert endoscopists, or participating in a live demonstration course for ESD. Procedure time allocated for one procedure in most international live demonstration courses of endoscopy is usually only around 15 minutes, which will not enable full understanding of the entire procedure for ESD, while the entire procedure for ESD is shown in ESD live demonstration seminars in Japan, which is very useful in training. DVDs of the procedure are also useful.

The basic technique for ESD is taught with a resected pig esophagus and stomach. Again, instruction by an expert during a hands-on seminar is preferable.

Beginners should start to use ESD for small one-quarter circumferential lesions rather than large ones, and larger lesions should be tried, depending on the skill of the endoscopists.

19.9 Conclusion

The incidence of lymph node metastasis of esophageal cancer relates closely to the depth of invasion, vascular invasion, and tissue type. *En bloc* resection is essential for investigating these parameters. Conventional EMR resects only a limited area in one piece, resulting in a high rate of piecemeal resection. Piecemeal resection may not enable sufficient histopathological examination, and may cause a high local recurrence rate. Although ESD enables us to perform *en bloc* resection of a given area, the procedure is more difficult to acquire than EMR. In this chapter, we have described the basic procedure and treatment results of ESD in the esophagus.

References

1 Hull MJ, Mino-Kenudson M, Nishioka NS, Ban S, Sepehr A, Puricelli W, *et al.* (2006). Endoscopic mucosal resection: an improved diagnostic procedure for early gastroesophageal epithelial neoplasms. *American Journal of Surgical Pathology* **30**(1), 114–8.

2 Farrell JJ, Lauwers GY, Brugge WR (2006). Endoscopic mucosal resection using a cap-fitted endoscope improves tissue resection and pathology interpretation: an animal study. *Gastric Cancer* **9**(1), 3–8.

3 Ahmad NA, Kochman ML, Long WB, Furth EE, Ginsberg GG (2002). Efficacy, safety, and clinical outcomes of endoscopic mucosal resection: a study of 101 cases. *Gastrointestinal Endoscopy* **55**(3), 390–6.

4 Makuuchi H, Yoshida T, Ell C (2004). Four-Step endoscopic esophageal mucosal resection (EEMR) tube method of resection for early esophageal cancer. *Endoscopy* **36**(11), 1013–8.

5 Inoue H, Kawano T, Tani M, Takeshita K, Iwai T (1999). Endoscopic mucosal resection using a cap: techniques for use and preventing perforation. *Canadian Journal of Gastroenterology* **13**(6), 477–80.

6 Tanabe S, Koizumi W, Mitomi H, Kitamura T, Tahara K, Ichikawa J, *et al.* (2004). Usefulness of EMR with an oblique aspiration mucosectomy device compared with strip biopsy in patients with superficial esophageal cancer. *Gastrointestinal Endoscopy* **59**(4), 558–63.

7 May A, Gossner L, Behrens A, Kohnen R, Vieth M, Stolte M, *et al.* (2003). A prospective randomized trial of two different endoscopic resection techniques for early stage cancer of the esophagus. *Gastrointestinal Endoscopy* **58**(2), 167–75.

8 Takeo Y, Yoshida T, Shigemitu T, Yanai H, Hayashi N, Okita K (2001). Endoscopic mucosal resection for early esophageal cancer and esophageal dysplasia. *Hepato-Gastroenterology* **48**(38), 453–7.

9 Nomura T, Boku N, Ohtsu A, Muto M, Matsumoto S, Tajiri H, *et al.* (2000). Recurrence after endoscopic mucosal resection for superficial esophageal cancer. *Endoscopy* **32**(4), 277–80.

10 Monma K, Yoshida M, Yamada Y, Amemiya K, Arakawa F, Ozawa H, *et al.* (2001). Endoscopic Mucosal Resection for Treatment of Superficial Esophageal Cancer – recent clinical results and extended indications. *Clinical Gastroenterology* **16**(12), 1601–8.

11 Ell C, May A, Gossner L, Gunter E, Mayer G, Henrich R, *et al.* (1998). Endoscopic mucosectomy of early adenocarcinoma in patients with Barrett's esophagus. *Gastroenterology* **114**(Suppl. 1), A589.

12 Eguchi T, Nakanishi Y, Shimoda T, Iwasaki M, Igaki H, Tachimori Y, *et al.* (2006). Histopathological criteria for additional treatment after endoscopic mucosal resection for esophageal cancer: analysis of 464 surgically resected cases. *Modern Pathology* **19**(3), 475–80.

13 Endo M, Yoshino K, Kawano T, Nagai K, Inoue H (2000). Clinicopathologic analysis of lymph node metastasis in surgically resected superficial cancer of the thoracic esophagus. *Diseases of the Esophagus* **13**(2), 125–9.

14 Oyama T, Miyata Y, Shimaya S, *et al.* (2002). Lymph nodal metastasis of m3, sm1 esophageal cancer. *Stomach and Intestine* **37**, 72–4.

15 The Japan Esophageal Society (2007). *Guidelines for the treatment of esophageal cancer.*

16 Soetikno RM, Gotoda T, Nakanishi Y, Soehendra N (2003). Endoscopic mucosal resection. *Gastrointestinal Endoscopy* **57**, 567–579.

17 Bollschweiler E, Baldus SE, Schroder W, Prenzel K, Gutschow C, Schneider PM, *et al.* (2006). High rate of lymph-node metastasis in submucosal esophageal squamous-cell carcinomas and adenocarcinomas. *Endoscopy* **38**(2), 149–56.

18 Dunbar KB, Spechler SJ (2012). The risk of lymph-node metastases in patients with high-grade dysplasia or intramucosal carcinoma in Barrett's esophagus: a systematic review. *American Journal of Gastroenterology* **107**(6), 850–62; quiz 63.

19 Yamamoto H, Yube T, Isoda N, Sato Y, Sekine Y, Higashizawa T, *et al.* (1999). A novel method of endoscopic mucosal resection using sodium hyaluronate. *Gastrointestinal Endoscopy* **50**(2), 251–6.

20 Yamamoto H, Yahagi N, Oyama T (2005). Mucosectomy in the colon with endoscopic submucosal dissection. *Endoscopy* **37**(8), 764–8.

21 Gotoda T, Yamamoto H, Soetikno RM (2006). Endoscopic submucosal dissection of early gastric cancer. *Journal of Gastroenterology* **41**(10), 929–42.

22 Oyama T, Kikuchi Y (2002). Aggressive endoscopic mucosal resection in the upper GI tract – Hook knife EMR method. *Minimally Invasive Therapy & Allied Technologies* **11**, 291–5.

23 Yamamoto H, Yahagi N, Oyama T, Gotoda T, Doi T, Hirasaki S, *et al.* (2007). Usefulness and safety of 0.4% sodium hyaluronate solution as a submucosal fluid "cushion" in endoscopic resection for gastric neoplasms: a prospective multicenter trial. *Gastrointestinal Endoscopy* **67**(6), 830–9.

24 Fujishiro M, Yahagi N, Kashimura K, Mizushima Y, Oka M, Enomoto S, *et al.* (2004). Comparison of various submucosal injection solutions for maintaining mucosal elevation during endoscopic mucosal resection. *Endoscopy* **36**(7), 579–83.

25 Yamamoto H, Kawata H, Sunada K, Sasaki A, Nakazawa K, Miyata T, *et al.* (2003). Successful *en-bloc* resection of large superficial tumors in the stomach and colon using sodium hyaluronate and small-caliber-tip transparent hood. *Endoscopy* **35**(8), 690–4.

26 Arantes V, Albuquerque W, Freitas Dias CA, Demas Alvares Cabral MM, Yamamoto H (2013). Standardized endoscopic submucosal tunnel dissection for management of early esophageal tumors (with video). *Gastrointestinal Endoscopy* **78**(6), 946–52.

27 Oyama T, Tomori A, Hotta K, Miyata Y (2006). Hemostasis with hook knife during Endoscopic submucosal dissection. *Digestive Endoscopy* **18**(Suppl. 1), S128–30.

28 Oyama T, Tomori A, Hotta K, Morita S, Kominato K, Tanaka M, *et al.* (2005). Endoscopic submucosal dissection of early esophageal cancer. *Clinical Gastroenterology and Hepatology* **3**(7 Suppl. 1), S67–70.

29 Fujishiro M, Yahagi N, Kakushima N, Kodashima S, Muraki Y, Ono S, *et al.* (2006). Endoscopic submucosal dissection of esophageal squamous cell neoplasms. *Clinical Gastroenterology and Hepatology* **4**(6), 688–94.

30 Choi IJ, Kim CG, Chang HJ, Kim SG, Kook MC, Bae JM (2005). The learning curve for EMR with circumferential mucosal incision in treating intramucosal gastric neoplasm. *Gastrointestinal Endoscopy* **62**(6), 860–5.

31 Gotoda T, Friedland S, Hamanaka H, Soetikno R (2005). A learning curve for advanced endoscopic resection. *Gastrointestinal Endoscopy* **62**(6), 866–7.

CHAPTER 20

Surgical therapy of early esophageal cancer

Toshitaka Hoppo & Blair A. Jobe

Esophageal & Lung Institute, Allegheny Health Network, Pittsburgh, PA, USA

20.1 Introduction

The incidence of esophageal cancer, especially esophageal adenocarcinoma, has been significantly increasing in the United States and Western countries over the last several decades, and overall prognosis remains lethal, with a five-year survival rate of approximately 15%, despite multidisciplinary approaches including surgical therapy and chemoradiation therapy [1, 2]. Only early esophageal cancers have a chance to be cured if complete resection is achieved.

With recent advances in endoscopic surveillance programs and optics technology, patients with high-grade dysplasia (HGD) and/or early esophageal cancer have been encountered more frequently [3, 4]. The advanced endoscopic techniques, with continuously refined endoscopic technology, have made esophageal-preserving endoscopic therapy (e.g., endoscopic ablation, endoscopic resection) a real option to treat highly selected patients with HGD and/or early esophageal cancer, with equivalent oncological outcomes as surgical resection [5, 6].

The guidelines put forth by the American College of Gastroenterology (2008) state that esophagectomy is no longer the necessary treatment response to HGD. However, the optimal management of HGD and/or early esophageal cancer remains controversial [7]. There is no doubt that surgical resection (esophagectomy) plays a major role as an essential component of treatment in patients with any "resectable" esophageal cancer, including early esophageal cancer, without evidence of metastatic disease. In this chapter, we focus on the role of surgical therapy to treat patients with HGD and/or early esophageal cancer in the era of endoscopic therapy.

20.2 "Early" esophageal cancer

In the American Joint Committee on Cancer (AJCC) staging system [8], HGD is termed carcinoma *in situ* (Tis), and is diagnosed when there is marked nuclear pleomorphism (compared to low-grade dysplasia) and a loss of cellular polarity. Invasive adenocarcinoma is diagnosed when neoplastic cells are found crossing the basement membrane of the epithelium. Early adenocarcinomas are defined as tumors that do not extend beyond the submucosal layer of the esophagus, and they are grouped as T1 tumors, which are further subdivided into intramucosal tumors (T1a) and submucosal tumors (T1b). T1a tumors are defined as tumors that are limited to the lamina propria or muscularis mucosae, while T1b tumors are defined as tumors that extend through the muscularis mucosae into the submucosal layer.

Previous studies have demonstrated that there is a significant difference in the risk of lymph node involvement between T1a and T1b tumors, although the differentiation between T1a and T1b does not change the final AJCC staging. The probability of lymph node involvement in patients with T1a tumors is low (<2%) [9–11]. However, the probability of lymph node involvement is increased to $\geq$ 20% once tumors extend into the submucosal layer (T1b) [12, 13]. For the purpose of more accurate staging, the mucosal and submucosal layers have been further subdivided into six planes, and T1 tumors have six different layers of invasion; T1m1 to T1m3 (m1 – limited to the epithelial layer; m2 – invades lamina propria; m3 – invades into but not through muscularis mucosa) and T1sm1 to T1sm3 (even thirds of the submucosa) [14].

Esophageal Cancer and Barrett's Esophagus, Third Edition. Edited by Prateek Sharma, Richard Sampliner and David Ilson.
© 2015 John Wiley & Sons, Ltd. Published 2015 by John Wiley & Sons, Ltd.

20.3 Indication of surgical resection for early esophageal adenocarcinoma

Surgical resection of the esophagus (esophagectomy) has been considered as a standard of care to treat HGD and/or early esophageal cancer, based on previous studies demonstrating that unexpected, concomitant invasive cancer was found in approximately 40% of surgically resected specimens from the patients with a pre-operative diagnosis of only HGD [15, 16]. The recent systematic review involving 1874 patients with HGD and/or T1a cancer who have undergone esophagectomy demonstrated that no metastatic disease was found in patients with HGD, and 1.93% of patients with T1a cancer had positive lymph nodes. This was lower than the rate of mortality and morbidity following esophagectomy [17].

The data suggest that the probability of lymph node involvement in patients with intramucosal adeno-carcinoma (T1a) is unlikely (<2%), but not zero. Surgical resection should be considered for any patients with potential lymph node involvement, although esophagectomy may be unnecessary for the majority of patients with HGD and/or T1a tumors with no risk of lymph node involvement. Therefore, it is crucial to understand the risk factors predicting lymph node involvement or tumor recurrence, in order to determine the optimal treatment options (surgical resection vs. endoscopic therapy). Several macro- and microscopic characteristics have been identified as such risk factors.

Multifocal HGD is a high risk factor for concomitant cancer, ranging from 60–78%, while limited or focal HGD less likely has concomitant cancer or progression to cancer [3, 4, 18, 19]. Submucosal invasion (T1b), squamous-type histology, lymphovascular invasion (L+ or V+), poor differentiation and a nodule > 3 cm in diameter are associated with an increased risk of lymph node involvement [20–23]. Based on these risk factors, surgical resection should be considered for patients with HGD and/or T1a cancer with any of risk factors listed above when patients' functional status is appropriate for surgery with no significant co-morbidities (Table 20.1). Note that the mortality rate of esophagectomy often exceeds 2%, and the balance of benefit between the risk of lymph node involvement associated with endoscopic therapy and the mortality and morbidity associated with esophagectomy should be considered and well discussed with patients, prior to the initiation of any treatment.

Table 20.1 Risk factors for lymph node involvement in patients with HGD and/or early esophageal cancer (T1).

Risk factors for lymph node involvement and/or recurrent cancer	
Macroscopic characteristics	*Microscopic characteristics*
1 Multifocal HGD	1 Submucosal invasion (T1b)
2 Non-ulcerated nodule > 3 cm in diameter	2 Lymphovascular invasion (L+ or V+)
3 Ulcerated lesion > 2 cm in diameter	3 Poor differentiation
	4 Squamous-type histology

Given that patients with T1b cancer have an increased risk of lymph node involvement, esophagectomy has been recommended as the first-line treatment for patients with T1b. A recent review, using the pooled data of 7645 patients with T1b cancer, demonstrated that there was a significant difference in lymph node involvement between T1sm1 and T1sm2/3 (6% vs. 23%/58%, respectively), although the overall rate of lymph node involvement was 37% [24].

Furthermore, the most recent study, involving 66 patients with low-risk T1sm1 (macroscopically polypoid or flat lesion, well-to-moderate differentiation and no lymphovascular invasion), demonstrated that 97% of patients with small nodules (=2 cm) achieved complete remission with endoscopic therapy, and 90% achieved long-term remission without the development of metachronous disease. Although one patient developed lymph node metastasis, no tumor-associated deaths were observed and the estimated five-year survival of this cohort was 84% [25].

These studies have suggested that patients with low-risk T1sm1 could be treated with endoscopic therapy, especially when poor functional status and co-morbid conditions make surgical resection too risky. It is important to note that these results were achieved within high-volume centers of excellence, and have not yet been generalized.

20.4 Strategy of surgical resection for early esophageal adenocarcinoma

The primary goal of surgical treatment for esophageal cancer is to achieve *en bloc* removal of tumor tissue and the accompanying lymphatic tissue with a margin of micro- and macroscopically uninvolved tissue (R0 resection). Esophagectomy is one of the most complicated, invasive surgeries in the upper gastrointestinal tract (GI), and involves subtotal removal of the esophagus, followed by reconstruction using other conduits such as the stomach, small intestine, and colon. Therefore, open esophagectomy requires both laparotomy and thoracotomy. This puts patients in increased risk of developing cardiopulmonary complications, potentially requiring mechanical ventilation and a prolonged stay in an intensive care unit. It has been reported that patients who develop pneumonia following esophageactomy face up to a 20% risk of death [26]. The majority of patients with HGD and/or intramucosal cancer can be cured with adequate surgical therapy. Especially for this population, it is therefore important to minimize post-operative mortality and complications and to maintain good quality of life, while achieving adequate complete resection of the disease.

One of the recent advances in the surgical therapy is the introduction of minimally invasive techniques into esophageal surgeries. Since Dallemange and colleagues described the first laparoscopic fundoplication in 1991 [27], several studies have demonstrated the benefits of minimally invasive surgery for the treatment of esophageal benign diseases, such as gastroesophageal reflux disease [28, 29] and achalasia [30, 31], including equivalent efficacy with decreased recovery times, compared with traditional open surgery. This experience and the techniques have been applied to esophagectomy, expecting the theoretical benefit of less trauma with an easier postoperative recovery, and with fewer wound and cardiopulmonary complications. This expectation has been supported by several, single-center, retrospective studies [32, 33]. Enhanced visualization may improve intra-operative procedure and decrease blood loss, potentially reducing complications.

20.5 Choice of surgical approach and outcomes

Ivor Lewis esophagectomy and transhiatal esophagectomy have been the most commonly performed surgeries for esophageal resection. Both procedures can be performed with a minimally invasive approach. Overall, esophagectomy is associated with a 30–50% risk of significant postoperative morbidity and a greater

than 5% risk of mortality. The mortality following esophagectomy has been shown to be highly dependent on the hospital volume for the procedure [34–36]. Dimick and colleagues have reported that there were significant differences in risk-adjusted mortality between high-volume (>12 esophagectomies per year) and low-volume (<5 esophagectomies per year) hospitals (24.3% vs. 11.4%, $p < 0.001$), and high-volume (>5 esophagectomies per year) and low-volume (<2 esophagectomies per year) surgeons (20.7% vs. 10–7%, $p < 0.001$).

Interestingly, special training as a thoracic surgeon appears to be less important to improve mortality, compared to the individual surgeon and hospital volumes [35]. This is further supported by several large, retrospective studies from high-volume esophageal surgery centers, demonstrating that esophagectomy, regardless of what approach is utilized, could be performed safely, and the mortality rate has been reduced to less than 2% [37, 38]. The surgical approaches are summarized in Table 20.2.

20.5.1 Ivor Lewis esophagectomy

Minimally invasive Ivor Lewis esophageactomy is indicated especially for distal esophageal cancer. It involves laparoscopic creation of the gastric conduit, followed by thoracoscopic removal of the thoracic esophagus and gastric pull-up, with high-intrathoracic anastomosis. Excellent thoracoscopic visualization of intrathoracic structures facilitates the safe mobilization of a thoracic esophagus and precious dissection of mediastinal lymph nodes. The additional advantages of this approach are that the neck is not violated, decreasing the risk of recurrent laryngeal nerve injury and eliminating a neck scar. Furthermore, several studies have demonstrated that the anastomotic leak rate is lower with the intrathoracic anastomosis than with the cervical anastomosis (2–10% vs. 5–30%, respectively).

The recent prospective comparison trial, involving 106 patients who had undergone either open ($n = 53$) or minimally invasive ($n = 53$) Ivor Lewis esophagectomy, demonstrated that blood loss was significantly reduced in minimally invasive approach, and there was no significant difference in outcome measures, including anastomotic leak rates (9% vs. 4%, $p = 0.241$), R0 resection (81% vs. 72%, $p = 0.253$), median lymph node yield (19 vs. 18, $p = 0.584$) and median length of hospital stay (12 vs. 12) between the minimally invasive

Table 20.2 Surgical approaches to HGD and/or early esophageal cancer.

	Ivor Lewis esophagectomy	Transhiatal esophagectomy	Vagal-sparing esophagectomy	Limited resection (Merendino)	3-field esophagectomy
Indication	Distal esophageal cancer	Lower-/middle-third early cancer and/or LSBE	HGD and/or T1a cancer (NO lymph node involvement)	Distal T1a cancer and/or HGD	Upper esophageal cancer or LSBE
Anastomosis	High intrathoracic	Neck	Neck	Jejunum interposition	Neck
Advantage	Lower leak or stricture rate, less recurrent nerve injury	No need for single-lung ventilation or patient repositioning during procedure	Reduction in post-op dumping and diarrhea	Less mortality and morbidity, reduction in post-op reflux symptoms	Removal of longer esophagus, more extensive lymph node dissection
Disadvantage	Leak could be fatal, not for upper-third cancer	Limited view of middle- and upper-third mediastinum (limited lymph node dissection)	No lymph node dissection	Limited lymph node dissection	High mortality/ morbidity, high recurrent nerve injury rate

LSBE – long-segment Barrett's esophagus; HGD – high-grade dysplasia.

and open approaches [39]. It has been noted that the intrathoracic anastomosis is technically more challenging than the cervical anastomosis, and a leak from an intrathoracic anastomosis is likely to prolong the hospital stay and could be fatal. This procedure should not be performed for upper-third esophageal cancers, because of potentially inadequate disease-free proximal margin.

20.5.2 Transhiatal esophagectomy

Transhiatal esophagectomy is indicated for patients who have lower- or middle-third early-stage tumors and/or long-segment Barrett's esophagus. This procedure uses a cervical anastomosis, thereby allowing the surgeons to maximize the proximal margin. However, this procedure is associated with a limited view of the middle- and upper-third of the mediastinum, thus causing technical difficulty in performing the mediastinal dissection and lymphadenectomy. Since the anastomosis is performed in the neck, there may be limitations on the length of the gastric conduit, potentially leading to anastomotic tension and an increased risk of leak, and the potential for recurrent laryngeal nerve injury.

To improve the mediastinal visualization, a laparoscopic transhiatal (inversion) esophagectomy (LIE) has been introduced and modified [40, 41], based on the open inversion technique previously described by Akiyama [42]. LIE has two approaches: retrograde and antegrade LIE [43]. Both approaches use the vein stripper to perform inversion of the esophagus (retrograde LIE – distal to proximal inversion, antegrade

LIE – proximal to distal inversion), thus providing an enhanced mediastinal working space with excellent counter traction between the esophagus and its surrounding mediastinal attachments, and facilitating a safe, thorough dissection of the distal periesophageal lymph nodes. Advantages of the transhiatal approach include no need for single-lung ventilation or patient repositioning during the procedure.

A case control study comparing retrograde LIE ($n = 21$) with open transhiatal esophagectomy ($n = 31$) demonstrated that intraoperative blood loss and the length of hospital stay were significantly reduced in the LIE group, compared with the open group (168 ml vs. 526 ml, $p < 0.001$; 10 days vs. 14 days, $p = 0.03$, respectively), although there was no significant difference in postoperative complications between the groups [44]. A recent review of patients ($n = 36$) with HGD and/or distal esophageal cancers who underwent antegrade LIE demonstrated that LIE was successfully completed in 34 (94%) patients, and R0 resection was achieved in 97% of cases, with a median harvest of 15 lymph nodes. Postoperative complications included anastomotic leak ($n = 11$), Stricture ($n = 18$), atrial arrhythmia ($n = 5$), pneumonia ($n = 4$) and tracheoesophageal fistula ($n = 2$) [45].

20.5.3 Vagal-sparing esophagectomy

Given that division of vagus nerve trunks during esophagectomy can lead to dumping and post-vagotomy diarrhea in up to 30% of patients [38], a vagal-sparing esophagectomy has been modified and adapted to a minimally invasive approach [46, 47]. In this procedure, used for high-grade dysplasia or early stage esophageal adenocarcinoma, the vagal innervation to the pylorus and the remaining GI tract is preserved, although no lymph node dissection is possible [48].

Previous studies have demonstrated that preservation of pyloric innervation leads to a significant reduction in the incidence of dumping and diarrhea and improved morbidity, compared with patients who had a standard esophagectomy with vagotomy [46, 47]. A retrospective review of patients with HGD and/or intramucosal adenocarcinoma who had undergone either a vagal-sparing ($n = 49$), transhital ($n = 39$) or *en bloc* ($n = 21$) esophagectomy, demonstrated that a vagal-sparing esophagectomy was associated with less postoperative morbidity, a shorter hospital stay and fewer late complication, such as weight loss, dumping and diarrhea, compared with transhiatal or *en bloc* esophagectomy. Furthermore, cancer-related five-year survival was 95%, regardless of which approach was used, suggesting that the survival of patients with HGD and/or intramucosal adenocarcinoma was independent of the type of resection and extent of lymph node dissection [49].

Based on this, vagal-sparing esophagectomy can be an option for patients with HGD and/or intramucosal cancer (no risk of lymph node involvement). It should be emphasized that this approach should be considered only when patients do not require lymph node dissection.

20.5.4   Limited resection (Merendino procedure)

For patients with T1a cancers with no risk or low risk of lymph node involvement, limited surgical resection of the gastroesophageal junction with regional lymphadenectomy may be sufficient, with reduced morbidity and mortality. Merendino and colleagues first described the vagal-sparing, transhiatal resection of the distal esophagus with proximal gastrectomy, followed by a reconstruction using the jejunum interposed in an isoperistaltic manner (Merendino procedure) [50]. Previous studies have demonstrated that the Merendino procedure is associated with less morbidity and mortality, equivalent oncologic outcomes, and superior quality of life in patients with T1N0 lesions, compared with radical esophagectomy, while preventing post-operative gastroesophageal reflux [51].

A retrospective study, involving 80 patients who had undergone the Merendino procedure, demonstrated that morbidity and mortality rates were as low as 16% and 0%, respectively, and the median number of harvested lymph nodes was 20. Quality of life assessed at one year following the surgery was comparable to a normal population. It is noted that the vagal-sparing technique may restrict lymphadenectomy and, therefore, the Merendino procedure should be considered for patients with HGD and/or T1a tumors [52].

20.5.5   Three-field esophagectomy

For patients who have the upper thoracic esophageal cancers or long-segment Barrett's esophagus extending to the proximal esophagus, a three-field esophagectomy can be an option, obtaining an adequate proximal resection margin. This approach was first described by McKeown in 1976 [53], and has been adopted to the minimally invasive approach [54]. This approach involves thoracoscopic esophageal mobilization and laparoscopic creation of a gastric conduit, followed by a gastric pull-up with a cervical anastomosis, in conjunction with three-field lymph node dissection.

The advantages of this approach include a longer segment of esophagus to be removed, and more extensive lymphadenectomy to be performed. Furthermore, the higher esophagogastrostomy appears to minimize post-operative gastroesophageal reflux symptoms. Since as many as 40% of patients with squamous cell carcinoma of the esophagus develop isolated cervical nodal metastases following an attempted curative resection [55], esophagectomy with three-field extensive lymph node dissection has been extensively performed by Japanese surgeons, with a potential improvement in five-year survival compared to esophagectomy with two-field lymph node dissection [56, 57]. However, the rate of recurrent nerve injury was reported to be unacceptably high (as many as 50%) and adenocarcinoma, the predominant cell type in Western countries, often develops in the distal esophagus from pre-existing Barrett's esophagus, and less likely spreads to cervical lymph nodes. Therefore, the benefit of three-field esophagectomy for the treatment of adenocarcinoma has not been widely accepted, especially in Western countries.

In a prospective observational study of patients who had undergone three-field esophagectomy ($n = 80$), Altorki and colleagues reported that overall hospital mortality and morbidity rates were 5% and 46%, respectively, and post-operative morbidities included pulmonary complications (26%, $n = 21$), anastomotic leak (11%, $n = 9$) and recurrent laryngeal nerve injury (9%, $n = 7$). No patients with T1a ($n = 8$) had nodal metastases, while 50% of patients with T1b ($n = 4$) had metastasis to cervicothoracic nodes [58]. This study concluded that three-field esophagectomy can be performed, with similar mortality and morbidity, as a less extensive esophagectomy, and the potential benefit of this approach is providing more accurate staging information, as 32% of patients were upstaged. However, the survival benefit of this approach, especially in patients with advanced esophageal cancers, has not been demonstrated in a well-controlled randomized clinical study. The three-field esophagectomy may clearly be too invasive for patients with HGD and/or early distal esophageal cancers.

20.6   Discussion

20.6.1   Surgical therapy vs. endoscopic therapy

The most recent population-based study to evaluate two-year and five-year outcomes in patients with early esophageal cancer (T0 and T1) who had undergone either endoscopic therapy ($n = 430$) or esophagectomy ($n = 1586$), demonstrated that there was no difference in the two-year (endoscopic therapy 10.5% vs. esophagectomy 12.7%; $p = 0.27$) and five-year (endoscopic therapy 36.7% vs. esophagectomy 42.8%; $p = 0.16$) cancer-related mortality between the groups. Interestingly, patients who had undergone endoscopic therapy had a higher five-year mortality rates attributed to non-cancer causes (46.6% vs. 20.6%; p <0.01) [59].

There were two retrospective reviews comparing endoscopic therapy with esophagectomy to treat patients with HGD and/or intramucosal (T1a) esophageal cancer, demonstrating that esophagectomy is associated with significantly higher morbidity (approximately 40%) compared with endoscopic therapy (0%). However, there was no metachronous cancer development after esophagectomy, compared with 6.6–18% in patients treated with endoscopic therapy, although the short- and mid-term survivals were comparable between the groups (94–100% at 3–5 years) [6, 60]. These data suggest that surgical resection for patients with HGD and/or T1a cancer can be one-time definitive therapy with excellent five-year survival, although esophagectomy is associated with higher morbidity, compared with endoscopic therapy.

20.6.2   Transhiatal vs. transthoracic approach

Esophagectomy is often performed on patients with locally advanced esophageal cancer, who are also likely to have significant co-morbidities and/or malnutrition. It is understandable that esophagectomy is associated with significant mortality and morbidity. Specifically for patients with early esophageal cancer (T1), the mortality and morbidity following esophagectomy appear to be slightly improved; the mortality rates range from 0–5% and the overall five-year survival ranges from 63–83%, depending on the extent of lymph node involvement [61–63]. Furthermore, there are no significant differences in oncologic outcomes, with comparable five-year survival in patient with T1 tumors treated by a transhiatal or a transthoracic approach [64, 65].

In a comparative study using a nationwide in-patient sample database involving 17,395 patients with any stage of esophageal cancer, who had undergone either transhiatal (THE) or transthoracic esophagectomy (TTE), overall morbidity was 50.7% and mortality was 8.8%. There was no significant difference in mortality between THE and TTE (8.47% vs. 8.91%, $p = $ ns), with similar complication rates [66]. In another nationwide study, using the Surveillance Epidemiology and End Results (SEER) database comparing THE and TTE, THE was associated with lower operative mortality compared with TTE (6.7 vs. 13.1%, p <0.01), with comparable five-year survival between the groups [67].

These observations were further supported by a meta-analysis which pooled data from 5905 patients (TTE, $n = 3389$; THE, $n = 2516$), demonstrating that TTE appeared to be associated with longer operative time, longer hospital stay, more respiratory complications, wound infections and early postoperative mortality, while THE had a higher risk of anastomotic leak and stricture and recurrent nerve palsy. However, there was no significant difference in five-year survival between the groups [68]. These data suggest that THE may be a better approach to treat HGD and/or early esophageal cancer, although the choice of surgical approach does not appear to affect five-year survival.

20.6.3   Open vs. minimally invasive approach

Minimally invasive esophagectomy (MIE), avoiding laparotomy and thoracotomy, is expected to be less traumatic, with an easier postoperative recovery and fewer wound and cardiopulmonary complications. There are two meta-analyses comparing MIE with open esophagectomy. Verhage and colleagues reported that MIE had less blood loss (312 ml vs. 577 ml), a shorter hospital (14.9 days vs. 19.6 days), and less ICU stay (4.5 days vs. 7.6 days), compared with open esophagectomy. Total complication rates were 60.4% for open esophagectomy and 43.8% for MIE. Pulmonary complications occurred in 22.9% for open and 15.1% for MIE [69]. In another meta-analysis, Biere and colleagues reported that MIE was associated with fewer incidences of major morbidity, pulmonary complications, anastomotic leakage and mortality, shorter length of hospital stay and operating time, and less blood loss [70].

These results are further supported by a recent multicenter, open-label, randomized controlled trial comparing open esophagectomy ($n = 56$) with MIE ($n = 59$), demonstrating that the rate of post-operative pulmonary infection both in-hospital, and within two weeks, was significantly less in the MIE group, compared with the open esophagectomy group (12% vs. 34%, 9% vs. 29%, respectively). However, there was no significant difference in the rate of R0 resection, the number of lymph nodes harvested, or the rate of mortality between the groups. The operative time was significantly longer for MIE (329 min vs. 299 min, $p = 0.002$), although blood loss was significantly less in MIE (200 ml vs. 475 ml, $p < 0.001$) compared with open esophagectomy [71].

20.7   Conclusion

The optimal management of patients with HGD and/or early esophageal cancer remains controversial. The majority of patients with HGD and/or intramucosal (T1a) cancer could be treated with endoscopic therapy; however, surgical resection should be considered for patients with potential lymph node involvement, which could be predicted based on the identified risk factors. Since patients with submucosal (T1b) cancer have an increased risk of lymph node involvement,

esophagectomy is currently considered as the first-line therapy for T1b cancer.

There are several surgical options available, but there has been no well-powered study to demonstrate the optimal surgical approach to treat patients with HGD and/or early esophageal cancer. Esophagectomy with minimally invasive technique appears to be associated with less mortality and morbidity, and shorter length of hospital stay, with oncological outcomes comparable to traditional open esophagectomy. A large, prospective, randomized controlled trial with long-term follow-up is required to evaluate the true benefit of each surgical approach, and to determine the optimal surgical therapy for the management of early esophageal cancer.

References

1 Pohl H, Sirovich B, Welch HG (2010). Esophageal adenocarcinoma incidence: are we reaching the peak? *Cancer Epidemiology, Biomarkers & Prevention* **19**(6), 1468–1470.

2 Siegel R, Naishadham D, Jemal A (2012). Cancer statistics, 2012. *CA: A Cancer Journal for Clinicians* **62**(1), 10–29.

3 Levine DS, Haggitt RC, Blount PL, Rabinovitch PS, Rusch VW, Reid BJ (1993). An endoscopic biopsy protocol can differentiate high-grade dysplasia from early adenocarcinoma in Barrett's esophagus. *Gastroenterology* **105**(1), 40–50.

4 Schnell TG, Sontag SJ, Chejfec G, *et al.* (2001). Long-term nonsurgical management of Barrett's esophagus with high-grade dysplasia. *Gastroenterology* **120**(7), 1607–1619.

5 Pech O, Behrens A, May A, *et al.* (2008). Long-term results and risk factor analysis for recurrence after curative endoscopic therapy in 349 patients with high-grade intraepithelial neoplasia and mucosal adenocarcinoma in Barrett's oesophagus. *Gut* **57**(9), 1200–1206.

6 Pech O, Bollschweiler E, Manner H, Leers J, Ell C, Holscher AH (2011). Comparison between endoscopic and surgical resection of mucosal esophageal adenocarcinoma in Barrett's esophagus at two high-volume centers. *Annals of Surgery* **254**(1), 67–72.

7 Wang KK, Sampliner RE (2008). Updated guidelines 2008 for the diagnosis, surveillance and therapy of Barrett's esophagus. *American Journal of Gastroenterology* **103**(3), 788–797.

8 Edge SB, Compton CC (2010). The American Joint Committee on Cancer: the 7th edition of the AJCC cancer staging manual and the future of TNM. *Annals of Surgical Oncology* **17**(6), 1471–1474.

9 Oh DS, Hagen JA, Chandrasoma PT, *et al.* (2006). Clinical biology and surgical therapy of intramucosal adenocarcinoma of the esophagus. *Journal of the American College of Surgeons* **203**(2), 152–161.

10 Rice TW, Blackstone EH, Adelstein DJ, *et al.* (2003). Role of clinically determined depth of tumor invasion in the treatment of esophageal carcinoma. *Journal of Thoracic and Cardiovascular Surgery* **125**(5), 1091–1102.

11 Rice TW, Zuccaro G, Jr., Adelstein DJ, Rybicki LA, Blackstone EH, Goldblum JR (1998). Esophageal carcinoma: depth of tumor invasion is predictive of regional lymph node status. *Annals of Thoracic Surgery* **65**(3), 787–792.

12 Rice TW (2006). Pro: esophagectomy is the treatment of choice for high-grade dysplasia in Barrett's esophagus. *American Journal of Gastroenterology* **101**(10), 2177–2179.

13 Sepesi B, Watson TJ, Zhou D, *et al.* (2010). Are endoscopic therapies appropriate for superficial submucosal esophageal adenocarcinoma? An analysis of esophagectomy specimens. *Journal of the American College of Surgeons* **210**(4), 418–427.

14 Shimada H, Nabeya Y, Matsubara H, *et al.* (2006). Prediction of lymph node status in patients with superficial esophageal carcinoma: analysis of 160 surgically resected cancers. *American Journal of Surgery* **191**(2), 250–254.

15 Falk GW, Rice TW, Goldblum JR, Richter JE (1999). Jumbo biopsy forceps protocol still misses unsuspected cancer in Barrett's esophagus with high-grade dysplasia. *Gastrointestinal Endoscopy* **49**(2), 170–176.

16 Collard JM (2002). High-grade dysplasia in Barrett's esophagus. The case for esophagectomy. *Chest Surgery Clinics of North America* **12**(1), 77–92.

17 Dunbar KB, Spechler SJ (2012). The risk of lymph-node metastases in patients with high-grade dysplasia or intramucosal carcinoma in Barrett's esophagus: a systematic review. *American Journal of Gastroenterology* **107**(6), 850–862; quiz 863.

18 Buttar NS, Wang KK, Sebo TJ, *et al.* (2001). Extent of high-grade dysplasia in Barrett's esophagus correlates with risk of adenocarcinoma. *Gastroenterology* **120**(7), 1630–1639.

19 Weston AP, Sharma P, Topalovski M, Richards R, Cherian R, Dixon A (2000). Long-term follow-up of Barrett's high-grade dysplasia. *American Journal of Gastroenterology* **95**(8), 1888–1893.

20 Bolton WD, Hofstetter WL, Francis AM, *et al.* (2009). Impact of tumor length on long-term survival of pT1 esophageal adenocarcinoma. *Journal of Thoracic and Cardiovascular Surgery* **138**(4), 831–836.

21 Ell C, May A, Pech O, *et al.* (2007). Curative endoscopic resection of early esophageal adenocarcinomas (Barrett's cancer). *Gastrointestinal Endoscopy* **65**(1), 3–10.

22 Pech O, May A, Gossner L, *et al.* (2007). Curative endoscopic therapy in patients with early esophageal squamous-cell carcinoma or high-grade intraepithelial neoplasia. *Endoscopy* **39**(1), 30–35.

23 Stein HJ, Feith M, Bruecher BL, Naehrig J, Sarbia M, Siewert JR (2005). Early esophageal cancer: pattern of lymphatic spread and prognostic factors for long-term survival after surgical resection. *Annals of Surgery* **242**(4), 566–573; discussion 573–565.

24 Gockel I, Sgourakis G, Lyros O, *et al.* (2011). Risk of lymph node metastasis in submucosal esophageal cancer: a review of surgically resected patients. *Expert Review of Gastroenterology & Hepatology* **5**(3), 371–384.

25 Manner H, Pech O, Heldmann Y, *et al.* (2013). Efficacy, Safety, and Long-term Results of Endoscopic Treatment for Early-stage Adenocarcinoma of the Esophagus With Low-risk sm1 Invasion. *Clinical Gastroenterology and Hepatology* **11**(6), 630–5; quiz e45.

26 Atkins BZ, Shah AS, Hutcheson KA, *et al.* (2004). Reducing hospital morbidity and mortality following esophagectomy. *Annals of Thoracic Surgery* **78**(4), 1170–1176; discussion 1170–1176.

27 Dallemagne B, Weerts JM, Jehaes C, Markiewicz S, Lombard R (1991). Laparoscopic Nissen fundoplication: preliminary report. *Surgical Laparoscopy & Endoscopy* **1**(3), 138–143.

28 Ackroyd R, Watson DI, Majeed AW, Troy G, Treacy PJ, Stoddard CJ (2004). Randomized clinical trial of laparoscopic versus open fundoplication for gastro-oesophageal reflux disease. *British Journal of Surgery* **91**(8), 975–982.

29 Hunter JG, Trus TL, Branum GD, Waring JP, Wood WC (1996). A physiologic approach to laparoscopic fundoplication for gastroesophageal reflux disease. *Annals of Surgery* **223**(6), 673–685; discussion 685–677.

30 Khajanchee YS, Kanneganti S, Leatherwood AE, Hansen PD, Swanstrom LL (2005). Laparoscopic Heller myotomy with Toupet fundoplication: outcomes predictors in 121 consecutive patients. *Archives of Surgery* **140**(9), 827–833; discussion 833–824.

31 Patti MG, Pellegrini CA, Horgan S, *et al.* (1999). Minimally invasive surgery for achalasia: an 8-year experience with 168 patients. *Annals of Surgery* **230**(4), 587–593; discussion 593–584.

32 Luketich JD, Alvelo-Rivera M, Buenaventura PO, *et al.* (2003). Minimally invasive esophagectomy: outcomes in 222 patients. *Annals of Surgery* **238**(4), 486–494; discussion 494–485.

33 Watson DI, Davies N, Jamieson GG (1999). Totally endoscopic Ivor Lewis esophagectomy. *Surgical Endoscopy* **13**(3), 293–297.

34 Birkmeyer JD, Siewers AE, Finlayson EV, *et al.* (2002). Hospital volume and surgical mortality in the United States. *New England Journal of Medicine* **346**(15), 1128–1137.

35 Dimick JB, Goodney PP, Orringer MB, Birkmeyer JD (2005). Specialty training and mortality after esophageal cancer resection. *Annals of Thoracic Surgery* **80**(1), 282–286.

36 Halm EA, Lee C, Chassin MR (2002). Is volume related to outcome in health care? A systematic review and methodologic critique of the literature. *Annals of Internal Medicine* **137**(6), 511–520.

37 Luketich JD, Pennathur A, Awais O, *et al.* (2012). Outcomes after minimally invasive esophagectomy: review of over 1000 patients. *Annals of Surgery* **256**(1), 95–103.

38 Orringer MB, Marshall B, Chang AC, Lee J, Pickens A, Lau CL (2007). Two thousand transhiatal esophagectomies:

39 Noble F, Kelly JJ, Bailey IS, Byrne JP, Underwood TJ (2013). A prospective comparison of totally minimally invasive versus open Ivor Lewis esophagectomy. *Diseases of the Esophagus* **26**(3), 263–271.

40 Jobe BA, Kim CY, Minjarez RC, O'Rourke R, Chang EY, Hunter JG (2006). Simplifying minimally invasive transhiatal esophagectomy with the inversion approach: Lessons learned from the first 20 cases. *Archives of Surgery* **141**(9), 857–865; discussion 865–856.

41 Perry KA, Enestvedt CK, Diggs BS, Jobe BA, Hunter JG (2009). Perioperative outcomes of laparoscopic transhiatal inversion esophagectomy compare favorably with those of combined thoracoscopic-laparoscopic esophagectomy. *Surgical Endoscopy* **23**(9), 2147–2154.

42 Akiyama H, Tsurumaru M, Kawamura T, Ono Y (1982). Esophageal stripping with preservation of the vagus nerve. *International Surgery* **67**(2), 125–128.

43 Hoppo T, Jobe BA, Hunter JG (2011). Minimally invasive esophagectomy: the evolution and technique of minimally invasive surgery for esophageal cancer. *World Journal of Surgery* **35**(7), 1454–1463.

44 Perry KA, Enestvedt CK, Pham T, *et al.* (2009). Comparison of laparoscopic inversion esophagectomy and open transhiatal esophagectomy for high-grade dysplasia and stage I esophageal adenocarcinoma. *Archives of Surgery* **144**(7), 679–684.

45 Perry KA, Funk LM, Muscarella P, Melvin WS (2013). Perioperative outcomes of laparoscopic transhiatal esophagectomy with antegrade esophageal inversion for high-grade dysplasia and invasive esophageal cancer. *Surgery* **154**(4), 901–908.

46 Banki F, Mason RJ, DeMeester SR, *et al.* (2002). Vagal-sparing esophagectomy: a more physiologic alternative. *Annals of Surgery* **236**(3), 324–335; discussion 335–326.

47 Peyre CG, DeMeester TR (2008). Vagal-sparing esophagectomy. *Advances in Surgery* **42**, 109–116.

48 Hermansson M, DeMeester SR (2012). Management of stage 1 esophageal cancer. *Surgical Clinics of North America* **92**(5), 1155–1167.

49 Peyre CG, DeMeester SR, Rizzetto C, *et al.* (2007). Vagal-sparing esophagectomy: the ideal operation for intramucosal adenocarcinoma and barrett with high-grade dysplasia. *Annals of Surgery* **246**(4), 665–671; discussion 671–664.

50 Merendino KA, Dillard DH (1955). The concept of sphincter substitution by an interposed jejunal segment for anatomic and physiologic abnormalities at the esophagogastric junction; with special reference to reflux esophagitis, cardiospasm and esophageal varices. *Annals of Surgery* **142**(3), 486–506.

51 Stein HJ, Feith M, Mueller J, Werner M, Siewert JR (2000). Limited resection for early adenocarcinoma in Barrett's esophagus. *Annals of Surgery* **232**(6), 733–742.

52 Stein HJ, Hutter J, Feith M, von Rahden BH (2007). Limited surgical resection and jejunal interposition for early adenocarcinoma of the distal esophagus. *Seminars in Thoracic and Cardiovascular Surgery* **19**(1), 72–78.

53 McKeown KC (1976). Total three-stage oesophagectomy for cancer of the oesophagus. *British Journal of Surgery* **63**(4), 259–262.

54 Luketich JD, Nguyen NT, Weigel T, Ferson P, Keenan R, Schauer P (1998). Minimally invasive approach to esophagectomy. *Journal of the Society of Laparoendoscopic Surgeons* **2**(3), 243–247.

55 Wright CD, Zeitels SM (2006). Recurrent laryngeal nerve injuries after esophagectomy. *Thoracic Surgery Clinics* **16**(1), 23–33.

56 Wani S, Drahos J, Cook MB, *et al.* (2013). Comparison of endoscopic therapies and surgical resection in patients with early esophageal cancer: a population-based study. *Gastrointestinal Endoscopy* **79**(2), 224–232.

57 Zehetner J, DeMeester SR, Hagen JA, *et al.* (2011). Endoscopic resection and ablation versus esophagectomy for high-grade dysplasia and intramucosal adenocarcinoma. *Journal of Thoracic and Cardiovascular Surgery* **141**(1), 39–47.

58 Pennathur A, Farkas A, Krasinskas AM, *et al.* (2009). Esophagectomy for T1 esophageal cancer: outcomes in 100 patients and implications for endoscopic therapy. *Annals of Thoracic Surgery* **87**(4), 1048–1054; discussion 1054–1045.

59 Reed MF, Tolis G, Jr., Edil BH, *et al.* (2005). Surgical treatment of esophageal high-grade dysplasia. *Annals of Thoracic Surgery* **79**(4), 1110–1115; discussion 1110–1115.

60 Saha AK, Sutton CD, Sue-Ling H, Dexter SP, Sarela AI (2009). Comparison of oncological outcomes after laparoscopic transhiatal and open esophagectomy for T1 esophageal adenocarcinoma. *Surgical Endoscopy* **23**(1), 119–124.

61 Grotenhuis BA, van Heijl M, Zehetner J, *et al.* (2010). Surgical management of submucosal esophageal cancer: extended or regional lymphadenectomy? *Annals of Surgery* **252**(5), 823–830.

62 Ikeguchi M, Maeta M, Kaibara N (2000). Limited operation for patients with T1 esophageal cancer. *Langenbecks Archives of Surgery* **385**(7), 454–458.

63 Connors RC, Reuben BC, Neumayer LA, Bull DA (2007). Comparing outcomes after transthoracic and transhiatal esophagectomy: a 5-year prospective cohort of 17,395 patients. *Journal of the American College of Surgeons* **205**(6), 735–740.

64 Chang AC, Ji H, Birkmeyer NJ, Orringer MB, Birkmeyer JD (2008). Outcomes after transhiatal and transthoracic esophagectomy for cancer. *Annals of Thoracic Surgery* **85**(2), 424–429.

65 Boshier PR, Anderson O, Hanna GB (2011). Transthoracic versus transhiatal esophagectomy for the treatment of esophagogastric cancer: a meta-analysis. *Annals of Surgery* **254**(6), 894–906.

changing trends, lessons learned. *Annals of Surgery* **246**(3), 363–372; discussion 372–364.

66 Verhage RJ, Hazebroek EJ, Boone J, Van Hillegersberg R (2009). Minimally invasive surgery compared to open procedures in esophagectomy for cancer: a systematic review of the literature. *Minerva Chirurgica* **64**(2), 135–146.

67 Biere SS, Cuesta MA, van der Peet DL (2009). Minimally invasive versus open esophagectomy for cancer: a systematic review and meta-analysis. *Minerva Chirurgica* **64**(2), 121–133.

68 Biere SS, van Berge Henegouwen MI, Maas KW, *et al.* (2012). Minimally invasive versus open oesophagectomy for patients with oesophageal cancer: a multicentre, open-label, randomised controlled trial. *Lancet* **379**(9829), 1887–1892.

CHAPTER 21

Chemoprevention: can we prevent esophageal cancer?

Janusz Jankowski & Mary Denholm

Centre for Digestive Diseases, Queen Mary University of London, London, UK

21.1 Overview

Over the past three decades, rates of esophageal cancer have continued to rise worldwide without corresponding improvements in prognosis, which has remained limited to five-year survival rates of 15–25% over the past 20 years [1]. Affecting over 450,000 people worldwide it is the sixth-leading cause of cancer-related mortality [2].

Despite extensive investigation, the cause of this ever-increasing incidence remains unclear, particularly with regard to esophageal adenocarcinoma. While squamous cell carcinoma continues to be the predominant histological subtype worldwide, rates of adenocarcinoma are rising at particularly unprecedented rates, and show no signs of abating.

The proportion of esophageal adenocarcinoma as a percentage of the total number of esophageal cancers among white men in the USA rose from 34% in the mid-1980s, to approximately 60% between 1992–1994, and had exceeded 70% by the year 2000 [3], with an overall 463% increase in esophageal adenocarcinoma between 1975–2004 [1]. This is reflected in other Western countries, with adenocarcinoma now the most prevalent esophageal tumor type in the UK, Australia, Finland, France and the Netherlands.

The importance of BE is related to its position as a precursor lesion of esophageal adenocarcinoma. It has previously been defined as:

> " … an esophagus in which any portion of the normal squamous lining has been replaced by a metaplastic columnar epithelium which is visible macroscopically." [4]

The chance of progression to esophageal adenocarcinoma from BE is approximated at 0.5% per year [5, 6]. With a reported prevalence of 1.6% in the general population and significantly higher in those undergoing endoscopy for reflux-related symptoms, it has proved challenging to produce an efficient and cost-effective surveillance strategy for those individuals with Barrett's.

The change from metaplasia to high-grade dysplasia within BE produces a marked increase in risk of adenocarcinoma. However, here again optimal therapy remains controversial – competing methods include esophagectomy, as well as newer approaches such as endoscopic resection and therapeutic ablation [7]. To date, there are no randomized controlled trials comparing these modalities. Current evidence suggests that, although minimally invasive approaches have better short-term morbidity and mortality profiles, the risk of recurrence following ablation and subsequent required surveillance schedule remains uncertain, and it remains particularly expensive [8, 9].

Given the ongoing controversy regarding optimal management, a focus has developed on possible methods of prevention. Lifestyle measures have been trialed, but interventions such as weight loss and diet alteration have no reliable evidence of efficacy as yet.

Chemoprevention with NSAID medications to prevent malignancy has already been investigated with regards to colorectal cancer, and high-risk populations show good responses to aspirin and other NSAIDs, including sulindac [10]. However, the role of aspirin in halting progress of the metaplastic-dysplastic sequence in BE and esophageal adenocarcinoma is yet to be fully characterized.

Esophageal Cancer and Barrett's Esophagus, Third Edition. Edited by Prateek Sharma, Richard Sampliner and David Ilson.
© 2015 John Wiley & Sons, Ltd. Published 2015 by John Wiley & Sons, Ltd.

Aspirin would be the NSAID of choice for mass chemoprevention, given its established cardioprotective effects and low cost. However, more information is needed regarding the exact populations who would benefit from this strategy, including genetic stratification. The role of aspirin in combination with proton-pump inhibitors (PPIs) also needs to be assessed. In addition, aspirin comes with significant side-effects, including gastrointestinal bleeds, and risk-benefit analyses continue. AspECT (Aspirin and Esomeprazole Chemoprevention Trial) will provide valuable epidemiological and biological information regarding the possible future use of aspirin as a chemopreventive agent in this setting.

21.2   The effect of aspirin on cancer prevention

Aspirin was developed in the 1890s by scientists in the German laboratories of Friederich Bayer and Co [11]. Initially developed as a more tolerable alternative to salicylic acid, its antipyretic and analgesic effects found it widespread use, even before its next revolutionary role in the prevention of cardiovascular events, including myocardial infarction and ischaemic stroke.

21.2.1   Mechanism of action of aspirin

Little was known about aspirin's exact mode of action until 1971, when Vane identified that aspirin and related compounds inhibited the production of prostaglandins [12, 13]. In 1975, Hemler and colleagues isolated the cyclo-oxygenase (COX) enzyme, found in greatest quantities in the endoplasmic reticulum of prostanoid-producing cells. Aspirin produces irreversible inhibition of the COX enzyme via selective acetylation of a serine residue (Ser 530), requiring new enzyme synthesis prior to more prostanoid production [14]. Later work further refined the knowledge of the COX family, and revealed that the COX-1 enzyme is involved in prostaglandin production for physiological processes, including platelet aggregation, protection of gastric mucosa and renal function, while COX-2 is induced by mediators such as mitogens, growth factors and tumor promoters, and is more specifically involved in prostaglandin-mediated inflammatory processes [12, 15].

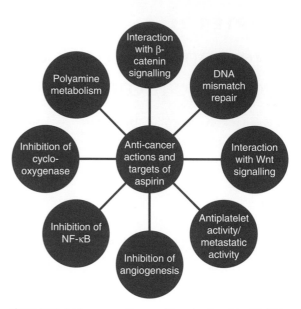

Figure 21.1 Anti-cancer actions and targets of aspirin [25–27].

21.2.2   Biological evidence for the anti-cancer action of aspirin

The first biological indication that aspirin could have anti-cancer properties (Figure 21.1) came from work by Gasic and colleagues, in which thrombocytopaenic rats were shown to have reduced levels of tumor metastases [16, 17]. Further work in rodents showed that raised levels of prostaglandins were present in rat colorectal tumor tissue, providing a viable mechanism for the action of aspirin [18, 19].

Forty years later, less than 1 mmol of aspirin was shown to induce apoptosis in human tumor-cell lines [20].

Some have suggested that the wide variety in the levels of naturally occurring salicylates in herbs and spices found internationally could even explain some regional differences in cancer incidence [21, 22]. Interestingly, serum and urinary concentrations of salicylates in vegetarians are higher than those in omnivores, reaching levels that correspond with those taking low-dose aspirin [23, 24].

21.2.3   Epidemiological evidence for the anti-cancer action of aspirin

Despite evidence from both human and animal experiments, it was from large-scale epidemiological studies monitoring aspirin's longer-term vascular effects that the notion of chemoprevention arose.

To date, the largest evidence base relates to aspirin's role as a putative chemopreventive agent for prevention of colorectal carcinoma (CRC). COX-2 is expressed in up to 90% of CRC and 40% of adenomas, with expression absent in non-malignant adenomas and normal colorectal tissue. The Melbourne Colorectal Cancer Study noted a highly significant 40% reduction in both the risk of colon and rectal cancer in both men and women using regular aspirin, compared with non-users [28, 29]. Both retrospective and prospective studies have shown that use of NSAIDs [30–35] and coxibs [36, 37] can bring about reductions in both size and number of adenomatous colorectal polyps.

The Women's Health Study, Physicians' Health Study, British Doctors Aspirin Trial and UK Transient Ischaemic Attack Aspirin Trial randomized participants to receive aspirin or placebo. The Women's Health Study showed no significant effect on the incidence of any cancer [38]. In the Physicians' Health Study, no protective effect was seen against colorectal cancer in the aspirin group [30]. Both the British Doctors Trial and the UK TIA Aspirin trial showed reduced incidence of colorectal carcinoma in their aspirin groups, with relative risks of 0.82 and 0.70 respectively [39, 40]. Follow-up was 23 years for both trials,. and a maximum chemopreventive effect was demonstrated after 10–19 years, whereas follow-up for the Women's Health Study was 10 years, and for the Physicians' Health Study it was12 years. Recent longer-term follow-up of the Women's Health Study has revealed a latent effect on colorectal cancer [41].

21.2.4 Reliability of the epidemiological evidence base

A meta-analysis by Rothwell and Algra revealed that those groups allocated to aspirin in randomized controlled trials experienced significant 20-year reductions in mortality for colorectal cancer, as well as a significant reduction in mortality from esophageal and other cancers [42].

Elwood et al. concluded that four factors increase the reliability of findings from observational studies in this field [27]. These are, namely, that cancer reduction appears similar in both genders; cessation of prophylaxis results in loss of protection; the effect of aspirin is replicated by other members of the NSAID family;

and, finally, analgesic agents aside from NSAIDs do not reduce cancer incidence [43].

However, even thorough meta-analyses of the subject have been criticized for sub-selecting trials likely to exaggerate the chemopreventive effect of aspirin [44, 45], and until definitive data is available from randomized controlled trials, this debate is likely to continue.

21.3 Risks and adverse effects of aspirin

Aspirin has been described as the "*most widely used drug in the world*" [13]. However, it does not come without serious potential side-effects, and the prevalence of aspirin intolerance is estimated at 5–7% [46], with aspirin resistance rates estimated at 10–25% [47].

21.3.1 Contraindications to aspirin

Aspirin is absolutely contraindicated in patients with active gastric ulceration, a history of recent gastrointestinal or intracranial bleeding, aspirin allergy or intolerance, renal failure, severe liver disease, thrombocytopenia and bleeding. Relative contraindications include concurrent use of anticoagulants or other NSAIDs, and poorly controlled hypertension [48].

21.3.2 Gastrointestinal bleeding and aspirin

The elevated risk of major gastrointestinal bleeding and NSAID-associated ulcers provides the main safety argument against use of aspirin as a chemopreventive agent. Most of the bleeding activity induced by aspirin is as a consequence of COX-1 inhibition, preventing platelet aggregation. Aspirin in high doses, and other non-selective inhibitors of COX-2, inhibit the production of prostaglandin E_2 (an anti-inflammatory prostaglandin) in gastric epithelium, increasing the risk of gastric ulceration and bleeding.

A meta-analysis by Derry and colleagues concluded that the risk of serious gastrointestinal bleeding in an untreated individual is 1% over 10 years, and increases to 2–3% in individuals taking regular aspirin [49]. This effect becomes more pronounced with age. Cuzick and colleagues found that the incidence of NSAID-induced ulcers increases linearly (although not exponentially), being approximately 10% in those under 45 years and

25% in patients over 75 years [50]. There is also considerable evidence that this risk is dose-dependent. A large meta-analysis of 192,036 patients in 31 clinical trials found that moderate (100–200 mg) doses had a relatively high hemorrhagic event rate, compared with low (less than 100 mg) doses [51].

21.3.3 Cranial hemorrhage and aspirin

Cranial hemorrhage in aspirin users is not as common as gastrointestinal hemorrhage, and exact rates can be difficult to estimate as differentiating between hemorrhagic cerebral events and occlusive stroke is sometimes challenging. A 2002 meta-analysis found that the proportional increase in the risk of an extra-cranial bleed was similar for all doses of aspirin less than 325 mg (range of doses from 75–325 mg) [52].

21.3.4 Asthma and aspirin

Aspirin-induced asthma (AIA) is the development of bronchoconstriction in asthmatic individuals following the ingestion of aspirin, symptoms usually developing within three hours. The syndrome may be precipitated by small amounts of aspirin or other NSAIDs, and typically presents with a triad of rhinoconjunctivitis, nasal polyps and asthma [53]; acute symptoms usually occur on a background of chronic, severe, asthma [46]. The COX inhibition produced by aspirin is thought to induce AIA by shifting the arachidonic acid metabolism pathway away from the COX pathway and towards the lipo-oxygenase pathway. In turn, this leads to decreased formation of prostaglandin E_2 and increased production of cysteinyl leukotrienes, leading to asthma-like inflammation in the airways. Management of AIA involves avoidance of aspirin and cross-reacting NSAIDs, and treatment with anti-leukotriene drugs, including monteleukast and zafirlukast. In those in whom aspirin treatment is considered essential, it is possible to conduct a process of aspirin desensitization using incremental doses of aspirin over the course of several days [54].

21.3.5 Significant drug interactions with aspirin

Despite its widespread use, aspirin has some notable interactions with other commonly used medications. Some are antagonistic (for example, the interaction between aspirin and NSAIDs such as ibuprofen), while others are additive (notably the reaction between aspirin and the coumarins including warfarin) (Table 21.1).

Table 21.1 Recognized drug interactions of aspirin (created using information from the British National Formulary.

Drug	Interaction/effects
Analgesics – NSAIDs	Side-effects of aspirin increased by NSAIDs Antiplatelet effects of aspirin possibly reduced by ibuprofen
Anticoagulants	Increased risk of bleeding with coumarins or phenidione due to antiplatelet effect. Aspirin enhances anticoagulant effect of heparins
Antidepressants	Increased risk of bleeding with SSRIs and venlafaxine
Antiepileptics	Effects of phenytoin and valproate enhanced by aspirin
Clopidogrel	Increased risk of bleeding in combination
Corticosteroids	Increased risk of gastrointestinal bleeding and ulceration with aspirin Corticosteroids reduce plasma concentration of salicylate
Cytotoxics	Aspirin reduces excretion of methotrexate
Diuretics	Diuretic effect of spironolactone antagonized Increased risk of toxicity between high-dose aspirin and carbonic anhydrase inhibitors
Iloprost	Increased risk of bleeding
Leukotriene receptor antagonists	Plasma concentrations of zafirlukast increased by aspirin
Metoclopramide	Enhances rate of absorption of aspirin
Drugs acting against hyperuricemia	Aspirin antagonizes probenecid Aspirin antagonizes sulfinpyrazone

21.3.6 Additional side-effects of alternative NSAIDs

The COX-2 selective agents of the coxib family were initially regarded with great promise, due to the hope that they would be less irritant to the gastrointestinal epithelium. However, analysis of large-scale trials revealed that the coxibs markedly increased the risk of cardiovascular events. High doses of the coxibs inhibit prostacyclin production in vascular endothelium without inhibiting thromboxane A_2, thereby predisposing certain groups to an increased risk of thrombotic cardiovascular events [55].

Bertagnolli and colleagues found a 33–45% colorectal polyp reduction in a large-scale randomized clinical trial

[56] of celecoxib for prevention of colorectal adenomas, but a dose-related increase was noted in severe cardiovascular events, including myocardial infarction, stroke and death, leading to early discontinuation of the trial drug [36].

21.4   The role of aspirin in reflux disease

While aspirin continues to emerge as a possible agent to prevent progression to esophageal adenocarcinoma, its role in the pathophysiology of adenocarcinoma's precursor lesions is less clear.

21.4.1   The role of aspirin in benign reflux disease

While the role of aspirin in the later stages of the dysplastic sequence is regarded as favorable, it may, in many instances, exacerbate the symptoms of benign reflux. Individuals with benign reflux make up the vast majority of those with GORD, only a small percentage progressing to Barrett's and OAC.

Work performed in the early 1980s found a significant association between the use of NSAIDs, including aspirin, and benign esophageal stricture [57]. Thrift and colleagues reported a positive association between use of low-dose aspirin and the development of Barrett's. However, the authors surmised that this effect was likely caused by confounding factors because, due to the fact that low-dose aspirin is used most frequently for prevention of cardiovascular disease, this group would likely have independent risk factors for Barrett's, including smoking, obesity and the metabolic syndrome [58].

A key question for future research is whether or not the incidence of gastric irritation and adverse events caused by aspirin could be tempered by the addition of a PPI. The AspECT trial is the world's third largest aspirin trial, and aims to address this question. Work by the Cancer Prevention Network showed that aspirin, combined with esomeprazole, reduced the concentration of prostaglandin E_2 in patients with BE [59].

21.4.2   Aspirin and BE

As previously mentioned, the clinical importance of BE relates mostly to its role as a precursor lesion for esophageal adenocarcinoma. Once BE is identified, endoscopic surveillance is costly and unwelcome for patients, which is why numerous chemopreventive agents have been proposed for this lesion (Box 21.1).

Box 21.1 Potential chemopreventive agents for BE.

Potential chemopreventive agents for BE
Aspirin/NSAIDs
Green tea polyphenol
Berries
Anti-oxidants
PPIs
Statins
Retinoids
Telomerase inhibitors
Curcumin
CDK inhibitors

Source: Jankowski and Hooper, 2011 [60]. Adapted with permission from Elsevier.

Overexpression of the COX-2 enzyme is seen in both adenocarcinoma and Barrett's [61, 62] but, to date, the risk reductions seen with the former and use of NSAIDs have not been as convincing for the precursor lesion. Anderson and colleagues found that the use of both aspirin and no-aspirin NSAIDs significantly reduced the risk of developing BE. In their FINBAR population-based case-control study, patients with Barrett's esophagus were 47% less likely to use aspirin on a regular basis than the control population [63], indicating that NSAIDs could potentially intervene in the inflammatory process prior to the development of metaplasia.

However, a subsequent population-based case-control study in Australia failed to reproduce this association. No inverse association between aspirin and non-aspirin NSAIDS and dysplastic Barrett's was noted. While non-aspirin NSAIDs were associated with a trend towards risk reduction in those patients with nondysplastic Barrett's, this was non-significant when the study's "inflammatory" control group was taken into account (a second control group of patients with acute inflammatory changes seen on endoscopy). Findings were consistent across classifications, according to frequency of GERD symptoms, gender, BMI, smoking history and PPI use [58]. This evidence reflects general trends that have failed to find an association between reduction or improvement of dysplastic lesions and aspirin.

21.4.3   The role of aspirin in progression to esophageal adenocarcinoma

Rat models of the metaplastic-dysplastic sequence have revealed that NSAIDs prevent the development of adenocarcinoma secondary to acid reflux [64, 65], and such studies are supported by the increasing body of epidemiological evidence that aspirin and other NSAIDs may have a chemopreventive role in esophageal cancer.

The anti-cancer properties of aspirin are believed to stem mainly from its inhibition of COX-2, which is known to inhibit apoptosis and promote tumor growth [66]. Similar to colorectal cancer, where COX-2 expression is up-regulated in adenoma tissue, enzyme expression is also seen in increased levels in BE in comparison to normal esophageal tissue [67, 68.]

To date, while the role of aspirin in preventing esophageal adenocarcinoma seems relatively well-supported by animal, human *in vitro* and epidemiological studies, its role in the prevention of progression to esophageal adenocarcinoma in patients with existing Barrett's is less clear. A range of studies have found mixed results, with some indicating that aspirin will slow the rate of progression to Barrett's [69–71], while others found negative results [72].

21.5   Risk-benefits of aspirin

Despite its proven benefits in cardiovascular prevention and its already long history, at the turn of the century, aspirin was still underused in an outpatient setting for those Americans with coronary artery disease [73]. Fear of its adverse effects were cited as a major factor in this. Its risk-benefit profile for chemoprevention is, as yet, not fully clear (Table 21.2).

21.5.1   Groups likely to benefit from aspirin

More work is needed to identify the precise groups who would benefit from chemoprevention with aspirin. It is possible to make some attempt to identify those at increased risk of bleeding on aspirin – risk factors include obesity, increasing age, smoking, *H. pylori* infection, diabetes, hypertension, male sex and excess alcohol consumption [74, 75].

Table 21.2 Summary of the advantages and disadvantages of aspirin as a chemopreventive agent.

Advantages of aspirin chemoprevention	Disadvantages of aspirin chemoprevention
Cheap	Gastrointestinal bleeding
Cost-effective	Intracranial hemorrhage
Acceptable to patients	Alternative bleeding sites e.g. conjunctival, genitourinary
Good alternative to endoscopic surveillance	Asthmatic reactions
20–50% reduced mortality risk from cancer	Drug interactions
Cardioprotective	Intolerance and resistance
Better safety profile than newer medications, could be used alongside PPI to ameliorate bleeding risks	Only certain groups likely to gain maximum benefits

Epidemiological evidence to date does not reveal a difference in effects of aspirin between male and female genders and between those over and under 60 years of age [42].

21.5.2   Dosage required and relationship to adverse effects

In a meta-analysis of six trials examining the use of low-dose aspirin (=325 mg) for secondary prevention of vascular events, aspirin reduced the number of strokes by 20%, the number of myocardial infarctions by 30% and, for the first time, demonstrated a significant decrease in all-cause mortality of 18%. The authors summarized that the number needed to treat in order for aspirin to prevent one death from any cause of mortality was 67 and, in terms of risk, 100 patients required to be treated to detect one non-fatal gastrointestinal bleed [76]. While the optimum dose for chemoprevention of cancer remains uncertain, estimates suggest that there is a strong possibility that doses in the category examined in this meta-analysis would be suitable. Baron and colleagues showed that doses of 81 mg daily produced greater reductions in all colorectal adenomas, including those of an advanced nature, than a higher 325 mg dose [31].

21.5.3   Duration of treatment required

The ever-growing literature on this topic suggests that chemopreventive actions of aspirin are only seen when the drug is used on a long-term basis. Meta-analysis of existing trials has reported that no effect on incidence or mortality is seen in years 0–3, with cancer incidence lower after three years, and mortality lower after five [42, 77].

Evidence from larger RCTs shows late effects, more marked in periods of time longer than ten years, raising further safety questions regarding long-term treatment with aspirin in older populations, given the linear relationship between adverse events and increasing age.

21.5.4 Cost-effectiveness analyses of aspirin as a chemopreventive agent

A Markov model analysis performed by Hur and colleagues indicated that aspirin, alongside recommended endoscopic surveillance strategies, was a cost-effective method for chemoprevention of esophageal cancer. They calculated an acceptable incremental cost-effectiveness ratio (ICER) with a cost per quality-adjusted life year (QALY) of $49,600. However, sensitivity analyses within their work suggested that the strategy did not display sufficient efficacy in more elderly populations. Additionally, they described that effects were not significant when the benefits of aspirin were " … *small or delayed considerably* … " [78].

21.5.5 Clinical recommendations

A meta-analysis and review by Sutcliffe and colleagues examined the use of aspirin in the primary prevention of CVD or cancer. They found a 6% reduction in all-cause mortality with aspirin, accompanied by a 10% reduction in major cardiovascular events. Pooled odds-ratios for the development of cancer ranged between 0.76–0.93. Absolute effects per 100,000 years of patient follow-up revealed a possible avoidance of 34 deaths from colorectal cancer. The authors concluded that the risk-benefit balance with aspirin was particularly fine, and that all absolute effects in relation to cancer prevention were small in comparison to the high disease burden. The report concluded that the use of aspirin as a chemopreventive agent for both cardiovascular disease and cancer should be a decision made between " … *each individual doctor and patient.*" [79]

In terms of patient choice compared with current standards, British patients have expressed a strong preference for chemoprevention over endoscopic surveillance, a preference mirrored by clinicians [80]. Further work with colorectal cancer also found that patients would prefer to take aspirin over selective COX-2 antagonists, including celecoxib, principally due to the different cardiovascular profiles of the two drugs [81].

21.5.6 International consensus of opinion on risk-benefit

A summary in 2009 concluded that "*….age-specific changes in the risk-benefit ratio of prophylactic treatment with aspirin to prevent premalignant lesions or cancer remain unclear.*" [10] Current re-assessment of the topic by the same group is at present considering a new consensus that " … *use of aspirin at a dose between 75–325 mg/day for at least five years appears to have a favorable benefit-harm ratio for most men and women aged between 50–65 years*" (Cuzick, 2013 – unpublished).

21.6 AspECT trial

In order to better investigate the possible role of aspirin in chemoprevention, a large Phase III randomized trial is underway. The Aspirin and Esomeprazole Chemoprevention Trial (AspECT) aims to ascertain whether aspirin reduces the rates of all causes of mortality, or conversion rate from Barrett's metaplasia to adenocarcinoma, or high grade dysplasia. A total of 2513 patients have been recruited and randomized to receive one of four regimens – symptomatic esomeprazole only (20 mg); high-dose esomeprazole (80 mg); and each of these respectively, combined with 300 mg aspirin. Thus, the trial will also provide more information regarding the role of high-dose PPI in preventing conversion and its effects on mortality. These primary outcome measures sit alongside secondary objectives, such as assessing whether further clinical or biological risk factors for progression to carcinoma can be identified, and assessing gender difference in outcomes. It will also add to the growing knowledge base surrounding the role of aspirin in preventing colorectal cancer, and its effects in relation to cardiac deaths.

Furthermore, the trial will provide a valuable resource in identifying genetic markers of progression towards adenocarcinoma, as a unique tissue bank will have been established containing full endoscopic, histological, physiological and pharmacological details.

This genetic information can then be used alongside other large genetic studies, such as the EAGLE (Esophageal Adenocarcinoma Genetic LinkagE) consortium, which aims to achieve genome-wide identification of inherited risk factors. Such information will prove highly valuable to ongoing research, as several recent surveys have shown a wide disparity in the sampling and histology practices internationally, and lack of adherence to international guidelines.

Presently, no specific trends have been demonstrated between the four treatment groups but interim analysis has shown a low-level rate of major side effects, and approximately 75% of patients have tolerated the medications well. Investigation continues, with the final data collection relating to primary outcome measures due in 2019.

References

1 Pennathur A, Gibson MK, Jobe BA, Luketich JD (2013). Oesophageal carcinoma. *Lancet* **381**(9864), 400–12.

2 Jemal A, Siegel R, Ward E, Hao Y, Xu J, Thun MJ (2009). Cancer statistics, 2009. *CA: A Cancer Journal for Clinicians* **59**(4), 225–49.

3 Blot WJ, McLaughlin JK, Fraumeni Jr JF (2006). Oesophageal cancer. In: Fraumeni JF, Schottenfeld D (eds). *Cancer epidemiology and prevention*, p. 1392. New York: Oxford University Press.

4 Bampton PA, Schloithe A, Bull J, Fraser RJ, Padbury RT, Watson DI (2006). Improving surveillance for Barrett's oesophagus. *BMJ* **332**(7553), 1320–3.

5 Voutilainen M, Sipponen P, Mecklin JP, Juhola M, Färkkilä M (2000). Gastroesophageal reflux disease: prevalence, clinical, endoscopic and histopathological findings in 1,128 consecutive patients referred for endoscopy due to dyspeptic and reflux symptoms. *Digestion* **61**(1), 6–13.

6 Ronkainen J, Aro P, Storskrubb T, Johansson SE, Lind T, Bolling–Sternevald E, *et al.* (2005). Prevalence of Barrett's esophagus in the general population: an endoscopic study. *Gastroenterology* **129**(6), 1825–31.

7 Pennathur A, Luketich JD (2008). Resection for esophageal cancer: strategies for optimal management. *Annals of Thoracic Surgery* **85**(2), S751–6.

8 Bennett C, Green S, Decaestecker J, Almond M, Barr H, Bhandari P, *et al.* (2012). Surgery versus radical endotherapies for early cancer and high-grade dysplasia in Barrett's oesophagus. *Cochrane Database of Systematic Reviews* **11**, CD007334.

9 Green S, Tawil A, Barr H, Bennett C, Bhandari P, Decaestecker J, *et al.* (2009). Surgery versus radical endotherapies for early cancer and high grade dysplasia in Barrett's oesophagus. *Cochrane Database of Systematic Reviews* **2**, CD007334.

10 Cuzick J, Otto F, Baron JA, Brown PH, Burn J, Greenwald P, *et al.* (2009). Aspirin and non-steroidal anti-inflammatory

drugs for cancer prevention: an international consensus statement. *Lancet Oncology* **10**(5), 501–7.

11 Sneader W (2000). The discovery of aspirin: a reappraisal. *BMJ* **321**(7276), 1591–4.

12 Vane JR, Botting RM (1998). Anti-inflammatory drugs and their mechanism of action. *Inflammation Research* **47**(Suppl 2), S78–87.

13 Vane JR, Botting RM (2003). The mechanism of action of aspirin. *Thrombosis Research* **110**(5–6), 255–8.

14 Botting RM (2006). Inhibitors of cyclooxygenases: mechanisms, selectivity and uses. *Journal of Physiology and Pharmacology* **57**(Suppl. 5), 113–24.

15 Xie WL, Chipman JG, Robertson DL, Erikson RL, Simmons DL (1991). Expression of a mitogen-responsive gene encoding prostaglandin synthase is regulated by mRNA splicing. *Proceedings of the National Academy of Sciences of the United States of America* **88**(7), 2692–6.

16 Gasic GJ, Gasic TB, Murphy S (1972). Anti-metastatic effect of aspirin. *Lancet* **2**(7783), 932–3.

17 Gasic GJ, Gasic TB, Galanti N, Johnson T, Murphy S (1973). Platelet-tumor-cell interactions in mice. The role of platelets in the spread of malignant disease. *International Journal of Cancer* **11**(3), 704–18.

18 Jaffe BM (1974). Prostaglandins and cancer: an update. *Prostaglandins* **6**(6), 453–61.

19 Bennett A, Del Tacca M (1975). Proceedings: Prostaglandins in human colonic carcinoma. *Gut* **16**(5), 409.

20 Mahdi JG, Alkarrawi MA, Mahdi AJ, Bowen ID, Humam D (2006). Calcium salicylate-mediated apoptosis in human HT-1080 fibrosarcoma cells. *Cell Proliferation* **39**(4), 249–60.

21 Swain AR, Dutton SP, Truswell AS (1985). Salicylates in foods. *Journal of the American Dietetic Association* **85**(8), 950–60.

22 Paterson JR, Srivastava R, Baxter GJ, Graham AB, Lawrence JR (2006). Salicylic acid content of spices and its implications. *Journal of Agricultural and Food Chemistry* **54**(8), 2891–6.

23 Blacklock CJ, Lawrence JR, Wiles D, Malcolm EA, Gibson IH, Kelly CJ, *et al.* (2001). Salicylic acid in the serum of subjects not taking aspirin. Comparison of salicylic acid concentrations in the serum of vegetarians, non-vegetarians, and patients taking low dose aspirin. *Journal of Clinical Pathology* **54**(7), 553–5.

24 Lawrence JR, Peter R, Baxter GJ, Robson J, Graham AB, Paterson JR (2003). Urinary excretion of salicyluric and salicylic acids by non-vegetarians, vegetarians, and patients taking low dose aspirin. *Journal of Clinical Pathology* **56**(9), 651–3.

25 Stark LA, Reid K, Sansom OJ, Din FV, Guichard S, Mayer I, *et al.* (2007). Aspirin activates the NF-kappaB signalling pathway and induces apoptosis in intestinal neoplasia in two in vivo models of human colorectal cancer. *Carcinogenesis* **28**(5), 968–76.

26 Jankowski JA, Anderson M (2004). Review article: management of oesophageal adenocarcinoma – control of

acid, bile and inflammation in intervention strategies for Barrett's oesophagus. *Alimentary Pharmacology & Therapeutics* **20**(Suppl. 5), 71–80; discussion 95–6.

27 Elwood PC, Gallagher AM, Duthie GG, Mur LA, Morgan G (2009). Aspirin, salicylates, and cancer. *Lancet* **373**(9671), 1301–9.

28 Kune GA, Kune S, Watson LF (1988). Colorectal cancer risk, chronic illnesses, operations, and medications: case control results from the Melbourne Colorectal Cancer Study. *Cancer Research* **48**(15), 4399–404.

29 Kune GA (2010). The Melbourne Colorectal Cancer Study: reflections on a 30-year experience. *Medical Journal of Australia* **193**(11–12), 648–52.

30 Gann PH, Manson JE, Glynn RJ, Buring JE, Hennekens CH (1993). Low-dose aspirin and incidence of colorectal tumors in a randomized trial. *Journal of the National Cancer Institute* **85**(15), 1220–4.

31 Baron JA, Cole BF, Sandler RS, Haile RW, Ahnen D, Bresalier R, *et al.* (2003). A randomized trial of aspirin to prevent colorectal adenomas. *New England Journal of Medicine* **348**(10), 891–9.

32 Benamouzig R, Deyra J, Martin A, Girard B, Jullian E, Piednoir B, *et al.* (2003). Daily soluble aspirin and prevention of colorectal adenoma recurrence: one-year results of the APACC trial. *Gastroenterology* **125**(2), 328–36.

33 Chan AT, Giovannucci EL, Schernhammer ES, Colditz GA, Hunter DJ, Willett WC, *et al.* (2004). A prospective study of aspirin use and the risk for colorectal adenoma. *Annals of Internal Medicine* **140**(3), 157–66.

34 García Rodríguez LA, Huerta-Alvarez C (2000). Reduced incidence of colorectal adenoma among long-term users of nonsteroidal antiinflammatory drugs: a pooled analysis of published studies and a new population-based study. *Epidemiology* **11**(4), 376–81.

35 Giovannucci E, Rimm EB, Stampfer MJ, Colditz GA, Ascherio A, Willett WC (1994). Aspirin use and the risk for colorectal cancer and adenoma in male health professionals. *Annals of Internal Medicine* **121**(4), 241–6.

36 Solomon SD, McMurray JJ, Pfeffer MA, Wittes J, Fowler R, Finn P, *et al.* (2005). Cardiovascular risk associated with celecoxib in a clinical trial for colorectal adenoma prevention. *New England Journal of Medicine* **352**(11), 1071–80.

37 Baron JA, Sandler RS, Bresalier RS, Quan H, Riddell R, Lanas A, *et al.* (2006). A randomized trial of rofecoxib for the chemoprevention of colorectal adenomas. *Gastroenterology* **131**(6), 1674–82.

38 Cook NR LI, Gaziano JM *et al.* (2005). Low-dose aspirin in the primary prevention of cancer: the Women's Health Study: a randomized controlled trial. *JAMA* **294**, 47–55.

39 Peto R, Gray R, Collins R, Wheatley K, Hennekens C, Jamrozik K, *et al.* (1988). Randomized trial of prophylactic daily aspirin in British male doctors. *British Medical Journal (Clinical Research Ed.)* **296**(6618), 313–6.

40 Farrell B, Godwin J, Richards S, Warlow C (1991). The United Kingdom transient ischaemic attack (UK-TIA) aspirin trial: final results. *Journal of Neurology, Neurosurgery & Psychiatry* **54**(12), 1044–54.

41 Cook NR, Lee IM, Zhang SM, Moorthy MV, Buring JE (2013). Alternate-day, low-dose aspirin and cancer risk: long-term observational follow-up of a randomized trial. *Annals of Internal Medicine* **159**(2), 77–85.

42 Algra AM, Rothwell PM (2012). Effects of regular aspirin on long-term cancer incidence and metastasis: a systematic comparison of evidence from observational studies versus randomized trials. *Lancet Oncology* **13**(5), 518–27.

43 Friis S, Nielsen GL, Mellemkjaer L, McLaughlin JK, Thulstrup AM, Blot WJ, *et al.* (2002). Cancer risk in persons receiving prescriptions for paracetamol: a Danish cohort study. *International Journal of Cancer* **97**(1), 96–101.

44 Rothwell PM, Wilson M, Elwin CE, Norrving B, Algra A, Warlow CP, *et al.* (2010). Long-term effect of aspirin on colorectal cancer incidence and mortality: 20-year follow-up of five randomized trials. *Lancet* **376**(9754), 1741–50.

45 Moayyedi P, Jankowski JA (2010). Does long term aspirin prevent cancer? *BMJ* **341**, c7326.

46 Babu KS, Salvi SS (2000). Aspirin and asthma. *Chest* **118**(5), 1470–6.

47 Hankey GJ, Eikelboom JW (2004). Aspirin resistance. *BMJ* **328**(7438), 477–9.

48 Miser WF (2011). Appropriate aspirin use for primary prevention of cardiovascular disease. *American Family Physician* **83**(12), 1380–6.

49 Derry S, Loke YK (2000). Risk of gastrointestinal hemorrhage with long term use of aspirin: meta-analysis. *BMJ* **321**(7270), 1183–7.

50 Cuzick J, Thorat MA, Bosetti C, Brown PH, Burn J, Cook NR, Ford LG, Jacobs EJ, Jankowski JA, La Vecchia C, Law M, Meyskens F, Rothwell PM, Senn HJ, Umar A (2015). Estimates of benefits and harms of prophylactic use of aspirin in the general population *Annals of Oncology* **26**(1), 47–57.

51 Serebruany VL, Steinhubl SR, Berger PB, Malinin AI, Baggish JS, Bhatt DL, *et al.* (2005). Analysis of risk of bleeding complications after different doses of aspirin in 192,036 patients enrolled in 31 randomized controlled trials. *American Journal of Cardiology* **95**(10), 1218–22.

52 Collaboration AT (2002). Collaborative meta-analysis of randomized trials of antiplatelet therapy for prevention of death, myocardial infarction, and stroke in high risk patients. *BMJ* **324**, 71–86.

53 Samter M, Beers RF (1968). Intolerance to aspirin. Clinical studies and consideration of its pathogenesis. *Annals of Internal Medicine* **68**(5), 975–83.

54 Pleskow WW, Stevenson DD, Mathison DA, Simon RA, Schatz M, Zeiger RS (1982). Aspirin desensitization in aspirin-sensitive asthmatic patients: clinical manifestations and characterization of the refractory period. *Journal of Allergy and Clinical Immunology* **69**(1 Pt 1), 11–9.

55 Fitzgerald GA (2004). Coxibs and cardiovascular disease. *New England Journal of Medicine* **351**(17), 1709–11.

56 Bertagnolli MM, Eagle CJ, Zauber AG, Redston M, Solomon SD, Kim K, *et al.* (2006). Celecoxib for the prevention of sporadic colorectal adenomas. *New England Journal of Medicine* **355**(9), 873–84.

57 Wilkins WE, Ridley MG, Pozniak AL (1984). Benign stricture of the oesophagus: role of non-steroidal anti-inflammatory drugs. *Gut* **25**(5), 478–80.

58 Thrift AP, Pandeya N, Smith KJ, Green AC, Webb PM, Whiteman DC (2011). The use of nonsteroidal anti-inflammatory drugs and the risk of Barrett's oesophagus. *Alimentary Pharmacology & Therapeutics* **34**(10), 1235–44.

59 Falk GW, Buttar NS, Foster NR, Ziegler KL, Demars CJ, Romero Y, *et al.* (2012). A combination of esomeprazole and aspirin reduces tissue concentrations of prostaglandin E(2) in patients with Barrett's esophagus. *Gastroenterology* **143**(4), 917–26.e1.

60 Jankowski JA, Hooper PA (2011). Chemoprevention in Barrett's esophagus: A pill a day? *Gastrointestinal Endoscopy Clinics of North America* **21**, 155–70.

61 Lagorce C, Paraf F, Vidaud D, Couvelard A, Wendum D, Martin A, *et al.* (2003). Cyclooxygenase-2 is expressed frequently and early in Barrett's oesophagus and associated adenocarcinoma. *Histopathology* **42**(5), 457–65.

62 Shirvani VN, Ouatu-Lascar R, Kaur BS, Omary MB, Triadafilopoulos G (2000). Cyclooxygenase 2 expression in Barrett's esophagus and adenocarcinoma: *Ex vivo* induction by bile salts and acid exposure. *Gastroenterology* **118**(3), 487–96.

63 Anderson LA, Johnston BT, Watson RG, Murphy SJ, Ferguson HR, Comber H, *et al.* (2006). Nonsteroidal anti-inflammatory drugs and the esophageal inflammation-metaplasia-adenocarcinoma sequence. *Cancer Research* **66**(9), 4975–82.

64 Buttar NS WK, Leontovich O *et al.* (2002). Chemoprevention of esophageal adenocarcinoma by COX-2 inhibitors in an animal model of Barrett's esophagus. *Gastroenterology* **122**, 1101–12.

65 Oyama K FT, Ninomiya I *et al.* (2005). A COX-2 inhibitor prevents the esophageal inflammation-metaplasia-adenocarcinoma sequence in rats *Carcinogenesis* **26**(565–570).

66 Hussain SS SI, Tamawski AS (2002). NSAID inhibition of GI cancer growth: clinical implications and molecular mechanisms of action. *American Journal of Gastroenterology* **97**(542–553).

67 Kandil HM TG, Smalley W *et al.* (2001). Cyclooxygenase-2 expression in Barrett's esophagus. *Digestive Diseases and Sciences* **46**, 785–789.

68 Morris CD, Armstrong GR, Bigley G, Green H, Attwood SE (2001). Cyclooxygenase-2 expression in the Barrett's metaplasia-dysplasia-adenocarcinoma sequence. *American Journal of Gastroenterology* **96**, 990–996.

69 Vaughan TL, Dong LM, Blount PL, Ayub K, Odze RD, Sanchez CA, *et al.* (2005). Non-steroidal anti-inflammatory drugs and risk of neoplastic progression in Barrett's oesophagus: a prospective study. *Lancet Oncology* **6**(12), 945–52.

70 Nguyen DM, Richardson P, El-Serag HB (2010). Medications (NSAIDs, statins, proton pump inhibitors) and the risk of esophageal adenocarcinoma in patients with Barrett's esophagus. *Gastroenterology* **138**(7), 2260–6.

71 Galipeau PC, Li X, Blount PL, Maley CC, Sanchez CA, Odze RD, *et al.* (2007). NSAIDs modulate CDKN2A, TP53, and DNA content risk for progression to esophageal adenocarcinoma. *PLoS Medicine* **4**(2), e67.

72 Gatenby PA, Ramus JR, Caygill CP, Winslet MC, Watson A (2009). Aspirin is not chemoprotective for Barrett's adenocarcinoma of the oesophagus in multicentre cohort. *European Journal of Cancer Prevention* **18**(5), 381–4.

73 Stafford RS, Radley DC (2003). The underutilization of cardiac medications of proven benefit, 1990 to 2002. *Journal of the American College of Cardiology* **41**(1), 56–61.

74 Baigent C, Blackwell L, Collins R, Emberson J, Godwin J, Peto R, *et al.* (2009). Aspirin in the primary and secondary prevention of vascular disease: collaborative meta-analysis of individual participant data from randomized trials. *Lancet* **373**(9678), 1849–60.

75 Kaufman DW, Kelly JP, Wiholm BE, Laszlo A, Sheehan JE, Koff RS, *et al.* (1999). The risk of acute major upper gastrointestinal bleeding among users of aspirin and ibuprofen at various levels of alcohol consumption. *American Journal of Gastroenterology* **94**(11), 3189–96.

76 Weisman SM, Graham DY (2002). Evaluation of the benefits and risks of low-dose aspirin in the secondary prevention of cardiovascular and cerebrovascular events. *Archives of Internal Medicine* **162**(19), 2197–202.

77 Rothwell PM, Fowkes FG, Belch JF, Ogawa H, Warlow CP, Meade TW (2011). Effect of daily aspirin on long-term risk of death due to cancer: analysis of individual patient data from randomized trials. *Lancet* **377**(9759), 31–41.

78 Hur C, Simon LS, Gazelle GS (2004). The cost-effectiveness of aspirin versus cyclooxygenase-2-selective inhibitors for colorectal carcinoma chemoprevention in healthy individuals. *Cancer* **101**(1), 189–97.

79 Sutcliffe P, Connock M, Gurung T, Freeman K, Johnson S, Kandala NB, *et al.* (2013). Aspirin for prophylactic use in the primary prevention of cardiovascular disease and cancer: a systematic review and overview of reviews. *Health Technology Assessment* **17**(43), 1–253.

80 Jankowski J, Moayyedi P (2004). Re: Cost-effectiveness of aspirin chemoprevention for Barrett's esophagus. *Journal of the National Cancer Institute* **96**(11), 885–7; author reply 7.

81 Hur C, Broughton DE, Kong CY, Ozanne EM, Richards EB, Truong T, *et al.* (2009). Patient preferences for the chemoprevention of colorectal cancer. *Digestive Diseases and Sciences* **54**(10), 2207–14.

CHAPTER 22

Selection of patients for cancer prevention and eradication

Aaron J. Small & Gary W. Falk

Division of Gastroenterology, University of Pennsylvania Perelman School of Medicine, Philadelphia, PA, USA

22.1   Introduction

The entire paradigm of Barrett's esophagus therapy has changed in recent years due to rapid advances in effective endoscopic ablative therapies. However, the decision to eradicate Barrett's esophagus is complex and involves a number of factors such as patient character- istics, grade of dysplasia, characteristics of the lesion in question, local expertise, and potential predictors of response to therapy (Table 22.1). Given the continued poor survival of advanced esophageal adenocarcinoma, it is essential to consider each of these variables in order to develop the best approach for each patient. This chapter will review the various factors to consider prior to embarking on endoscopic eradication of Barrett's esophagus.

22.2   Patient factors

A variety of patient related factors enter into decision-making for ablation. These include: age and, hence, life expectancy; co-morbidities; cancer fears; and an understanding of the risks; as well as the benefits, of ablation therapy. Additional patient factors include the need for compliance with rigorous endoscopic follow-up, including touch-up ablation, as well as a clear understanding of the evolving failure rate data for ablation therapy. Patients also should be counseled that the esophageal milieu that led to the development of Barrett's esophagus and esophageal cancer is still present after any endoscopic ablative therapy. Finally, patients need to clearly understand that ablative therapies represent an ongoing treatment, not a guarantee of a cure of Barrett's esophagus and its complications. As such, patients should also be aware of the pros and cons of other approaches to the disease, including surgery or continued surveillance.

22.2.1   Pre-procedural risk assessment

Many patients with intraepithelial neoplasia are elderly, with multiple co-morbidities. As such, careful risk assessment may help identify individuals who are poor surgical candidates, thereby making the choice for endoscopic ablation for intraepithelial neoplasia much simpler. A variety of studies have identified patient fac- tors that may predict complications and mortality from esophagectomy. These factors include: increasing age; co-morbidities (i.e. pulmonary hypertension, heart fail- ure, liver disease, chronic lung disease, anemia, diabetes, history of cerebro-vascular accident/transient ischemic attack or myocardial infarction, renal disease); smoking; and pre-operative chemo-radiation [1–4]. In a similar manner, older patients with multiple co-morbidities and, consequently, a shorter life expectancy, may be considered higher risk when deciding between endo- scopic therapy, continued surveillance, or simply doing nothing, compared with younger, healthier patients [5].

22.2.2   Patient perception of cancer risk and ablative therapy

Next, the patient's perceptions of cancer risk and com- mitment to therapy must be considered. It is currently unknown how perception of cancer risk enters into the patient's decision-making for surgical versus endoscopic approaches to dysplasia and early cancer. Intuitively,

Esophageal Cancer and Barrett's Esophagus, Third Edition. Edited by Prateek Sharma, Richard Sampliner and David Ilson.
© 2015 John Wiley & Sons, Ltd. Published 2015 by John Wiley & Sons, Ltd.

Table 22.1 Selection of patients for eradication: variables to consider.

Patient	Age
	Co-morbidities
	Compliance with endoscopic surveillance
	Cancer fears
Lesion	Length
	Nodularity
	Dysplasia
	Grade
	Extent
Local quality measures	Endoscopist
	Pathologist

one would believe that in a patient who is cancer "phobic," surgery would be the preferred approach, given its potential for definitive cure, whereas, for those less concerned about the development of cancer, an endoscopic approach would be more appealing.

Unfortunately, we do not know how these perceptions enter into a patient's decision-making process. We do know that choice of treatment may be influenced by whether the initial evaluation is performed by a gastroenterologist or a surgeon [6]. We also know that patient perception of cancer risk in Barrett's esophagus surveillance programs is not accurate. Shaheen *et al.* found that 68% of such patients overestimated their one-year risk of cancer, and 38% overestimated their lifetime risk [7]. On the other hand, work from the Netherlands found just the opposite: 69% of patients underestimated their risk of developing adenocarcinoma [8]. Thus, it appears that patients really do not have a good estimate of their own cancer risk.

Nonetheless, patients who undergo ablative therapy report an improved health-related quality of life that is likely secondary to a perceived reduction in cancer risk [9]. The impact of carrying a "premalignant" condition for a lethal disease and instituting "watchful waiting" can incur high psychological stress, despite the actual low risk of malignant potential in most patients.

Patients who decide to undergo endoscopic therapy should have a clear understanding of the risks and benefits of this approach. While the benefits of a minimally invasive approach to eradicate early neoplasia

are evident, ablation is not failure-proof. The ability to achieve a durable remission depends on many factors, including optimization of technique, potent acid suppression, and other predictors discussed later in this chapter. Eradication therapy alone offers no guarantee for sustained remission and, thus, it should be viewed as a treatment and not a cure [10].

As such, it is important for patients to realize that ablation requires a long-term commitment to continued endoscopic surveillance. Patients should not undergo ablation if they are unwilling to undergo continued and regular surveillance. In addition, patients should remain informed about evolving data on endoscopic ablation, in order to optimize their expectations and long-term management.

22.3 Cancer risk and grade of dysplasia

The grade of dysplasia remains the best available marker of cancer risk in Barrett's esophagus, and is considered a histologic expression of genetic alterations that lead to unregulated cell growth [11]. Dysplasia is defined by morphologic changes in tissue that a pathologist recognizes by cytologic and architectural abnormalities in esophageal biopsy specimens. Patients with Barrett's esophagus can progress through the phenotypic sequence of no dysplasia, low-grade dysplasia, high-grade dysplasia, and adenocarcinoma. However, this stepwise sequence, while appealing, is not predetermined and is not always seen [11].

Any decision about eradication must weigh the risk of developing cancer prior to embarking on an endoscopic intervention. Recent studies consistently show that the risk of developing cancer in patients without dysplasia is lower than previously thought, and is approximately 0.1–0.5% per year [12–16]. Furthermore, large studies from Denmark and Northern Ireland demonstrate that the risk of cancer does not increase over time [17, 18]. A Danish population-based study estimated that the absolute annual risk of developing cancer in Barrett's esophagus patients without dysplasia was 0.12% [17]. Similarly, a longitudinal study of a large Irish Barrett's esophagus registry found a 0.22% annual risk of progression from non-dysplastic Barrett's esophagus to high-grade dysplasia or esophageal cancer, a risk that did not increase over time [18].

Other modern studies find similar low rates of progression for non-dysplastic Barrett's esophagus, and most patients remain cancer-free during five and ten years of follow-up (98.6% and 97.1%, respectively) [12]. Persistence of non-dysplastic Barrett's over time may also identify patients who are at an even lower risk for development of esophageal adenocarcinoma [19, 20]. In addition, the vast majority of patients with Barrett's esophagus will never develop cancer and will die from other causes [21–24]. Thus, despite the ready availability of a variety of different ablation techniques, it is difficult to justify a decision to embark on endoscopic therapy for patients without dysplasia at present, for the following reasons:

1 Lack of proof of efficacy in a randomized controlled trial.
2 Cancer risk for a given patient is low, and there are no yet proven predictors of high-risk patients.
3 Lack of data on cancer prevention benefit.
4 The need for surveillance is not changed.
5 Long-term durability is imperfect and need for retreatment may be necessary.
6 All of the techniques involve considerable financial cost (i.e. upper endoscopy, anesthesia support, capital equipment, frequent biopsies).
7 Adverse events, while rare may still occur.

Lastly, a recent economic analysis demonstrated that ablation of non-dysplastic Barrett's may not be cost-effective and may actually be prohibitively expensive [25].

On the other hand, the evidence for proceeding with ablation is stronger for low-grade dysplasia. The natural history of low-grade dysplasia is highly variable; some patients clearly progress to high-grade dysplasia or adenocarcinoma, whereas "regression" is seen in many of these individuals. However, "regression", in many cases, could be related to diagnostic accuracy and/or sampling error. Interobserver variability in the interpretation of low-grade dysplasia remains problematic, even among expert GI pathologists, and may explain the highly variable natural history of this lesion [26].

Although the precise risk is difficult to determine, due to pathology interpretation, several recent studies suggest that the risk of low-grade dysplasia progressing to cancer is 0.5–13% per year [19, 27–29]. Two key studies suggest that low-grade dysplasia increases the risk for developing cancer. Hvid-Jensen et al. determined the incidence of adenocarcinoma among Barrett's patients with low-grade dysplasia in Denmark was increased by five-fold, compared with patients with non-dysplastic Barrett's esophagus [17]. Curvers et al., in the Netherlands, found an incidence rate of high-grade dysplasia/adenocarcinoma of 13.4% per year for patients with low-grade dysplasia when the diagnosis was confirmed by expert pathologists at university centers [28]. Finally, the interim results from a European randomized controlled trial of ablation for low-grade dysplasia (SURF) support an evolving body of evidence that ablation of low-grade dysplasia reduces the risk of developing high-grade dysplasia and/or cancer [32]. Furthermore, a recent decision analysis suggests that ablation of confirmed low-grade dysplasia may be cost-effective, given the newer assumptions cited above [25].

On the other hand, other studies suggest that progression rates of low-grade dysplasia may be overestimated. Wani et al. found a much lower rate of progression to high-grade dysplasia, with an incidence of only 1.6% per year and 0.44% per year for adenocarcinoma [29]. In this large multicenter cohort of patients with low-grade dysplasia, it was estimated that over 97% of patients were cancer free at five-year follow-up. The incidence rate of neoplasia development was comparable to patients with no dysplasia, at less than 1% per year, despite concordance among three expert pathologists. However, this study has been criticized, based on the duration of follow-up, the inclusion of dysplasia cases that were indefinite for dysplasia, and the low pathologist interobserver agreement, all of which can underestimate the actual low-grade dysplasia progression risk [33]. Given that the risk of progression of low-grade dysplasia remains unclear, the current American Gastroenterological Association (AGA) guidelines suggest that patients with confirmed low-grade dysplasia should be given the option to undergo either strategy: endoscopic eradication or close endoscopic surveillance every 6–12 months [34].

The evidence to ablate high-grade dysplasia is more convincing. High-grade dysplasia is a well-recognized risk factor for the development of adenocarcinoma [35, 36]. The risk of cancer progression in patients with high-grade dysplasia ranges from approximately 6–20% per year [34, 35, 37]. Unsuspected carcinoma has been detected at esophagectomy in approximately 40% of patients with high-grade dysplasia in older series, although this misclassification is decreased with the use of endoscopic mucosal resection in conjunction with a rigorous biopsy protocol [38, 39]. The AIM dysplasia trial demonstrated a reduction in the annual progression rates for high-grade dysplasia in the ablation cohort, compared with the untreated cohort (0.60% vs. 16.3% per patient per year) [32]. High-grade dysplasia remains a worrisome lesion, although progression to carcinoma may take many years, and is not seen in all patients.

The AGA medical position statement endorses endoscopic eradication therapy for confirmed high-grade dysplasia rather than endoscopic surveillance [34]. An international consensus statement (BADCAT) also recommends that endoscopic therapy, including resection of any mucosal nodularity, is preferred to surgery or surveillance for patients with high-grade dysplasia [40]. Radiofrequency ablation, with or without endoscopic mucosal resection, can achieve long-term remission for high-grade dysplasia [41]. Nonetheless, the promising remission rates should not absolve the patient from continued surveillance, given the risk of recurrence [42, 43].

Overall, the benefits of ablation of high-grade dysplasia appear to outweigh the risks, especially when considering the morbidity of an operative approach. Furthermore, the risk of lymph node metastases in high-grade dysplasia is nil and only 1.93% for intramucosal carcinoma. Given that esophagectomy carries an operative mortality of > 2% [44], the decision to proceed with endoscopic ablation of high-grade dysplasia rather than surgery is relatively clear-cut.

However, dysplasia remains an imperfect biomarker of increased cancer risk. It is often indistinguishable endoscopically and frequently focal in nature, thus making targeting of biopsies problematic. There is considerable interobserver variability in the grading of dysplasia in both community and academic settings, and the ability of pathologists to distinguish between intramucosal carcinoma and high-grade dysplasia is problematic, even in esophagectomy specimens [26, 45, 46]. For these reasons, the current guidelines recommend that the diagnosis of dysplasia should be confirmed by at least one additional pathologist, preferably one who is an expert in esophageal histopathology [34]. A less subjective marker for cancer risk that could supplement or replace the current dysplasia grading system remains an unmet need.

22.4 Baseline quality measures

Selection of patients for endoscopic ablation therapy is also dependent on the available local expertise in endoscopy and pathology. Prior to embarking on endoscopic therapy, a number of baseline quality measures need to be addressed regarding both endoscopy and pathology.

22.4.1 Endoscopic quality measures

Several endoscopic quality benchmarks should be met prior to embarking on ablation. First, the baseline endoscopy prior to ablation should include careful visual inspection with high-resolution endoscopy of the Barrett's segment, and should describe any mucosal abnormalities identified. The Prague classification, a well-validated international endoscopic grading tool, should be utilized to accurately define the segment length [47, 48].

Second, the endoscopist should commit an adequate amount of time to carefully visualize and biopsy any mucosal abnormalities. Taking additional time to inspect the Barrett's mucosa is an easy method to increase the yield of surveillance. A recent study suggests that longer inspection time of the Barrett's segment results in higher detection rates of high-grade dysplasia and adenocarcinoma [49].

Third, the endoscopist should employ a rigorous biopsy protocol. Systematic biopsies every 1–2 cm of the Barrett's segment should occur, in conjunction with additional biopsies of any mucosal abnormalities, as per the current AGA guidelines [34]. Adherence to systematic surveillance biopsy protocols is associated with increased detection of dysplasia and cancer [50–52]. Unfortunately, adherence to this biopsy protocol decreases as the length of the Barrett's segment increases [50]. If dysplasia is suspected or detected, surveillance biopsies should occur more frequently, at every 1 cm, in order to minimize sampling error [34].

Another key quality metric prior to commencing endoscopic eradication of Barrett's esophagus is proficiency in endoscopic mucosal resection. Endoscopic mucosal resection of mucosal abnormalities permits more accurate histological staging of neoplasia when compared to esophageal biopsy specimens. It may also change the diagnosis in approximately 50% of patients and, therefore, may lead to a change in treatment plan [34, 45, 53, 54]. Negative margins on endoscopic mucosal resection specimens correlate well with the absence of residual disease at the time of surgery [55]. Furthermore, endoscopic mucosal resection, with or without ablation, can achieve effective outcomes for selected patients with high-grade dysplasia or early superficial neoplasia [56–58]. Endoscopic mucosal resection specimens with submucosal involvement are associated both with residual disease at the time of surgery, and with lymph node metastases. The issue of submucosal cancer limited to the superficial layer is an evolving area of debate (as discussed in a later section).

Taken together, the endoscopist should be committed to several quality measures to facilitate accuracy of diagnosis and staging. Time spent on meticulous inspection for mucosal irregularities, Prague grading of the Barrett's segment, adherence to a rigorous surveillance biopsy protocol, and endoscopic mucosal resection of any visible nodularity are essential baseline components.

22.4.2 Pathology quality measures

Of equal importance to endoscopic quality measures, pathology expertise is critical in decision making for patients with intraepithelial neoplasia. It is well recognized that pathologic interpretation of Barrett's esophagus specimens is problematic in the community as well as in academic centers. There are clear problems with interobserver agreement among pathologists in the interpretation of dysplasia in the Barrett's specimen. Alikhan et al. found that only 30% of a group of community pathologists correctly identified high-grade dysplasia, and non-dysplastic Barrett's was interpreted as invasive carcinoma by 5% of these same pathologists [46].

Pathologic interpretation is also problematic for expert gastrointestinal pathologists, where interobserver reproducibility is substantial at the ends of the spectrum of Barrett's esophagus, namely negative for dysplasia and high-grade dysplasia/carcinoma but not especially good for low-grade dysplasia or indefinite for dysplasia [26]. Interobserver variation is particularly challenging for low-grade dysplasia among community pathologists as, often, low-grade dysplasia is over-diagnosed. Work by Curvers et al. found that low-grade dysplasia diagnosed by community pathologists was downgraded to non-dysplastic Barrett's esophagus in 77% of cases after review by expert gastrointestinal pathologists. However, in the cases where low-grade dysplasia was confirmed, the cumulative progression rate to high-grade dysplasia/cancer was 85% over a nine-year period, compared with 4.6% for those downgraded, thereby demonstrating the importance of expert pathology review for optimal risk stratification [28].

Taken together, these findings point out some of the problems in pathologic interpretation: experience of the pathologist; quality of the slides; size of the specimens; and the difficulties for all pathologists in interpreting dysplasia. Endoscopic mucosal resection clearly enhances the ability of pathologists to establish a more accurate diagnosis than mucosal biopsies [45, 56]. Mino-Kenudson et al. found that the interobserver agreement for Barrett's associated neoplasia on endoscopic mucosal resection specimens was higher than that for mucosal biopsies [59]. Resection specimens afford a larger amount of tissue that provides details on tumor grade, depth, and vascular invasion.

In a Dutch study, endoscopic mucosal resection changed the biopsy diagnosis in 49% of lesions, thereby leading to a change in treatment plan in 30% of patients [45]. Other studies confirm these findings; endoscopic mucosal resection results in upstaging of histology in 40% to 50% of patients with visible lesions within the Barrett's segment [60]. This is especially important for an accurate diagnosis for intramucosal and submucosal carcinoma.

22.5 The lesion

After baseline quality measures are met, it is important to define the characteristics of the Barrett's segment. Factors involving the Barrett's epithelium may impact the decision to eradicate, the most important of which is the grade of dysplasia (Table 22.2). However, other characteristics include the presence and appearance of any focal lesions, and length of the Barrett's segment.

22.5.1 Macroscopic and microscopic features of the lesion

Mucosal nodularity in patients with high-grade dysplasia is associated with an increased risk of subsequent adenocarcinoma. Buttar et al. found that there is an association between the presence of nodularity and

Table 22.2 Selection for endoscopic eradication based on grade of dysplasia/neoplasia.

Patients that should be treated	Patients that should not be treated	Patients that should possibly be treated
High-grade dysplasia Intramucosal adenocarcinoma	No dysplasia Invasive adenocarcinoma (extending into the middle submucosal layer – sm2)	Low-grade dysplasia Invasive adenocarcinoma (confined to upper submucosal layer – sm1)

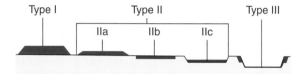

Figure 22.1 Paris classification of the endoscopic appearance of superficial neoplastic lesions of the digestive tract mucosa.

risk of developing adenocarcinoma. Up to 60% of high-grade dysplasia patients with visible nodularity went on to develop cancer, compared to 23% in patients without a nodule [35].

The Paris classification of superficial neoplastic lesions (Figure 22.1) was initially developed to help predict the extent of invasion into the submucosa of gastric cancer and as such, the choice between endoscopic versus surgical approaches [61]. It has subsequently been adopted for esophageal lesions as well. Furthermore, deep invasion can be suspected by the presence of the "non-lifting" sign, whereby a lesion fails to lift after injection of saline into the submucosa.

Work by the Wiesbaden group has defined low-risk lesions amenable to endoscopic approaches as having the following characteristics [62]:

- Lesion diameter < 2 cm and macroscopically Paris type I (polypoid), IIa (flat and slightly elevated), or IIb (flat and level).
- IIc (flat and depressed < 10 mm).
- Well- or moderately differentiated histologic grade.
- Lesions limited to the mucosa proven by histology of the resected specimens.
- Absence of either blood vessel or lymphatic invasion.

Peters *et al.* further refined our understanding of the Paris classification in this setting by examining the endoscopic features that predicted favorable pathologic characteristics. They found that well-differentiated (grade 1) lesions were associated with submucosal

cancer in only 6% of cases, whereas submucosal cancer was encountered in 44% of moderately differentiated (grade 2) lesions and 50% of poorly differentiated (grade 3) lesions, based on histologic review of resection specimens [45]. The endoscopic lesions most predictive of submucosal cancer were Paris type 0-I and 0-IIc. All other Paris type lesions were associated with submucosal cancer in ≤ 10% of cases. Others have confirmed a high rate of concurrent submucosal invasion in patients with an endoscopically visible lesion [63, 64].

Dysplasia at multiple different levels of the esophagus may also be a risk factor for underlying adenocarcinoma or progression to cancer [65]. The Mayo Clinic group found that the extent of high-grade dysplasia predicted risk of progression to adenocarcinoma [35]. Patients with diffuse high-grade dysplasia were at higher risk of progression, compared with those with focal high-grade dysplasia (56% vs. 14% at three years follow-up). Multifocal low-grade dysplasia may also be a risk factor for progression to neoplasia [66]. Thus, multilevel dysplasia should be approached with heightened caution.

In summary, mucosal nodularity and multifocal dysplasia are associated with an increased risk of progression to cancer over time. Paris Type 0-I and 0-IIc lesions are especially worrisome for submucosal cancer at the time of endoscopic mucosal resection, and patients with moderate or poor differentiation, lesions > 2 cm and evidence of lymphatic or vascular invasion on endoscopic mucosal resection are poor candidates for continued endoscopic therapies.

22.5.2 Tumor depth

Early invasive cancer may be classified as intramucosal when neoplastic cells penetrate through the basement membrane to the lamina propria or muscularis mucosa and submucosal when neoplastic cells infiltrate into the submucosa [67]. The prognosis for these two lesions is very different. Recent data show that the risk of lymph node metastases is approximately 1.93% for intramucosal cancer [44]. However, that risk increases for submucosal cancer with a range of 21% to 50% [68–71]. Given the fact that lymph node metastases are a clear risk factor for decreased survival, tumor depth is perhaps one of the most significant factors in decision making for the approach to superficial neoplasia [70].

The issue of endoscopic therapy for submucosal lesions is currently evolving. Until recently, submucosal cancer was viewed as a contraindication to ablative therapies. This is based on prior data demonstrating lymph node metastasis as high as approximately 45% to 50% for neoplasia that invaded deep into the submucosa [69, 71]. Recent work from the Mayo Clinic confirmed that both superficial and deep submucosal invasion had worrisome rates of metastatic lymphadenopathy of 12.9% and 20.4%, respectively, which negatively impacted survival [72].

On the other hand, a surgical group evaluated the outcome of submucosal cancers by classifying invasion as limited to the upper third (sm1), middle third (sm2) and lower third of the submucosa (sm3), and found that lymph node metastases were found in 0/25 sm1, lesions in contrast to 6/23 sm2 lesions and 12/18 sm3 lesions [73]. The outcome (very low risk of lymphatic dissemination and 97% remained free of recurrence on five-year follow-up) for patients with sm1 disease was no different than that for patients with intramucosal carcinoma.

This has led some to now extend indications of endoscopic mucosal resection to low-risk submucosal cancer characterized by the following criteria: sm1 invasion; absence of infiltration into lymphatics or veins; and histology characterized by well or moderate grades of differentiation [53]. Indeed, the Wiesbaden group achieved complete endoluminal eradication using endoscopic mucosal resection for patients with sm1 invasion (T1b) deemed "low risk" based on the above criteria. Complete remission was achieved in 87%, and only one patient (1.9%) had lymph node metastases [74]. Patients in this study had a five-year survival of 84%. However, 19% of treated subjects were found to have metachronous neoplasia.

The Mayo Clinic group has also investigated the outcome of their cohort of Barrett's patients with submucosal cancer treated surgically or endoscopically, and found no difference in survival with either approach.

Both groups had a median survival of less than four years [75]. Given the issues outlined above, endoscopic therapy of superficial submucosal cancer remains an area of active study.

22.5.3 Segment length

Esophageal cancer develops in both short and long segments of Barrett's esophagus. Prior studies have yielded mixed results for length as a risk factor, in part because of the low incidence of progression to cancer in cohort studies. It now appears that the prevalence of cancer and dysplasia is higher in longer lengths of Barrett's epithelium [76]. Several recent studies have also found that the longer the segment length, the higher the risk of progression [20, 77, 78]. The Kansas City group demonstrated that the likelihood of progression was directly related to Barrett's length, with a 28% increase in risk of progression for every 1 cm increase in Barrett's length [78].

Taken together, these data suggest that there is a relationship between segment length and cancer risk. However, it is important to keep in mind that the longer the Barrett's segment length, the higher the probability of sampling error with endoscopic surveillance. Other decisions regarding endoscopic ablation based on segment length include the threshold for performing focal versus circumferential endoscopic mucosal resection and thermal ablation alone, or in combination with endoscopic mucosal resection.

22.6 Predictors of response

Although the data to date, regarding efficacy and durability of radiofrequency ablation with and without endoscopic mucosal resection, have been encouraging, not all patients respond initially, and recurrences may occur. As such, it would be important to develop predictors of response to help guide therapy. There are emerging data that begin to shed light on this issue.

22.7 Predictors of initial response to therapy

Some patients may fail to achieve complete regression of Barrett's epithelium despite ablation. The Amsterdam group recently identified factors associated with a poor response to circumferential radiofrequency ablation [79]. Evidence of active reflux esophagitis, scar regeneration with Barrett's epithelium instead of squamous epithelium after endoscopic resection, relative esophageal narrowing, and duration of neoplasia were found to be predictors of poor response to ablation. The proportion of non-responders increased in conjunction with the number of independent risk factors present.

Acid suppression is key to optimizing the success of ablation, and all patients are placed on high-dose proton pump inhibitor therapy. However, complete acid suppression is well recognized to be problematic in Barrett's esophagus patients, even with high-dose PPI therapy [80]. This issue has led to the question of whether uncontrolled reflux impacts the outcome of radiofrequency ablation. Krishnan et al. found that uncontrolled, weakly acidic reflux, despite twice daily proton pump inhibitor therapy, was associated with persistent intestinal metaplasia after ablation [81]. They also found that the presence and size of a hiatal hernia and length of Barrett's segment were associated with persistent intestinal metaplasia. With the exception of acid suppression, it remains unclear whether intervening on any other patient factors truly improves outcomes.

Numerous molecular markers may define patients at increased risk for progression to esophageal adenocarcinoma and potentially identify poor responders to endoscopic ablation. To date, one study has evaluated biomarkers to predict response to ablation. Prasad et al. found that loss of p16, detected by fluorescence in situ hybridization of cytology specimens, obtained prior to photodynamic therapy for high-grade dysplasia or intramucosal carcinoma, predicted a reduced response to photodynamic therapy [82]. Studies are currently under way to determine if similar findings are seen in patients undergoing ablation with radiofrequency ablation along, or in combination, with endoscopic mucosal resection. Future studies will need to examine biomarkers, or other patient factors that predict response, carefully. Similarly, there is a growing body of evidence that demonstrates the potential for biomarkers to enhance early detection and predict risk of neoplastic progression and response to therapy [83–85]. However, the use of biomarkers to predict response to ablation therapy is not yet ready for clinical practice.

22.7.1 Predictors of recurrence

Few studies to date have examined predictors of recurrent dysplasia and/or early cancer following endoscopic therapy. Data on these predictors are based on the endoscopic modality utilized. For photodynamic therapy, these include advanced age, smoking, and persistent intestinal metaplasia. For radiofrequency ablation, incomplete mucosal healing between treatment sessions is a predictor for recurrent dysplasia and/or cancer [86, 87].

Pech et al. found that recurrence is higher if ablation of residual Barrett's is not performed following endoscopic mucosal resection [88]. In that same study, long-segment Barrett's esophagus, multifocal neoplasia, piecemeal resection, and longer time to achieve complete eradication were all associated with higher recurrence rates. In our experience, multifocal dysplasia and advanced age are associated with recurrent dysplasia/neoplasia when using a combination of endoscopic resection and thermal ablative therapies [89].

Patients should be informed, and the endoscopist should be aware, of the factors associated with treatment failure, the risk of recurrence, and the need for continued surveillance following remission. A multicenter study by Gupta et al. analyzed data on 592 patients treated with radiofrequency ablation, 71% of whom had high-grade dysplasia or adenocarcinoma, almost half of whom had undergone endoscopic mucosal resection prior to ablation [43]. Recurrence of intestinal metaplasia was seen in 33% two years after complete eradication was achieved. Dysplasia or neoplasia was found in nearly a quarter of all recurrences. Recurrence rates reported have been variable in other series, with a pooled estimate of 13% in a recent meta-analysis [90]. These findings reinforce the importance of long-term, continued surveillance post-eradication therapy.

22.7.2 Compliance with endoscopic follow-up protocols

Given the problems with recurrence following therapy, any decision to treat intraepithelial neoplasia endoscopically requires compliance by both the patient and the physician, with continued endoscopic follow-up. There are currently no established guidelines for the ideal surveillance intervals following endoscopic eradication of dysplasia/early cancer. For example, the Wiesbaden group protocol for follow-up after endoscopic mucosal resection of intraepithelial neoplasia involves follow-up endoscopy at 1, 2, 3, 6, 9, and 12 months after treatment, then at six-month intervals up to five years, and annual endoscopy thereafter [62]. At our institution and other high-volume centers, post-ablation surveillance for high-grade dysplasia and intramucosal cancer is characterized by at least eight biopsies every 1–2 cm of the neosquamous Barrett's segment carried out at three-month intervals for year one, followed by six-month intervals for year two, then annually thereafter [91]. Inability to comply with a rigorous endoscopic follow-up protocol should be considered a contraindication to endoscopic approaches to intraepithelial neoplasia.

22.8 Future considerations

Despite the many recent advances in therapies for Barrett's esophagus, many unresolved questions remain. Can we better predict treatment responders and failures? Is there a practical role for molecular markers to improve risk stratification? What are the optimal surveillance intervals post-ablation, and can these techniques be improved? What is the natural history of less recognized histologic lesions, such as subsquamous intestinal metaplasia, how can we better detect it, and what is the significance of buried intestinal metaplasia?

22.9 Conclusions

Patient selection for endoscopic ablation starts with patient education regarding cancer risk, a review of the risks and benefits of endoscopic therapy, and emphasis on the concept that endoscopic therapy represents a treatment, not a cure, of the problem at hand. Furthermore, endoscopic therapy requires adherence to a variety of quality metrics in both endoscopy and pathology. Endoscopic therapy is problematic for intestinal metaplasia negative for dysplasia, and is currently not advisable. There are evolving data on the utility of endoscopic therapy for confirmed low-grade dysplasia, but overall endoscopic therapy appears to be a reasonable option for this patient group.

Endoscopic eradication, using the combination of endoscopic mucosal resection and radiofrequency ablation, is the preferred strategy for high-grade dysplasia and intramucosal carcinoma. Endoscopic therapy requires a commitment to meticulous staging, and likely ongoing lifelong surveillance. Lastly, predictors of response and failure to achieve sustained eradication is an area in which data are slowly emerging.

References

1 Steyerberg EW, Neville BA, Koppert LB, *et al.* (2006). Surgical mortality in patients with esophageal cancer: development and validation of a simple risk score. *Journal of Clinical Oncology* **24**, 4277–84.

2 Lagarde SM, Reitsma JB, Maris AK, *et al.* (2008). Pre-operative prediction of the occurrence and severity of complications after esophagectomy for cancer with use of nomogram. *Annals of Thoracic Surgery* **85**, 1938–45.

3 Yoshida N, Watanabe M, Baba Y, *et al.* (2014). Risk factors for pulmonary complications after esophagectomy for esophageal cancer. *Surgery Today* **44**(3), 526–32.

4 Bhayani NH, Gupta A, Dunst CM, *et al.* (2013). Esophagectomies With Thoracic Incisions Carry Increased Pulmonary Morbidity. *JAMA Surgery* **148**, 733–8.

5 Enestvedt BK, Eisen GM, Holub J, *et al.* (2013). Is the American Society of Anesthesiologists classification useful in risk stratification for endoscopic procedures? *Gastrointestinal Endoscopy* **77**, 464–71.

6 Yachimski P, Nishioka NS, Richards F, Hur C (2008). Treatment of Barrett's esophagus with high-grade dysplasia or cancer: predictors of surgical versus endoscopic therapy. *Clinical Gastroenterology and Hepatology* **6**, 1206–11.

7 Shaheen NJ, Green B, Medapalli RK, *et al.* (2005). The perception of cancer risk in patients with prevalent Barrett's esophagus enrolled in an endoscopic surveillance program. *Gastroenterology* **129**, 429–36.

8 Kruijshaar ME, Siersema PD, Janssens AC, Kerkhof M, Steyerberg EW, Essink-Bot ML; CYBAR Study Group (2007). Patients with Barrett's esophagus perceive their risk of developing esophageal adenocarcinoma as low. *Gastrointestinal Endoscopy* **65**, 26–30.

9 Shaheen NJ, Peery AF, Hawes RH, *et al*; AIM Dysplasia Trial Investigators (2010). Quality of life following radiofrequency ablation of dysplastic Barrett's esophagus. *Endoscopy* **42**, 790–9.

10 Bergman JJ, Corley DA (2012). Barrett's esophagus: who should receive ablation and how can we get the best results? *Gastroenterology* **143**, 524–6.

11 Spechler SJ, Fitzgerald RC, Prasad GA, Wang KK (2010). History, molecular mechanisms, and endoscopic treatment of Barrett's esophagus. *Gastroenterology* **138**, 854–69.

12 Wani S, Falk G, Hall M, *et al.* (2011). Patients with nondysplastic Barrett's esophagus have low risks for developing dysplasia or esophageal adenocarcinoma. *Clinical Gastroenterology and Hepatology* **9**, 220–7.

13 Shaheen NJ, Crosby MA, Bozymski EM, *et al.* (2000). Is there publication bias in the reporting of cancer risk in Barrett's esophagus? *Gastroenterology* **119**, 333–8.

14 Shields HM, Nardone G, Zhao J, *et al.* (2011). Barrett's esophagus: prevalence and incidence of adenocarcinomas. *Annals of the New York Academy of Sciences* **1232**, 230–47.

15 van der Burgh A, Dees J, Hop WC, *et al.* (1996). Oesophageal cancer is an uncommon cause of death in patients with Barrett's oesophagus. *Gut* **39**, 5–8.

16 Desai TK, Krishnan K, Samala N, *et al.* (2012). The incidence of oesophageal adenocarcinoma in non-dysplastic Barrett's oesophagus: a meta-analysis. *Gut* **61**, 970–6.

17 Hvid-Jensen F, Pedersen L, Drewes AM, *et al.* (2011). Incidence of adenocarcinoma among patients with Barrett's esophagus. *New England Journal of Medicine* **365**, 1375–83.

18 Bhat S, Coleman HG, Yousef F, *et al.* (2011). Risk of malignant progression in Barrett's esophagus patients: results from a large population-based study. *Journal of the National Cancer Institute* **103**(13), 1049–57.

19 Gaddam S, Singh M, Balasubramanian G, *et al.* (2013). Persistence of Non-Dysplastic Barrett's Esophagus Identifies Patients at Lower Risk for Esophageal Adenocarcinoma-Results from a Large Multicenter Cohort. *Gastroenterology* **145**, 548–53.

20 Sikkema M, Looman CW, Steyerberg EW, *et al.* (2011). Predictors for neoplastic progression in patients with Barrett's Esophagus: a prospective cohort study. *American Journal of Gastroenterology* **106**, 1231–8.

21 Moayyedi P, Burch N, Akhtar-Danesh N, *et al.* (2008). Mortality rates in patients with Barrett's oesophagus. *Alimentary Pharmacology & Therapeutics* **27**, 316–20.

22 Anderson LA, Murray LJ, Murphy SJ, *et al.* (2003). Mortality in Barrett's oesophagus: results from a population based study. *Gut* **52**, 1081–4.

23 Solaymani-Dodaran M, Card TR, West J (2013). Cause-specific mortality of people with Barrett's esophagus compared with the general population: a population-based cohort study. *Gastroenterology* **144**, 1375–83.

24 Sikkema M, de Jonge PJ, Steyerberg EW, *et al.* (2010). Risk of esophageal adenocarcinoma and mortality in patients with Barrett's esophagus: a systematic review and meta-analysis. *Clinical Gastroenterology and Hepatology* **8**, 235–44.

25 Hur C, Choi SE, Rubenstein JH, *et al.* (2012). The cost effectiveness of radiofrequency ablation for Barrett's esophagus. *Gastroenterology* **143**, 567–75.

26 Montgomery E, Bronner MP, Goldblum JR, *et al.* (2001). Reproducibility of the diagnosis of dysplasia Barrett esophagus: a reaffirmation. *Human Pathology* **32**, 368–78.

27 Sharma P (2004). Low-grade dysplasia in Barrett's esophagus. *Gastroenterology* **127**, 1233–8.

28 Curvers WL, ten Kate FJ, Krishnadath KK, *et al.* (2010). Low-grade dysplasia in Barrett's esophagus: overdiagnosed and underestimated. *American Journal of Gastroenterology* **105**, 1523–30.

29 Wani S, Falk GW, Post J, *et al.* (2011). Risk factors for progression of low-grade dysplasia in patients with Barrett's esophagus. *Gastroenterology* **141**, 1179–86.

30 Phoa KY, van Vilsteren FG, Pouw RE, *et al* (2013). Radiofrequency ablation in Barrett's esophagus with confirmed low-grade dysplasia: Interim results of a European multicenter randomized controlled trial (SURF). *Gastroenterology* **144**(5), S–187.

31 Shaheen NJ, Sharma P, Overholt BF, *et al.* (2009). Radiofrequency ablation in Barrett's esophagus with dysplasia. *New England Journal of Medicine* **360**, 2277–88.

32 Shaheen NJ, Overholt BF, Sampliner RE, *et al.* (2011). Durability of radiofrequency ablation in Barrett's esophagus with dysplasia. *Gastroenterology* **141**, 460–8.

33 Bergman JJ, Vieth M, Fitzgerald RC. (2012). Let's not jump to conclusions regarding low-grade dysplasia in Barrett's esophagus. *Gastroenterology* **142**, e18–9.

34 Spechler SJ, Sharma P, Souza RF, *et al.* (2011). American Gastroenterological Association medical position statement on the management of Barrett's esophagus. *Gastroenterology* **140**, 1084–91.

35 Buttar NS, Wang KK, Sebo TJ, *et al.* (2001). Extent of high-grade dysplasia in Barrett's esophagus correlates with risk of adenocarcinoma. *Gastroenterology* **120**, 1630–9.

36 Schnell TG, Sontag SJ, Chejfec G, *et al.* (2001). Long-term nonsurgical management of Barrett's esophagus with high-grade dysplasia. *Gastroenterology* **120**, 1607–19.

37 Verbeek RE, van Oijen MG, ten Kate FJ, *et al.* (2012). Surveillance and follow-up strategies in patients with high-grade dysplasia in Barrett's esophagus: a Dutch population-based study. *American Journal of Gastroenterology* **107**, 534–42.

38 Pellegrini CA, Pohl D. (2000). High-grade dysplasia in Barrett's esophagus: surveillance or operation? *Journal of Gastrointestinal Surgery* **4**, 131–4.

39 Prasad GA, Wang KK, Buttar NS, *et al.* (2007). Long-term survival following endoscopic and surgical treatment of high-grade dysplasia in Barrett's esophagus. *Gastroenterology* **132**, 1226–33.

40 Bennett C, Vakil N, Bergman J, *et al.* (2012). Consensus statements for management of Barrett's dysplasia and early-stage esophageal adenocarcinoma, based on a Delphi process. *Gastroenterology* **143**, 336–46.

41 Leggett CL, Prasad GA (2012). High-grade dysplasia and intramucosal adenocarcinoma in Barrett's esophagus: the role of endoscopic eradication therapy. *Current Opinion in Gastroenterology* **28**, 354–61.

42 Wang KK, Tian JM, Gorospe E, *et al.* (2012). Medical and endoscopic management of high-grade dysplasia in Barrett's esophagus. *Diseases of the Esophagus* **25**, 349–55.

43 Gupta M, Iyer PG, Lutzke L, *et al.* (2013). Recurrence of Esophageal Intestinal Metaplasia After Endoscopic Mucosal Resection and Radiofrequency Ablation of Barrett's Esophagus: Results From a US Multicenter Consortium. *Gastroenterology* **145**, 79–86.

44 Dunbar KB and Spechler SJ (2012). The risk of lymph-node metastases in patients with high-grade dysplasia or intramucosal carcinoma in Barrett's esophagus: a systematic review. *American Journal of Gastroenterology* **J107**, 850–62.

45 Peters FP, Brakenhoff KP, Curvers WL, *et al.* (2008). Histologic evaluation of resection specimens obtained at 293 endoscopic resections in Barrett's esophagus. *Gastrointestinal Endoscopy* **67**, 604–9.

46 Alikhan M, Rex D, Khan A, *et al.* (1999). Variable pathologic interpretation of columnar lined esophagus by general pathologists in community practice. *Gastrointestinal Endoscopy* **50**, 23–6.

47 Sharma P, Dent J, Armstrong D, *et al.* (2006). The development and validation of an endoscopic grading system for Barrett's esophagus: the Prague C & M criteria. *Gastroenterology* **131**, 1392–9.

48 Anand O, Wani S, Sharma P (2008). When and how to grade Barrett's columnar metaplasia: the Prague system. *Best Practice & Research Clinical Gastroenterology* **22**, 661–9.

49 Gupta N, Gaddam S, Wani SB, *et al.* (2012). Longer inspection time is associated with increased detection of high-grade dysplasia and esophageal adenocarcinoma in Barrett's esophagus. *Gastrointestinal Endoscopy* **76**, 531–8.

50 Abrams JA, Kapel RC, Lindberg GM, *et al.* (2009). Adherence to biopsy guidelines for Barrett's esophagus surveillance in the community setting in the United States. *Clinical Gastroenterology and Hepatology* **7**, 736–42.

51 Abela JE, Going JJ, Mackenzie JF, McKernan M, O'Mahoney S, Stuart RC (2008). Systematic four-quadrant biopsy detects Barrett's dysplasia in more patients than nonsystematic biopsy. *American Journal of Gastroenterology* **103**, 850 5.

52 Fitzgerald RC, Saeed IT, Khoo D, Farthing MJ, Burnham WR (2001). Rigorous surveillance protocol increases detection of curable cancers associated with Barrett's esophagus. *Digestive Diseases and Sciences* **46**, 1892–8.

53 Manner H, May A, Pech O, *et al.* (2008). Early Barrett's carcinoma with "low-risk" submucosal invasion: long-term results of endoscopic resection with a curative intent. *American Journal of Gastroenterology* **103**, 2589–97.

54 Mino-Kenudson M, Brugge WR, Puricelli WP, *et al.* (2005). Management of superficial Barrett's epithelium-related neoplasms by endoscopic mucosal resection: clinicopathologic analysis of 27 cases. *American Journal of Surgical Pathology* **29**, 680–6.

55 Prasad GA, Buttar NS, Wongkeesong LM, *et al.* (2007). Significance of neoplastic involvement of margins obtained by endoscopic mucosal resection in Barrett's esophagus. *American Journal of Gastroenterology* **102**, 2380–6.

56 Pouw RE, Seewald S, Gondrie JJ, *et al.* (2010). Stepwise radical endoscopic resection for eradication of Barrett's oesophagus with early neoplasia in a cohort of 169 patients. *Gut* **59**, 1169–77.

57 van Vilsteren FG, Pouw RE, Seewald S, *et al.* (2011). Stepwise radical endoscopic resection versus radiofrequency ablation for Barrett's oesophagus with high-grade dysplasia or early cancer: a multicentre randomised trial. *Gut* **60**, 765–73.

58 Bulsiewicz WJ, Kim HP, Dellon ES, *et al.* (2013). Safety and efficacy of endoscopic mucosal therapy with radiofrequency ablation for patients with neoplastic Barrett's esophagus. *Clinical Gastroenterology and Hepatology* **11**, 636–42.

59 Mino-Kenudson M, Hull MJ, Brown I, *et al.* (2007). EMR for Barrett's esophagus-related superficial neoplasms offers better diagnostic reproducibility than mucosal biopsy. *Gastrointestinal Endoscopy* **66**, 660–6.

60 Hull MJ, Mino-Kenudson M, Nishioka NS, *et al.* (2006). Endoscopic mucosal resection: an improved diagnostic procedure for early gastroesophageal epithelial neoplasms. *American Journal of Surgical Pathology* **30**, 114–8.

61 Endoscopic Classification Review Group (2005). Update on the Paris classification of superficial neoplastic lesions in the digestive tract. *Endoscopy* **37**, 570–8.

62 Ell C, May A, Pech O, *et al.* (2007). Curative endoscopic resection of early esophageal adenocarcinomas (Barrett's cancer). *Gastrointestinal Endoscopy* **65**, 3–10.

63 Konda VJ, Ross AS, Ferguson MK, *et al.* (2008). Is the risk of concomitant invasive esophageal cancer in high-grade dysplasia in Barrett's esophagus overestimated? *Clinical Gastroenterology and Hepatology* **6**, 159–64.

64 Wang VS, Hornick JL, Sepulveda JA, *et al.* (2009). Low prevalence of submucosal invasive carcinoma at esophagectomy for high-grade dysplasia or intramucosal adenocarcinoma in Barrett's esophagus: a 20-year experience. *Gastrointestinal Endoscopy* **69**, 777–83.

65 Tharavej C, Hagen JA, Peters JH, *et al.* (2006). Predictive factors of coexisting cancer in Barrett's high-grade dysplasia. *Surgical Endoscopy* **20**, 439–43.

66 Srivastava A, Hornick JL, Li X, *et al.* (2007). Extent of low-grade dysplasia is a risk factor for the development of esophageal adenocarcinoma in Barrett's esophagus. *American Journal of Gastroenterology* **102**, 483–93.

67 Ormsby AH, Petras RE, Henricks WH, *et al.* (2002). Observer variation in the diagnosis of superficial oesophageal adenocarcinoma. *Gut* **51**, 671–6.

68 Stein HJ, Feith M, Bruecher BL, Naehrig J, Sarbia M, Siewert JR. (2005). Early esophageal cancer: pattern of lymphatic spread and prognostic factors for long-term survival after surgical resection. *Annals of Surgery* **242**, 566–73.

69 Bollschweiler E, Baldus SE, Schröder W, *et al.* (2006). High rate of lymph-node metastasis in submucosal esophageal squamous-cell carcinomas and adenocarcinomas. *Endoscopy* **38**, 149–56.

70 Ancona E, Rampado S, Cassaro M, *et al.* (2008). Prediction of lymph node status in superficial esophageal carcinoma. *Annals of Surgical Oncology* **15**, 3278–88.

71 Sepesi B, Watson TJ, Zhou D, *et al.* (2010). Are endoscopic therapies appropriate for superficial submucosal esophageal adenocarcinoma? An analysis of esophagectomy specimens. *Journal of the American College of Surgeons* **210**, 418–27.

72 Badreddine RJ, Prasad GA, Lewis JT, *et al*. (2010). Depth of submucosal invasion does not predict lymph node metastasis and survival of patients with esophageal carcinoma. *Clinical Gastroenterology and Hepatology* **8**, 248–53.

73 Westerterp M, Koppert LB, Buskens CJ, *et al*. (2005). Outcome of surgical treatment for early adenocarcinoma of the esophagus or gastro-esophageal junction. *Virchows Archiv* **446**, 497–504.

74 Manner H, Pech O, Heldmann Y, *et al*. (2013). Efficacy, safety, and long-term results of endoscopic treatment for early stage adenocarcinoma of the esophagus with low-risk sm1 invasion. *Clinical Gastroenterology and Hepatology* **11**, 630–5.

75 Tian J, Prasad GA, Lutzke LS, *et al*. (2011). Outcomes of T1b esophageal adenocarcinoma patients. *Gastrointestinal Endoscopy* **74**, 1201–6.

76 Weston AP, Sharma P, Mathur S, *et al*. (2004). Risk stratification of Barrett's esophagus: updated prospective multivariate analysis. *American Journal of Gastroenterology* **99**, 1657–66.

77 Avidan B, Sonnenberg A, Schnell TG, *et al*. (2002). Hiatal hernia size, Barrett's length, and severity of acid reflux are all risk factors for esophageal adenocarcinoma. *American Journal of Gastroenterology* **97**, 1930–6.

78 Anaparthy R, Gaddam S, Kanakadandi V, *et al*. (2013). Association between length of Barrett's esophagus and risk of high-grade dysplasia or adenocarcinoma in patients without dysplasia. *Clinical Gastroenterology and Hepatology* **11**(11), 1430–6.

79 van Vilsteren FG, Alvarez Herrero L, Pouw RE, *et al*. (2013). Predictive factors for initial treatment response after circumferential radiofrequency ablation for Barrett's esophagus with early neoplasia: a prospective multicenter study. *Endoscopy* **45**, 516–25.

80 Spechler SJ, Sharma P, Traxler B, *et al*. (2006). Gastric and esophageal pH in patients with Barrett's esophagus treated with three esomeprazole dosages: a randomized, double-blind, crossover trial. *American Journal of Gastroenterology* **101**, 1964–71.

81 Krishnan K, Pandolfino JE, Kahrilas PJ, *et al*. (2012). Increased risk for persistent intestinal metaplasia in patients with Barrett's esophagus and uncontrolled reflux exposure before radiofrequency ablation. *Gastroenterology* **143**, 576–81.

82 Prasad GA, Wang KK, Halling KC, *et al*. (2008). Utility of biomarkers in prediction of response to ablative therapy in Barrett's esophagus. *Gastroenterology* **135**, 370–9.

83 Bird-Lieberman EL, Dunn JM, Coleman HG, *et al*. (2012). Population-based study reveals new risk-stratification biomarker panel for Barrett's esophagus. *Gastroenterology* **143**, 927–35.

84 Kastelein F, Biermann K, Steyerberg EW, *et al*; on behalf of the ProBar-study group (2013). Aberrant p53 protein expression is associated with an increased risk of neoplastic progression in patients with Barrett's oesophagus. *Gut* **62**(12), 1676–83.

85 Fels Elliott DR, Fitzgerald RC. (2013) Molecular markers for Barrett's esophagus and its progression to cancer. *Current Opinion in Gastroenterology* **29**, 437–45.

86 Badreddine RJ, Prasad GA, Wang KK, *et al*. (2010). Prevalence and predictors of recurrent neoplasia after ablation of Barrett's esophagus. *Gastrointestinal Endoscopy* **71**, 697–703.

87 Orman ES, Kim HP, Bulsiewicz WJ, *et al*. (2013). Intestinal metaplasia recurs infrequently in patients successfully treated for Barrett's esophagus with radiofrequency ablation. *American Journal of Gastroenterology* **108**, 187–95.

88 Pech O, Behrens A, May A, *et al*. (2008). Long-term results and risk factor analysis for recurrence after curative endoscopic therapy in 349 patients with high-grade intraepithelial neoplasia and mucosal adenocarcinoma in Barrett's oesophagus. *Gut* **57**, 1200–6.

89 Guarner-Argente C, Buoncristiano T, Furth EE, *et al*. (2013). Long-term outcomes of patients with Barrett's esophagus and high-grade dysplasia or early cancer treated with endoluminal therapies with intention to complete eradication. *Gastrointestinal Endoscopy* **77**, 190–9.

90 Orman ES, Li N, Shaheen NJ (2013). Efficacy and Durability of Radiofrequency Ablation for Barrett's Esophagus: Systematic Review and Meta-analysis. *Clinical Gastroenterology and Hepatology* **11**, 1245–55.

91 Bedi AO, Kwon RS, Rubenstein JH, *et al*. (2013). A survey of expert follow-up practices after successful endoscopic eradication therapy for Barrett's esophagus with high-grade dysplasia and intramucosal adenocarcinoma. *Gastrointestinal Endoscopy* **78**(5), 696–701.

CHAPTER 23

Combined modality therapy in locally advanced esophageal cancer

Geoffrey Y. Ku & David H. Ilson

Gastrointestinal Oncology Service, Department of Medicine, Memorial Sloan-Kettering Cancer Center, New York, NY, USA

23.1 Introduction

In the United States, cancers of the esophagus and gastroesophageal (GE) junction are uncommon but aggressive. In 2013, an estimated 17,990 patients will be diagnosed, with an estimated 15,210 deaths from this disease [1].

Squamous cell carcinoma (SCC) and adenocarcinoma account for 98% of all cases of esophageal cancer. While cases of SCC have steadily declined, the incidence of adenocarcinoma of the distal esophagus, GE junction and gastric cardia has increased by 4% to 10% per year among men in the USA since 1976, so that it is now the most common histology [2, 3].

In comparison to its relative rarity in the US, esophageal cancer (predominantly SCC) is endemic in parts of East Asia, which account for more than half of the approximately 500,000 cases that develop per year (this number does not fully take into account GE junction tumors, which may variously be categorized as gastric cancers) [4].

For locally advanced esophageal cancer, surgery remains the mainstay of treatment. Various reviews have reported five-year overall survival (OS) rates from 10% up to 30–40% with surgical resection alone [5, 6]. Numerous studies, which have included both adenocarcinoma and SCC histologies and focused on tumors from the esophagus and GE junction, have evaluated pre-operative strategies for locally advanced disease, including chemotherapy or chemoradiation, followed by surgery. Relatively few esophageal cancer-specific studies have focused on an adjuvant (post-operative) approach.

23.2 Pre-operative chemotherapy

Benefit for this approach has been mixed. The North American Intergroup 113 trial failed to show a survival benefit for three pre- and two post-operative cycles of peri-operative 5-fluorouracil (5-FU)/cisplatin plus surgery vs. surgery alone, in 440 patients with adenocarcinoma and SCC [7, 8]. Pathologic complete responses (pCR) were seen in only 2.5% of patients receiving pre-operative chemotherapy, and there was no improvement in the R0 resection rate. The median overall survival (OS) was not significantly different in the two groups, and the five-year OS with or without chemotherapy was 20%. Outcome also did not differ by histology, with no benefit seen for either adenocarcinoma or SCC.

On the other hand, the OEO2 trial, performed by the Medical Research Council Oesophageal Cancer Working Group, revealed a small benefit [9]. This study randomized 802 patients (nearly double the number of patients in the INT 113 trial) to surgery alone vs. two cycles of pre-operative 5-FU/cisplatin. It reported a modest improvement in five-year OS with chemotherapy (23% vs. 17%, $p = 0.03$) [10]. Two-thirds of patients had adenocarcinomas, and three-quarters of tumors were in the lower esophagus or gastric cardia. The limited benefit in this trial was purportedly because of improvements in the R0 resection rate from pre-operative chemotherapy, with no impact of chemotherapy on distant recurrence. This observation is also at odds with the INT 113 trial, where pre-operative chemotherapy failed to improve either R0 resection rates or survival.

Esophageal Cancer and Barrett's Esophagus, Third Edition. Edited by Prateek Sharma, Richard Sampliner and David Ilson.
© 2015 John Wiley & Sons, Ltd. Published 2015 by John Wiley & Sons, Ltd.

It may be that the larger sample size of the OEO2 study, compared with the Intergroup trial, facilitated the detection of a small improvement with chemotherapy. In addition, a larger proportion of patients on this trial had adenocarcinoma histology compared with the INT 113 trial (66% vs. 54%). An updated meta-analysis by Sjoquist *et al.* suggests a potentially greater survival benefit from pre-operative chemotherapy for patients with adenocarcinoma (hazard ratio or HR 0.83, 95% CI 0.71–0.95, $p = 0.01$) than SCC (HR 0.92, 0.81–1.04, $p = 0.07$) [11].

Other studies of pre- or peri-operative chemotherapy have enrolled gastric cancer patients but have also included patients with GE junction adenocarcinomas, which may be relevant to this patient population. The most prominent of these studies is the UK MAGIC (Medical Research Council Adjuvant Gastric Infusional Chemotherapy) trial [12]. This trial randomized 503 patients with gastric adenocarcinomas (26% of whom had tumors in the lower esophagus/GE junction) to three cycles each of pre- and post-operative ECF (epirubicin/cisplatin/5-FU) and surgery or surgery alone. Peri-operative chemotherapy resulted in significant improvement in five-year OS (36% vs. 23%, $p = 0.009$), establishing this regimen as a standard of care. On this trial, however, there was no improvement in the rate of R0 resection with preoperative chemotherapy.

A similar degree of benefit was also noted in the contemporaneous French FFCD 9703 trial, of 224 patients with esophagogastric adenocarcinoma (75% had tumors in the lower esophagus/GE junction) [13]. Patients were randomized to three cycles each of peri-operative 5-FU/cisplatin followed by surgery vs. surgery alone. Peri-operative chemotherapy on this trial was associated with a significant improvement in five-year disease-free survival (DFS; 34% vs. 19%, $p = 0.003$) and OS (38% vs. 24%, $p = 0.02$). Although comparisons between different clinical trials must be made cautiously, the survival benefit seen with 5-FU/cisplatin on this trial appears to be nearly identical to that seen with ECF in the MAGIC study. On this trial, R0 resection rate was superior on the preoperative chemotherapy arm.

In contrast, and most recently, the European EORTC 40954 trial evaluated a strategy of pre-operative 5-FU/leucovorin/cisplatin in 144 patients with GE junction and gastric adenocarcinoma [14]. The trial was stopped because of poor accrual, which limits the power of the study, and no differences in survival were detected. An improvement in the R0 resection rate in the pre-operative chemotherapy group in this trial failed to translate into any survival benefit.

These data are summarized in Table 23.1.

23.3 Post-operative therapy

Combined modality therapy in esophageal SCC has long focused on pre-operative strategies. The role of adjuvant therapy has not been studied extensively, and the data that are available suggest no clear benefit for such an approach.

Post-operative chemotherapy without pre-operative therapy was studied in two Japanese randomized trials, where patients with SCC histology were randomized to receive two cycles of chemotherapy with cisplatin/vindesine [15]. or 5-FU/cisplatin [16], respectively. While the trial with cisplatin/vindesine did not show any survival benefit, an unplanned subset analysis of the trial with 5-FU/cisplatin revealed a survival benefit for patients with lymph node involvement (five-year DFS 52% vs. 38%).

The possible benefit for post-operative therapy suggested by the above trial led to a subsequent Japanese trial that randomized 330 patients with SCC histology to surgery and either two cycles of pre- vs. post-operative 5-FU/cisplatin [17]. The results showed improved five-year OS for the pre-operative chemotherapy group (55% vs. 43%, $p = 0.04$), further raising questions about the value of adjuvant chemotherapy for these patients.

However, interpretation of these results is confounded by the fact that only 96 of the 166 patients randomized to post-operative chemotherapy received any treatment. 38 patients who had pN0 disease were not treated per protocol, because of the prior observation that adjuvant chemotherapy only benefited patients with lymph node involvement. Furthermore, this study observed that a survival benefit for pre-operative chemotherapy was seen only in N0 patients, which contrasted with the prior post-operative adjuvant study that claimed a benefit only in N1 patients.

In comparison, there have been no randomized evaluations of adjuvant chemotherapy for resected esophageal adenocarcinoma. However, two large phase

Table 23.1 Results of phase III peri-operative chemotherapy trials in esophageal and gastric cancer.

Treatment	Histology	No. of patients	R0 resection rate	Pathologic CR rate	Survival Median	Overall	Local failure*	Reference
Peri-op 5FU/Cis + surgery	Adeno (54%) + SCC	213	62%	2.5%	14.9 months	3-year 23%	32%	Kelsen et al. [7]
Surgery		227	59%	N/A	16.1 months	3-year 26%	31%	
Pre-op 5FU/Cis + surgery	Adeno (66%) + SCC	400	**60%**	NS	**16.8 months**	5-year **23%**	19%	Medical Research Council, [9] Allum et al. [10]
Surgery		402	**54%**	N/A	**13.3 months**	5-year **17%**	17%	
Peri-op ECF + surgery	Adeno	250	69%	0%	**24 months**	5-year **36%**	14%	Cunningham et al. [12]
Surgery		253	66%	N/A	**20 months**	5-year **23%**	21%	
Peri-op 5FU/Cis + surgery	Adeno	109	**87%**	NS	NS	5-year **38%**	24%	Ychou et al. [13]
Surgery		110	**74%**	N/A	NS	5-year **24%**	26%	
Pre-op 5FU/LV/Cis + surgery	Adeno (66%) + SCC	72	**82%**	7.1%	64.6 months	2-year 73%	NS	Schumacher et al. [14]
Surgery		72	**67%**	N/A	52.5 months	2-year 70%	NS	
Surgery	SCC	100	N/A		NS	5-year 45%	30%	Ando et al. [15]
Surgery + Cis/vindesine		105			NS	5-year 48%	30%	
Surgery	SCC	122	N/A		NS	5-year 52%	**46%**	Ando et al. [16]
Surgery + 5FU/Cis		120			NS	5-year 61%	**8%**	
5FU/Cis + Surgery	SCC	164	**90%**	2.4%	NS	5-year **55%**	NS	Ando et al. [17]
Surgery + 5FU/Cis		166	**88%**	N/A	NS	5-year **43%**	NS	
Surgery	Adeno (gastric)	530	N/A		NR	5-year **61%**	2.8%	Sakuramoto et al. [18], Sasako et al. [19]
Surgery +S-1		529			NR	5-year **72%**	1.3%	
Surgery	Adeno (gastric)	515	N/A		NR[+]	3-year[+] **59%**	44%	Bang et al. [20]
Surgery + Capeox		520			NR[+]	3-year[+] **74%**	21%	

Adeno – adenocarcinoma; cis – cisplatin; Capeox – capecitabine/oxaliplatin; CR – complete response; ECF – epirubicin, cisplatin, 5-fluoruoracil; 5FU – 5-fluorouracil; N/A – not applicable; NR – not reached; NS – not stated; RT – radiotherapy; SCC – squamous cell carcinoma.
*Local failure with or without distant recurrence; Numbers in bold indicate statistically significant differences.
[+]disease-free survival

III trials from East Asia have demonstrated a benefit for this approach in resected gastric cancer. These data support the use of adjuvant fluoropyrimidines as monotherapy [18, 19] and combination chemotherapy, with a fluoropyrimidine plus platinum agent [20]. The results should be interpreted with considerable caution, as these trials have exclusively enrolled patients with gastric adenocarcinoma. In East Asia, < 10% of tumors occur in the proximal stomach/GE junction, making it unclear if they are applicable to the patient population discussed in this review article.

In the US, a standard of care is adjuvant chemoradiation for resected GE junction adenocarcinomas, based primarily on the results of the Intergroup 116 trial [21]. This trial randomized 556 patients with gastric adenocarcinomas (20% of whom had tumors that involved the GE junction) to adjuvant chemotherapy and chemoradiation with bolus 5-FU/leucovorin vs. observation alone following surgery. Patients who received adjuvant chemoradiation had an improvement in relapse-free survival (three-year RFS 48% vs. 31%, $p < 0.001$) and OS (three-year OS 51% vs. 40%, $p = 0.005$).

Despite these positive results, this trial is frequently criticized because of the relatively inadequate surgical resections that were performed; 54% of patients had less than a D1 or D2 resection, which is less than a complete dissection of the involved lymph nodes. It has been argued that radiation in this setting compensated for inadequate surgery, because the greatest impact of adjuvant chemoradiation was a reduction in local recurrence of cancer. Such benefits may not be seen for radiotherapy if a more complete D1 or D2 surgical resection is undertaken. The size of the radiotherapy field for GE junction cancers, extending from the surgical bed high into the mediastinum to cover the anastamosis, is likely to exacerbate toxicity, and reinforces the application of pre- rather than post-operative chemoradiation for these patients.

23.4 Chemoradiation for medically inoperably patients

The seminal phase III US Radiation Therapy Oncology Group (RTOG) trial 85-01 demonstrated the superiority of chemoradiation over radiation alone [22]. This non-operative study compared radiation to 64 Gy with radiation (50 Gy) plus concurrent 5-FU/cisplatin. The trial was stopped when data from 121 patients showed an improved OS in favor of chemoradiation (12.5 months vs. 8.9 months), which was confirmed in longer follow-up confirmed (five-year OS 21% vs. 0%) [23]. Although the majority of patients treated on this trial had SCC, long-term survival was also seen in the small

number of adenocarcinoma patients on the trial, with 13% of patients alive at five years.

In addition to a survival benefit, disease recurrence was significantly reduced by the addition of chemotherapy to radiation. At one year, recurrent disease was observed in 62% of the group that received radiation vs. 44% in the chemoradiation arm. Distant recurrence rates were 38% and 22%, respectively. Based on this study, chemoradiation was established as the standard of care in the non-surgical management of locally advanced esophageal cancer.

23.5 Pre-operative chemoradiation

Six contemporary randomized trials subsequently compared chemoradiation followed by surgery vs. surgery alone [24–29]. The results are summarized in Table 23.2.

Overall, many of these trials are associated with methodological concerns (including the lack of rigorous pre-therapy staging with endoscopic ultrasound and/or laparoscopy), are significantly smaller than randomized preoperative chemotherapy trials, and produce conflicting results. Three each have been positive and negative.

A potential new standard of care was established by the rigorously conducted Dutch CROSS trial [29]. In this study of 366 evaluable patients with esophageal tumors (of which 75% and 65% respectively were adenocarcinomas and lymph node positive by endoscopic ultrasound), patients were randomized to pre-operative carboplatin/paclitaxel combined with 41.4 Gy of radiation vs. surgery alone. Pre-operative chemoradiation resulted in an improvement in R0 resection rates (92% vs. 67%, $p < 0.001$), in a pCR rate of 29% (23% for adenocarcinoma and 49% for SCC) and in improved OS compared to surgery alone (median OS 49.4 vs. 24.0 months, three-year OS 58% vs. 44%, $p = 0.003$). Pre-operative therapy was also relatively well-tolerated, with mostly grade 3 toxicities noted in only 20% of patients (13% non-hematologic, 7% hematologic). There did appear to be a greater degree of benefit for patients with SCC vs. adenocarcinoma histology (univariate HR for death 0.45 vs. 0.73), but all patients derived benefit.

While this study demonstrates a clear benefit for chemoradiation, it is not possible to conclude definitively that carboplatin/paclitaxel is the preferred

Table 23.2 Results of phase III pre-operative chemoradiation trials in esophageal cancer.

Treatment	Histology	No. of patients	R0 resection rate	Pathologic CR rate	Survival Median	Overall	Local failure*	Reference
Pre-op CRT	Adeno (76%) +	50	45%	24%	16.9 months	3-yr 30%	19%	Urba *et al.* [24]
Surgery	SCC	50	45%	N/A	17.6 months	3-yr 16%	42%	
Pre-op CRT	Adeno	58	NS	25%	**16 months**	3-yr **32%**	NS	Walsh *et al.* [25]
Surgery		55		N/A	**11 months**	3-yr **6%**		
Pre-op CRT	SCC	143	81%	26%	18.6 months	5-yr 26%	NS	Bosset *et al.* [26]
Surgery		139	69%	N/A	18.6 months	5-yr 26%		
Pre-op CRT	Adeno (63%) +	128	**80%**	9%	22.2 months	NS	15%	Burmeister *et al.* [27]
Surgery	SCC + other	128	**59%**	N/A	19.3 months	NS	26%	
Pre-op CRT	Adeno (75%) +	30	NS	40%	**4.5 years**	5-yr **39%**	NS	Tepper *et al.* [28
Surgery	SCC	26		N/A	**1.8 years**	5-yr **16%**		
Pre-op CRT	Adeno (74%) +	178	**92%**	29%	**49.4 months**	3-yr **58%**	NS	Van Hagen *et al.* [29]
Surgery	SCC	188	**69%**	N/A	**24.0 months**	3-yr **44%**		

Adeno – adenocarcinoma; CR – complete response; NS – not stated; Pre-op CRT – preoperative chemoradiation; SCC – squamous cell carcinoma

regimen combined with radiation relative to standard fluoropyrimidine/platinum doublet utilized in other trials. Nevertheless, the pCR rate of 49% in SCC is the highest ever reported in a phase III trial, while the pCR rate of 23% for adenocarcinomas compares favorably to other phase II/III studies. Coupled with the ease of administration and tolerability, carboplatin/paclitaxel may be considered the new standard of care and the reference regimen for future trial design.

23.6 Pre-operative chemoradiation vs. chemotherapy

The possible superiority of pre-operative chemoradiation over chemotherapy was suggested by the German POET (PreOperative Chemotherapy or Radiochemotherapy in Esophagogastric Adenocarcinoma Trial) study, in which patients with GE junction adenocarcinomas were randomized to either 5-FU/leucovorin/cisplatin followed by surgery vs. 5-FU/leucovorin/cisplatin followed by chemoradiation with cisplatin/etoposide and then surgery [30]. 119 eligible patients were randomized before the trial was

closed, due to poor accrual, limiting the power of this study to detect a difference between the treatment groups. Nevertheless, patients who received pre-operative chemoradiation had a higher pCR rate (15.6% vs. 2%, $p = 0.03$) and tumor-free lymph node status (ypN0 64.4% vs. 36.7%, $p = 0.01$) than those who received pre-operative chemotherapy. There were also trends toward an improvement in local control (76.5% vs. 59%, $p = 0.06$) and in three-year OS (47.4% vs. 27.7%, $p = 0.07$) for the chemoradiation group.

A similar non-significant trend toward improved outcomes with pre-operative chemoradiation over chemotherapy was also suggested by the meta-analysis by Sjoquist *et al*, which revealed an all-cause mortality HR of 0.88 (95% CI 0.76-1.01, $p = 0.07$).

23.7 Definitive vs. pre-operative chemoradiation

Two randomized European trials have compared definitive chemoradiation vs. chemoradiation followed by surgery in esophageal SCC patients [31, 32]. Taken together, both studies suggest that local control is improved by subsequent surgery but that there is no clear improvement in survival.

An interesting question that arises from one of these studies (the FFCD 9102 trial), is whether patients who do not respond to initial therapy benefit from subsequent surgery. In this study, patients received initial treatment with 5-FU/cisplatin and radiation, and only responders were subsequently randomized to surgery vs. more chemoradiation. In an abstract presentation, the authors discussed the outcome of the 192 of the 451 registered patients who were not randomized to further protocol therapy after initial chemoradiation, primarily because of a lack of response, but also because of medical contraindication or patient refusal [33]. Of these non-randomized patients, 112 subsequently underwent surgery, with 80 undergoing R0 resections.

The median OS for the patients who underwent surgery was significantly superior to the median OS of those who did not (17.3 vs. 6.1 months), and was comparable to the median OS of the patients who were randomized. While there are clear limitations and potential strong confounders to such an analysis, these data suggest that salvage esophagectomy may be beneficial for a subset of patients who do not respond to initial therapy.

23.8 Newer chemoradiation regimens

Although the CROSS study established that carboplatin/paclitaxel and radiation is a new standard of care, the question of whether this chemotherapy regimen is superior to the traditional 5-FU/cisplatin doublet remains unanswered. In fact, the few studies that have directly compared different chemotherapy regimens with radiation suggest that no specific regimen is clearly superior to 5-FU/cisplatin, in terms of toxicity or efficacy.

Paclitaxel-based chemotherapy was compared in the randomized phase II RTOG trial 0113, where a regimen of induction 5-FU/cisplatin/paclitaxel, followed by weekly 5-FU/paclitaxel and radiation, was compared to induction cisplatin/paclitaxel and weekly cisplatin/paclitaxel with radiation as definitive therapy in locally advanced disease [34]. Neither arm achieved the pre-specified one-year survival rate, although there appeared to be a non-significant trend towards improved survival in the 5-FU-containing arm (median

OS 29 vs. 15 months). Both arms were also associated with a grade 3/4 toxicity rate of > 80%. The authors concluded that neither arm was sufficiently superior to historical cisplatin/5-FU and radiation to warrant further investigation.

The Eastern Cooperative Oncology Group 1201 trial compared two non-5-FU based regimens – weekly cisplatin/irinotecan vs. weekly cisplatin/paclitaxel – with concurrent radiation, followed by surgery and adjuvant therapy, with the respective pre-operative regimens in patients with esophageal adenocarcinoma [35]. The results – so far presented only in abstract form – revealed a disappointingly low pCR rate of 15% and 16%, respectively, with a toxicity profile comparable to that historically noted with standard 5-FU/cisplatin and radiation. Median OS in the cisplatin/irinotecan arm was 34.9 months, while median OS in the cisplatin/paclitaxel arm was 21 months (with overlapping confidence intervals for both arms) [36]. The conclusion is that neither regimen is clearly superior to conventional 5-FU/cisplatin and radiation.

Most recently, the French PRODIGE 5/ACCORD 17 study randomized 267 patients (86% with SCC) to 5-FU/cisplatin or FOLFOX (infusional 5-FU/leucovorin/oxaliplatin) and radiation [37]. Data presented in abstract form indicate, once again, comparable toxicities and outcomes for these regimens. Nevertheless, there were fewer toxic deaths seen on the FOLFOX arm, supporting the use of infusional 5-FU and oxaliplatin as an alterative to 5-FU/cisplatin.

23.9 Targeted therapies

The UK MAGIC-B trial is randomizing patients with locally advanced gastric and GE junction cancer to perioperative ECX chemotherapy (epirubicin/cisplatin/capecitabine) with or without bevacizumab, a monoclonal antibody against vascular endothelial growth factor. However, two single-arm phase II trials combining bevacizumab (alone [38], or with erlotinib [39], an oral tyrosine kinase inhibitor against epidermal growth factor receptor or EGFR) with pre-operative chemoradiation have failed to show an improvement in outcomes, compared with historical controls.

Recently, the results of the UK SCOPE 1 study, a phase III evaluation of the anti-EGFR antibody cetuximab with chemoradiation, actually revealed inferior outcomes for its addition to standard therapy [40]. No benefit for the addition of cetuximab to chemoradiation was also recently reported on the RTOG 0436 study, a phase III evaluation of cisplatin/paclitaxel and radiation, with or without cetuximab, enrolling SCC and adenocarcinoma patients [41].

The RTOG 1010 study (NCT01196390) is an ongoing phase III evaluation of carboplatin/paclitaxel and radiation, with or without trastuzumab, an antibody against Her2, for patients with Her2 positive esophageal and GE junction tumors. Patients randomized to receive trastuzumab will also receive it as monotherapy for one year following surgery. Trastuzumab is currently the only Food and Drug Administration-approved targeted agent for advanced esophagogastric adenocarcinoma that is Her2 positive.

23.10 Positron emission tomography-directed therapy

[^{18}F]2-fluoro-deoxy-D-glucose positron emission tomography (FDG-PET) scanning is emerging as an important tool to investigate response to therapy. Several studies in esophagogastric tumors have demonstrated that the degree of response detected by PET, following preoperative chemoradiation [42, 43] or chemotherapy [44, 45], is highly correlated with pathologic response at surgery and with patient survival.

The German MUNICON trial evaluated the strategy of taking patients with locally advanced GE junction adenocarcinomas with a suboptimal response to two weeks of induction chemotherapy with 5-FU/cisplatin – as determined by serial PET scans – directly to immediate surgery, instead of continuing with presumably ineffective chemotherapy. Patients with a metabolic response by PET (defined as = 35% reduction in standard uptake value between baseline and repeat PET scan) continued with an additional 12 weeks of chemotherapy prior to surgery [46].

This trial revealed a significantly improved R0 resection rate (96% vs. 74%, $p = 0.002$), major pathologic response rate (58% vs. 0%, $p = 0.001$ and median OS (median not reached vs. 25.8 months, $p = 0.015$) for PET responders vs. PET non-responders. The outcome for PET non-responders referred for immediate surgery was similar to the outcome of such patients in an earlier trial who completed three months of pre-operative chemotherapy [44], indicating that non-responding patients were not compromised by referral to immediate surgery. These results, therefore, support the early discontinuation of inactive pre-operative chemotherapy in PET non-responder patients.

Building on the results of the MUNICON trial, the MUNICON-2 trial attempted to improve outcome in the PET non-responders to the same regimen of pre-operative 5-FU/cisplatin by treating them with "salvage" chemoradiation prior to surgery [47]. When compared to the PET responders who completed three months of 5-FU/cisplatin before surgery, the PET non-responders had inferior two-year PFS (64% vs. 33%, $p = 0.035$) and a trend toward inferior two-year OS (71% vs. 42%, $p = 0.10$). These results likely speak to the underlying unfavorable biology of the tumors of PET non-responders, but do not rule out the possibility that such patients can receive effective salvage therapy. In this trial, the chemotherapy (cisplatin), administered with an unusually low dose of 32 Gy of radiation, had already been assessed to be associated with sub-optimal outcomes by PET when administered as induction therapy.

As such, another possible strategy would be to use PET assessment after induction chemotherapy to dictate subsequent chemotherapy during concurrent radiation. Our group has reported long-term disease-free survival in patients who progressed on induction chemotherapy but were changed to alternative chemotherapy during subsequent combined chemoradiation [48].

Based on this concept, the Cancer and Leukemia Group B has launched the 80803 trial (NCT01333033), which is enrolling patients with esophageal and GE junction adenocarcinomas. They are randomized to receive induction chemotherapy with either carboplatin/paclitaxel, or a modification of the FOLFOX6 regimen. Responses to induction chemotherapy are then adjudicated with an early PET scan performed after induction chemotherapy. While PET responders continue with the same regimen during concurrent radiation, PET non-responders are changed to the alternative regimen with radiation prior to surgery. The primary endpoint is to improve the rate of pathologic response in PET non-responder patients, by changing chemotherapy during combined chemoradiation.

23.11 Conclusion

While the treatment of esophageal cancer presents a great challenge to medical, surgical, and radiation oncologists, completed trials over the last decade now indicate that more than surgery alone should be offered to patients.

Primary chemoradiation remains the standard of care in the treatment of inoperable, localized disease. The large and well-conducted CROSS study demonstrates clear benefit for pre-operative chemoradiation, which is associated with a significant pCR rate and improvement in R0 resection. For patients undergoing primary resection of lower esophageal and GE junction adenocarcinoma, post-operative chemoradiation may improve survival, compared with surgery alone.

In SCC patients, definitive chemoradiation is an accepted approach, especially for patients who achieve a clinical CR. For patients with locally persistent disease after chemoradiation, surgery may be an effective salvage option.

Several recent trials have suggested that pre-, peri- or post-operative chemotherapy is also a valid strategy in adenocarcinoma, although the benefits in SCC are much less clear. Based on the POET study and a large meta-analysis, pre-operative chemoradiation may be superior to chemotherapy.

Investigational approaches continue to focus on the addition of targeted agents. However, phase II evaluations of bevacizumab and chemoradiation have been disappointing, and the SCOPE 1 study actually showed a detriment for adding cetuximab to chemoradiation, while RTOG 0436 also failed to improve outcome with the use of cetuximab. Ongoing efforts include the RTOG 1010 study (which is adding trastuzumab to chemoradiation for Her2 positive tumors) and the CALGB 80803 study (which uses PET scans to assess response to chemotherapy and to guide treatment during concurrent radiation).

References

1 Siegel R, Naishadham D, Jemal A (2013). Cancer statistics. *CA: A Cancer Journal for Clinicians (2013)* **63**(1), 11–30.

2 Crew KD, Neugut AI (2004). Epidemiology of upper gastrointestinal malignancies. *Seminars in Oncology* **31**(4), 450–64.

3 Devesa SS, Fraumeni JF, Jr. (1999). The rising incidence of gastric cardia cancer. *Journal of the National Cancer Institute* **91**(9), 747–9.

4 Ferlay J, Shin HR, Bray F, Forman D, Mathers C, Parkin DM (2008). Estimates of worldwide burden of cancer in 2008: GLOBOCAN 2008. *International Journal of Cancer* **127**(12), 2893–917.

5 Muller JM, Erasmi H, Stelzner M, Zieren U, Pichlmaier H (1990). Surgical therapy of oesophageal carcinoma. *British Journal of Surgery* **77**(8), 845–57.

6 Hulscher JB, van Sandick JW, de Boer AG, Wijnhoven BP, Tijssen JG, Fockens P, *et al.* (2002). Extended transthoracic resection compared with limited transhiatal resection for adenocarcinoma of the esophagus. *New England Journal of Medicine* **347**(21), 1662–9.

7 Kelsen DP, Ginsberg R, Pajak TF, Sheahan DG, Gunderson L, Mortimer J, *et al.* (1998). Chemotherapy followed by surgery compared with surgery alone for localized esophageal cancer. *New England Journal of Medicine* **339**(27), 1979–84.

8 Kelsen DP, Winter KA, Gunderson LL, Mortimer J, Estes NC, Haller DG, *et al.* (2007). Long-term results of RTOG trial 8911 (USA Intergroup 113), a random assignment trial comparison of chemotherapy followed by surgery compared with surgery alone for esophageal cancer. *Journal of Clinical Oncology* **25**(24), 3719–25.

9 Medical Research Council Oesophageal Cancer Working Group (2002). Surgical resection with or without preoperative chemotherapy in oesophageal cancer: a randomised controlled trial. *Lancet* **359**(9319), 1727–33.

10 Allum WH, Stenning SP, Bancewicz J, Clark PI, Langley RE (2009). Long-term results of a randomized trial of surgery with or without preoperative chemotherapy in esophageal cancer. *Journal of Clinical Oncology* **27**(30), 5062–7.

11 Sjoquist KM, Burmeister BH, Smithers BM, Zalcberg JR, Simes RJ, Barbour A, *et al.* (2011). Survival after neoadjuvant chemotherapy or chemoradiotherapy for resectable oesophageal carcinoma: an updated meta-analysis. *The Lancet Oncology* **12**(7), 681–92.

12 Cunningham D, Allum WH, Stenning SP, Thompson JN, Van de Velde CJ, Nicolson M, *et al.* (2006). Perioperative chemotherapy versus surgery alone for resectable gastroesophageal cancer. *New England Journal of Medicine* **355**(1), 11–20.

13 Ychou M, Boige V, Pignon JP, Conroy T, Bouche O, Lebreton G, *et al.* (2011), Perioperative chemotherapy compared with surgery alone for resectable gastroesophageal adenocarcinoma: an FNCLCC and FFCD multicenter phase III trial. *Journal of Clinical Oncology* **29**(13), 1715–21.

14 Schuhmacher C, Gretschel S, Lordick F, Reichardt P, Hohenberger W, Eisenberger CF, *et al.* (2010)Neoadjuvant chemotherapy compared with surgery alone for locally advanced cancer of the stomach and cardia: European Organisation for Research and Treatment of Cancer randomized trial 40954. *Journal of Clinical Oncology* **28**(35), 5210–8.

15 Ando N, Iizuka T, Kakegawa T, Isono K, Watanabe H, Ide H, *et al.* (1997). A randomized trial of surgery with and without chemotherapy for localized squamous carcinoma of the thoracic esophagus: the Japan Clinical Oncology Group Study. *Journal of Thoracic and Cardiovascular Surgery* **114**(2), 205–9.

16 Ando N, Iizuka T, Ide H, Ishida K, Shinoda M, Nishimaki T, *et al.* (2003). Surgery plus chemotherapy compared with surgery alone for localized squamous cell carcinoma of the thoracic esophagus: a Japan Clinical Oncology Group Study – JCOG9204. *Journal of Clinical Oncology* **21**(24), 4592–6.

17 Ando N, Kato H, Igaki H, Shinoda M, Ozawa S, Shimizu H, *et al.* (2012). A randomized trial comparing postoperative adjuvant chemotherapy with cisplatin and 5-fluorouracil versus preoperative chemotherapy for localized advanced squamous cell carcinoma of the thoracic esophagus (JCOG9907). *Annals of Surgical Oncology* **19**(1), 68–74.

18 Sakuramoto S, Sasako M, Yamaguchi T, Kinoshita T, Fujii M, Nashimoto A, *et al.* (2007). Adjuvant chemotherapy for gastric cancer with S-1, an oral fluoropyrimidine. *New England Journal of Medicine* **357**(18), 1810–20.

19 Sasako M, Sakuramoto S, Katai H, Kinoshita T, Furukawa H, Yamaguchi T, *et al.* (2011). Five-year outcomes of a randomized phase III trial comparing adjuvant chemotherapy with S-1 versus surgery alone in stage II or III gastric cancer. *Journal of Clinical Oncology* **29**(33), 4387–93.

20 Bang YJ, Kim YW, Yang HK, Chung HC, Park YK, Lee KH, *et al.* (2012). Adjuvant capecitabine and oxaliplatin for gastric cancer after D2 gastrectomy (CLASSIC): a phase 3 open-label, randomised controlled trial. *Lancet* **379**(9813), 315–21.

21 Macdonald JS, Smalley SR, Benedetti J, Hundahl SA, Estes NC, Stemmermann GN, *et al.* (2001). Chemoradiotherapy after surgery compared with surgery alone for adenocarcinoma of the stomach or gastroesophageal ction. *New England Journal of Medicine* **345**(10), 725–30.

22 Herskovic A, tz K, al-Sarraf M, Leichman L, Brindle J, Vaitkevicius V, *et al.* (1992). Combined chemotherapy and radiotherapy compared with radiotherapy alone in patients with cancer of the esophagus. *New England Journal of Medicine* **326**(24), 1593–8.

23 Cooper JS, Guo MD, Herskovic A, Macdonald JS, tenson JA, Jr., Al-Sarraf M, *et al.* (1999). Chemoradiotherapy of locally advanced esophageal cancer: long-term follow-up of a prospective randomized trial (RTOG 85-01). Radiation Therapy Oncology Group. *JAMA* **281**(17), 1623–7.

24 Urba SG, Orringer MB, Turrisi A, Iannettoni M, Forastiere A, Strawderman M (2001). Randomized trial of preoperative chemoradiation versus surgery alone in patients with locoregional esophageal carcinoma. *Journal of Clinical Oncology* **19**(2), 305–13.

25 Walsh TN, Noonan N, Hollywood D, Kelly A, Keeling N, Hennessy TP (1996). A comparison of multimodal therapy and surgery for esophageal adenocarcinoma. *New England Journal of Medicine* **335**(7), 462–7.

26 Bosset JF, Gignoux M, Triboulet JP, Tiret E, Mantion G, Elias D, *et al.* (1997). Chemoradiotherapy followed by surgery compared with surgery alone in squamous-cell cancer of the esophagus. *New England Journal of Medicine* **337**(3), 161–7.

27 Burmeister BH, Smithers BM, Gebski V, Fitzgerald L, Simes RJ, Devitt P, *et al.* (2005). Surgery alone versus chemoradiotherapy followed by surgery for resectable cancer of the oesophagus: a randomised controlled phase III trial. *The Lancet Oncology* **6**(9), 659–68.

28 Tepper J, Krasna MJ, Niedzwiecki D, Hollis D, Reed CE, Goldberg R, *et al.* (2008). Phase III trial of trimodality therapy with cisplatin, fluorouracil, radiotherapy, and surgery compared with surgery alone for esophageal cancer: CALGB 9781. *Journal of Clinical Oncology* **26**(7), 1086–92.

29 van Hagen P, Hulshof MC, van Lanschot JJ, Steyerberg EW, van Berge Henegouwen MI, Wijnhoven BP, *et al.* (2012). Preoperative chemoradiotherapy for esophageal or ctional cancer. *New England Journal of Medicine* **366**(22), 2074–84.

30 Stahl M, Walz MK, Stuschke M, Lehmann N, Meyer HJ, Riera-Knorrenschild J, *et al.* (2009). Phase III comparison of preoperative chemotherapy compared with chemoradiotherapy in patients with locally advanced adenocarcinoma of the esophagogastric ction. *Journal of Clinical Oncology* **27**(6), 851–6.

31 Stahl M, Stuschke M, Lehmann N, Meyer HJ, Walz MK, Seeber S, *et al.* (2005). Chemoradiation with and without surgery in patients with locally advanced squamous cell carcinoma of the esophagus. *Journal of Clinical Oncology* **23**(10), 2310–7.

32 Bedenne L, Michel P, Bouche O, Milan C, iette C, Conroy T, *et al.* (2007). Chemoradiation Followed by Surgery Compared With Chemoradiation Alone in Squamous Cancer of the Esophagus: FFCD 9102. *Journal of Clinical Oncology* **25**(10), 1160–8.

33 Jouve J, Michel P, Mariette C, Bonnetain F, Bouché O, Conroy T, *et al.* (eds, 2008). Outcome of the nonrandomized patients in the FFCD 9102 trial: Chemoradiation followed by surgery compared with chemoradiation alone in squamous cancer of the esophagus. *Journal of Clinical Oncology* **26**(Suppl), 4555 [abstr].

34 Ajani JA, Winter K, Komaki R, Kelsen DP, Minsky BD, Liao Z, *et al.* (2008). Phase II randomized trial of two nonoperative regimens of induction chemotherapy followed by chemoradiation in patients with localized carcinoma of the esophagus: RTOG 0113. *Journal of Clinical Oncology* **26**(28), 4551–6.

35 Kleinberg L, Powell M, Forastiere A, Keller S, Anne P, Benson A (eds, 2007). E1201: An Eastern Cooperative Oncology Group (ECOG) randomized phase II trial of neoadjuvant preoperative paclitaxel/cisplatin/RT or irinotecan/cisplatin/RT in endoscopy with ultrasound (EUS) staged adenocarcinoma of the esophagus. *Journal of Clinical Oncology* **25**, 4533 [abstr].

36 Kleinberg L, Powell M, Forastiere A, Keller S, Anne P, Benson A (eds, 2008). Survival outcome of E1201: An Eastern Cooperative Oncology Group (ECOG) randomized phase II trial of neoadjuvant preoperative paclitaxel/cisplatin/radiotherapy (RT) or irinotecan/cisplatin/RT in endoscopy with ultrasound (EUS) staged esophageal adenocarcinoma. *Journal of Clinical Oncology* **26**, 4532 [abstr].

37 Conroy T, Galais M-P, Raoul J, Bouche O, Gourgou-Bourgade S, Douillard J-Y, *et al.* (eds, 2012). Phase III randomized trial of definitive chemoradiotherapy (CRT) with FOLFOX or cisplatin and fluorouracil in esophageal *Cancer* (EC): Final results of the PRODIGE 5/ACCORD 17 trial. *Journal of Clinical Oncology* **30**, LBA4003 [abstr].

38 Ilson D, Goodman K, jigian Y, Shah M, Kelsen D, Rizk N, *et al.* (eds, 2012). Phase II trial of bevacizumab, irinotecan, cisplatin, and radiation as preoperative therapy in esophageal adenocarcinoma. *Journal of Clinical Oncology* **30**, 67 [abstr].

39 Bendell JC, Meluch A, Peyton J, Rubin M, Waterhouse D, Webb C, *et al.* (2012). A phase II trial of preoperative concurrent chemotherapy/radiation therapy plus bevacizumab/erlotinib in the treatment of localized esophageal cancer. *Clinical Advances in Hematology and Oncology* **10**(7), 430–7.

40 Crosby T, Hurt CN, Falk S, Gollins S, Mukherjee S, Staffurth J, *et al.* (2013). Chemoradiotherapy with or without cetuximab in patients with oesophageal *Cancer* (SCOPE1): a multicentre, phase 2/3 randomised trial. *The Lancet Oncology* **14**(7), 627–37.

41 Ilson D, Moughan J, Suntharalingam M, Dicker A, Kachnic L, Konski A, *et al.* (eds, 2014). RTOG 0436: A phase III trial evaluating the addition of cetuximab to paclitaxel, cisplatin, and radiation for patients with esophageal cancer treated without surgery. *Journal of Clinical Oncology* **32**, 4007 [abstr].

42 Downey RJ, Akhurst T, Ilson D, Ginsberg R, Bains MS, Gonen M, *et al.* (2003). Whole body 18FDG-PET and the response of esophageal cancer to induction therapy: results of a prospective trial. *Journal of Clinical Oncology* **21**(3), 428–32.

43 Flamen P, Van Cutsem E, Lerut A, Cambier JP, Haustermans K, Bormans G, *et al.* (2002). Positron emission tomography for assessment of the response to induction radiochemotherapy in locally advanced oesophageal cancer. *Annals of Oncology* **13**(3), 361–8.

44 Ott K, Weber WA, Lordick F, Becker K, Busch R, Herrmann K, *et al.* (2006). Metabolic imaging predicts response, survival, and recurrence in adenocarcinomas of the esophagogastric ction. *Journal of Clinical Oncology* **24**(29), 4692–8.

45 Weber WA, Ott K, Becker K, Dittler HJ, Helmberger H, Avril NE, *et al.* (2001). Prediction of response to preoperative chemotherapy in adenocarcinomas of the esophagogastric ction by metabolic imaging. *Journal of Clinical Oncology* **19**(12), 3058–65.

46 Lordick F, Ott K, Krause BJ, Weber WA, Becker K, Stein HJ, *et al.* (2007). PET to assess early metabolic response and to guide treatment of adenocarcinoma of the oesophagogastric ction: the MUNICON phase II trial. *The Lancet Oncology* **8**(9), 797–805.

47 zum Buschenfelde CM, Herrmann K, Schuster T, Geinitz H, Langer R, Becker K, *et al.* (2011). (18)F-FDG PET-guided salvage neoadjuvant radiochemotherapy of adenocarcinoma of the esophagogastric action: the MUNICON II trial. *Journal of Nuclear Medicine* **52**(8), 1189–96.

48 Ilson DH, Minsky BD, Ku GY, Rusch V, Rizk N, Shah M, *et al.* (2012). Phase 2 trial of induction and concurrent chemoradiotherapy with weekly irinotecan and cisplatin followed by surgery for esophageal cancer. *Cancer* **118**(11), 2820–7.

CHAPTER 24

Surgery in locally advanced esophageal cancer

Nabil Rizk

Department of Surgery, Memorial Sloan Kettering Cancer Center, New York, NY, USA

24.1 Introduction

In the present era, surgery in patients with locally advanced esophageal cancer implies surgery after pre-operative therapy, most typically after chemoradiation. Esophagectomy for esophageal cancers remains a highly complex, high-risk operation, fraught with high complication rates. However, these issues are more germane after pre-operative therapy, especially when radiation therapy is used, due to a perception that the risks are accentuated after such therapies. This chapter reviews the available literature, in an effort to identify true concerns and considerations when performing esophagectomy after pre-operative therapy. The specific issues which will be addressed, concerning esophagectomy after chemoradiation, will include:

1 the relative incidence of technical and post-operative complications, with a focus on anastomotic leaks;

2 technical intra-operative considerations, including the need for an adequate lymph node resection as dictated by the operative approach, and achieving a clear surgical margin;

3 the added risks of salvage surgery after definitive chemoradiotherapy.

24.2 Chemotherapy, chemoradiation and surgical complications

The impact on surgical risks of chemoradiation prior to an esophagectomy has been a highly debated topic during the course of the past two decades. In fact, a large part of the resistance to evaluating, and even adopting, this approach was the perception that pre-operative chemoradiation added significantly to surgical morbidity and mortality [1, 2]. Some prospective and retrospective studies showed a significant increase in mortality [3], and some specifically noted an increase in respiratory complications, anastomotic leak, thoracic duct leaks, and thromboembolic events [4]. Other studies showed that an increase in these risks was present mainly in older patients, variably defined as patients older than 70 [5, 6] or older than 80 [7].

The increase in these risks was attributed to radiation, in particular post-operative pneumonitis [8], and the effect of radiation on the ability of the gastric conduit to heal properly at the anastomotic site, due to the potential radiation-induced tissue ischemia and damaged microvasculature. This increased anastomotic leak risk was noted in situations where there was significant radiation targeted to the gastric conduit beyond the site of the resected stomach [9]. The potential deleterious impact of radiation, leading to conduit ischemia, was reinforced in studies where the anastomoses were performed in the neck, with the implication that more damaged, irradiated stomach was retained in these patients [4]. The attribution of increased risk of radiation was also reinforced by clinical trials of pre-operative chemotherapy alone, without radiotherapy, where the peri-operative risks appeared no greater than in those who did not receive any therapy prior to surgery [10, 11].

Many of the concerns regarding the impact of chemoradiation prior to surgery have been allayed by the recent results of the CROSS trial [12]. No differences were noted in morbidity or mortality in

Esophageal Cancer and Barrett's Esophagus, Third Edition. Edited by Prateek Sharma, Richard Sampliner and David Ilson.
© 2015 John Wiley & Sons, Ltd. Published 2015 by John Wiley & Sons, Ltd.

the chemoradiation arm, relative to the surgery-only group. The lack of any significant impact on complications noted in this trial has been attributed to modern radiation planning, which spared the gastric conduit by limiting the radiation fields to less than 4 cm above and below the tumor, as well as the improved tolerability of the chemotherapy regimen used in this trial. What this trial did not fully resolve, however, is whether or not concerns of multimodality therapy remain relevant in "older" patients, since the CROSS population median age was 60, and no site-specific breakdown of complications by age was provided. Likewise, in the CROSS trial, anastomoses were done both in the chest and in the neck, but no breakdown was provided regarding the leak rate (22–30%) relative to the anastomotic site. It is conceivable that there was a differential impact on leaks, based on the site of the anastomosis.

24.3 Technical considerations

A fundamental surgical dictum, based on little supporting data, is that a planned surgical resection after chemotherapy or chemoradiotherapy should incorporate all known sites of disease present *prior to* the pre-operative treatment, rather than those visibly present after tumor regression has occurred. One reason for this assumption is that it is not possible definitively to prove the lack of viable disease in a regressed, previously tumor-bearing area without actually removing it. This assumption has important implications when considering a surgical approach in pre-treated patients, especially regarding issues of the extent of lymphadenectomy and pathologic margins.

24.3.1 Lymphadenectomy
There are convincing data, both retrospective [13–16] and prospective [17–19], supporting an association between a more aggressive lymphadenectomy and improved survival in surgically treated patients with esophageal cancer. Furthermore, these data show that this association is most relevant in patients who are at the highest risk of having nodal disease [15]. Similar lymphadenectomy data are not available in patients who received pre-operative therapy, where the expected number of involved lymph nodes may be less due to nodal down-staging [12] and the expected overall yield of lymph nodes removed at the time of

surgery on average is less than in untreated patients [12]. However, the assumption remains that there are potential benefits to removing more lymph nodes in these patients.

The goal of an adequate lymphadenectomy after pre-operative therapy should, in part, dictate the surgical approach. Since most patients who receive pre-operative therapy have locally advanced disease (i.e. T2–3), an appropriate lymphadenectomy should include 30 nodes or more removed. While there have been various cut-off values presented in the literature regarding an adequate lymphadenectomy, and while the AJCC staging system requires 15 nodes to be removed, the best available data was derived from the WECC analysis [15], wherein the extent of lymphadenectomy was correlated to the risk of nodal disease. In this analysis, untreated patients with T2–3 tumors had the best survival when more than a total of 30 lymph nodes were removed.

In most patients, an intra-abdominal and intra-thoracic lymphadenectomy (i.e. two-field) should be done. The intra-abdominal component should include celiac, splenic, and common hepatic lymph nodes [20], and the intra-thoracic lymphadenectomy should include all the lymph nodes from the sub-carinal space down to the hiatus. Because of these requirements, an intra-thoracic approach is necessary to remove all potentially involved lymph nodes, and an approach such as a trans-hiatal esophagectomy might be considered inadequate in these patients. This can be achieved with either an open or a minimally invasive approach.

24.3.2 Margins
A key goal of esophagectomy, and an indication of good surgical planning and surgical technique, is the achievement of margins free of disease (R0 resection). The presence of uninvolved surgical resection margins, both proximal-distal and radial, has been associated with improved survival in surgically treated patients [21–23]. With regard to radial margins, many studies have shown that pre-operative chemoradiotherapy significantly increases the likelihood of achieving an R0 resection when compared to either surgery alone [12, 24] or chemotherapy alone [11], without any alteration of surgical technique. Presumably, this is due to the sterilization of the tumor's radial margins. Because of this sterilization of the margins, however, some have questioned whether pre-operative radiation is

used by some to supplement a poor surgical technique. These critics cite data showing that a more aggressive resection, such as an *en bloc* esophagectomy, which includes resection of the thoracic duct, pericardium, and contralateral pleura, can achieve R0 resection rates equivalent to those in patients undergoing pre-operative chemoradiotherapy [25, 26].

Proximal and distal margins are rarely positive if appropriate surgical planning is done, which should include careful pre- and post-treatment endoscopic evaluation. A particular issue that arises in previously treated patients, however, is establishing the extent of tumor extension after pre-operative therapy, both in regards to the initial extent of disease and also distinguishing treated normal tissue from disease. The latter problem is particularly relevant in patients who received a wider radiation field than usual. As a result of the uncertainty in distinguishing treated disease, extent of original disease, and treatment effect on normal tissue, it is often difficult intra-operatively to decide how proximal and distal the resection needs to be. While technically one can usually remove additional esophagus and obtain true negative proximal margins, this issue is more problematic in patients with disease extension into the gastric cardia and sub-cardia regions. In these patients, if a gastric conduit is to be used, the extent of a possible distal resection is limited, due to technical considerations (conduit size, vascular supply).

A reasonable solution to these proximal and distal margin issues is for the surgeon to carefully perform a pre-treatment endoscopy, in order to carefully map out the extent of disease prior to treatment, and to plan the ultimate surgical approach and extent of resection based on this original endoscopy. This would include, for instance, adhering to a pre-treatment planned gastrectomy and esophagectomy, despite clinical evidence of disease regression, which would otherwise seem to permit performing a lesser resection.

A separate technical issue, which arises more commonly in previously treated patients, is an intra-operative finding of an involved proximal or distal resection margin on frozen section. In these patients, if achieving negative margins requires a significant extension of the procedure, one reasonable approach is to defer the extended procedure until the final pathology is available. If the patient's prognosis based on the pathology is poor [27], then a more

extensive, and likely morbid, procedure is likely to be of little benefit to the patient.

24.4 Risks of salvage surgery

The approach of definitive chemoradiation, with salvage esophagectomy when needed, is increasingly used in patients with squamous cell carcinoma, given the vigorous clinical response seen in these patients [28]. Salvage esophagectomy is defined as a surgical resection in patients who develop recurrent esophageal cancer, following a clinical complete response after definitive non-surgical treatment with chemoradiation. There is no defined time for this intervention after chemoradiation is completed, although the length of time after completion of radiation is frequently cited as a risk factor for complications.

While salvage esophagectomy has appeal, in that it could possibly avoid an "unnecessary" esophagectomy in patients deemed to have a complete clinical response, there are significant concerns regarding the potential for added surgical risks. Data supporting these concerns are typically from retrospective surgical series, in which patients undergo a salvage esophagectomy only because they were not deemed to be a surgical candidate in the first place. As such, these data should be considered highly biased. There are several series in the literature that claim that complication rates are significantly higher in patients who undergo a salvage esophagectomy [29–32]. The potential delayed effect of radiation, including the impact on healing of the anastomosis and the higher risks of pneumonitis, is frequently cited.

An additional concern expressed by some is the increased technical difficulty encountered when resecting these patients, in whom the esophagus can be densely adherent (either with scar or with tumor) to surrounding structures, including the aorta and the airway. In these patients, if intra-operatively they are found to be technically unresectable, the only potentially palliative surgical options available are either an esophageal diversion or a bypass – potentially avoidable morbid scenarios, had the patients undergone a resection after initial completion of pre-operative therapy. A reasonable approach, if contemplating a salvage esophagectomy, is to use it selectively in patients in whom a planned post-treatment esophagectomy is felt to be more morbid than the risks associated with a possible salvage esophagectomy. This should also take into consideration the experience of the institution where the esophagectomy would be performed.

24.5 Conclusion

Many of the concerns regarding an increased risk of complications after esophagectomy which have been attributed to pre-operative chemoradiation appear to have been unfounded, based on recent randomized data, where no association was seen. There remain, however, particular technical considerations, which should be incorporated into the surgical approach, including the extent of lymphadenectomy and the achievement of negative surgical margins. Lastly, the association between complications and salvage esophagectomy remains unresolved. Many surgeons express particular concern about the delayed impact of radiation on tissue healing and the increased likelihood of unresectability due to the obliteration of tissue planes.

References

1 Walsh TN, Noonan N, Hollywood D, Kelly A, Keeling N, Hennessy TP (1996). A comparison of multimodal therapy and surgery for esophageal adenocarcinoma. *New England Journal of Medicine* **335**(7), 462–7.

2 Bosset JF, Gignoux M, Triboulet JP, Tiret E, Mantion G, Elias D, Lozach P, Ollier JC, Pavy JJ, Mercier M, Sahmoud T (1997). Chemoradiotherapy followed by surgery compared with surgery alone in squamous-cell cancer of the esophagus. *New England Journal of Medicine* **337**(3), 161–7.

3 Stahl M, Stuschke M, Lehmann N, Meyer HJ, Walz MK, Seeber S, Klump B, Budach W, Teichmann R, Schmitt M, Schmitt G, Franke C, Wilke H (2005). Chemoradiation with and without surgery in patients with locally advanced squamous cell carcinoma of the esophagus. *Journal of Clinical Oncology* **23**(10), 2310–7. Erratum in: *Journal of Clinical Oncology*.

4 Rizk N, Bach P, Schrag D, Bains M, Turnbull A, Karpeh M, Brennan M, Rusch VW (2004). The impact of complications on outcomes after resection for esophageal and gastroesophageal junction carcinoma. *Journal of the American College of Surgeons* **98**(1), 42–50.

5 Griffin S, Desai J, Charlton M, Townsend E, Fountain SW (1989). Factors influencing mortality and morbidity following oesophageal resection. *European Journal of Cardio-Thoracic Surgery* **3**, 419–424.

6 Naunheim KS, Hanosh J, Zwischenberger J, Turrentine MW, Kesler KA, Reeder LB, Ferguson MK, Baue AE (1993). Esophagectomy in the septuagenarian. *Annals of Thoracic Surgery* **56**, 880–884.

7 Moskovitz AH, Rizk NP, Venkatraman E, Bains MS, Flores RM, Park BJ, Rusch VW (2006). Mortality increases for octogenarians undergoing esophagogastrectomy for esophageal cancer. *Annals of Thoracic Surgery* **82**(6), 2031–6; discussion 2036.

8 Reynolds JV, Ravi N, Hollywood D, Kennedy MJ, Rowley S, Ryan A, Hughes N, Carey M, Byrne P (2006). Neoadjuvant chemoradiation may increase the risk of respiratory complications and sepsis after transthoracic esophagectomy. *Journal of Thoracic and Cardiovascular Surgery* **132**(3), 549–55.

9 Vande Walle C, Ceelen WP, Boterberg T, Vande Putte D, Van Nieuwenhove Y, Varin O, Pattyn P (2012). Anastomotic complications after Ivor Lewis esophagectomy in patients treated with neoadjuvant chemoradiation are related to radiation dose to the gastric fundus. *International Journal of Radiation Oncology * Biology * Physics* **82**(3), e513–9.

10 Medical Research Council Oesophageal Cancer Working Group (2002). Surgical resection with or without preoperative chemotherapy in oesophageal cancer: a randomised controlled trial. *Lancet* **359**(9319), 1727–33.

11 Kelsen DP, Ginsberg R, Pajak TF, Sheahan DG, Gunderson L, Mortimer J, Estes N, Haller DG, Ajani J, Kocha W, Minsky BD, Roth JA (1998). Chemotherapy followed by surgery compared with surgery alone for localized esophageal cancer. *New England Journal of Medicine* **339**(27), 1979–84.

12 van Hagen P, Hulshof MC, van Lanschot JJ, Steyerberg EW, van Berge Henegouwen MI, Wijnhoven BP, Richel DJ, Nieuwenhuijzen GA, Hospers GA, Bonenkamp JJ, Cuesta MA, Blaisse RJ, Busch OR, ten Kate FJ, Creemers GJ, Punt CJ, Plukker JT, Verheul HM, Spillenaar Bilgen EJ, van Dekken H, van der Sangen MJ, Rozema T, Biermann K, Beukema JC, Piet AH, van Rij CM, Reinders JG, Tilanus HW, van der Gaast A; CROSS Group (2012). Preoperative chemoradiotherapy for esophageal or junctional cancer. *New England Journal of Medicine* **366**(22), 2074–84.

13 Stiles BM, Mirza F, Coppolino A, Port JL, Lee PC, Paul S, Altorki NK (2011). Clinical T2-T3N0M0 esophageal cancer: the risk of node positive disease. *Annals of Thoracic Surgery* **92**(2), 491–6; discussion 496–8.

14 Peyre CG, Hagen JA, DeMeester SR, Altorki NK, Ancona E, Griffin SM, Hölscher A, Lerut T, Law S, Rice TW, Ruol A, van Lanschot JJ, Wong J, DeMeester TR (2008). The number of lymph nodes removed predicts survival in esophageal cancer: an international study on the impact of extent of surgical resection. *Annals of Surgery* **248**(4), 549–56.

15 Rizk NP, Ishwaran H, Rice TW, Chen LQ, Schipper PH, Kesler KA, Law S, Lerut TE, Reed CE, Salo JA, Scott WJ, Hofstetter WL, Watson TJ, Allen MS, Rusch VW, Blackstone EH (2010). Optimum lymphadenectomy for esophageal cancer. *Annals of Surgery* **251**(1), 46–50.

16 Rizk N, Venkatraman E, Park B, Flores R, Bains MS, Rusch V; American Joint Committee on Cancer staging system (2006). The prognostic importance of the number of involved lymph nodes in esophageal cancer: implications for revisions of the American Joint Committee on Cancer staging system. *Journal of Thoracic and Cardiovascular Surgery* **132**(6), 1374–81.

17 Nishihira T, Hirayama K, Mori S (1998). A prospective randomized trial of extended cervical and superiormediastinal lymphadenectomy for carcinoma of the thoracic esophagus. *American Journal of Surgery* **175**(1), 47–51.

18 Hulscher JB, van Sandick JW, de Boer AG, Wijnhoven BP, Tijssen JG, Fockens P, Stalmeier PF, ten Kate FJ, van Dekken H, Obertop H, Tilanus HW, van Lanschot JJ (2002). Extended transthoracic resection compared with limited transhiatal resection for adenocarcinoma of the esophagus. *New England Journal of Medicine* **347**(21), 1662–9.

19 Omloo JM, Lagarde SM, Hulscher JB, Reitsma JB, Fockens P, van Dekken H, Ten Kate FJ, Obertop H, Tilanus HW, van Lanschot JJ (2007). Extended transthoracic resection compared with limited transhiatal resection for adenocarcinoma of the mid/distal esophagus: five-year survival of a randomized clinical trial. *Annals of Surgery* **246**(6), 992–1000; discussion 1000–1.

20 Feith M, Stein HJ, Siewert JR (2003). Pattern of lymphatic spread of Barrett's cancer. *World Journal of Surgery* **27**(9), 1052–7.

21 Suttie SA, Nanthakumaran an S, Mofidi R, Rapson T, Gilbert FJ, Thompson AM, Park KG (2012). The impact of operative approach for oesophageal cancer on outcome: the transhiatal approach may influence circumferential margin involvement. *European Journal of Surgical Oncology* **38**(2), 157–65.

22 Dexter SP, Sue-Ling H, McMahon MJ, Quirke P, Mapstone N, Tin IG (2001). Circumferential resection margin involvement: an independent predictor of survival following surgery for oesophageal cancer. *Gut* **48**(5), 667–70.

23 Sagar PM, Johnston D, McMahon MJ, Dixon MF, Quirke P (1993). Significance of circumferential resection margin involvement after oesophagectomy for cancer. *British Journal of Surgery* **80**(11), 1386–8.

24 Mariette C, Piessen G, Lamblin A, Mirabel X, Adenis A, Triboulet JP (2006). Impact of preoperative radiochemotherapy on postoperative course and survival in patients with locally advanced squamous cell oesophageal carcinoma. *British Journal of Surgery* **93**(9), 1077–83.

25 Smit JK, Pultrum BB, van Dullemen HM, Van Dam GM, Groen H, Plukker JT (2010). Prognostic factors and patterns of recurrence in esophageal cancer assert arguments for extended two-field transthoracic esophagectomy. *American Journal of Surgery* **200**(4), 446–53.

26 Rizzetto C, DeMeester SR, Hagen JA, Peyre CG, Lipham JC, DeMeester TR (2008). *En bloc* esophagectomy reduces local recurrence and improves survival compared with transhiatal resection after neoadjuvant therapy for esophageal adenocarcinoma. *Journal of Thoracic and Cardiovascular Surgery* **135**(6), 1228–36.

27 Kim SH, Karpeh MS, Klimstra DS, Leung D, Brennan MF (1999). Effect of microscopic resection line disease on gastric cancer survival. *Journal of Gastrointestinal Surgery* **3**(1), 24–33.

28 Bedenne L, Michel P, Bouché O, Milan C, Mariette C, Conroy T, Pezet D, Roullet B, Seitz JF, Herr JP, Paillot B, Arveux P, Bonnetain F, Binquet C (2007). Chemoradiation followed by surgery compared with chemoradiation alone in squamous cancer of the esophagus: FFCD 9102. *Journal of Clinical Oncology* **25**(10), 1160–8.

29 Tachimori Y, Kanamori N, Uemura N, Hokamura N, Igaki H, Kato H (2009). Salvage esophagectomy after high-dose chemoradiotherapy for esophageal squamous cell carcinoma. *Journal of Thoracic and Cardiovascular Surgery* **137**(1), 49–54.

30 Yoo C, Park JH, Yoon DH, Park SI, Kim HR, Kim JH, Jung HY, Lee GH, Choi KD, Song HJ, Song HY, Shin JH, Cho KJ, Kim YH, Kim SB (2012). Salvage esophagectomy for locoregional failure after chemoradiotherapy in patients with advanced esophageal cancer. *Annals of Thoracic Surgery* **94**(6), 1862–8.

31 Morita M, Kumashiro R, Hisamatsu Y, Nakanishi R, Egashira A, Saeki H, Oki E, Ohga T, Kakeji Y, Tsujitani S, Yamanaka T, Maehara Y (2011). Clinical significance of salvage esophagectomy for remnant or recurrent cancer following definitive chemoradiotherapy. *Journal of Gastroenterology* **46**(11), 1284–91.

32 Miyata H, Yamasaki M, Takiguchi S, Nakajima K, Fujiwara Y, Nishida T, Mori M, Doki Y (2009). Salvage esophagectomy after definitive chemoradiotherapy for thoracic esophageal cancer. *Journal of Surgical Oncology* **100**(6), 442–6.

CHAPTER 25

Radiation therapy for locally advanced esophageal cancer

Heath D. Skinner & Bruce D. Minsky

Department of Radiation Oncology, The University of Texas MD Anderson Cancer Center, Houston, TX, USA

25.1 Introduction

Locally advanced esophageal cancer (LAEC) is broadly defined as clinical stage III or IVa (T3–4 and/or N+) disease. Therapeutic approaches commonly include pre-operative concurrent chemotherapy plus radiation (chemoradiation), or primary chemoradiation alone. There is controversy as to the ideal therapeutic approach to this disease. The US Patterns of Care Study offers a historical perspective. A total of 414 patients (51% adenocarcinoma and 49% squamous cell carcinoma (SCC)) received radiation therapy as part of definitive or adjuvant management at 59 institutions from 1996–1999 [1, 2].

Overall, patients who received chemoradiation followed by surgery had a significant decrease in locoregional recurrence (HR, 0.40, $p < 0.0001$) and improved survival (HR, 0.32, $p < 0.001$), compared with those who did not undergo surgery. A similar significant decrease in locoregional recurrence (HR, 1.36, $p = 0.01$) and improved survival (HR 1.32, $p < 0.03$) were seen in those patients who received their care at large radiation oncology centers (treating ≥ 500 new cancer patients/year), compared with small centers (treating < 500 new cancer patients/year).

25.2 Definitive therapy in unresectable locally advanced esophageal cancer

25.2.1 Radiation monotherapy

In LAEC, radiation therapy alone should be reserved for palliation, or for patients who are medically unable to receive chemotherapy. The five-year survival rate for patients treated with conventional doses of radiation therapy alone is 0–10% [3–5]. In the radiation therapy alone arm of the RTOG 85-01 trial, in which patients received 64 Gy at 2 Gy/day with conventional techniques, all patients were all dead of disease by three years [6, 7]. Shi and colleagues reported a 33% five-year survival rate with the use of late course accelerated fractionation to a total dose of 68.4 Gy [8].

Primary radiation is more successful in patients with cT1N0 disease. Sai and colleagues from Kyoto University treated 34 patients who were either medically inoperable or who refused surgery with either external beam alone (64 Gy) or external beam (52 Gy) plus 8–12 Gy with brachytherapy [9]. The five-year results included 59% overall survival, 68% local relapse-free survival, and 80% cause specific survival. Yamada and colleagues reported the results in a similar group of 63 patients treated with chemoradiation plus brachytherapy [10]. The five-year results included 66% overall survival, 64% disease-free survival, and 76% cause-specific survival.

25.2.2 Brachytherapy boost

Brachytherapy can be delivered by low- or high-dose rates, and has previously been used as a boost following external beam radiation therapy or chemoradiation [11–16]. This technique is limited by the effective treatment distance. The primary isotope is ^{192}Ir, which is usually prescribed to treat to a distance of 1 cm from the source. Therefore, as confirmed by pathologic analysis of treated specimens, any portion of the tumor which is > 1 cm from the source will receive a suboptimal radiation dose [17].

Esophageal Cancer and Barrett's Esophagus, Third Edition. Edited by Prateek Sharma, Richard Sampliner and David Ilson.
© 2015 John Wiley & Sons, Ltd. Published 2015 by John Wiley & Sons, Ltd.

There does not appear to be an advantage of adding brachytherapy to external beam radiation. One series reported a local failure rate of 57% and a five-year actuarial survival of 28% in 46 patients with stage T2-3N0-1M0 disease [18]. Even in patients with earlier stage disease (clinical T1-2), brachytherapy likely does not offer an advantage. Yorozu et al. reported a local failure rate of 44% and a five-year survival of 26% [19], while Pasquier and associates reported local failure of 23%, and the five-year survival was 36% [20].

However, in an updated series by Ishikawa et al, 59 patients with submucosal esophageal cancer received external beam followed by brachytherapy in a subset of 36 patients with either low-dose rate ^{137}Cs (17 pts) or high-dose rate ^{192}Ir (19 pts) [21]. Patients selected to receive a brachytherapy boost had a significantly higher five-year cause-specific survival (86% vs. 62%, $p = 0.04$).

Chemoradiation plus brachytherapy was tested prospectively by the RTOG 92-07 trial. A total of 75 patients with cancers of the of the thoracic esophagus (92% squamous cell, 8% adenocarcinoma) received the RTOG 85-01 50 Gy chemoradiation regimen, followed by a boost during cycle 3 of chemotherapy, with either low-dose rate or high-dose rate intraluminal brachytherapy [22]. Due to low accrual, the low-dose rate option was discontinued, and the analysis was limited to patients who received the high-dose rate treatment. High-dose rate brachytherapy was delivered in weekly fractions of 5 Gy during weeks 8, 9, and 10. Several patients developed fistulas, and the fraction delivered at week 10 was discontinued. The complete response rate was 73%.

With a median follow-up of only 11 months, local failure as the first site of failure was 27%. Acute toxicities were high. These included 58% grade 3, 26% grade 4, and 8% grade 5 (treatment-related death). The cumulative incidence of fistula was 18% per year, and the crude incidence was 14%. Of the six treatment-related fistulas, three were fatal. Significant toxicity, combined with the lack of dramatic efficacy and the labor-intensive nature of brachytherapy, has resulted in limited interest in developing this technique further in esophageal cancer.

If brachytherapy is to be used, guidelines for esophageal brachytherapy, published by the American Brachytherapy Society, are available [23]. For patients treated in the curative setting, brachytherapy should be limited to tumors ≤ 10 cm with no evidence of distant metastasis. Contraindications include tracheal or bronchial involvement, cervical esophagus location, or stenosis which cannot be bypassed. The applicator should have an external diameter of 6–10 cm. If chemoradiation is used (defined as 5-FU based chemotherapy plus 45–50 Gy) the recommended doses of brachytherapy are 10 Gy in two weekly fractions of 5 Gy each for high-dose rate, and 20 Gy in a single fraction at 4–10 Gy/hr for low-dose rate. The doses should be prescribed to 1 cm from the source. Lastly, brachytherapy should be delivered after the completion of external beam, not concurrently with chemotherapy.

25.2.3 Definitive chemoradiation

Although there are six randomized trials comparing definitive radiation therapy alone with chemoradiation, the only trial which designed to deliver adequate doses of systemic chemotherapy with concurrent radiation therapy was the RTOG 85-01 trial reported by Herskovic and colleagues [24–26]. As was common in the 1980s, most patients had SCC. Treatment included four cycles of 5-FU (1000 mg/m^2/24 hr × 4 days) and Cisplatin (75 mg/m^2, day 1). Radiation therapy (50 Gy at 2 Gy/day) was given concurrently with the first day of cycle 1 of chemotherapy. Cycles 3 and 4 of chemotherapy were delivered every three weeks rather than every four weeks. Only 50% of the patients finished all four cycles of the chemotherapy. The control arm was radiation therapy alone, albeit at a higher dose (64 Gy) than the chemoradiation arm.

Patients treated with chemoradiation had a significant improvement in both median (14 months vs. 9 months), and five-year survival (27% vs. 0%, $p < 0.0001$) [25]. The eight-year survival was 22% [26]. Histology did not significantly influence the results. The five-year survival was 21% for the 107 patients with SCC vs. 13% of the 23 patients with adenocarcinoma ($p =$ NS). Local failure (defined as local persistence plus recurrence) was also lower in the chemoradiation arm (47% vs. 65%). Although African-Americans had larger primary tumors, of which all were SCC, there was no difference in survival rate compared with Caucasians [27].

25.2.4 Dose escalation – 2D and 3D techniques

These promising results led to Intergroup 0122, a phase II trial of dose-escalated chemoradiation to 64.8 Gy delivered concurrently with cisplatin and 5-FU [28]. This regimen appeared to have acceptable toxicity, and formed the experimental arm of INT 0123 (RTOG 9405) [29]. In this trial, patients selected for a non-surgical approach were randomized to a slightly modified RTOG 85-01 chemoradiation regimen, with 50.4 Gy, versus the same chemotherapy with 64.8 Gy, based on INT 0122. As with RTOG 85-01, the majority of patients (85%) had SCC.

There were a number of modifications to the original RTOG 85-01 chemoradiation arm. These included using 1.8 Gy fractions to 50.4 Gy, rather than 2 Gy fractions to 50 Gy, treating with 5 cm proximal and distal margins for 50.4 Gy, rather than treating the whole esophagus for the first 30 Gy followed by a cone down with 5 cm margins to 50 Gy. Cycle 3 of 5-FU/cisplatin also did not begin until four weeks following the completion of radiation therapy, rather than three weeks and, lastly, cycles 3 and 4 of chemotherapy were delivered every four weeks rather than every three weeks. The trial opened in late 1994 and was closed in 1999, when an interim analysis revealed that it was unlikely that the high dose arm would achieve a superior survival compared to the standard dose arm.

For the 218 eligible patients, there was no significant difference in median survival (13.0 months vs. 18.1 months), two-year survival (31% vs. 40%), or local/regional failure and/or local/regional persistence of disease (56% vs. 52%) between the high dose and standard dose arms. Although 11 treatment-related deaths occurred in the high-dose arm, compared with two in the standard dose arm, seven of the 11 occurred in patients who had received ≤ 50.4 Gy.

An alternative approach to dose escalation is altered fractionation. This has been investigated in LAEC, with modest results. Zaho and colleagues treated 201 patients with squamous cell cancer using 41.4 Gy, followed by late-course accelerated hyperfractionation to 68.4 Gy [30]. The results were similar to RTOG 85-01 (38% local failure and 26% five-year survival). Choi and colleagues treated 46 patients with 5-FU/cisplatin and BID radiation using a concurrent boost technique, and reported a 37% five-year survival [31]. Additionally, Lee *et al* reported on a trial of 102 patients with LAEC, limited to SCC, randomized to surgery alone, versus preoperative therapy with 45.6 Gy (1.2 Gy BID) plus 5-FU/cisplatin [32]. There was no difference in median survival (28 vs. 27 months). Thus, although these approaches may appear to be reasonable, there appears to be a significant increase in acute toxicity without any clear therapeutic benefit.

25.2.5   Dose escalation – IMRT and protons

A criticism of many dose escalation trials in the definitive management of LAEC is the use of conventional 2D and 3D radiation techniques. Trials using newer techniques, such as IMRT and protons, may be able to deliver higher doses of radiation with a more tolerable toxicity profile. Multiple dosimetric studies comparing standard 3D-conformal radiotherapy and IMRT generally have found improved sparing of the heart, lung or both, using either static field or arc-based IMRT [33–44]. This has led multiple clinical centers to begin the routine use of IMRT in this disease.

Retrospective analysis of these data does not suggest inferior outcome and may provide decreased toxicity vs. non-IMRT treatment techniques [45 47]. Investigators at the MD Anderson reported the results of 676 patients with LAEC treated with either IMRT (263) or 3DCRT (413) [45]. On multivariate analysis, IMRT was associated with improved survival ($p = 0.004$), but not cancer-specific survival ($p = 0.86$). The survival difference between 3DCRT and IMRT was thought to be due to a higher level of cardiac ($p = 0.05$) and unexplained deaths ($p = 0.003$) in the 3DCRT patients, suggesting that decreased cardiac dose may have a direct impact on patient outcome. Although this and other comparisons between 3DCRT and IMRT in LAEC are retrospective, a randomized trial is unlikely, so therefore the available data may represent the best comparison.

Another theoretical advantage of IMRT is the possibility of dose escalation. With the use of IMRT, a simultaneous integrated boost (SIB) may be performed while maintaining commonly used lung and heart dosimetric constraints. Retrospective data from Zhang and colleagues suggest a positive correlation between radiation dose and locoregional control [48]. This has led to a Phase I study examining this approach in LAEC at MD Anderson. However, at this point, based on results of the INT 0123 trial, the standard dose of external beam radiation remains 50.4 Gy.

25.2.6   Induction chemotherapy

A potential advantage of neoadjuvant chemotherapy is the early identification of those patients who may or may not respond to the chemotherapeutic regimen being delivered concurrently with chemoradiation. Ilson *et al.* have shown that the change in SUV on FDG-PET scan was able to predict which patients showed a response to the full course of chemotherapy [49]. Weider and associates reported similar findings in 38 patients with squamous cell cancers [50]. Although this approach is investigational, if the non-responders can be identified early, then changing the chemotherapeutic regimen may be helpful.

However, in the context of induction chemotherapy prior to definitive chemoradiation, the data do not support its routine use. For example, Ruhstaller and colleagues report the outcomes from a phase II trial using cisplatin/docetaxel followed by chemoradiation in unresectable LAEC [51]. In this study, median survival was 16 months, with 29% of patients surviving long-term, suggesting no benefit over chemoradiation alone. A prospective trial, using PET scan after induction chemotherapy to direct the choice of subsequent chemotherapy during radiation therapy, is now under way in the USA (CALGB Trial 80803 (NCT01333033)).

25.2.7 Tracheoesophageal fistula

A malignant tracheoesophageal (TE) fistula is an unfavorable prognostic feature, and its management deserves special attention. Although the survival of such patients is low, occasionally they may have long-term survival. Historically, the use of radiation therapy was contraindicated, due to the concern of exacerbating the fistula as the tumor responded. However, some data suggest that this is not the case. At the Mayo Clinic, ten patients with a malignant TE fistula received 30–66 Gy, and their median survival was five months [52]. None of the patients experienced an enlarging or more debilitating fistula, following radiation. Rueth and colleagues showed improved survival with a palliative course of radiation, compared to stent placement alone (3.3 vs. one month), and no significant difference in complications [53]. Finally, in a series of 24 patients with TE fistulae, Muto and colleagues found a 71% TE fistula closure rate following chemoradiation, with a median survival time of 6.7 months [54].

The data, albeit limited, suggest that radiation does not necessarily increase the severity of a malignant TE fistula and is not a contraindication to its use. However, given the overall poor prognosis of this subset of patients, the impact on outcome is not clear.

25.3 Trimodality therapy

25.3.1 Pre-operative chemoradiation

There are seven randomized trials comparing preoperative combined modality therapy with surgery alone in patients with clinically resectable disease, the most recent being the CROSS trial [32, 55–60].

The CROSS trial randomized 366 patients with LAEC (75% adenocarcinoma, 23% SCC) to receive either neoadjuvant chemoradiation with 41.4 Gy and carboplatin/paclitaxel followed by surgical resection, versus surgical resection alone [60]. In this trial, median survival was effectively doubled by the addition of chemoradiation (49.4 vs. 24 months, $p = 0.003$). Improved survival was seen in both adenocarcinoma and SCC, although the magnitude was slightly greater in SCC. The R0 resection was 93% in the chemoradiation arm, compared to 69% in the surgery-alone arm ($p < 0.001$). Despite concerns that a lower radiation dose combined with carboplatin and paclitaxel may not be as effective, the pCR rate was 29%. This is comparable to most previous trials and retrospective reviews [61]. Additionally, no significant difference in perioperative complications was seen between treatment arms.

Prior to the publication of the CROSS trial, the role of preoperative chemoradiation was controversial. The first six trials (Urba [55], Walsh [56], EORTC [57], Australasian [58], Korea [32], and CALGB 9781 [59]) had limited patient numbers, heterogeneous treatment regimens and, in some, the dose of radiation was insufficient, based on a dose response analysis by Geh *et al.* [62] (see Table 25.1). Despite all of these limitations, a meta-analysis did suggest a survival benefit [63]. However, with the publication of the CROSS trial, pre-operative chemoradiation is now a standard of care for patients with locally advanced but medically resectable adenocarcinoma of the esophagus.

25.3.2 Necessity for surgery following chemoradiation

Because of the known response of LAEC to chemoradiation, as well as the significant morbidity of an esophagectomy, questions arise as to the necessity of surgery after chemoradiation. Two randomized trials examined whether surgery is necessary after chemoradiation.

In the Federation Francaise de Cancerologie Digestive (FFCD) 9102 trial, 445 patients with clinically resectable

Table 25.1 Randomized trials of neoadjuvant chemoradiation in LAEC.

Trial	n	Patients	Comparison	Concurrent Chemotherapy	Outcome	Comments
Urba et al. [55]	100	Adenocarcinoma: 75% SCC: 25%	Arm 1: surgery Arm 2: 45 Gy/1.5 Gy BID → surgery	CDDP, 5-FU and vinblastine	MS: 17.6 months Arm 2 vs. 16.9 months Arm 1 (NS) LRF: 19% Arm 2 vs. 42% Arm 1 ($p = 0.02$)	Small study, required a greater than 1 year improvement in MS to be significant
Walsh et al. [56]	113	Adenocarcinoma: 100%	Arm 1: surgery Arm 2: 40 Gy/2.67 Gy QD → surgery	CDDP and 5-FU	MS: 16 months Arm 2 vs. 11 months Arm 1 ($p = 0.01$)	Low survival rate in Arm 1 compared to other trials
FFCD 8805/EORTC 40881 [57]	282	SCC: 100%	Arm 1: surgery Arm 2: 18.5 Gy/3.7 QD → 2 wk break → 18.5 Gy/3.7 QD → surgery	CDDP	MS: 18.6 for both arms (NS) DFS: 40% Arm 2 vs. 28% Arm 1 ($p = 0.003$)	Unconventional radiotherapy
TTROG/AGITG [58]	128	Adenocarcinoma: 63% SCC: 35%	Arm 1: surgery Arm 2: 30 Gy/3 Gy QD → surgery	CDDP and 5-FU	MS: 22.2 months Arm 2 vs. 19.3 months Arm 1 (NS)	R0 80% in Arm 2 vs. 59% Arm 1
Lee et al. [32]	101	SCC: 100%	Arm 1: surgery Arm 2: 45.6 Gy/1.2 Gy BID → surgery	CDDP and 5-FU	MS: 28.2 months Arm 2 vs. 27.3 months Arm 1 (NS)	31% of patients in Arm 2 did not have a surgical resection
CALGB 9781 [59]	56	Adenocarcinoma: 75% SCC: 25%	Arm 1: surgery Arm 2: 50.4 Gy/1.8 Gy QD → surgery	CDDP and 5-FU	MS: 53.8 months Arm 2 vs. 21.5 months Arm 1 ($p = 0.002$)	Closed early due to poor accrual
CROSS [60]	366	Adenocarcinoma: 75% SCC: 23%	Arm 1: surgery Arm 2: 41.4 Gy/1.8 Gy QD → surgery	Carboplatin and paclitaxel	MS: 49.4 months Arm 2 vs. 24 months Arm 1 ($p = 0.003$)	R0: 93% in Arm 2 vs. 69% in Arm 1

MS – median survival; QD – Daily; BID – twice daily; CDDP – cisplatin; 5-FU – 5-Flurouracil; NS – not significant; SCC – squamous cell carcinoma.

T3-4N0-1M0 SCC or adenocarcinoma of the esophagus received initial chemoradiation [64], with the vast majority of patients treated on this trial having SCC. Patients initially received two cycles of 5-FU, cisplatin, and concurrent radiation (either 46 Gy at 2 Gy/day or split course 15 Gy weeks 1 and 3). The 259 patients who had at least a partial response were then randomized to surgery versus additional chemoradiation which included three cycles of 5-FU, cisplatin, and concurrent radiation (either 20 Gy at 2 Gy/day or split course 15 Gy). There was no significant difference in two-year survival (34% vs. 40%, $p = 0.56$) or median survival (18 months vs. 19 months) in patients who underwent surgery versus additional chemoradiation.

These data suggest that patients with squamous cancer, who initially respond to chemoradiation, should complete chemoradiation, rather than stop and undergo surgery. Using the Spitzer index, there was no difference in global quality of life, although a significantly greater decrease in quality of life was observed in the surgery arm during the postoperative period (7.52 vs. 8.45, $p < 0.01$, respectively) [65]. A separate analysis revealed that, compared with split-course radiation, patients who received standard course radiation had improved two-year local relapse-free survival rates (77% vs. 57%, $p = 0.002$), but no significant difference in overall survival (37% vs. 31%) [66].

The German Oesophageal Cancer Study Group compared preoperative chemoradiation followed by surgery, versus chemoradiation alone [67]. In this trial, 172 eligible patients < 70 years old with uT3-4N0-1M0 SCC were randomized to preoperative therapy (three cycles of 5-FU, leucovorin, etoposide, and cisplatin, followed by concurrent etoposide, cisplatin, plus 40 Gy) followed by surgery, versus chemoradiation alone (the same chemotherapy but the radiation dose was increased to 60–65 Gy ± brachytherapy). The pCR rate was 33%. Although there was a decrease in two-year local failure (36% vs. 58%, $p = 0.003$), there was no significant difference in three-year survival (31% vs. 24%) for those who were randomized to preoperative chemoradiation followed by surgery vs. chemoradiation alone.

Despite the above data, the current standard of care is to perform esophagectomy following chemoradiation in patients that can tolerate this approach. However, it is known that a subset of patients will have a complete response to chemoradiation. Furthermore, it is known that patients with pCR have improved survival. Data from both Berger *et al.* [68] and Rohatgi *et al.* [69] suggest that patients who achieve a pCR had an improvement in survival, compared with those who do not (five-year: 48% vs. 15%, and median: 133 months vs. 34 months, respectively). In these patients, surgical resection may not be necessary, and this has led to the concept of "selective" surgery after preoperative chemoradiation.

Swisher and colleagues reported a retrospective analysis of patients who underwent a salvage compared with a planned esophagectomy [70]. The operative mortality was higher in those who underwent salvage vs. planned surgery (15% vs. 6%), but there was no difference in survival (25%). However, only 13 patients were identified who had salvage, limiting the broad interpretation of these findings.

However, a recent phase II trial, RTOG 0246, prospectively examined the approach of preoperative paclitaxel/CDDP and 50.4 Gy followed by selective surgery in patients with either residual disease or recurrent disease in the absence of distant metastasis. In this trial of 43 patients with LAEC, 21 patients required surgical resection after chemoradiation, due to residual (17 patients) or recurrent (three patients) disease [71]. This approach led to a one-year overall survival of 71% – lower than the desired predetermined survival rate (77.5%).

25.3.3 Evaluation of response to chemoradiation

To further pursue the selective surgical approach as a treatment modality, it will be critical to establish the definition of an adequate response. However, the ability to predict a pCR prior to surgery is variable.

Yang and associates found that patients with a negative post-treatment biopsy had a higher chance of achieving a pCR (33%), compared with those who did not have a negative biopsy (7%). A multivariate analysis by Gaca and colleagues reported that post-treatment nodal status ($p = 0.03$), not the degree of primary tumor response, predicted disease-free survival [72].

Current available imaging modalities and/or post-chemoradiation biopsies are also of limited value in predicting a pCR. Bates *et al.* noted a 41% false-negative rate with preoperative endoscopy and biopsy [73]. Jones *et al.* reported that CT had a sensitivity of 65%, a specificity of 33%, a positive predictive value of 58%, and a negative predictive value of 41% in evaluating pathologic response after preoperative chemoradiation [74]. Many studies show that EUS performed after chemoradiation is a suboptimal predictor of complete response, because of the inability to distinguish post-irradiation fibrosis and inflammation from residual tumor. Reported accuracy is generally at or below 50% [75]. For example, Sarkaria and colleagues found that in 165 patients, a negative endoscopic biopsy was not a useful predictor of a pCR after chemoradiation (31% negative predictive value), final nodal status, or overall survival [76].

The value of FDG-PET for staging after chemoradiation is unclear. Several studies of esophageal cancer patients show that an early decrease in FDG uptake after chemotherapy can predict clinical response [77, 78]. Additionally, multiple studies have evaluated the ability of FDG-PET to predict a pCR following chemoradiation [79–84]. Flamen *et al.* evaluated the predictive value of PET after chemoradiation in patients receiving preoperative treatment [80]. The sensitivity and positive predictive value of PET for identifying a pCR were 67% and 50%, respectively. Both false-positive PET findings (residual FDG activity in an area of intense inflammatory activity on histopathologic analysis) and false-negative findings occurred at the primary tumor site.

Vallbohmer *et al* treated 119 patients with preoperative chemoradiation, and reported a non-significant association between major responders and FDG-PET results ($p = 0.056$). There was no clear SUV threshold which predicted response [79]. The inflammatory effect of chemoradiation, as well as a lack of standardization of FDG-PET protocols and techniques and definitions of a pathologic response, may be responsible for the variation in results [85]. Thus, although most studies investigating the role of post-treatment FDG-PET in evaluating pCR found some correlation between the two, a wide array of SUV threshold values and a lack of specificity preclude its use as a surrogate marker of pCR.

25.3.4 Biomarkers of response

Because of the marginal results of using clinical variables to predict and assess pCR following chemoradiation, attention has been given to the use of pathologic or molecular markers to this end. Studies have linked tumor lymphocytic infiltration, as well as apoptotic index, with response to chemoradiation [86]. Additional studies have linked a large number of proteins and genes involved in a wide array of signaling cascades with response to chemoradiation. Examples include alterations in diverse signaling cascades involving PI3 kinase, p53, EGFR and HIF-1α [87–96]. Unfortunately, the vast majority of these studies lack validation and the specificity required to be used clinically. One recent study generated a micro-RNA signature to predict pCR from LAEC tumors in 52 patients treated uniformly with chemoradiation [97]. This signature was then validated in a separate cohort of 72 patients treated similarly. When combined with clinical stage, the AUC for pCR was 0.77 ($p = 2 \times 10^{-41}$). These validated data argue for further investigation, possibly within the context of a clinical trial.

25.4 Techniques of radiation therapy

25.4.1 Radiation dose and fractionation

Historically, the standard radiation dose, based on INT 0123, for patients selected for chemoradiation, is 50.4 Gy at 1.8 Gy per fraction [29]. However, recent data from the CROSS trial suggest that 41.4 Gy in the same fractionation may be sufficient to treat in the preoperative setting [60]. As previously described, some investigators have performed dose escalation. However, based on INT 0113, dose escalation above 50.4 Gy should not be performed off-protocol. Additionally, radiation should be delivered without treatment breaks, as randomized data from France reveal a higher local control (57% vs. 29%) and two-year survival rate (37% vs. 23%) with continuous course, compared with split course radiation [98].

The radiation field should include the primary tumor, with 5 cm superior and inferior margins and 2 cm lateral margins. The primary local/regional lymph nodes should receive the same dose. For cervical (proximal) primary tumors (defined as at or proximal to the carina), the treatment volume includes the bilateral supra-clavicular nodes and, for GE junction (distal) primaries, the celiac axis nodes should be included.

25.4.2 Treatment modality

At many centers, the standard of care in radiotherapy for LAEC is 3D conformal radiotherapy using a beam arrangement optimized via CT based planning. However, as mentioned previously, many clinicians have used IMRT, with a possible benefit in regards to toxicity and no apparent compromise in oncologic outcome [45]. A comparison of three techniques is shown in Figure 25.1: see also Plate 25.1. If IMRT is to be used, careful attention should be given to target delineation. In addition, particularly in the case of distal/GEJ tumors, 4D CT or other forms of motion management should be considered.

Recently, proton radiotherapy has become move available as a treatment modality. By virtue of its physical characteristics, proton radiotherapy is thought to decrease dose to critical structures, in large part by minimizing the low dose "bath" often seen with IMRT. This is shown to some degree in dosimetric studies, with V5, V10 and V20 to the lung and heart with protons, compared to IMRT in Figure 25.1 [99].

Several studies have examined patient outcome after treating with proton radiotherapy. Sugahara and colleagues examined outcomes in 46 patients with SCC treated with protons, with or without photons, to a median total dose of 76 Gy [100]. The five-year local control rate was T1: 83%, T2–4: 29%, and survival, T1: 55% and T2–4: 13%. Koyama and Tsujii reported mean actuarial survival rates of 60% for patients with superficial and 39% for those with advanced disease, treated to mean total doses of 78–81 Gy [101]. The incidence of esophageal ulcer was 67%. In the US, Lin and colleagues retrospectively reviewed 62 patients treated with proton radiotherapy for LAEC [102]. Overall, 47% were treated with surgical resection following chemoradiation, with a pCR rate in these patients of 28%. In this series, two patients (3.2%) developed symptomatic pneumonitis, and an additional two patients died due to treatment-related factors. Proton therapy for LAEC remains experimental, and it is currently being evaluated in a randomized trial.

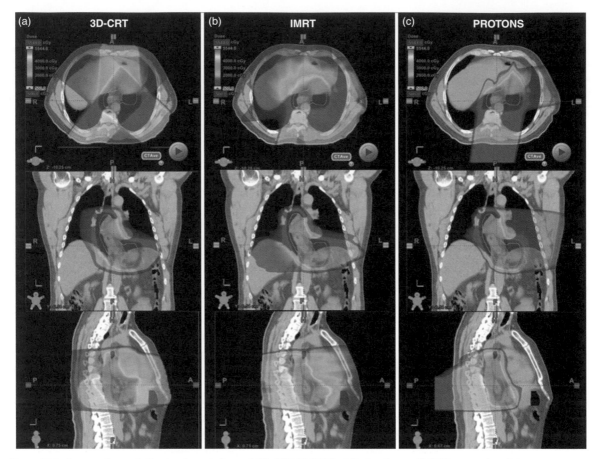

Figure 25.1 Comparative radiation treatment plans. a) 3D-CRT; b) IMRT; c) Proton beam; d) DVH comparison between treatment modalities. In this case, both IMRT and protons provide improved lung and cardiac sparing compared with 3D-CRT. Proton beam decreases liver dose compared to other modalities. *(See insert for color representation of this figure.)*

25.4.3 Target delineation

Although CT can identify adjacent organs and structures, it may be limited in defining the extent of the primary tumor. Leong and colleagues have demonstrated that the addition of PET/CT information for treatment planning improved the identification of the gross tumor volume (GTV) [103]. The GTV based on CT information alone excluded PET-avid disease in 11 of 16 patients (69%), five of whom would have resulted in a geographic miss of gross tumor. Thus, in many centers, it is customary to obtain pretreatment FDG-PET scans, not only to identify patients with occult metastatic disease, but also to assist in target delineation. Conversely, MRI has also been suggested to delineate esophageal tumors, although initial studies showed limited benefit in tumor or positive lymph node delineation [104]. Thus, the use of MRI in this context remains experimental. The current recommendation for target delineation includes using contrasted CT and EGD/EUS findings, as well as FDG-PET, if available.

25.4.4 Limiting toxicity of chemoradiation

Depending on the location of the primary tumor, there are a number of sensitive organs which will be in the radiation field. Specifically, the most well-studied organs at risk in the context of treating LAEC include the lungs and heart. Radiation pneumonitis is clearly linked to the dose and volume of lung treated. Various single dosimetric parameters have been proposed to estimate the probability of developing radiation pneumonitis after radiotherapy [105–111].

Investigators from the Netherlands [109] compared different normal tissue complication probability (NTCP) models to predict radiation pneumonitis. Using the observed incidence of radiation pneumonitis among breast cancer, malignant lymphoma, and inoperable non-small cell lung cancer (NSCLC) patients, they found that the underlying local dose-effect relation for radiation pneumonitis was linear. This was better represented by the mean lung dose (MLD) model, rather than a step function model represented by a threshold dose such as V20. In their patient population, the MLD was the most accurate predictor for the incidence of radiation pneumonitis.

Willner and colleagues performed an analysis of pneumonitis risk from DVH parameters among patients treated with 3D conformal radiotherapy [106]. Their data indicated that it is reasonable to disperse the dose outside the target volume over large areas, in order to reduce the volumes of lung receiving > 40 Gy. They found that reducing the high-dose volume reduces the pneumonitis rate more than a corresponding reduction in the low-dose regions of the DVH. Additionally, Konski and colleagues were able to correlate cardiac toxicity to dosimetric and patient factors [112]. Specifically, they recommended a threshold of V20, V30 and V40 below 70%, 65% and 60%, respectively, to decrease symptomatic cardiac toxicity. In general practice, a MLD < 20 Gy is standard. Cardiac dose constraints are not as clearly defined but, at our institution, a V30 < 35% is reasonable.

25.5 Conclusions

The management of esophageal cancer continues to evolve. General guidelines for therapy of LAEC include both preoperative and non-operative approaches, predicated upon resectability, histology and location. In patients with resectable disease, who are medically fit for this procedure, we recommend preoperative chemoradiation to 50.4 Gy, with consideration of a lower dose (41.4 Gy) based on the CROSS trial. One possible exception to this recommendation is SCC of the cervical esophagus, for which definitive chemoradiation should be considered. Additionally, in non-operative patients, definitive chemoradiation to 50.4 Gy is standard, although enrollment of these patients on dose-escalation or other protocols is encouraged.

Clinicians should make use of all available imaging modalities to delineate tumor and involved lymphadenopathy. Motion management should be considered, particularly if the tumor is distal and IMRT is the preferred treatment modality. Reasonable goal dose constraints for treatment planning include a MLD < 20 Gy and heart V30 < 45%. Future directions include evaluation of tumor biomarkers of response to chemoradiation, with a goal of possibly omitting surgery in favorable patients, while targeting non-responders for protocol-based chemo and radiosensitizers.

References

1 Kenjo M, Uno T, Murakami Y, Nagata Y, Oguchi M, Saito S, et al. (2009). Radiation therapy for esophageal cancer in Japan: results of the patterns of care study 1999–2001. International Journal of Radiation Oncology*Biology*Physics **75**, 357–63.

2 Suntharalingam M, Moughhan J, Coia LR, Krasna MJ, Kachnic L, Haller DG, et al. (2005). Outcome results of the 1996–1999 patterns of care survey of the national practice for patients receiving radiation therapy for carcinoma of the esophagus. Journal of Clinical Oncology **23**, 2325–31.

3 De-Ren S (1989). Ten-year follow-up of esophageal cancer treated by radical radiation therapy: analysis of 869 patients. International Journal of Radiation Oncology*Biology*Physics **16**, 329–34.

4 Newaishy GA, Read GA, Duncan W, Kerr GR (1982). Results of radical radiotherapy of squamous cell carcinoma of the esophagus. Clinical Radiology **33**, 347–52.

5 Okawa T, Kita M, Tanaka M, Ikeda M (1989). Results of radiotherapy for inoperable locally advanced esophageal cancer. International Journal of Radiation Oncology*Biology*Physics **17**, 49–54.

6 Smyth E, Schoder H, Strong VE, Capanu M, Kelsen DP, Coit DG, et al. (2012). A prospective evaluation of the utility of 2-deoxy-2-18F Fluoro-D-Glucose Positron Emission Tomography and computed tomography in staging locally advanced gastric cancer. Cancer **118**, 5481–8.

7 Kozak KR, Moody JS (2008). The survival impact of the Intergroup 0116 trial on patients with gastric cancer. International Journal of Radiation Oncology*Biology*Physics **72**, 517–21.

8 Shi X, Yao W, Liu T (1999). Late course accelerated fractionation in radiotherapy of esophageal carcinoma. Radiotherapy and Oncology **51**, 21–6.

9 Sai H, Mitsumori M, Arai K, Mizowaki T, Nagata Y, Nishimura Y, et al. (2005). Long-term results of definitive radiotherapy for stage I esophageal cancer. International Journal of Radiation Oncology*Biology*Physics **62**, 1339–44.

10 Yamada K, Murakami M, Okamoto Y, Okuno Y, Nakajima T, Kusumi F, et al. (2006). Treatment results

of chemoradiotherapy for clinical stage I (T1N0M0) esophageal carcinoma. *International Journal of Radiation Oncology*Biology*Physics* **64**, 1106–11.

11 Moni J, Armstrong JG, Minsky BD, Bains MS, Harrison LB (1996). High dose rate intraluminal brachytherapy for carcinoma of the esophagus. *Diseases of the Esophagus* **9**, 123–7.

12 Calais G, Dorval E, Louisot P, Bourlie P, Klein V, Chapet S, *et al.* (1997). Radiotherapy with high dose rate brachytherapy boost and concomitant chemotherapy for stages IIB and III esophageal carcinoma: results of a pilot study. *International Journal of Radiation Oncology*Biology*Physics* **38**, 769–75.

13 Schraube P, Fritz P, Wannenmacher MF (1997). Combined endoluminal and external irradiation of inoperable oesophageal carcinoma. *Radiotherapy and Oncology* **44**, 45–51.

14 Akagi Y, Hirokawa Y, Kagemoto M, Matsuura K, Ito A, Fujita K, *et al.* (1999). Optimum fractionation for high-dose-rate endoesophageal brachytherapy following external irradiation of early stage esophageal cancer. *International Journal of Radiation Oncology*Biology*Physics* **43**, 525–30.

15 Okawa T, Dokiya T, Nishio M, Hishikawa Y, Morita K (1999). Multi-institutional randomized trial of external radiotherapy with and without intraluminal brachytherapy for esophageal cancer in Japan. *International Journal of Radiation Oncology*Biology*Physics* **45**, 623–8.

16 Caspers RJL, Zwinderman AH, Griffioen G, Welvaart K, Sewsingh EN, Davelaar J, *et al.* (1993). Combined external beam and low dose rate intraluminal radiotherapy in oesophageal cancer. *Radiotherapy and Oncology* **27**, 7–12.

17 Sur M, Sur R, Cooper K, Levin V, Bizos D, Dubazana N (1996). Morphologic alterations in esophageal squamous cell carcinoma after preoperative high dose rate intraluminal brachytherapy. *Cancer* **77**, 2200–5.

18 Yorozu A, Toya K, Dokiya T (2006). Long-tern results of concurrent chemoradiotherapy followed by high dose rate brachytherapy for T2-3N0-1M0 esophageal cancer. *Esophagus* **3**, 1–5.

19 Yorozu A, Dokiya T, Oki Y, Suzuki T (1999). Curative radiotherapy with high-dose-rate brachytherapy boost for localized esophageal carcinoma: dose-effect relationship of brachytherapy with the balloon type applicator system. *Radiotherapy and Oncology* **51**, 133–9.

20 Pasquier D, Mirabel X, Adenis A, Rezvoy N, Hecquet G, Fournier C, *et al.* (2006). External beam radiation therapy followed by high-dose-rate brachytherapy for inoperable superficial esophageal carcinoma. *International Journal of Radiation Oncology*Biology*Physics* **65**, 1456–61.

21 Ishikawa H, Nonaka T, Sakurai H, Tamaki Y, Kitamoto Y, Ebara T, *et al.* (2010). Usefulness of intraluminal brachytherapy combined with external beam radiation therapy for submucosal esophageal cancer: long-term follow-up results. *International Journal of Radiation Oncology*Biology*Physics* **76**, 452–9.

22 Gaspar LE, Qian C, Kocha WI, Coia LR, Herskovic A, Graham M (1995). A phase I/II study of external beam radiation, brachytherapy, and concurrent chemotherapy in localized cancer of the *Esophagus* (RTOG 9207): Preliminary toxicity report. *International Journal of Radiation Oncology*Biology*Physics* **32**, 160.

23 Gaspar LE, Nag S, Herskovic A, Mantravadi R, Speiser B (1997). American Brachytherapy Society (ABS) consensus guidelines for brachytherapy of esophageal cancer. *International Journal of Radiation Oncology*Biology*Physics* **38**, 127–32.

24 Herskovic A, Martz LK, Al-Sarraf M, Leichman L, Brindle J, Vaitkevicius V, *et al.* (1992). Combined chemotherapy and radiotherapy compared with radiotherapy alone in patients with cancer of the esophagus. *New England Journal of Medicine* **326**, 1593–8.

25 Al-Sarraf M, Martz K, Herskovic A, Leichman L, Brindle JS, Vaitkevicius VK, *et al.* (1997). Progress report of combined chemoradiotherapy versus radiotherapy alone in patients with esophageal cancer: An intergroup study. *Journal of Clinical Oncology* **15**, 277–84.

26 Cooper JS, Guo MD, Herskovic A, Macdonald JS, Martenson JA, Al-Sarraf M, *et al.* (1999). Chemoradiotherapy of locally advanced esophageal cancer. Long-term follow-up of a prospective randomized trial (RTOG 85-01). *JAMA* **281**, 1623–7.

27 Streeter OE, Martz KL, Gaspar LE, Delrowe JD, Asbell SO, Salter MM, *et al.* (1999). Does race influence survival for esophageal cancer patients treated on the radiation and chemotherapy arm of RTOG # 85-01? *International Journal of Radiation Oncology*Biology*Physics* **44**, 1047–52.

28 Minsky BD, Neuberg D, Kelsen DP, Pisansky TM, Ginsberg RJ, Pajak T, *et al.* (1999). Final report of intergroup trial 0122 (ECOG PE-289, RTOG 90-12): Phase II trial of neoadjuvant chemotherapy plus concurrent chemotherapy and high-dose radiation for squamous cell carcinoma of the esophagus. *International Journal of Radiation Oncology*Biology*Physics* **43**, 517–23.

29 Minsky BD, Pajak T, Ginsberg RJ, Pisansky TM, Martenson JA, Komaki R, *et al.* (2002). INT 0123 (RTOG 94-05) phase III trial of combined modality therapy for esophageal cancer: high dose (64.8 Gy) vs. standard dose (50.4 Gy) radiation therapy. *Journal of Clinical Oncology* **20**, 1167–74.

30 Zaho KL, Shi XH, Jiang GL, Wang Y. (2004) Late course accelerated hyperfractionated radiotherapy for localized esophageal carcinoma. *International Journal of Radiation Oncology*Biology*Physics* **60**, 123–9.

31 Choi N, Park SD, Lynch T, Wright C, Ancukiewicz M, Wain J, *et al.* (2004). Twice-daily radiotherapy as concurrent boost technique during chemotherapy cycles in neoadjuvant chemoradiotherapy for resectable esophageal carcinoma: mature results of a phase II study. *International Journal of Radiation Oncology*Biology*Physics* **60**, 111–22.

32 Lee JL, Kim SB, Jung HY, Lee GH, Park SI, Kim JH, *et al.* (2004). A single institutional phase III trial of preoperative

chemotherapy with hyperfractionation radiotherapy plus surgery versus surgery alone for resectable esophageal squamous cell carcinoma. *Annals of Oncology* **15**, 947–54.

33 Wu VWC, Sham JST, Kwong DLW (2004). Inverse planning in three-dimensional conformal and intensity-modulated radiotherapy of mid-thoracic oesophageal cancer. *British Journal of Radiology* **77**(919), 568–72.

34 Woudstra E, Heijmen BJM, Storchi PRM (2005). Automated selection of beam orientations and segmented intensity-modulated radiotherapy (IMRT) for treatment of oesophagus tumors. *Radiotherapy and Oncology* **77**(3), 254–61.

35 Chandra A, Guerrero TM, Liu HH, Tucker SL, Liao Z, Wang X, *et al.* (2005). Feasibility of using intensity-modulated radiotherapy to improve lung sparing in treatment planning for distal esophageal cancer. *Radiotherapy and Oncology* **77**, 247–53.

36 Fenkell L, Kaminsky I, Breen S, Huang S, Van Prooijen M, Ringash J (2008). Dosimetric comparison of IMRT vs. 3D conformal radiotherapy in the treatment of cancer of the cervical esophagus. *Radiotherapy and Oncology* **89**(3), 287–91.

37 Kole TP, Aghayere O, Kwah J, Yorke ED, Goodman KA (2012). Comparison of heart and coronary artery doses associated with intensity-modulated radiotherapy versus three-dimensional conformal radiotherapy for distal esophageal cancer. *International Journal of Radiation Oncology*Biology*Physics* **83**(5), 1580–6.

38 Yin L, Wu H, Gong J, Geng J-H, Jiang F, Shi A-H, *et al.* (2012). Volumetric-modulated arc therapy vs. c-IMRT in esophageal cancer: a treatment planning comparison. *World Journal of Gastroenterology* **18**(37), 5266–75.

39 Nicolini G, Ghosh-Laskar S, Shrivastava SK, Banerjee S, Chaudhary S, Agarwal JP, *et al.* (2012). Volumetric modulation arc radiotherapy with flattening filter-free beams compared with static gantry IMRT and 3D conformal radiotherapy for advanced esophageal cancer: a feasibility study. *International Journal of Radiation Oncology*Biology*Physics* **84**(2), 553–60.

40 Martin S, Chen JZ, Rashid Dar A, Yartsev S (2011). Dosimetric comparison of helical tomotherapy, RapidArc, and a novel IMRT & Arc technique for esophageal carcinoma. *Radiotherapy and Oncology* **101**(3), 431–7.

41 Vivekanandan N, Sriram P, Kumar SAS, Bhuvaneswari N, Saranya K (2012). Volumetric modulated arc radiotherapy for esophageal cancer. *Medical Dosimetry* **37**(1), 108–13.

42 Yin Y, Chen J, Xing L, Dong X, Liu T, Lu J, *et al.* (2011). Applications of IMAT in cervical esophageal cancer radiotherapy: a comparison with fixed-field IMRT in dosimetry and implementation. *Journal of Applied Clinical Medical Physics* **12**(2), 3343.

43 Van Benthuysen L, Hales L, Podgorsak MB (2011). Volumetric modulated arc therapy vs. IMRT for the treatment of distal esophageal cancer. *Medical Dosimetry* **36**(4), 404–9.

44 Gong Y, Wang S, Zhou L, Liu Y, Xu Y, Lu Y, *et al.* (2010). Dosimetric comparison using different multileaf collimeters in intensity-modulated radiotherapy for upper thoracic esophageal cancer. *Radiation Oncology* **5**, 65.

45 Lin SH, Wang L, Myles B, Thall PF, Hofstetter WL, Swisher SG, *et al.* (2012). Propensity score-based comparison of long-term outcomes with 3-dimensional conformal radiotherapy vs intensity-modulated radiotherapy for esophageal cancer. *International Journal of Radiation Oncology*Biology*Physics* **84**(5), 1078–85.

46 Wang S-L, Liao Z, Liu H, Ajani J, Swisher S, Cox JD, *et al.* (2006). Intensity-modulated radiation therapy with concurrent chemotherapy for locally advanced cervical and upper thoracic esophageal cancer. *World Journal of Gastroenterology* **12**(34), 5501–8.

47 La TH, Minn AY, Su Z, Fisher GA, Ford JM, Kunz P, *et al.* (2010). Multimodality treatment with intensity modulated radiation therapy for esophageal cancer. *Diseases of the Esophagus* **23**(4), 300–8.

48 Zhang Z, Liao Z, Jin J, Ajani J, Chang JY, Jeter M, *et al.* (2005). Dose response relationship in locoregional control for patients with stage II-III esophageal cancer treated with concurrent chemotherapy and radiotherapy. *International Journal of Radiation Oncology*Biology*Physics* **61**, 656–64.

49 Ilson DH, Bains M, Rizk NP, Shah MA, Rusch V, Capanu M, *et al.* (2006). Phase II trial of preoperative cisplatin-irinotecan followed by concurrent cisplatin-irinotecan and radiotherapy: PET scan after induction therapy may identify early treatment failure. *Proceedings of the American Society of Clinical Oncology* **24**, 184s.

50 Wieder HA, Brucher BLDM, Zimmermann F, Becker K, Lordick F, Beer A, *et al.* (2004). Time course of tumor metabolic activity during chemoradiotherapy of esophageal squamous cell carcinoma and response to treatment. *Journal of Clinical Oncology* **22**, 900–8.

51 Ruhstaller T, Templeton A, Ribi K, Schuller JC, Borner M, Thierstein S, *et al.* (2010). Intense therapy in patients with locally advanced esophageal cancer beyond hope for surgical cure: a prospective, multicenter phase II trial of the Swiss Group for Clinical Cancer Research (SAKK 76/02). *Onkologie* **33**(5), 222–8.

52 Gschossmann JM, Bonner JA, Foote RL, Shaw EG, Martenson JA, Su J (1993). Malignant tracheoesophageal fistula in patients with esophageal cancer. *Cancer* **72**, 1513–21.

53 Rueth NM, Shaw D, D'Cunha J, Cho C, Maddaus MA, Andrade RS (2012). Esophageal stenting and radiotherapy: a multimodal approach for the palliation of symptomatic malignant dysphagia. *Annals of Surgical Oncology* **19**, 4223–8.

54 Muto M, Ohtsu A, Miyamoto S, Muro K, Boku N, Ishikura S, *et al.* (1999). Concurrent chemoradiotherapy for esophageal carcinoma patients with malignant fistulae. *Cancer* **86**, 1406–13.

55 Urba SG, Orringer MB, Turrisi A, Iannettoni M, Forastiere A, Strawderman M (2001). Randomized trial of

preoperative chemoradiation versus surgery alone in patients with locoregional esophageal carcinoma. *Journal of Clinical Oncology* **19**, 305–13.

56 Walsh TN, Noonan N, Hollywood D, Kelly A, Keeling N, Hennessy TPJ (1996). A comparison of multimodal therapy and surgery for esophageal adenocarcinoma. *New England Journal of Medicine* **335**, 462–7.

57 Bosset JF, Gignoux M, Triboulet JP, Tiret E, Mantion G, Elias D, *et al.* (1997). Chemoradiotherapy followed by surgery compared with surgery alone in squamous cell cancer of the esophagus. *New England Journal of Medicine* **337**, 161–7.

58 Burmeister BH, Smithers BM, Fitzgerald L, Simes R, Devitt S, Ackland S, *et al.* (2005). Surgery alone versus chemora-diotherapy followed by surgery for resectable cancer of the oesophagus: a randomised controlled phase III trial. *The Lancet Oncology* **6**, 659–68.

59 Tepper JE, Krasna MJ, Niedzwiecki D, Hollis D, Reed CE, Goldberg R, *et al.* (2008). Phase III trial of trimodality therapy with cisplatin, fluorouracil, radiotherapy, and surgery compared with surgery alone for esophageal cancer: CALGB 9781. *Journal of Clinical Oncology* **26**, 1086–92.

60 Van Hagen P, Hulshof MCCM, Van Lanschot JJB, Steyerberg EW, Van Berge Henegouwen MI, Wijnhoven BPL, *et al.* (2012). Preoperative chemoradiotherapy for esophageal or junctional cancer. *New England Journal of Medicine* **366**(22), 2074–84.

61 Scheer RV, Fakiris AJ, Johnstone PAS (2011). Quantifying the Benefit of a Pathologic Complete Response After Neoadjuvant Chemoradiotherapy in the Treatment of Esophageal Cancer. *International Journal of Radiation Oncology*Biology*Physics* **80**(4), 996–1001.

62 Geh JI, Bond SJ, Bentzen SM, Glynne-Jones R (2006). Systematic overview of preoperative (neoadjuvant) chemoradiotherapy trials in oesophageal cancer: evidence of a radiation and chemotherapy dose response. *Radiotherapy and Oncology* **78**, 236–44.

63 Urschel JD, Vasan H (2002). A meta-analysis of random-ized controlled clinical trials that compared neoadjuvant chemoradiation and surgery to surgery alone for resectable esophageal cancer. *American Journal of Surgery* **185**, 538–43.

64 Bedenne L, Michel P, Bouche O, Milan C, Mariette C, Con-roy T, *et al.* (2007). Chemoradiation followed by surgery compared with chemoradiation alone in squamous cell cancer of the esophagus: FFCD 9102. *Journal of Clinical Oncology* **25**, 1160–8.

65 Bonnetain F, Bouche O, Michel P, Mariette C, Conroy T, Pezet D, *et al.* (2006). A comparative longitudinal quality of life study using the spitzer quality of life index in a randomized multicenter phase III trial (FFCD 9102): chemoradiation followed by surgery compared with chemoradiation alone in locally advanced squamous resectable thoracic esophageal cancer. *Annals of Oncology* **17**, 827–34.

66 Crehange G, Maingon P, Peignaux K, N'guyen TD, Mirabel X, Marchal C, *et al.* (2007). Phase III trial of protracted compared with split-course chemoradiation for esophageal cancer: Federation Francophone de Cancerologie Digestive 9102. *Journal of Clinical Oncology* **25**, 4895–901.

67 Stahl M, Stuschke M, Lehmann N, Meyer HJ, Walz MK, Seeber S, *et al.* (2005). Chemoradiation with and without surgery in patients with locally advanced squamous cell carcinoma of the esophagus. *Journal of Clinical Oncology* **23**, 2310–7.

68 Berger AC, Farma J, Scott WJ, Freedman G, Weiner L, Cheng JD, *et al.* (2005). Complete response to neoadjuvant chemoradiotherapy in esophageal carcinoma is associated with significantly improved survival. *Journal of Clinical Oncology* **23**(19), 4330–7.

69 Rohatgi P, Swisher S, Correa AM, Wu TT, Liao Z, Komaki R, *et al.* (2005). Characterization of pathologic complete response after preoperative chemoradiotherapy in car-cinoma of the esophagus and outcome after pathologic response. *Cancer* **104**, 2365–72.

70 Swisher SG, Hofsetter W, Wu TT, Correra AM, Ajani JA, Komaki RR, *et al.* (2005). Proposed revision of the esophageal cancer staging system to accommodate patho-logic response (pP) following preoperative chemoradiation (CRT). *Annals of Surgery* **241**, 810–20.

71 Swisher SG, Winter KA, Komaki RU, Ajani JA, Wu TT, Hofstetter WL, *et al.* (2012). A phase II study of a paclitaxel-based chemoradiation regimen with selective surgical salvage for resectable locoregionally advanced esophageal cancer: initial reporting of RTOG 0246. *Inter-national Journal of Radiation Oncology*Biology*Physics* **82**, 1967–72.

72 Gaca JG, Petersen RP, Peterson BL, Harpole DH, D'Amico TA, Pappas TN, *et al.* (2006). Pathologic nodal status predicts disease-free survival after neoadjuvant chemora-diation for gastroesophageal junction carcinoma. *Annals of Surgical Oncology* **13**, 340–6.

73 Bates BA, Detterbeck FC, Bernard SA, Qaqish BF, Tepper JE (1996). Concurrent radiation therapy and chemother-apy followed by esophagectomy for localized esophageal carcinoma. *Journal of Clinical Oncology* **14**, 156–63.

74 Jones DR, Parker LA, Detterbeck FC, Egan TM (1999). Inadequacy of computed tomography in assessing patients with esophageal carcinoma after induction chemoradiotherapy. *Cancer* **85**, 1026–32.

75 Lightdale CJ, Kulkarni KG (2005). Role of Endoscopic Ultrasonography in the Staging and Follow-Up of Esophageal Cancer. *Journal of Clinical Oncology* **23**(20), 4483–9.

76 Sarkaria IS, Rizk NP, Bains MS, Tang LH, Ilson DH, Min-sky BD, *et al.* (2009). Post-treatment endoscopic biopsy is a poor-predictor of pathologic response in patients undergo-ing chemoradiation therapy for esophageal cancer. *Annals of Surgery* **249**, 764–7.

77 Wieder HA, Ott K, Lordick F, Becker K, Stahl A, Herrmann K, *et al.* (2007). Prediction of tumor response by FDG-PET: comparison of the accuracy of single and sequential studies in patients with adenocarcinomas of the esophagogastric junction. *European Journal of Nuclear Medicine and Molecular Imaging* **34**(12), 1925–32.

78 Ott K, Weber WA, Lordick F, Becker K, Busch R, Herrmann K, *et al.* (2006). Metabolic imaging predicts response, survival, and recurrence in adenocarcinomas of the esophagogastric junction. *Journal of Clinical Oncology* **24**(29), 4692–8.

79 Vallbohmer D, Holscher AH, Dietlein M, Bollschweiler E, Baldus SE, Monig SP, *et al.* (2009). [18F] fluorodeoxy-glucose-positron emission tomography for the assessment of histologic response and prognosis after completion of neoadjuvant chemoradiation in esophageal cancer. *Annals of Surgery* **250**, 888–94.

80 Flamen P, Van Cutsem E, Lerut T, Cambier JP, Hustermans K, Bormans G, *et al.* (2002). Positron emission tomography for assessment of the response to induction radiochemotherapy in locally advanced oesophageal cancer. *Annals of Oncology* **13**, 361–8.

81 Klayton T, Li T, Yu JQ, Keller L, Cheng J, Cohen SJ, *et al.* (2012). The role of qualitative and quantitative analysis of F18-FDG positron emission tomography in predicting pathologic response following chemoradio-therapy in patients with esophageal carcinoma. *Journal of Gastrointestinal Cancer* **43**(4), 612–8.

82 Swisher SG, Erasmus J, Maish M, Correa AM, Macapinlac H, Ajani JA, *et al.* (2004). 2-Fluoro-2-deoxy-D-glucose positron emission tomography imaging is predictive of pathologic response and survival after preoperative chemoradiation in patients with esophageal carcinoma. *Cancer* **101**(8), 1776–85.

83 Monjazeb AM, Riedlinger G, Aklilu M, Geisinger KM, Isom S, Clark P, *et al.* (2010). Outcomes of patients with esophageal cancer staged with [18F] fluorodeoxyglu-cose positron emission tomography (FDG-PET): can postradiochemotherapy FDG-PED predict the utility of resection? *Journal of Clinical Oncology* **28**, 4714–21.

84 Eng CW, Fuqua JL 3rd, Grewal R, Ilson D, Messiah ACD, Rizk N, *et al.* (2013). Evaluation of response to induction chemotherapy in esophageal cancer: is barium esophagog-raphy or PET-CT useful? *Clinical Imaging* **37**(3), 468–74.

85 Erasmus JJ, Munden RF, Truong MT, Ho JJ, Hofstet-ter WL, Macapinlac HA, *et al.* (2006). Preoperative chemo-radiation-induced ulceration in patients with esophageal cancer: a confounding factor in tumor response assessment in integrated computed tomographic-positron emission tomographic imaging. *Journal of Thoracic Oncology* **1**(5), 478–86.

86 Morita M, Kuwano H, Araki K, Egashira A, Kawaguchi H, Saeki H, *et al.* (2001). Prognostic significance of lymphocytic infiltration following preoperative chemora-diotherapy and hyperthermia for esophageal cancer. *International Journal of Radiation Oncology*Biology*Physics* **49**, 1259–66.

87 Alexander BM, Wang XZ, Niemierko A, Weaver DT, Mak RH, Roof KS, *et al.* (2012). DNA repair biomarkers predict response to neoadjuvant chemoradiotherapy in esophageal cancer. *International Journal of Radiation Oncology*Biology*Physics* **83**(1), 164–71.

88 Kuwahara A, Yamamori M, Fujita M, Okuno T, Tamura T, Kadoyama K, *et al.* (2010). TNFRSF1B A1466G geno-type is predictive of clinical efficacy after treatment with a definitive 5-fluorouracil/cisplatin-based chemoradiother-apy in Japanese patients with esophageal squamous cell carcinoma. *Journal of Experimental & Clinical Cancer Research* **29**, 100.

89 Yi Y, Li B, Sun H, Zhang Z, Gong H, Li H, *et al.* (2010). Pre-dictors of sensitivity to chemoradiotherapy of esophageal squamous cell carcinoma. *Tumor Biology* **31**(4), 333–40.

90 Gotoh M, Takiuchi H, Kawabe S, Ohta S, Kii T, Kuwakado S, *et al.* (2007). Epidermal growth factor receptor is a possible predictor of sensitivity to chemoradiotherapy in the primary lesion of esophageal squamous cell carcinoma. *Japanese Journal of Clinical Oncology* **37**(9), 652–7.

91 Luthra R, Luthra MG, Izzo J, Wu T-T, Lopez-Alvarez E, Malhotra U, *et al.* (2006). Biomarkers of response to pre-operative chemoradiation in esophageal cancers. *Seminars in Oncology* **33**(6, Suppl 11), S2–5.

92 Izzo JG, Correa AM, Wu T-T, Malhotra U, Chao CKS, Luthra R, *et al.* (2006). Pretherapy nuclear factor-kappaB status, chemoradiation resistance, and metastatic progres-sion in esophageal carcinoma. *Molecular Cancer Therapeutics* **5**(11), 2844–50.

93 Wu X, Gu J, Wu T-T, Swisher SG, Liao Z, Correa AM, *et al.* (2006). Genetic variations in radiation and chemother-apy drug action pathways predict clinical outcomes in esophageal cancer. *Journal of Clinical Oncology* **24**(23), 3789–98.

94 Okumura H, Natsugoe S, Matsumoto M, Mataki Y, Takatori H, Ishigami S, *et al.* (2005). The predictive value of p53, p53R2, and p21 for the effect of chemoradiation therapy on oesophageal squamous cell carcinoma. *British Journal of Cancer* **92**(2), 284–9.

95 Sohda M, Ishikawa H, Masuda N, Kato H, Miyazaki T, Nakajima M, *et al.* (2004). Pretreatment evaluation of combined HIF-1alpha, p53 and p21 expression is a useful and sensitive indicator of response to radiation and chemotherapy in esophageal cancer. *International Journal of Cancer* **110**(6), 838–44.

96 Harpole DH Jr, Moore MB, Herndon JE 2nd, Aloia T, D'Amico TA, Sporn T, *et al.* (2001). The prognostic value of molecular marker analysis in patients treated with trimodality therapy for esophageal cancer. *Clinical Cancer Research* **7**(3), 562–9.

97 Skinner HD, Xu E, Lee JH, Bhutani MS, Weston B, Suzuki A, *et al.* (2013). A validated miRNA expression profile for response to neoadjuvant therapy in esophageal cancer.

Journal of Clinical Oncology **31**(suppl; abstr 4078). Available from: http://meetinglibrary.asco.org/content/82991

98 Jacob JH, Seitz JF, Langlois C, Raoul JL, Bardet E, Bouche O, *et al.* (1999). Definitive concurrent chemo-radiation therapy (CRT) in squamous cell carcinoma of the *Esophagus* (SCCE): preliminary results of a French randomized trial comparing standard vs. split course irradiation (FNCLCC-FFCD 9305). *Proceedings of the American Society of Clinical Oncology* **18**, 270a.

99 Zhang X, Zhao K, Guerrero TM, McGuire SE, Yaremko B, Komaki R, *et al.* (2008). Four-dimensional computed tomography-based treatment planning for intensity-modulated radiation therapy and proton therapy for distal esophageal cancer. *International Journal of Radiation Oncology*Biology*Physics* **72**(1), 278–87.

100 Sugahara S, Tokuuye K, Okumura T, Nakahara A, Saida Y, Kagei K, *et al.* (2005). Clinical results of proton beam therapy for cancer of the esophagus. *International Journal of Radiation Oncology*Biology*Physics* **61**, 76–84.

101 Koyama S, Hirohiko T (2003). Proton beam therapy with high dose irradiation for superficial and advanced esophageal carcinomas. *Clinical Cancer Research* **9**(3571), 3577.

102 Lin SH, Komaki R, Liao Z, Wei C, Myles B, Guo X, *et al.* (2012). Proton beam therapy and concurrent chemotherapy for esophageal cancer. *International Journal of Radiation Oncology*Biology*Physics* **83**(3), e345–351.

103 Leong T, Everitt C, Yuen K, Condron S, Hui A, Ngan SY, *et al.* (2006). A prospective study to evaluate the impact of FDG-PET on CT-based radiotherapy treatment planning for oesophageal cancer. *Radiotherapy and Oncology* **78**, 254–61.

104 Sakurada A, Takahara T, Kwee TC, Yamashita T, Nasu S, Horie T, *et al.* (2009). Diagnostic performance of diffusion-weighted magnetic resonance imaging in esophageal cancer. *European Radiology* **19**(6), 1461–9.

105 Seppenwoolde Y, Lebesque JV, De Jaeger K, *et al.* (2003). Comparing different NTCP models that predict the incidence of radiation pneumonitis. Normal tissue complication probability. *International Journal of Radiation Oncology*Biology*Physics* **55**, 724–35.

106 Willner J, Jost A, Baier K, *et al.* (2003). A little to a lot or a lot to a little? An analysis of pneumonitis risk from dose-volume histogram parameters of the lung in patients with lung cancer treated with 3-D conformal radiotherapy. *Strahlentherapie und Onkologie* **179**, 548–56.

107 Yorke ED, Jackson A, Rosenzweig KE, *et al.* (2002). Dose-volume factors contributing to the incidence of radiation pneumonitis in non-small-cell lung cancer patients treated with three-dimensional conformal radiation therapy. *International Journal of Radiation Oncology*Biology*Physics* **54**, 329–39.

108 Kwa SL, Lebesque JV, Theuws JC, *et al.* (1998). Radiation pneumonitis as a function of mean lung dose: an analysis of pooled data of 540 patients. *International Journal of Radiation Oncology*Biology*Physics* **42**, 1–9.

109 Schallenkamp J, Miller R, Brinkmann D, *et al.* (2007). Incidence of radiation pneumonitis after thoracic irradiation; Dose-Volume correlates. *International Journal of Radiation Oncology*Biology*Physics* **67**, 410–6.

110 Wang S, Liao Z, Wej X, *et al.* (2006). Analysis of clinical and dosimetric factors associated with treatment-related pneumonitis (TRP) in patients with non-small-cell lung *Cancer* (NSCLC) treated with concurrent chemotherapy and three-dimensional conformal radiotherapy (3D-CRT). *International Journal of Radiation Oncology*Biology*Physics* **66**, 1399–407.

111 Kong F-M, Hayman JA, Griffith KA, Kalemkerian GP, Arenberg D, Lyons S, *et al.* (2006). Final toxicity results of a radiation-dose escalation study in patients with non-small-cell lung *Cancer* (NSCLC): predictors for radiation pneumonitis and fibrosis. *International Journal of Radiation Oncology*Biology*Physics* **65**(4), 1075–86.

112 Konski A, Li T, Christensen M, Cheng JD, Yu JQ, Crawford K, *et al.* (2012). Symptomatic cardiac toxicity is predicted by dosimetric and patient factors rather than changes in 18F-FDG PET determination of myocardial activity after chemoradiotherapy for esophageal cancer. *Radiotherapy and Oncology* **104**, 72–7.

CHAPTER 26

Systemic therapy and targeted agents in advanced esophageal cancer

Mark A. Lewis[1] & Harry H. Yoon[2]

[1]General Oncology and Gastrointestinal Medical Oncology, The University of Texas MD Anderson Cancer Center, Houston, TX, USA
[2]Medical Oncology, Mayo Clinic, Rochester, MN, USA

26.1 Introduction

Cancers of the esophagus, gastroesophageal junction (GEJ), and gastric cardia are highly fatal: 17,990 new cases of esophageal cancer are expected in the United States in 2013, with nearly as many (15,210) anticipated deaths; 21,600 cases of stomach cancer (including non-cardia sites) are projected, with 10,990 expected deaths [1]. The incidence of these malignancies is also rising, primarily due to an increase in adenocarcinoma, which surpassed squamous cell carcinoma as the dominant histology in esophageal cancer in about 1990 [2]. With considerable efforts to enhance patient outcomes, survival rates from esophagogastric cancers are improving modestly. The philosophy of care for unresectable and/or metastatic disease is palliative, and chemotherapy can be given with the intent of controlling tumor growth, improving quality of life, or extending survival [3]. We will review the current standard of care for the use of systemic chemotherapy in advanced esophagogastric adenocarcinoma, with a focus on recent developments in targeted therapies.

26.2 Chemotherapy

26.2.1 First-line therapy

26.2.1.1 Chemotherapy vs. best supportive care

For fit patients, systemic chemotherapy is generally recommended for the treatment of advanced disease. A recent meta-analysis of randomized controlled trials evaluating chemotherapy vs. best supportive care (BSC), in treatment-naïve patients with advanced adenocarcinoma of the stomach or GEJ, found that chemotherapy was associated with longer overall survival (OS) compared with BSC alone (median OS 11.0 vs. 4.3 months, respectively; hazard ratio (HR) 0.37; 95% confidence interval (CI) 0.24, 0.55) [4].

26.2.1.2 Combination chemotherapy

Chemotherapy for esophagogastric cancer has evolved from using cytotoxic drugs as single agents, including 5-fluorouracil (5FU), platinums, taxanes, irinotecan, and anthracyclines [5], toward regimens that combine these agents and others in doublets or triplets. In the aforementioned meta analysis, a survival benefit was observed for combination vs. single-agent chemotherapy (HR 0.82; 95% CI 0.74, 0.90), with median survivals of 8.3 vs. 6.7 months, respectively [4]. A standard regimen for the treatment of advanced disease has not been established in the first-line setting, and a variety of agents are used (Table 26.1). Recognition has increased that esophageal adenocarcinoma and squamous cell carcinoma represent distinct diseases [6, 7], yet clear differences in the efficacy of various chemotherapy agents have not yet been observed for advanced disease and, therefore, similar agents are used to treat each subtype.

Whether triplet combination regimens offer more overall benefit over doublets remains controversial, given that triplets can cause greater toxicity and only modestly enhance efficacy, and also given the importance of quality of life in these patients, who generally die within one year, utilizing any therapy [8, 9]. Whereas the triplet regimen of docetaxel, added

Esophageal Cancer and Barrett's Esophagus, Third Edition. Edited by Prateek Sharma, Richard Sampliner and David Ilson.
© 2015 John Wiley & Sons, Ltd. Published 2015 by John Wiley & Sons, Ltd.

Table 26.1 Efficacy of combination chemotherapy regimens for the treatment of advanced esophagogastric cancer.

Trial	N	Design	Regimen	Primary endpoint
Cunningham *et al.* [13]	1002	Phase 3	ECF vs. ECX vs. EOF vs. EOX	OS: 9.9 mo vs. 9.9 mo vs. 9.3 mo vs. 11.2 mo
Al-Batran *et al.* [10]	220	Phase 3	FLO vs. FLP	PFS: 5.8 mo vs. 3.9 mo $p = 0.077$
Boku *et al.* [18]	704	Phase 3	CI vs. 5FU vs. S1	OS: 12.3 mo vs. 10.8 mo vs. 11.4 mo; $p = 0.0005$ for non-inferiority
Van Cutsem *et al.* [8]	445	Phase 2–3	DCF vs. CF	OS: 9.2 mo vs. 8.6 mo; $p = 0.02$

OS – overall survival; PFS – progression-free survival; ORR – objective response rate; ECF – epirubicin, cisplatin, 5FU; ECX – epirubicin, cisplatin, capecitabine; EOF – epirubicin, oxalipatin, 5FU; EOX – epirubicin, oxaliplatin, capecitabine, FLO – 5FU, leucovorin, oxaliplatin; FLP – 5FU, leucovorin, cisplatin; DF – docetaxel, 5FU; CI – cisplatin/irinotecan; DCF – docetaxel, cisplatin, 5FU; CF – cisplatin, 5FU.

to infusional 5FU and cisplatin, modestly improved response, progression-free and overall survival, thc severe toxicity of this regimen has limited its application to younger, high functional status patients without medical co-morbidities, and with access to frequent assessments for toxicity. Randomized trials and meta-analyses have shown a modest survival benefit of anthracycline-containing triplets over 5FU/cisplatin doublets, albeit with increased toxicity, leading to the common use of triplets in Europe [4].

However, newer doublet regimens that combine short-term high-dose infusional 5FU with oxaliplatin, or capecitabine plus cisplatin, may be more effective than older regimens in which cisplatin was combined with 4–5 day infusions of 5FU [10].

In a randomized Phase 2 trial patients received cetuximab plus one of three chemotherapy regimens: ECF (epirubicin, cisplatin, 5FU), irinotecan plus cisplatin, or FOLFOX. The clinical outcome measures (response rates, progression-free survival (PFS), OS) were similar in the ECF and FOLFOX groups [11], raising the question of whether the anthracycline added benefit to the ECF regimen. The uncertain contribution from an anthracycline is supported by results from a small randomized Phase 2 study in which patients received ECF vs. DF (docetaxel, 5FU), which found similar outcomes between the two arms [12].

Recent data support oxaliplatin as a reasonable replacement for cisplatin in the advanced setting. An oxaliplatin doublet compared favorably to a cisplatin doublet in a recent Phase 3 trial [10], in which chemotherapy-naive patients with advanced esophageal or GEJ adenocarcinoma ($n = 220$) were randomized to receive 5FU, leucovorin, and either oxaliplatin (FLO) or cisplatin (FLP). The study had 80% power to detect an improvement in median progression-free survival (PFS) from 3.5 to 5.0 months (one-sided alpha 0.05). Patients treated with FLO had higher median PFS compared with those treated with FLP (5.8 vs. 3.9 months), and higher OS (10.7 vs. 8.8 months), but neither finding reached statistical significance. Bearing in mind the problems inherent with cross-trial comparisons, median survivals with FLO compare favorably with other large trials in the disease, including those utilizing anthracycline-containing triplet regimens [8, 13]. Moreover, overall serious adverse events were reduced in FLO patients (9%) compared with FLP patients (19%), though FLO treatment was associated with increased peripheral neuropathy.

Non-inferiority of oxaliplatin compared to cisplatin was further demonstrated in a recent Phase 3 study performed in the UK (REAL-2). In a two-by-two non-inferiority design ($n = 1002$), patients with advanced esophageal, GEJ, or gastric cancer were treated with one of four regimens: ECF, ECX (epirubicin, cisplatin, capecitabine), EOF (epirubicin, oxaliplatin, 5FU), or EOX (epirubicin, oxaliplatin, capecitabine) [13]. The HR for death (primary endpoint) non-significantly favored oxaliplatin over cisplatin (HR 0.92; 95% CI 0.80, 1.10). Comparing capecitabine (ECX or EOX) against 5FU (ECF or EOF), the HR for death non-significantly favored capecitabine (HR 0.86; 95% CI 0.80, 0.99). Among the four treatments, EOX had the longest median survival at 11.2 months (9.3 months for EOF, 9.9 months for ECF or ECX).

In a secondary analysis, EOX showed improved OS compared with ECF (HR 0.80; 95% CI 0.66, 0.97). Oxaliplatin was associated with higher rates of grade 3–4 neuropathy and diarrhea but lower rates of neutropenia, nephrotoxicity, and thromboembolism, when compared with cisplatin [13]. These data demonstrated that oxaliplatin and capecitabine could be routinely included in combination regimens. The substitution of capecitabine for 5FU was also supported in a meta-analysis [14, 15].

While toxicity has sometimes been prohibitive, significant responses have been observed by combining irinotecan with taxanes [16, 17] or cisplatin [18]. Attempts have been made to replace infusional 5FU with the oral fluoropyrimidine, S-1, which has been tested in Asia in gastric cancers [19, 20].

In summary, an abundance of combination therapies have been tested in advanced esophagogastric cancers, but the superiority of an anthracycline-containing triplet over an oxaliplatin-containing doublet in the first-line setting has not been shown. Either can serve as a chemotherapeutic backbone in future clinical trials. Anthracycline-containing triplet regimens, often including epirubicin, tend to form the chemotherapeutic backbone of trials in the UK (e.g., REAL-3), whereas the oxaliplatin doublets are used in ongoing trials in the USA and elsewhere (e.g., LOGiC, EXPAND).

26.2.2   Subsequent therapy

The clinical benefit of second-line chemotherapy has been demonstrated in two Phase 3 trials. In COUGAR-02, docetaxel showed enhanced quality of life and survival, compared with best supportive care alone, when given after first-line progression on fluoropyrimidines or platinums. Patients with esophagogastric cancer ($n = 168$) whose disease had progressed within six months of initial therapy were randomized to receive active symptom control (ASC), with or without docetaxel [21]. The trial demonstrated that docetaxel plus ASC prolonged median OS to 5.2 months vs. 3.6 months in the control arm ($p = 0.01$). Symptom scores, including pain, were significantly better in the chemotherapy arm. Salvage chemotherapy was also found to increase OS compared with BSC alone in a Korean study restricted to advanced gastric cancer (5.3 vs. 3.8 months; HR 0.657; 95% CI 0.485, 0.891) [22].

Single-agent administration of a targeted therapy, ramucirumab, was recently shown to improve OS over BSC alone (REGARD; see section on Angiogenesis below).

26.3   Targeted therapy

Recent advances in the treatment of metastatic esophagogastric cancer have occurred in the development of biologic agents, particularly by targeting members of the HER/ErbB family of growth factor receptors and tumor-related angiogenesis.

26.3.1   HER2

The HER family consists of four closely related transmembrane tyrosine kinase receptors: epidermal growth factor receptor (EGFR; also known as HER1), HER2, HER3, and HER4. After ligand binding to the extracellular domain, the receptor undergoes homo- or hetero-dimerization, leading to autophosphorylation of the kinase and activation of downstream growth signals. EGFR and HER4 have active tyrosine kinase domains and known ligands, and HER3 can bind to several ligands (but lacks intrinsic tyrosine kinase activity). HER2 possesses an active tyrosine kinase domain, but no direct ligand has been identified, and HER2 is constitutively available for dimerization [23]. Approximately 20% of esophagogastric cancers over-express HER2 [24], which usually results from amplification of its gene, *her2-neu*. This frequency is similar to that found in breast cancers, where the demonstrated clinical activity of HER2-targeted therapy has led to FDA approvals for multiple indications.

HER2 status in clinical specimens can be assessed by measuring protein expression via immunohistochemistry (IHC) or gene amplification via fluorescence *in situ* hybridization (FISH). IHC is scored on a four-point scale (0, 1+, 2+, 3+) based on the intensity of expression and the percentage of cells with a particular staining intensity. FISH is scored by counting the number of HER2 signals as compared to its centromere (CEP17), with a ratio of 2.0 or more generally considered gene-amplified.

26.3.1.1   Trastuzumab

Trastuzumab is a humanized monoclonal antibody which binds to the extracellular domain of HER2. Postulated mechanisms of action include inhibition of HER2-mediated cell signaling and triggering of apoptosis via the phosphatidylinositol-3-kinase (PI3K)/AKT/mammalian target of rapamycin (mTOR) pathways, as well as antibody-dependent cellular cytotoxicity [25].

Trastuzumab was found to improve OS in patients with advanced HER2-positive GEJ or gastric adeno-carcinoma in a landmark Phase 3 trial (ToGA), where patients were randomized 1 : 1 to trastuzumab plus chemotherapy (fluoropyrimidine plus cisplatin) or to chemotherapy alone [26]. To be eligible, patient tumors were required to show strong HER2 protein expression by IHC (3+) or gene amplification by FISH. Almost all tumors were HER2-amplified, whereas HER2 expression rates varied. Of 584 patients in the primary analysis, median OS was 13.8 months for trastuzumab plus chemotherapy, vs. 11.1 months for chemotherapy alone (HR 0.74; 95% CI 0.60, 0.91; $p = 0.0046$) (Figure 26.1). Rates of overall grade 3–4 adverse events and cardiac adverse events did not differ between the groups. This trial established the addition of trastuzumab to cytotoxic chemotherapy as a standard of care for advanced HER2-positive GEJ or gastric cancer. The ToGA findings have been extended in practice to include esophageal adenocarcinomas, given that rates of HER2 overexpression and/or gene amplification are the same or higher in these tumors [27].

HER2 has distinct expression patterns in esopha-gogastric cancer tissues, compared with breast cancers [28, 29]. As a result, HER2 interpretive criteria spe-cific to upper gastrointestinal tumors were developed and utilized in the ToGA trial, and they are required in clinical practice [28, 29]. These modified criteria account for unique patterns of HER2 membrane stain-ing and reportedly more pronounced intra-tumor HER2 heterogeneity in esophagogastric vs. breast tumors.

In an exploratory analysis of the ToGA study, trastuzumab benefit appeared to increase as HER2 protein expression level increased, regardless of the presence of gene amplification. In patients with low HER2-expressing tumors (IHC0–1+ with FISH-positive), trastuzumab was associated with no benefit. By con-trast, in patients high HER2-expressing tumors (IHC3+ or IHC2+ with FISH-positive), trastuzumab therapy was associated with a 35% relative risk reduction in death (median OS of 16 vs. 11.8 months in the trastuzumab vs. non-trastuzumab arms; interaction $p = 0.036$).

While questions remain as to why trastuzumab benefit was not observed in HER2-amplified low

expressors, the complex interpretation of the ToGA subgroup analysis has led to geographic regulatory differences in the HER2 criteria that are used to identify patients for trastuzumab therapy. The FDA in the US approved trastuzumab for IHC3+ or FISH-positive cases (i.e., all ToGA-eligible patients, including those who are IHC0–1+ with FISH-positive). In contrast, the European Medicine Agency has approved trastuzumab only for cases showing IHC3+ expression or IHC2+ expression with FISH-positivity, consistent with results from the subgroup analysis [30]. The concordance of HER2 results between IHC and FISH is high in the IHC0–1+ and 3+ groups, but variable in the IHC2+ group [31–34]. While not universally accepted, it is generally recommended that IHC be used as the initial screening test to determine HER2 status, with FISH restricted to equivocal (IHC2+) cases [35].

In contrast to breast cancer, the association between HER2 expression/amplification and prognosis in esoph-agogastric cancer remains unknown, with conflicting data reported in gastric cancers [33, 36–41]. HER2 positivity has been associated with intestinal-type (vs. diffuse or mixed/anaplastic) histology [27, 42]. In esophageal adenocarcinoma, prognostic data are also conflicting [27, 43–46]. In the largest evaluation to date in esophageal adenocarcinoma, we examined HER2 expression and amplification in 713 tumors and did not find an association with survival in the overall cohort [27]. However, we found that HER2 positivity was more common in adenocarcinomas with adjacent Barrett's metaplasia and, within this subgroup, was significantly associated with longer overall survival [27], suggesting the existence of distinct HER2-based molecular subtypes that may differ based on etiology.

26.3.1.2 Lapatinib

Lapatinib, a small-molecule TKI that targets EGFR (HER1) and HER2, was evaluated in a Phase 3 study of advanced *HER2*-amplified gastric cancer (Tytan), in which Asian patients ($n = 261$) who progressed on prior chemotherapy were randomized to second-line treatment with lapatinib plus paclitaxel, or paclitaxel alone [47]. The study did not meet its primary endpoint; median OS was 11.0 vs. 8.9 months for lapatinib vs. paclitaxel alone ($p = 0.2088$). Subgroup analysis showed that lapatinib may have benefitted patients with IHC3+ HER2 expression; median OS 14.0 vs. 7.6 months for lapatinib vs. paclitaxel monotherapy ($p = 0.0176$).

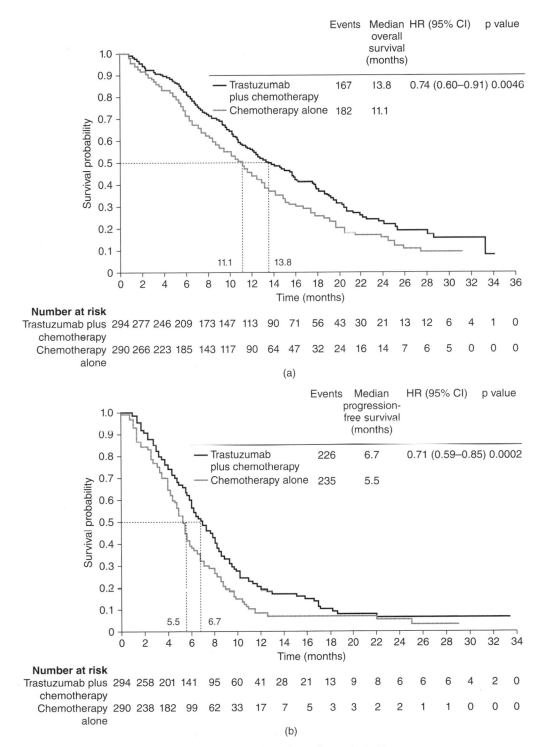

Figure 26.1 (a) OS and (b) PFS of chemotherapy + trastuzumab vs. chemotherapy in ToGA.

Diarrhea (19.1% vs. 2.3%) and febrile neutropenia (6.9% vs. 1.6%) were more common on combination therapy.

Likewise, the TRIO-013/LOGiC trial was a Phase 3 study evaluating lapatinib in advanced HER2-positive adenocarcinomas of the upper gastrointestinal tract in the first-line setting. HER2 inclusion criteria were IHC3+ or HER2 amplification [48]. In LOGiC, 545 patients inside and outside Asia were randomized to capecitabine/oxaliplatin, with or without lapatinib. The primary endpoint of OS was not reached (HR 0.91; $p = 0.35$). Though there was no association between IHC status and OS, pre-planned subgroup analysis showed significantly improved OS in Asian patients (HR 0.68) and patients younger than 60 (HR 0.69).

While lapatinib is not recommended for use outside of a clinical trial, it is possible that responsive subpopulations may be identified in the future.

26.3.2 EGFR

The epidermal growth factor receptor (EGFR) is overexpressed in 50-70% of esophageal cancers and 60-86% of gastric tumors [49]. Compared with non-small cell lung cancer, activating mutations in *EGFR* are uncommon in esophageal cancer. Downstream *KRAS* or *BRAF* mutations, which are known or suspected markers of resistance to anti-EGFR antibodies, are also rare [50]. Research efforts have focused on the potential role for targeted agents against EGFR, including monoclonal antibodies and small-molecule TKIs.

26.3.2.1 Cetuximab and panitumumab

Cetuximab is a chimeric monoclonal antibody directed against the external domain of EGFR, which then inhibits the activity of the tyrosine kinase located on the inner surface of the cell membrane [51]. The clinical efficacy of cetuximab was evaluated in EXPAND, an open-label, randomized Phase 3 trial, in which 904 patients with unresectable locally advanced or metastatic adenocarcinoma of the stomach or GEJ were randomized to capecitabine and cisplatin, with or without weekly cetuximab [37]. There was no significant difference in the primary endpoint of PFS, which was actually shorter in cetuximab recipients (4.4 months) than in those only given capecitabine/cisplatin (5.6 months, $p = 0.32$). Grade 3–4 adverse events, which included neutropenia and acneiform skin reactions,

were also more common in the cetuximab (83%) vs. control (77%) group.

Similarly negative results were reported for panitumumab, a fully humanized IgG2 monoclonal antibody against EGFR. In a Phase 2–3 trial (REAL-3) panitumumab was added to EOX [38]. Median OS was 11.3 months for EOX patients vs. 8.8 months for the panitumumab arm (HR 1.37; $p = 0.013$), again demonstrating that the addition of an anti-EGFR monoclonal antibody may decrease efficacy. EOX plus panitumumab was also associated with increased incidence of grade 3–4 diarrhea, mucositis, and hypomagnesemia.

Together, these data demonstrate that anti-EGFR monoclonal antibody therapy does not add benefit to cytotoxic chemotherapy in patients with advanced esophagogastric adenocarcinoma.

In advanced esophageal squamous cell carcinoma, which is distinct epidemiologically from esophageal adenocarcinoma, preliminary data suggest that anti-EGFR therapy may have activity [52–54]. The addition of panitumumab to chemotherapy is being evaluated in a Phase 3 trial of patients with advanced esophageal squamous cell cancer [53].

26.3.2.2 Gefitinib and erlotinib

Gefitinib, a small molecule inhibitor of EGFR, failed to demonstrate meaningful clinical activity in esophageal cancer [55]. In a Phase 3 trial (Cancer Oesophagus Gefitinib (COG)), 450 unselected patients with esophageal/GEJ adenocarcinoma or squamous cell carcinoma who had progressed after one prior chemotherapy regimen were randomized to receive gefitinib 500 mg daily or placebo. There was no significant OS benefit for gefitinib (3.7 vs. 3.6 months), and the statistically significant improvement in PFS was two weeks in duration (median 49 vs. 35 days, $p = 0.017$). Patients receiving gefitinib had better quality of life, but more diarrhea [55]. These data are insufficient to conclude that gefitinib has meaningful activity in esophageal cancer. Erlotinib has not been studied as extensively [56–58].

26.3.3 cMET

The cell surface receptor c-MET (mesenchymal-epithelial transition factor) and its ligand hepatocyte growth factor (HGF) are therapeutic targets of interest in esophagogastric cancer. Activation of the MET tyrosine kinase is mediated by binding of HGF, leading to signal transduction down multiple pathways, including Ras, mTOR, and PI3K [59, 60] . As such, MET/HGF can regulate cell proliferation, invasion, and angiogenesis [61]. MET amplification has been identified in a small subset of esophageal adenocarcinomas and associated with adverse prognosis [62, 63]. High levels of c-MET protein expression have been described in gastric cancers, and may be associated with a poorer prognosis [64].

Rilotumumab, a fully human monoclonal antibody against HGF, was examined in a Phase 2 three-arm trial, in which 121 patients with locally advanced or metastatic esophagogastric cancers were randomized 1 : 1 : 1 to ECX (epirubicin, cisplatin, and capecitabine), in combination with two different doses of rilotumumab (7.5 mg/kg or 15 mg/kg every three weeks), or placebo. The addition of rilotumumab to chemotherapy improved median PFS from 4.2 months to 5.6 months (HR 0.64; 80% CI 0.48, 0.85). Median OS increased from 8.9 months to 11.1 months (HR 0.73; 80% CI 0.53, 1.01) [65].

In an exploratory analysis of 90 patients with immunohistochemically measured MET levels, the addition of rilotumumab to chemotherapy in patients with high MET expression improved median OS from 5.7 months to 11.1 months (HR 0.29; 95% CI 0.11, 0.76). Conversely, in patients with low MET expression, adding rilotumumab to chemotherapy trended towards a less favorable OS (HR 1.84; 95% CI 0.78, 4.34) [66]. A global Phase 3 trial of ECX with or without rilotumumab in high MET-expressing patients is near completion.

An anti-MET antibody, onartuzumab, is being examined in combination with chemotherapy in ongoing Phase 3 trials in previously untreated patients with MET-expressing adenocarcinomas of the GEJ or stomach. Tivantinib, a small molecule with reported activity against cMET, is also under clinical development.

26.3.4 Angiogenesis

The therapeutic value of disrupting tumor-related angiogenesis in GEJ/gastric adenocarcinoma was demonstrated recently, utilizing ramucirumab, a monoclonal antibody against vascular endothelial growth factors receptor-2 (VEGFR-2). The principal force driving angiogenesis is the interaction between VEGFs and vascular endothelial growth factor receptors (VEGFRs), with persistent upregulation affecting cancer growth, metastases, and vascular permeability

of tumors. VEGFR-2 is the critical receptor involved in malignant angiogenesis, with its activation inducing a number of other cellular modifications, resulting in tumor growth and metastases. The progression from normal esophagus to Barrett's metaplasia and to esophageal adenocarcinoma is characterized by neovascularization [67]. VEGFR-2 is highly expressed in gastrointestinal malignancies, including esophageal adenocarcinomas [68].

Ramucirumab is a recombinant human monoclonal antibody that targets VEGFR-2 and inhibits VEGF activities, including receptor phosphorylation and signaling pathway activation [69]. A murine version (DC-101) has shown activity in a gastric cancer model [70].

Ramucirumab has demonstrated improved OS in two Phase 3 trials (REGARD, RAINBOW) in previously treated patients with advanced gastric/GEJ adenocarcinoma. In REGARD, 355 patients with metastatic cancer and progression after first-line platinum- and/or fluoropyrimidine-containing regimens were randomized in a double-blinded, 2 : 1 fashion, to receive ramucirumab or placebo. In this study, which primarily consisted of patients from North America, Europe, and Australia, median OS was significantly higher in ramucirumab-treated patients (5.2 vs. 3.8 months, respectively; HR 0.776; 95% CI 0.603, 0.998; $p = 0.0473$) [71]. While overall response rates were similar between arms, ramucirumab-treated patients had significantly improved median PFS (2.1 vs. 1.3 months; HR 0.483; $p < 0.0001$) and disease control rate (49% vs. 23%; $p < 0.0001$). Ramucirumab was well-tolerated, and no unexpected safety findings were noted [71].

RAINBOW evaluated the benefit of adding ramucirumab to cytotoxic chemotherapy, again in the second-line setting. In this recently reported Phase 3 study, 665 patients with metastatic GEJ or gastric adenocarcinoma were randomized, within four months of progression on first-line platinum- and fluoropyrimidine-containing regimens, to paclitaxel (80 mg/m^2 days 1, 8, 15 of a four-week cycle), in combination with either ramucirumab (8 mg/kg IV q2weeks) or placebo. Ramucirumab-treated patients showed an improvement in the primary endpoint, with a median OS of 9.6 vs. 7.4 months in the ramucirumab vs. placebo arm (HR 0.81; 95% CI: 0.68–0.96; $p = 0.017$). Improvements in PFS and ORR were also statistically significant. Neutropenia was more frequently reported with ramucirumab, but the incidence of febrile neutropenia was comparable between treatment arms [72].

Ramucirumab is the second biologic agent to improve OS in a Phase 3 trial in this malignancy. The survival benefit of ramucirumab over BSC, as shown in REGARD, was comparable to that demonstrated by second-line cytotoxic chemotherapy over BSC in Phase 3 trials [21, 22]. However, detailed cost-effective analysis has not been performed for REGARD data. Though cross-trial comparisons should be interpreted with caution, it is noteworthy that the OS shown in RAINBOW is among the highest reported in a second-line Phase 3 trial of advanced gastric/GEJ adenocarcinoma in which the patient population was predominantly non-Asian. The results of REGARD and RAINBOW validate the role of therapeutically targeting the VEGFR2 signaling pathway in gastric/GEJ adenocarcinoma, and offer a new therapeutic option in previously treated patients with advanced disease.

The effect of adding ramucirumab to cytotoxic chemotherapy in the front line setting was evaluated in a randomized Phase 2 study, whose preliminary results were presented at the 2014 ASCO meeting. In this multicenter US trial, 168 patients with untreated metastatic or locally advanced esophageal, GEJ, or gastric adenocarcinoma were randomly assigned to mFOLFOX6, in combination with either ramucirumab (8 mg/kg IV) or placebo, every 14 days. Unlike REGARD or RAINBOW, which did not include esophageal cancer patients, the primary tumors of approximately half of the patients in the US trial were located in the esophagus. Though the disease-control rate was significantly higher in the ramucirumab group, median PFS did not differ between the arms (6.4 vs. 6.7 months in ramucirumab vs. placebo, respectively; HR 0.98 (95% CI 0.69, 1.37)). However, the analysis of efficacy results may have been affected by a higher treatment discontinuation rate that was observed in the ramucirumab group.

In an exploratory analysis that attempted to control for these discontinuations via on-treatment censoring, a longer PFS favoring ramucirumab was observed in the subset of patients with gastric or GEJ cancer, whereas no benefit was seen in the esophageal cancer subset [73]. Biomarker analyses are ongoing in order to understand these potential tumor site differences further. Overall, these Phase 2 results have raised questions regarding the synergy between ramucirumab and FOLFOX in

this disease and, to date, ramucirumab can only be recommended for use in previously treated patients with gastric or GEJ adenocarcinoma.

The potential activity of an anti-angiogenesis monoclonal antibody in pan-American patients with GEJ or gastric cancer was suggested by results from a recent Phase 3 trial (AVAGAST) [74]. In this international trial, 774 patients with advanced gastric or GEJ cancer were randomized to bevacizumab (an anti-VEGF-A antibody) or placebo, utilizing a fluoropyrimidine-cisplatin backbone. Approximately < 15% of patients had GEJ tumors. A trend toward benefit was observed for its primary endpoint, OS (12.1 vs. 10.1 months in the bevacizumab vs. non-bevacizumab arms; $p = .1002$) (Figure 26.2).

Bevacizumab significantly improved median PFS ($p = .0037$) and ORR ($p = .0315$) over placebo. Subgroup analyses revealed that bevacizumab effect differed by geographic region (with a significant benefit in the pan-American subgroup) and by other variables, suggesting potential patient subgroups where anti-angiogenesis therapy may be efficacious. The much higher rate of utilization of second line chemotherapy in Asian, compared with Western, patients likely undercut the potential survival benefit for the addition of bevacizumab to first line chemotherapy.

Of various biomarkers evaluated in AVAGAST, high-circulating VEGF-A and low tumor expression of neuropilin-1 were identified as potential predictors of improved bevacizumab efficacy. For both biomarkers, subgroup analyses demonstrated significance only in patients from non-Asian regions [75]. Further efforts are ongoing to identify predictive biomarkers for anti-angiogenesis therapy.

26.4 Future directions

Poly-ADP ribose polymerase (PARP) inhibitors are being combined with cytotoxic agents to hinder the ability of esophagogastric cancer cells to repair DNA strand breaks. A Phase 2 randomization of 124 patients to paclitaxel, vs. paclitaxel plus olaparib, was recently reported, and showed an OS benefit for the taxane/PARP inhibitor combination, with enhanced benefit in tumors with low levels of ataxia telangiectasia mutated (ATM) protein [76].

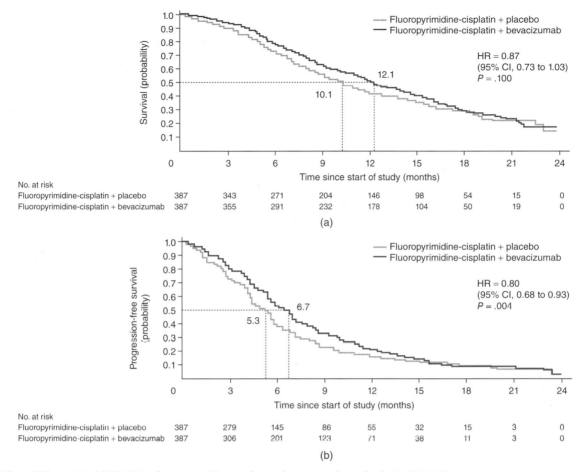

Figure 26.2 (a) OS and (b) PFS in fluoropyrimidine-cisplatin + bevacizumab vs. placebo in AVAGAST.

Further improvement of outcomes in advanced esophagogastric cancers depends on a deeper understanding of disease biology and identification of new targets in therapy. To this end, whole-exome sequencing of nearly 150 tumor-normal pairs recently identified 26 significantly mutated genes in treatment-naïve samples of esophageal adenocarcinoma, only five of which have previously been implicated in tumorigenesis. Among the many novel mutations, ELMO1 and DOCK2, upstream modulators of the RAC1 GTPase and its signaling pathway, are potentially actionable candidates for biologic therapy in the future [77, 78]. Four potentially targetable receptor-associated tyrosine kinase pathways showed more common gene amplification, including EGFR, HER2, MET, and FGF. KRAS also showed gene amplification.

26.5 Conclusions

Although progress has been modest, recent advances in the treatment of metastatic esophageal or GEJ adenocarcinoma have been made through the development of biologic agents. To date, monoclonal antibodies targeting HER2 (trastuzumab) and tumor-related angiogenesis (ramucirumab) have been shown to improve OS in Phase 3 trials of GEJ or gastric adenocarcinoma, whereas EGFR-targeted monoclonal antibodies (cetuximab, panitumumab) and small molecule inhibitors (gefitinib) have failed to show efficacy. Benefit from the dual EGFR/HER2-targeted tyrosine kinase inhibitor, lapatinib, appears to be limited, though responsive subpopulations may be identified. Success in further development of anti-cancer therapies in advanced disease will likely rely on focusing patient enrollment on those with actionable molecular targets.

References

1 Siegel R, Naishadham D, Jemal A (2013). Cancer statistics, 2013. *CA: A Cancer Journal for Clinicians* **63**(1), 11–30.

2 Devesa SS, Blot WJ, Fraumeni JF, Jr. (1998). Changing patterns in the incidence of esophageal and gastric carcinoma in the United States. *Cancer* **83**(10), 2049–53.

3 Homs MY, v d Gaast A, Siersema PD, Steyerberg EW, Kuipers EJ (2006). Chemotherapy for metastatic carcinoma of the esophagus and gastro-esophageal junction. *Cochrane Database of Systematic Reviews* (**4**), CD004063.

4 Wagner AD, Unverzagt S, Grothe W, Kleber G, Grothey A, Haerting J, et al. (2010). Chemotherapy for advanced gastric cancer. *Cochrane Database of Systematic Reviews* (**3**), CD004064.

5 Ezdinli EZ, Gelber R, Desai DV, Falkson G, Moertel CG, Hahn RG (1980). Chemotherapy of advanced esophageal carcinoma: Eastern Cooperative Oncology Group experience. *Cancer* **46**(10), 2149–53.

6 Kleinberg L, Forastiere AA (2007). Chemoradiation in the management of esophageal cancer. *Journal of Clinical Oncology* **25**(26), 4110–7.

7 Agrawal N, Jiao Y, Bettegowda C, Hutfless SM, Wang Y, David S, et al. (2012). Comparative genomic analysis of esophageal adenocarcinoma and squamous cell carcinoma. *Cancer Discovery* **2**(10), 899–905.

8 Van Cutsem E, Moiseyenko VM, Tjulandin S, Majlis A, Constenla M, Boni C, et al. (2006). Phase III study of docetaxel and cisplatin plus fluorouracil compared with cisplatin and fluorouracil as first-line therapy for advanced gastric cancer: a report of the V325 Study Group. *Journal of Clinical Oncology* **24**(31), 4991–7.

9 Ajani JA, Moiseyenko VM, Tjulandin S, Majlis A, Constenla M, Boni C, et al. (2007). Clinical benefit with docetaxel plus fluorouracil and cisplatin compared with cisplatin and fluorouracil in a phase III trial of advanced gastric or gastroesophageal cancer adenocarcinoma: the V-325 Study Group. *Journal of Clinical Oncology* **25**(22), 3205–9.

10 Al-Batran SE, Hartmann JT, Probst S, Schmalenberg H, Hollerbach S, Hofheinz R, et al. (2008). Phase III trial in metastatic gastroesophageal adenocarcinoma with fluorouracil, leucovorin plus either oxaliplatin or cisplatin: a study of the Arbeitsgemeinschaft Internistische Onkologie. *Journal of Clinical Oncology* **26**(9), 1435–42.

11 Enzinger P, Burtness B, Hollis D, et al. (2010). CALGB 80403/ECOG 1206: A randomized phase II study of three standard chemotherapy regimens (SCF, IC, FOLFOX) plus cetuximab in metastatic esophageal and GE junction cancer. *Journal of Clinical Oncology* **28**, 302s.

12 Thuss-Patience PC, Kretzschmar A, Repp M, Kingreen D, Hennesser D, Micheel S, et al. (2005). Docetaxel and continuous-infusion fluorouracil versus epirubicin, cisplatin, and fluorouracil for advanced gastric adenocarcinoma: a randomized phase II study. *Journal of Clinical Oncology* **23**(3), 494–501.

13 Cunningham D, Starling N, Rao S, Iveson T, Nicolson M, Coxon F, et al. (2008). Capecitabine and oxaliplatin for advanced esophagogastric cancer. *New England Journal of Medicine* **358**(1), 36–46.

14 Kang YK, Kang WK, Shin DB, Chen J, Xiong J, Wang J, et al. (2009). Capecitabine/cisplatin versus 5-fluorouracil/cisplatin as first-line therapy in patients with advanced gastric cancer: a randomised phase III noninferiority trial. *Annals of Oncology* **20**(4), 666–73.

15 Okines AF, Norman AR, McCloud P, Kang YK, Cunningham D (2009). Meta-analysis of the REAL-2 and ML17032 trials: evaluating capecitabine-based combination chemotherapy and infused 5-fluorouracil-based combination chemotherapy for the treatment of advanced oesophago-gastric cancer. *Annals of Oncology* **20**(9), 1529–34.

16 Enzinger PC, Ryan DP, Clark JW, Muzikansky A, Earle CC, Kulke MH, et al. (2009). Weekly docetaxel, cisplatin, and irinotecan (TPC): results of a multicenter phase II trial in patients with metastatic esophagogastric cancer. *Annals of Oncology* **20**(3), 475–80.

17 Di Lauro L, Nunziata C, Arena MG, Foggi P, Sperduti I, Lopez M (2007). Irinotecan, docetaxel and oxaliplatin combination in metastatic gastric or gastroesophageal junction adenocarcinoma. *British Journal of Cancer* **97**(5), 593–7.

18 Boku N, Yamamoto S, Fukuda H, Shirao K, Doi T, Sawaki A, et al. (2009). Fluorouracil versus combination of irinotecan plus cisplatin versus S-1 in metastatic gastric cancer: a randomised phase 3 study. *The Lancet Oncology* **10**(11), 1063–9.

19 Koizumi W, Narahara H, Hara T, Takagane A, Akiya T, Takagi M, et al. (2008). S-1 plus cisplatin versus S-1 alone for first-line treatment of advanced gastric cancer (SPIRITS trial): a phase III trial. *The Lancet Oncology* **9**(3), 215–21.

20 Ajani JA, Rodriguez W, Bodoky G, Moiseyenko V, Lichinitser M, Gorbunova V, et al. (2010). Multicenter phase III comparison of cisplatin/S-1 with cisplatin/infusional fluorouracil in advanced gastric or gastroesophageal adenocarcinoma study: the FLAGS trial. *Journal of Clinical Oncology* **28**(9), 1547–53.

21 Cook N, Marshall A, Blazeby JM, et al. (2013). Cougar-02: A randomized phase III study of docetaxel versus active symptom control in patients with relapsed esophago-gastric adenocarcinoma. *Journal of Clinical Oncology* **31**(suppl; abstr 4023).

22 Kang JH, Lee SI, Lim do H, Park KW, Oh SY, Kwon HC, et al. (2012). Salvage chemotherapy for pretreated gastric cancer: a randomized phase III trial comparing chemotherapy plus best supportive care with best supportive care alone. *Journal of Clinical Oncology* **30**(13), 1513–8.

23 Baselga J, Swain SM (2009). Novel anticancer targets: revisiting ERBB2 and discovering ERBB3. *Nature Reviews Cancer* **9**(7), 463–75.

24 Liang Z, Zeng X, Gao J, Wu S, Wang P, Shi X, *et al.* (2008). Analysis of EGFR, HER2, and TOP2A gene status and chromosomal polysomy in gastric adenocarcinoma from Chinese patients. *BMC Cancer* **8**, 363.

25 Bang YJ (2012). Advances in the management of HER2-positive advanced gastric and gastroesophageal junction cancer. *Journal of Clinical Gastroenterology* **46**(8), 637–48.

26 Bang YJ, Van Cutsem E, Feyereislova A, Chung HC, Shen L, Sawaki A, *et al.* (2010). Trastuzumab in combination with chemotherapy versus chemotherapy alone for treatment of HER2-positive advanced gastric or gastro-oesophageal junction cancer (ToGA): a phase 3, open-label, randomised controlled trial. *Lancet* **376**(9742), 687–97.

27 Yoon HH, Shi Q, Sukov WR, Wiktor AE, Khan M, Sattler CA, *et al.* (2012). Association of HER2/ErbB2 expression and gene amplification with pathologic features and prognosis in esophageal adenocarcinomas. *Clinical Cancer Research* **18**(2), 546–54.

28 Ruschoff J, Dietel M, Baretton G, Arbogast S, Walch A, Monges G, *et al.* (2010). HER2 diagnostics in gastric cancer-guideline validation and development of standardized immunohistochemical testing. *Virchows Archiv* **457**(3), 299–307.

29 Hofmann M, Stoss O, Shi D, Buttner R, van de Vijver M, Kim W, *et al.* (2008). Assessment of a HER2 scoring system for gastric cancer: results from a validation study. *Histopathology* **52**(7), 797–805.

30 NCI (2010). *FDA Approval for Trastuzumab:HER2-overexpressing Metastatic Gastric or Gastroesophageal (GE) Junction Adenocarcinoma* [cited 2010 Nov 5]. Available from: http://www.cancer.gov/canccrtopics/druginfo/fda-trastuzumab.

31 Kim MA, Lee HJ, Yang HK, Bang YJ, Kim WH (2011). Heterogeneous amplification of ERBB2 in primary lesions is responsible for the discordant ERBB2 status of primary and metastatic lesions in gastric carcinoma. *Histopathology* **59**(5), 822–31.

32 Park YS, Hwang IIS, Park IIJ, Ryu MH, Chang HM, Yook JH, *et al.* (2012). Comprehensive analysis of HER2 expression and gene amplification in gastric cancers using immunohistochemistry and in situ hybridization: which scoring system should we use? *Human Pathology* **43**(3), 413–22.

33 Terashima M, Kitada K, Ochiai A, Ichikawa W, Kurahashi I, Sakuramoto S, *et al.* (2012). Impact of expression of human epidermal growth factor receptors EGFR and ERBB2 on survival in stage II/III gastric cancer. *Clinical Cancer Research* **18**(21), 5992–6000.

34 Yoon HH, Shi Q, Sukov WR, Sattler CA, Wiktor AE, Wu T-T, *et al.* (2012). HER2 testing in esophageal adenocarcinoma (EAC) using parallel tissue-based methods. *Journal of Clinical Oncology* **30**(suppl 34, abstr 2).

35 European Medicines Agency (2009). *Post-authorisation summary of positive opinion for Herceptin.* Available at: http://www.emea.europa.eu/docs/en_GB/document_library/Summary_of_opinion/human/000278/WC500059913.pdf (accessed April 9, 2012).

36 Janjigian YY, Werner D, Pauligk C, Steinmetz K, Kelsen DP, Jager E, *et al.* (2012). Prognosis of metastatic gastric and gastroesophageal junction cancer by HER2 status: a European and USA International collaborative analysis. *Annals of Oncology* **23**(10), 2656–62.

37 Lordick F, Kang YK, Chung HC, Salman P, Oh SC, Bodoky G, *et al.* (2013). Capecitabine and cisplatin with or without cetuximab for patients with previously untreated advanced gastric cancer (EXPAND): a randomised, open-label phase 3 trial. *The Lancet Oncology* **14**(6), 490–9.

38 Waddell T, Chau I, Cunningham D, Gonzalez D, Frances A, Okines C, *et al.* (2013). Epirubicin, oxaliplatin, and capecitabine with or without panitumumab for patients with previously untreated advanced oesophagogastric cancer (REAL3): a randomised, open-label phase 3 trial. *The Lancet Oncology* **14**(6), 481–9.

39 Okines AF, Thompson LC, Cunningham D, Wotherspoon A, Reis-Filho JS, Langley RE, *et al.* (2012). Effect of HER2 on prognosis and benefit from peri-operative chemotherapy in early oesophago-gastric adenocarcinoma in the MAGIC trial. *Annals of Oncology* **24**(5), 1253–61.

40 Gordon MA, Gundacker HM, Benedetti J, Macdonald JS, Baranda JC, Levin WJ, *et al.* (2013). Assessment of HER2 gene amplification in adenocarcinomas of the stomach or gastroesophageal junction in the INT-0116/SWOG9008 clinical trial. *Annals of Oncology* **24**(7), 1754–61.

41 Chua TC, Merrett ND (2011). Clinicopathologic factors associated with HER2-Positive gastric cancer and its impact on survival outcomes – a systematic review. *International Journal of Cancer* **130**(12), 2845–56.

42 Reddy D, Wainberg ZA (2011). Targeted therapies for metastatic esophagogastric cancer. *Current Treatment Options in Oncology* **12**(1), 46–60.

43 Brien TP, Odze RD, Sheehan CE, McKenna BJ, Ross JS (2000). HER-2/neu gene amplification by FISH predicts poor survival in Barrett's esophagus-associated adenocarcinoma. *Human Pathology* **31**(1), 35–9.

44 Schoppmann SF, Jesch B, Friedrich J, Wrba F, Schultheis A, Pluschnig U, *et al.* (2010). Expression of Her-2 in carcinomas of the esophagus. *American Journal of Surgical Pathology* **34**(12), 1868–73.

45 Hu Y, Bandla S, Godfrey TE, Tan D, Luketich JD, Pennathur A, *et al.* (2011). HER2 amplification, overexpression and score criteria in esophageal adenocarcinoma. *Modern Pathology* **24**(7), 899–907.

46 Thompson SK, Sullivan TR, Davies R, Ruszkiewicz AR (2011). HER-2/neu Gene Amplification in Esophageal Adenocarcinoma and Its Influence on Survival. *Annals of Surgical Oncology* **18**(7), 2010–7.

47 Bang YJ (2012). A randomized o-l, phase III study of lapatinib in combination with weekly paclitaxel versus weekly paclitaxel alone in the second-line treatment of HER2 amplified advanced gastric cancer (AGC) in Asian population: Tytan study. *Journal of Clinical Oncology* **30**(suppl 34, abstr 11).

48 Hecht JR, Bang Y-J, Qin S, Chung H-C, Xu J-M, *et al.* (2013). Lapatinib in combination with capecitabine plus oxaliplatin (CapeOx) in HER2-positive advanced or metastatic gastric, esophageal, or gastroesophageal adenocarcinoma (AC): The TRIO-013/LOGiC Trial. *Journal of Clinical Oncology* **31**(suppl; abstr LBA4001).

49 Norguet E, Dahan L, Seitz JF (2012). Targetting esophageal and gastric cancers with monoclonal antibodies. *Current Topics in Medicinal Chemistry* **12**(15), 1678–82.

50 Xu Y, Sheng L, Mao W (2013). Role of epidermal growth factor receptor tyrosine kinase inhibitors in the treatment of esophageal carcinoma and the suggested mechanisms of action. *Oncology Letters* **5**(1), 19–24.

51 Tomblyn MB, Goldman BH, Thomas CR, Jr., Benedetti JK, Lenz HJ, Mehta V, *et al.* (2012). Cetuximab plus cisplatin, irinotecan, and thoracic radiotherapy as definitive treatment for locally advanced, unresectable esophageal cancer: a phase-II study of the SWOG (S0414). *Journal of Thoracic Oncology* **7**(5), 906–12.

52 Lorenzen S, Schuster T, Porschen R, Al-Batran SE, Hofheinz R, Thuss-Patience P, *et al.* (2009). Cetuximab plus cisplatin-5-fluorouracil versus cisplatin-5-fluorouracil alone in first-line metastatic squamous cell carcinoma of the esophagus: a randomized phase II study of the Arbeitsgemeinschaft Internistische Onkologie. *Annals of Oncology* **20**(10), 1667–73.

53 Moehler MH, Ringshausen I, Hofheinz R, Al-Batran S-E, Mueller L, Thuss-Patience PC, *et al.* (2013). POWER: An open-label, randomized phase III trial of cisplatin and 5-FU with or without panitumumab (P) for patients (pts) with nonresectable, advanced, or metastatic esophageal squamous cell cancer (ESCC). *Journal of Clinical Oncology* **31**(suppl; abstr TPS4158).

54 Zhang X, Lu M, Wang X, Li J, Li Y, Li J, *et al.* (2013). Nimotuzumab plus paclitaxel and cisplatin as first-line treatment for esophageal squamous cell cancer: A single center prospective clinical trial. *Journal of Clinical Oncology* **31**(suppl, abstr 4097).

55 Dutton SJ, Blazeby JM, Petty RD, Mansoor W, *et al.* (2013). Patient-reported outcomes from a phase III multicenter, randomized, double-blind, placebo-controlled trial of gefitinib versus placebo in esophageal cancer progressing after chemotherapy: Cancer Oesophagus Gefitinib (COG). *Journal of Clinical Oncology* **30**(suppl 34; abstr 6).

56 Dragovich T, McCoy S, Fenoglio-Preiser CM, Wang J, Benedetti JK, Baker AF, *et al.* (2006). Phase II trial of erlotinib in gastroesophageal junction and gastric adenocarcinomas: SWOG 0127. *Journal of Clinical Oncology* **24**(30), 4922–7.

57 Personeni N (2007). Outcome prediction to erlotinib in gastroesophageal adenocarcinomas: can we improve epidermal growth factor receptor and phospho-AKT testing? *Journal of Clinical Oncology* **25**(7), 910; author reply 1.

58 Wainberg ZA, Lin LS, DiCarlo B, Dao KM, Patel R, Park DJ, *et al.* (2011). Phase II trial of modified FOLFOX6 and erlotinib in patients with metastatic or advanced adenocarcinoma of the oesophagus and gastro-oesophageal junction. *British Journal of Cancer* **105**(6), 760–5.

59 Trusolino L, Bertotti A, Comoglio PM (2010). MET signalling: principles and functions in development, organ regeneration and cancer. *Nature Reviews Molecular Cell Biology* **11**(12), 834–48.

60 Eder JP, Vande Woude GF, Boerner SA, LoRusso PM (2009). Novel therapeutic inhibitors of the c-Met signaling pathway in cancer. *Clinical Cancer Research* **15**(7), 2207–14.

61 Xin X, Yang S, Ingle G, Zlot C, Rangell L, Kowalski J, *et al.* (2001). Hepatocyte growth factor enhances vascular endothelial growth factor-induced angiogenesis *in vitro* and *in vivo*. *American Journal of Pathology* **158**(3), 1111–20.

62 Lennerz JK, Kwak EL, Ackerman A, Michael M, Fox SB, Bergethon K, *et al.* (2011). MET amplification identifies a small and aggressive subgroup of esophagogastric adenocarcinoma with evidence of responsiveness to crizotinib. *Journal of Clinical Oncology* **29**(36), 4803–10.

63 Miller CT, Lin L, Casper AM, Lim J, Thomas DG, Orringer MB, *et al.* (2006). Genomic amplification of MET with boundaries within fragile site FRA7G and upregulation of MET pathways in esophageal adenocarcinoma. *Oncogene* **25**(3), 409–18.

64 Tsugawa K, Yonemura Y, Hirono Y, Fushida S, Kaji M, Miwa K, *et al.* (1998). Amplification of the c-met, c-erbB-2 and epidermal growth factor receptor gene in human gastric cancers: correlation to clinical features. *Oncology* **55**(5), 475–81.

65 Iveson T, Donehower RC, Davidenko I, *et al.* (2011). *Safety and efficacy of epirubicin, cisplatin, and capecitabine (ECX) plus rilotumumab (R) as first-line treatment for unresectable locally advanced (LA) or metastatic (M) gastric or esophagogastric junction (EGJ) adenocarcinoma.* Program and abstracts of the 2011 European Multidisciplinary Cancer Congress, September 23–27, 2011, Stockholm, Sweden. Abstract 6504.

66 Oliner KS, Tang R, Anderson A, Lan Y, Iveson T, Donehower RC, Jiang Y, Dubey S, Loh E (2012). Evaluation of MET pathway biomarkers in a phase II study of rilotumumab (R, AMG 102) or placebo (P) in combination with epirubicin, cisplatin, and capecitabine (ECX) in patients (pts) with locally advanced or metastatic gastric (G) or esophagogastric junction (EGJ) cancer. *Journal of Clinical Oncology* **30**(suppl; abstr 4005).

67 Auvinen MI, Sihvo EI, Ruohtula T, Salminen JT, Koivistoinen A, Siivola P, *et al.* (2002). Incipient angiogenesis in Barrett's epithelium and lymphangiogenesis in Barrett's adenocarcinoma. *Journal of Clinical Oncology* **20**(13), 2971–9.

68 Gockel I, Moehler M, Frerichs K, Drescher D, Trinh TT, Duenschede F, *et al.* (2008). Co-expression of receptor tyrosine kinases in esophageal adenocarcinoma and squamous cell cancer. *Oncology Reports* **20**(4), 845–50.

69 Spratlin J. Ramucirumab (2011). (IMC-1121B): Monoclonal antibody inhibition of vascular endothelial growth factor receptor-2. *Current Oncology Reports* **13**(2), 97–102.

70 Jung YD, Mansfield PF, Akagi M, Takeda A, Liu W, Bucana CD, *et al.* (2002). Effects of combination anti-vascular endothelial growth factor receptor and anti-epidermal growth factor receptor therapies on the growth of gastric cancer in a nude mouse model. *European Journal of Cancer* **38**(8), 1133–40.

71 Fuchs CS, Tomasek J, Cho JY, Dumitru F, *et al.* (2012). REGARD: A phase III, randomized, double-blinded trial of ramucirumab and best supportive care (BSC) versus placebo and BSC in the treatment of metastatic gastric or gastroesophageal junction (GEJ) adenocarcinoma following disease progression on first-line platinum- and/or fluoropyrimidine-containing combination therapy. *Journal of Clinical Oncology* **30**(suppl 34, abstr LBA5).

72 Wilke H, Van Cutsem E, Oh SC, *et al.* (2014). RAINBOW: A global, phase III, randomized, double-blind study of ramucirumab plus paclitaxel versus placebo plus paclitaxel in the treatment of metastatic gastroesophageal junction (GEJ) and gastric adenocarcinoma following disease progression on first-line platinum- and fluoropyrimidine-containing combination therapy rainbow IMCL CP12-0922 (I4T-IE-JVBE). *Journal of Clinical Oncology* **32**(suppl 3, abstr LBA7).

73 Yoon HH, Bendell JC, Braiteh FS, *et al.* (2014). Ramucirumab (RAM) plus FOLFOX as front-line therapy (Rx) for advanced gastric or esophageal adenocarcinoma (GE-AC): Randomized, double-blind, multicenter phase 2 trial. *Journal of Clinical Oncology* **32**(5s) (suppl; abstr 4004).

74 Ohtsu A, Shah MA, Van Cutsem E, Rha SY, Sawaki A, Park SR, *et al.* (2011). Bevacizumab in combination with chemotherapy as first-line therapy in advanced gastric cancer: a randomized, double-blind, placebo-controlled phase III study. *Journal of Clinical Oncology* **29**(30), 3968–76.

75 Van Cutsem E, de Haas S, Kang YK, Ohtsu A, Tebbutt NC, Ming Xu J, *et al.* (2012). Bevacizumab in combination with chemotherapy as first-line therapy in advanced gastric cancer: a biomarker evaluation from the AVAGAST randomized phase III trial. *Journal of Clinical Oncology* **30**(17), 2119–27.

76 Bang Y-J, Im S-A, Lee K-W, *et al.* (2013). Olaparib plus paclitaxel in patients with recurrent or metastatic gastric cancer: A randomized, double-blind phase II study. *Journal of Clinical Oncology* **31**(suppl; abstr 4013).

77 Dulak AM, Stojanov P, Peng S, Lawrence MS, Fox C, Stewart C, *et al.* (2013). Exome and whole-genome sequencing of esophageal adenocarcinoma identifies recurrent driver events and mutational complexity. *Nature Genetics* **45**(5), 478–86.

78 Dulak AM, Schumacher SE, van Lieshout J, Imamura Y, Fox C, Shim B, *et al.* (2012). Gastrointestinal adenocarcinomas of the esophagus, stomach, and colon exhibit distinct patterns of genome instability and oncogenesis. *Cancer Research* **72**(17), 4383–93.

CHAPTER 27

Role of endoscopy and nutritional support in advanced esophageal cancer

Manol Jovani, Andrea Anderloni & Alessandro Repici

Digestive Endoscopy Unit, Division of Gastroenterology, Humanitas Research Hospital, Rozzano, Milan, Italy

27.1 Introduction

Esophageal cancer is the eighth most common malignant disorder and sixth on the list of cancer-related mortality with a five-year survival rate of 10–15% [1]. Despite recent advances in curative treatment, more than 50% of patients have inoperable disease at presentation, due to local tumor infiltration and/or distant metastases (stage III or IV disease), or other poor general conditions that make them unsuitable candidates for surgery [2].

Dysphagia is the most common clinical manifestation, scored in ascending order according to its severity: 0 = ability to eat a normal diet; 1 = ability to eat some solid food; 2 = ability to eat some semi-solids only; 3 = ability to swallow liquids only; and 4 = complete dysphagia [3]. The inevitable result of dysphagia is weight loss, which has an estimated global incidence at the diagnosis of esophageal cancer of approximately 80% [1, 4]. Another important complication of advanced dysphagia is aspiration pneumonia.

The mechanisms of weight loss are multifaceted. Reduced or annulled oral food intake, mostly due to the mechanical obstruction of the tumor mass, obviously plays an important role. The side-effects of administered radiochemotherapy, such as nausea, vomiting, diarrhea, mucositis, pharyngodynia and pain in swallowing, fatigue and loss of appetite, also may worsen oral nutrient intake and, hence, malnutrition [5].

Metabolism alteration is another important component of the weight loss. A systemic inflammatory response determining an increase in the catabolism of proteins and fats, increased energy expenditure, and modified hormonal secretions, is observed in these patients, and underpins the manifestation of cachexia [6]. Increased pro-inflammatory cytokines, such as IL-1β, IL-6, TNFα, as well as C reactive protein (CRP) levels have been constantly observed in patients affected by neoplasia [7]. In obese patients, who are at increased risk of developing esophageal cancer, weight loss is not always clinically discernible, particularly in the early stages of the disease, since sarcopenia is usually the first alteration of body composition [5, 6]. Eventually, however, the disease, if not treated, progresses inexorably toward cachexia.

Cancer cachexia is associated with poor health-related quality of life (HRQoL), reduced performance status with decline in motor and mental function, lower response rates to treatment, increased morbidity, prolonged hospital stays and overall poorer clinical outcome [5, 6, 8]. Weight loss exceeding 15% has been found to be an independent predictive factor of survival and response to radiochemotherapy in different studies [6, 9]. The Glasgow Prognostic score, which takes into account the levels of albumin (as a nutritional marker) and CRP (as an inflammatory marker), has been associated with cancer-specific survival, independent of stage and type of treatment received, in patients with inoperable gastroesophageal cancer [6, 10]. Hence, nutritional support is of paramount importance in this setting.

Esophageal Cancer and Barrett's Esophagus, Third Edition. Edited by Prateek Sharma, Richard Sampliner and David Ilson.
© 2015 John Wiley & Sons, Ltd. Published 2015 by John Wiley & Sons, Ltd.

27.2 Nutritional support in advanced esophageal cancer

The average time of survival from diagnosis for patients affected by inoperable esophageal cancer is 4–6 months. When interventions aimed at the radical cure of the disease are not feasible, palliation and improvement of the HRQoL come next on the priority scale. In this setting, they are achieved by providing adequate nourishment to the patient. Both enteral and parenteral nutrition have been used for nutritional support and, overall, seem to be equally effective. The enteral route is, however, preferable to the parenteral one, since it is more physiologic. Enteral nutrition, in fact, stimulates the intestinal mucosa and, hence, preserves gut function and integrity, reducing thus the risk of bacterial translocation and septic complications. Furthermore, it reduces the risk of aspiration pneumonia and is less expensive [4, 5]. Early dysphagia relief and restored oral food intake has the crucial benefit of providing the physiologically needed enteral nutritional support. It has substantial additional psychological, spiritual, social, and cultural benefits as well, since patients can taste food and follow social customs and life which often revolves around food. Dysphagia relief is, therefore, pivotal for a good HRQoL for both patients and caregivers [11].

Yet, reducing/annulling dysphagia and restoring oral intake may often, in itself, be insufficient to sustain an adequate weight, since metabolic factor are at play as well. In fact, in two retrospective studies with patients affected by IEC palliated with stent placement, cachexia was not reversed and overall survival was not significantly altered. This implies that simple dysphagia relief may not, in itself, be sufficient for sustaining the metabolic needs of the patients [8, 12].

Additional means of nutritional support are therefore needed [5], including diet modification and oral supplementation. It has been shown that regular interventions, in particular dietary counseling, aid in improving nutritional status and, therefore, HRQoL, as well as tolerance to palliative radiochemotherapy and survival [5, 11]. Dietary counseling by a professional dietitian is useful for developing a healthier diet, with the addition of specific supplements designed to reduce oxidative stress and inflammation, as a part of the overall palliative care plan. Dietary alteration may also be psychologically helpful for both the patient and the caregiver, as they feel more in control of their circumstances and active in the management of the disease, thereby increasing their HRQoL [11].

27.3 Palliative endoscopy in inoperable esophageal cancer

27.3.1 Introduction

As mentioned, cachexia may be countered by antagonizing both its main arms: metabolic alterations and dysphagia. The former is beyond the scope of this chapter, whose focus is the role of endoscopy in relieving dysphagia. To date, the best efforts of clinical research have focused on this aspect. Historically, surgery (either resection, by-pass or surgical jejunostomy) has been the cornerstone of palliative interventions aimed at dysphagia relief. Other, non-endoscopic, palliative treatments include palliative external beam radiation therapy and/or systemic chemotherapy. These treatments are usually plagued by long hospitalization stay and high costs, important complications and co-morbidities [13].

The advent of endoscopy has radically changed this scenario. Generally speaking, the endoscopic palliation consists of the elimination, reduction or bypass of the mechanic obstruction caused by the tumor, with the reconstitution of a normal, or almost normal, oral nutrition. Ideally, palliative interventions should provide an early and easy symptomatic relief, with a minimal number of interventions, minimal morbidity and reduced hospital stay and costs. Endoscopic palliation performs better than surgery in all of these aspects [13, 14].

Stent placement and brachytherapy are currently the two most evidence-based palliative options. Other techniques include dilatation, photodynamic therapy, APC, laser and cryotherapy, injection of ethanol and chemotherapeutic agents, and PEG placement, or any combination of these [14]. We will now briefly review each of these modalities, mention both pros and cons of each, and prospect future directions in the palliative care of inoperable esophageal cancer.

27.3.2 Endoscopic dilatation

Both methods of dilatation – mechanic polyvinyl bougie or pneumatic balloon dilatation – offer an immediate, easy-to-perform and cheap relief of dysphagia. Recurrence, however, is often the rule, with a need for new interventions from a few days to at least every few weeks, with an important risk of perforation [14, 15]. In clinical practice, dilation is rarely performed alone. Its main role is that of adjunct treatment to facilitate stent [16] or PEG [17] placement.

27.3.3 Endoscopic stent placement

Stent placement has become the most frequent endoscopic method of palliation in inoperable esophageal cancer, since it allows an immediate relief of dysphagia with an acceptable rate of complications.

Stents may be placed with radiologic guidance or under direct endoscopic guidance. Some of the technical aspects of stent placement are as follows. The correct length and diameter of the stent should be selected before insertion, to ensure optimal results. Barium swallow and endoscopic estimation of tumor length are necessary to select proper stent length because, ideally, the prosthesis should be long enough to completely cover the tumor, with 2–3 cm projecting both distally and proximally to the borders of the tumor.

The procedure is usually performed under deep sedation. After the patient is placed into the left lateral position and the bite block is inserted, a standard or a small-caliber gastroscope is advanced to the upper margin of the stricture. If the procedure is performed with radiologic guidance, an internal marker (injection of contrast or placement of endoscopic clips) should be placed, using fluoroscopy, to allow for precise location of the tumor upper margin. Once the location and the length of the tumor have been defined, the stricture is crossed with a guidewire. A super-stiff metallic guidewire or a soft or hydrophilic guidewire is used, depending on the type of strictures. After stent deployment, contrast medium is injected through the working channel of the scope to confirm correct position and expansion of the stent, and to exclude complications such as perforation. Although there is little evidence, dilation of the stricture before esophageal stent placement should be discouraged, unless the severity of the stricture precludes the advancement of the stent catheter.

The stent can be also placed under endoscopic guidance. A small-diameter endoscope is used to traverse the stricture. A guidewire is passed into the stomach or proximal duodenum. The scope is reinserted first into the esophagus, and the stent is advanced over the guidewire under endoscopic visualization. With the scope alongside the pre-deployed stent delivery system, direct observation of the proximal end of the stent and its precise location can be maintained and monitored. The stent can be advanced or withdrawn, as necessary, based upon the relationship of the stent to the stricture. Although the distal end is not seen (if fluoroscopy is not used at all during the procedure), this should not be a concern, assuming that a stent of appropriate length has been chosen.

The advantage of SEMS placement by direct vision is that it allows stent deployment in the endoscopy room at the time of assessment, thereby minimizing the number of interventions required. The length of the stent is chosen so that at least 2 cm of the normal esophagus is covered by the stent above and below the tumor. Long strictures may require more than one stent, with one-third overlap between the stents. Stent placement is technically feasible in over 95% of cases, and dysphagia relief has been reported in 90–100% of patients in most studies. Technical failure, such as stent misplacement, failed expansion, and/or failed deployment, are quite rare [16, 18, 19].

A great variety of stents exist and have been employed in the palliation of malignant dysphagia [19–29]. Self-expanding metal stents (SEMS) are the most common, both uncovered and covered, either fully-covered (FC) or partially-covered (PC). Nowadays, the majority of stents are made of nitinol, an alloy of nickel and titanium, which carries the unique properties of superelasticity and shape memory [16]. Other types of stents include rigid stents, self-expanding plastic stents (SEPS) and biodegradable stents. All of these stents come in different designs, diameters and compositions, but all have the same basic trait – that of creating an artificial lumen across the stenosis caused by the exophytic neoplasia (Figure 27.1: see also Plate 27.1). Stents are easily visualized with plain radiography, and the luminal patency is easily evaluated by fluoroscopy (Figure 27.2: see also Plate 27.2). Most of these stents can be removed and replaced, if necessary [16, 18].

Rigid stent placement has fallen out of favor because of higher complication rates and morbidity and lower dysphagia relief, compared to SEMS, and are currently seldom, if ever, used [16, 30, 31]. SEMS and SEPS seem to be equally effective in relieving dysphagia, but SEPS are more difficult to place and more prone to migration and are, therefore, less preferable [28, 29]. In the family of SEMS, the uncovered stents have been almost universally abandoned, because of the high rates

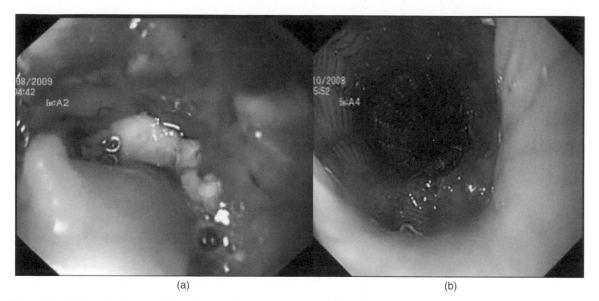

Figure 27.1   (a) Stenosis from esophageal cancer. (b) Reconstruction of luminal perviety with placement of an esophageal stent. *(See insert for color representation of this figure.)*

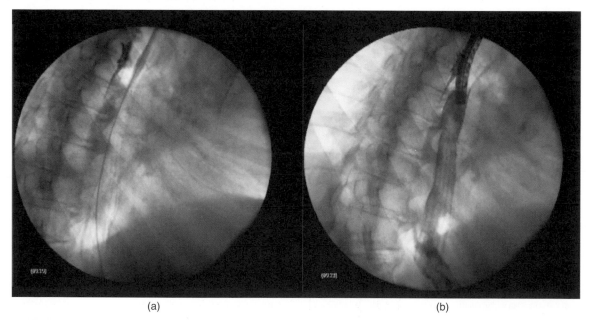

Figure 27.2   (a) Plain radiography after stent placement. (b) Fluoroscopy after stent placement. *(See insert for color representation of this figure.)*

of recurrent dysphagia from tumor ingrowth through the bare metal mesh [16, 18]. In the covered family of SEMS, the FC design seems preferable to the PC design, because PC-SEMS stents develop recurrent dysphagia from strictures of the uncovered stent ends, by tissue reaction/tumor invasion of the bare metal mesh, in up to 31% of patients, with consequent unsafe stent removal [19, 21, 22].

The FC-SEMS have been designed to overcome such shortcomings, with the assumption that the complete covering would greatly reduce, if not annul, tissue/tumor ingrowth and, consequently, reduce recurrent dysphagia and facilitate removal [18, 21]. A well-known, and predictable, drawback of the FC design has, however, been an increase in the rate of migration, ranging from 20–39% in most studies, especially when placed across the gastroesophageal junction (GEJ) [18–21]. Migration rates of PC-SEMS are generally lower, ranging 2–17% in most studies, because the same tissue reaction that may cause dysphagia recurrence also serves to anchor the stent and prevent migration [3, 18, 23, 24, 26]. Newer FC-SEMS designs or refinement of old FC designs, seem, however, to have lowered the rates of migration, making them similar to the PC designs, on the order of 7–12% [21, 25, 26].

While the FC design has greatly reduced tissue ingrowth, tissue overgrowth is still a problem [18, 21, 25]. Both tissue in- and overgrowth may be treated by placing another FC-SEMS across the grown tissue/neoplasia, thus causing mechanical necrosis of that tissue – so that, successively, both stents may be removed if necessary ("stent-in-stent" technique) – or else by argon plasma coagulation or laser therapy [32]. Fully-covered SEMS are the treatment of choice for malignant tracheo-esophageal fistula, or for perforation following endoscopic treatment [33].

There is very little experience with the newly introduced biodegradable stents in esophageal cancer, and this is mostly in a bridge-to-surgery setting [34]. To date, there is only one study using biodegradable stents in inoperable esophageal tumor in combination to brachytherapy, and it did not perform well [35].

Even though placement of stents for the palliation of neoplasia close (<2 cm) to the upper esophageal sphincter is more problematic, because of increased risk of perforation, airway compression, aspiration pneumonia and pain and globus sensation, it is nevertheless feasible. Two studies have shown that it is safe and effective for dysphagia relief and fistula closure, with acceptable rates of complications [27, 36]. Airway compression may be avoided by using small-diameter stents, or by stenting the airway as well [18]. When stenting is not feasible, other palliative techniques can be used [37, 38].

Apart from the aforementioned tissue/tumor in- and overgrowth, there can be other complications from stent placement in up to 50% of patients [39]. Serious or life-threatening complications from stent placement are relatively rare, in the order of 5–15%, although higher rates, sometimes up to 40% [23], have been reported

in some studies. Such complications include early or late perforation, early or late bleeding, formation of tracheoesophageal fistula, tracheal compression, fever and pneumonia, or procedure-related death. These may be managed with medical therapy, such as antibiotics, and with other endoscopic interventions, such as removal of the stent or placement of another.

Prior or concomitant radiochemotherapy may increase the risk of these complications, especially for patients with a T4 neoplasia [40–42], though not all data from the literature concur [43]. Most complications are, however, minor, such as mild chest pain or gastroesophageal reflux disease, which are usually managed with medical therapy. Some stents have also an antireflux valve, particularly stents placed across the GEJ, which seem to offer little or no additional benefit [33, 44]. Food impaction is another complication easily treated with endoscopic cleansing.

It is our practice to give to the patients some useful dietary instructions to avoid food impaction. Starting from 2–3 hours after stent placement, up to the first 24 hours, we advise a liquid diet. After that, for the successive 24–48 hours, we advise semi-solid soft diet, and free diet afterward. We further advise the patient to eat small quantities of food frequently, and to masticate well, to eat in an upright position and to drink small quantities of carbonated sparkling beverages frequently during and after meals (e.g. cola or similar). We would, furthermore, advise them to reduce or avoid certain foods which may predispose to food impaction, such as fresh bread and fibrous meat (poultry, fowl) and, in their place, to use more toasted bread and minced meat (e.g. hamburger). Such dietary instruction, together with the amelioration of the stent designs, has greatly reduced the rate of dysphagia recurrence from food impaction [18].

Placement of SEMS has become the mainstay palliative option in inoperable esophageal cancer, and is widespread in clinical practice, particularly for patients with relatively poor prognosis [45]. The challenge for the future is that of creating a stent design which minimizes both tissue in- and overgrowth, as well as migration. Stent insertion has also been combined with other palliative modalities, as we shall discuss below.

27.3.4 Intraluminal radiotherapy (brachytherapy)

Intraluminal radiotherapy (brachytherapy) is performed by placing the radiation source directly onto the site of the esophageal cancer, temporarily exposing it to high amounts of radiation from a short distance. Iridium (^{192}I) is the most common radioactive source utilized [15]. Brachytherapy may be applied either as single-fraction treatment, usually 12 Gy per hour, or multi-fraction treatment, usually 16 Gy in two fractions or 18 Gy in three fractions. These last options seems to offer the better results [46]. Here, in contrast to external beam radiotherapy, the radiation affects just a localized area around the source, and the dose decreases rapidly in the surrounding normal tissue, sparing the lungs, heart and liver. Brachytherapy is used as palliation in obstructing and bleeding tumors, with an overall dysphagia relief rate of nearly 90%. The offset of this effect is, however, delayed in time, and it usually becomes significant after 4–6 weeks [15, 46].

One important study compared single-dose brachytherapy with stent placement [47]. Stents offered an immediate and better dysphagia relief during the first month, while the offset of dysphagia relief with brachytherapy was slower. This difference, however, tended to disappear by the third month, and brachytherapy showed a more durable long-term relief. Nearly 45% of patients allocated to brachytherapy also received SEMS during follow-up, which may explain, in part, the positive long-term effects observed in this group. Complication rates were higher on the stent group, mostly owing to late bleeding. Overall, HRQoL was better in the brachytherapy-treated patients. No difference, in terms of persistent or recurrent dysphagia, as well as median survival and costs, was observed [47]. Similar results were seen in another, smaller trial, that compared stenting with three-dose fractionated brachytherapy [48]. In this case, however, cost-effectiveness favored stenting [49].

Since stent placement offers an immediate relief of dysphagia, and brachytherapy offers a better long-term dysphagia relief, combining these two techniques may prove to be the best choice for patients with an expected survival of more than three months. This hypothesis was recently evaluated in two studies. One was a single-arm safety study, in which no major complications were reported with the combination therapy [50]. The other was a comparative study, in which patients were randomized to receive either SEMS plus brachytherapy, or brachytherapy alone. Combination therapy offered a more prolonged dysphagia-free period and prolonged survival, compared

with stent alone, with a relatively low rate of major complications [51].

However, another recent, single-arm safety study using biodegradable stents did not support the use of combined treatment. The procedure was technically feasible and luminal patency was restored in all patients. The study was, nevertheless, prematurely interrupted, because of the high early intervention-related major complication rates (47%), such as severe retrosternal pain, nausea, vomiting, hematemesis and recurrent dysphagia. The authors concluded that the BS design was probably responsible for such outcomes [52].

Another interesting way to associate stents with brachytherapy is that of loading stents with radioactive iodine 125 seeds (^{125}I). One study compared this association with conventional stent treatment in advanced esophageal cancer. Both treatments performed equally in terms of dysphagia relief in the first month. By the second month, however, dysphagia improvement was significantly better in the combination group, as was overall survival, with equal major complication rates [53]. Combination of brachytherapy with other techniques – such as laser [54], PDT [55] or APC [56] – is feasible, too, and adds to their palliative potential.

Advantages of brachytherapy include short treatment sessions performed in an outpatient setting, thus allowing a greater number of patients to receive it, and its local nature avoids radiation of surrounding tissue and of health-care professionals. Complications of brachytherapy are relatively rare, in the order of 10–20%, and include fistula formation, pain, radiation esophagitis and esophageal strictures [15]. Brachytherapy is considered the first treatment choice in patients with inoperable esophageal cancer with expected survival of more than three months [45]. Ongoing studies will reveal whether the association of brachytherapy with stents, or other palliative modalities, will become the new standard of care in palliative treatments.

27.3.5 Other techniques
27.3.5.1 Photodynamic therapy (PDT)
PDT is a non-thermal endoscopic ablative technique that makes use of photo-sensible molecules which accumulate in malignant cells, such as porfimer sodium. Twenty-four hours after intravenous administration of the agent, endoscopy is performed and the photosensitizer-carrying malignant cells are selectively exposed to a red light with a specific

wavelength. This, in turn, induces the production of highly reactive oxygen molecules that destroy the host cells [55]. By carefully and specifically limiting the area exposed to the red light, it is possible to ablate only the neoplastic mass without damaging the surrounding tissue. A repeat endoscopy is usually necessary 48 hours later, for tumor response assessment, mechanical or pneumatic dilation of the esophageal lumen to avoid post-PDT stricture formation, debridement of necrotic tumor and administration of additional laser therapy, if necessary.

Initial studies have shown significant improvement of the HRQoL and dysphagia score [37, 57]. In a minority of cases, it has been used for treating tumor-related bleeding, pain or poor appetite. PDT may be useful as a palliative treatment in patients with cancer at the cervical esophagus, where the placement of stents is problematic, as well as salvage therapy in cases of dysphagia recurrence from in-or-overgrowth after stent placement, locally recurrent neoplasia after resection and/or failure of other palliative techniques [37, 57].

PDT may be also combined with other endoscopic techniques, such as laser therapy [58], brachytherapy [55] or stent placement [57]. Complications are usually rare, in the order of 2–8%, and include esophagitis, stricture formation, aspiration pneumonia and perforation [55]. Combination with pneumatic/mechanical dilation increase the risk of perforation, and PDT-related death has been reported in up to 1.8% of patients [57].

One of the main disadvantages of PDT is skin photosensitivity, which obliges the patient to avoid sunlight for the subsequent 4–6 weeks. Other disadvantages include the need for repeat session in 6–8 weeks for tumor regrowth, and expensive device and special skills required for its administration. This technique is still considered experimental, and current guidelines do not recommend it for routine palliation of inoperable esophageal cancer [33, 58].

27.3.5.2 Neodymium-doped yttrium aluminum garnet (Nd:YAG) laser

Laser therapy is a thermal ablative technique, during which esophageal neoplasia is vaporized or coagulated under direct endoscopic vision, obtaining recanalization of the lumen in over 90% of cases [54]. This procedure may be unsafe for submucosal tumors or angulated ones, and also it may cause important esophageal stenosis if administered to circumferential lesions.

Hence, small (<6 cm), exophytic, mid-esophageal tumors are most amenable to this kind of treatment [15]. Nd:YAG laser can also be used for the treatment of recurrent dysphagia in obstructed stents from tumor in- or overgrowth [57].

Thermal therapy (Nd:YAG laser or APC) performs well compared to stent placement in terms of dysphagia relief rates, with better HRQoL but higher costs [59]. An important disadvantage is that repeat sessions, often every few weeks, become necessary as the neoplasia re-grows. The combination with brachytherapy was shown to reduce tumor regrowth and, therefore, enhance the palliative effect of Nd:YAG [33, 54].

Complications are relatively rare, and include perforation and/or fistula formation, hemorrhage and sepsis in 5–10% of patients, more so in non-experienced hands [15]. Nd:YAG seems to perform equally to PDT in terms of dysphagia relief, but it has higher perforation rates, lower duration of response, and higher patient discomfort. However, it lacks photo-sensibility [57, 60]. Other disadvantages of Nd:YAG laser therapy include high costs and the necessity of special equipments and technical skill. It is, therefore, only available in specialized centers [14, 15].

27.3.5.3 Argon plasma coagulation (APC)

APC is an easy-to-apply, safe and cheap method of tumor thermal ablation, with an overall rate of recanalization of nearly 90% [33]. A trial with a new high-power system of APC showed good dysphagia relief rates with a low number of treatments (2.3 treatments per patient; range 1–5) and low complication rates. These characteristics allowed the authors to propose that it could be used as an alternative to Nd:YAG in this setting [61]. A recent randomized trial compared APC treatment alone with combined treatments (APC + PDT and APC + brachytherapy) as palliative interventions. Both combination treatments almost doubled the dysphagia-free period, compared to APC treatment alone, with only slightly higher minor complication rates. The best HRQoL was achieved by combining APC with brachytherapy [56].

Serious complications of APC are relatively rare, in the order of 5–10%, and include perforation and/or fistula formation. The main role of APC at the moment remains that of treating neoplastic bleeding and/or tumor in- or overgrowth after stent placement [30, 33]. Future studies will determine whether it can enter routine use in the palliation of esophageal cancer, most likely in combination with other modalities.

27.3.5.4 Cryospray ablation (CSA)

CSA is a novel technique of local tissue ablation which makes use of liquid nitrogen sprayed under endoscopic visualization directly onto the dysplastic/neoplastic tissue by specially designed catheters, followed by slow warming of the tissue. It induces apoptosis and cryonecrosis at very cold temperatures (up to −158°C), by direct tissue injury, transient ischemia and cryo-induced inflammation. Initial studies have already shown good results in the treatment of Barrett's esophagus with or without high-grade dysplasia [62]. In one case report, palliation of inoperable esophageal cancer with this technique was feasible [63]. CSA is promising, but it is at its earliest stages of development and, hence, thus far it may be considered only fit for clinical trials in specialized centers.

27.3.5.5 Percutaneous endoscopic gastrostomy (PEG)

In patients with head and neck cancers, including those with inoperable upper esophageal cancer, which are unfit for stent placement, PEG and nasogastric tube (NGT) feeding have been used for nutritional support [5, 38]. The main advantage of these methods is that a fixed and adjustable amount of calories may be given, even to patients with tumor-related anorexia, who would not benefit much from oral nutrition. NGT is usually placed in patients with a life expectancy of one month, with PEG being preserved for those with a predicted better prognosis. A recent study, however, suggests that PEG placement may be acceptable, even in patients with worse prognosis, though it must be evaluated on a case-to-case basis. In this study, PEG placement was associated with stability of body weight and markers of nutritional parameters [64].

In a large retrospective study, PEG was placed in patients with esophageal neoplasia of all types and stages, both for palliation and as bridge-to-surgery. PEG placement was safe and feasible in 97% of patients, and provided good nutritional support and HRQoL. Prior endoscopic dilation was necessary in nearly half the patients, and side-effects were very few [17]. Patients usually prefer PEG to NGT, since it is easier to manage, is cosmetically more acceptable, it allows more flexibility in social interaction and it can easily

be utilized during sleep for nutritional support, thus producing an overall better HRQoL. Furthermore, PEG is usually more stable over time than NGT [5, 38]. Disadvantages or complications of PEG include patient discomfort, episodes of blockage, leakage or dislodgement, needing replacement, local skin infection and, more rarely, injury of the blood vessels of the stomach, implantation metastases and perforation. Moreover, PEG placement has no effect on local pain or risk of aspiration pneumonia. Overall, PEG placement is safe and effective and should be considered for nutritional support where other techniques are unfeasible, or in combination to them.

27.3.5.6 Local injection of chemotherapeutic agents

Direct local injection of antiblastic agents into exophytic tumor tissue debulks the neoplastic nodule that causes obstruction and thereby relieves dysphagia. The local nature of this treatment, unlike conventional chemotherapy, has the theoretical advantage of inducing little or no systemic side effects, such as nephrotoxicity, nausea and/or vomiting. Furthermore, no special skills or equipments are required for its administration.

In a small pilot study, a gel containing cysplatin/epinephrine was used. It showed good results in terms of tumor mass reduction and dysphagia relief, with no systemic side effects. The only major complication was the creation of a tracheoesophageal fistula [65]. Combination with radiotherapy, especially brachytherapy may, theoretically, further enhance the ablative effects of such treatment, since cysplatin is a radiosensitizer. This method seems an effective and safe palliative option, but more studies will be necessary to establish its role in this setting.

27.3.5.7 Ethanol injection

Ethanol-induced tumor necrosis (ETN) is a simple, cheap and readily available palliative treatment. Aliquots of 100% ethanol are injected into the visible neoplasia under direct endoscopic visualization, causing tissue necrosis. However, the procedure needs to be repeated after an interval of 3–7, days and the pattern of tumor necrosis is unpredictable. Overall, it seems no different from dilation treatment in terms of dysphagia relief and recurrence, but with a high rate of analgesia use. Therefore, it is not recommended as a primary treatment [30, 33].

27.3.6 Which option is best?

The existence of so many options makes this question irresistible. Stent placement and brachytherapy are currently the most widely used, and the best, evidence-based options. Stent placement offers a more rapid dysphagia relief, while brachytherapy proffers a slower but more durable effect, together with an overall better HRQoL and survival. Evidence is, however, mounting that the other modalities may have a similar efficacy, though it seems that the rate of required re-interventions with them is higher [14].

Since no single modality can be considered ideal for every single patient, the choice of the best treatment option should be tailored on the basis of patient characteristics, as well as local expertise and availability. Some authors have proposed a prognostic score which could help guide the choice [45]. This takes into account age, gender, tumor length, WHO performance score, and the presence of metastases. The score differentiates between patients with good, poor or intermediate prognosis. The authors propose that for patients with expected survival of $\geq$ 3 months, brachytherapy offers the best results while, for patients with expected survival of $\leq$ 3 months, as well as for those not adequately responding to brachytherapy, stent placement may be the best choice. In patients with very bad prognosis and expected survival of $\leq$ 2 weeks, only dilation may be sufficient [15]. It is, therefore, best that patients affected by inoperable esophageal cancer are managed with a multidisciplinary approach in specialist centers which offer a wide range of therapeutic options [14, 31].

Finally, a combination of different palliative modalities is feasible and, probably, preferable to each single intervention, since complementary techniques may enhance the efficacy, and make up for the shortcomings, of each other. Results from recent studies allow us to prospect that, in the future, combination treatment may become more common.

27.4 Conclusion

More than half of patients affected by esophageal cancer have inoperable disease at presentation. Dysphagia relief and nutritional support assume a primary importance in this setting. Palliation has become, for the most part, an area of endoscopic pertinence. Stent placement and brachytherapy are currently the first choices, but other options are also gaining popularity.

A combination of different palliative options is feasible, and may enhance the efficacy of each technique. The management of patients affected by inoperable esophageal cancer should be personalized, to offer the best palliative treatment to each patient.

References

1 Parkin DM, Bray F, Ferlay J, *et al.* (2005). Global cancer statistic, 2002. *CA: A Cancer Journal for Clinicians* **55**, 74–108

2 Stein HJ, Siewert JR (2004). Improved prognosis of resected esophageal cancer. *World Journal of Surgery* **28**, 520–5

3 van Boeckel PG, Siersema PD, Sturgess R, *et al.* (2010). A new partially covered metal stent for palliation of malignant dysphagia: a prospective follow-up study. *Gastrointestinal Endoscopy* **72**, 1269–73.

4 Riccardi D, Allen K (1999). Nutritional Management of Patients With Esophageal and Esophagogastric Junction Cancer. *Cancer Control* **6**(1), 64–72.

5 Bozzetti F (2010). Nutritional support in patients with oesophageal cancer. *Support Care Cancer* **18**(Suppl 2), S41–50.

6 Douglas E, McMillan DC (2013). Towards a simple objective framework for the investigation and treatment of cancer cachexia: The Glasgow Prognostic Score. *Cancer Treatment Reviews* **40**(6), 685–91.

7 Argilés JM, López-Soriano FJ (1999). The role of cytokines in cancer cachexia. *Medicinal Research Reviews* **19**, 223–48.

8 Lecleire S, Di Fiore F, Antonietti M, *et al.* (2006). Undernutrition is predictive of early mortality after palliative self-expanding metal stent insertion in patients with inoperable or recurrent esophageal cancer. *Gastrointestinal Endoscopy* **64**(4), 479–84.

9 DiFiore F, Lecleire S, Pop D, *et al.* (2007). Baseline nutritional status is predictive of response to treatment and survival in patients treated by definitive chemoradiotherapy for a locally advanced esophageal cancer. *American Journal of Gastroenterology* **102**, 2557–2563.

10 Crumley ABC, McMillan M, McKennanM, *et al.* (2006). Evaluation of an inflammation-based prognostic score in patients with inoperable gastro-oesophageal cancer. *British Journal of Cancer* **94**, 437–441

11 Bazzan AJ, Newberg AB, Cho WC, Monti DA (2013). Diet and Nutrition in Cancer Survivorship and Palliative Care. *Evidence-Based Complementary and Alternative Medicine* **2013**; 917647.

12 Gray RT, O'donnell ME, Scott RD, *et al.* (2011). Impact of nutritional factors on survival in patients with inoperable oesophageal cancer undergoing self-expanding metal stent insertion. *European Journal of Gastroenterology & Hepatology* **23**(6), 455–60.

13 Aoki T, Osaka Y, Takagi Y, *et al.* (2001). Comparative study of self-expandable metallic stent and bypass surgery for inoperable esophageal cancer. *Diseases of the Esophagus* **14**, 208–11.

14 Sreedharan A, Harris K, Crellin A, *et al.* (2009). Interventions for dysphagia in oesophageal cancer. *Cochrane Database of Systematic Reviews* **7**(4), CD005048.

15 Siersema PD, Vleggaar FP (2010). Esophageal strictures, tumors, and fistulae: alternative techniques for palliating primary esophageal cancer. *Techniques in Gastrointestinal Endoscopy* **12**(4), 203–209

16 Repici A, Rando G (2008). Expandable stent for malignant dysphagia. *Techniques in Gastrointestinal Endoscopy* **10**, 175–183.

17 Stockeld D, Fagerberg J, Granström L, Backman L (2001). Percutaneous endoscopic gastrostomy for nutrition in patients with oesophageal cancer. *European Journal of Surgery* **167**(11), 839–44.

18 Vleggaar FP, Siersema PD (2011). Expandable stents for malignant esophageal disease. *Gastrointestinal Endoscopy Clinics of North America* **21**(3), 377–88.

19 Seven G, Irani S, Ross AS, *et al.* (2013). Partially versus fully covered self-expanding metal stents for benign and malignant esophageal conditions: a single center experience. *Surgical Endoscopy* **27**(6), 2185–92.

20 Uitdehaag MJ, Siersema PD, Spaander MC, *et al.* (2010). A new fully covered stent with antimigration properties for the palliation of malignant dysphagia: a prospective cohort study. *Gastrointestinal Endoscopy* **71**, 600–5.

21 Hirdes MM, Siersema PD, Vleggaar FP (2012). A new fully covered metal stent for the treatment of benign and malignant dysphagia: a prospective follow-up study. *Gastrointestinal Endoscopy* **75**(4), 712–8.

22 van Heel NC, Haringsma J, Boot H, *et al.* (2012). Comparison of 2 expandable stents for malignant esophageal disease: a randomized controlled trial. *Gastrointestinal Endoscopy* **76**(1), 52–8.

23 Verschuur EM, Steyerberg EW, Kuipers EJ, Siersema PD (2007). Effect of stent size on complications and recurrent dysphagia in patients with esophageal or gastric cardia cancer. *Gastrointestinal Endoscopy* **65**(4), 592–601.

24 van Boeckel PG, Repici A, Vleggaar FP, *et al.* (2010). A new metal stent with a controlled-release system for palliation of malignant dysphagia: a prospective, multicenter study. *Gastrointestinal Endoscopy* **71**, 455–60.

25 Lazaraki G, Katsinelos P, Nakos A, *et al.* (2011). Malignant esophageal dysphagia palliation using insertion of a covered Ultraflex stent without fluoroscopy: a prospective observational study. *Surgical Endoscopy* **25**(2), 628–35.

26 Verschuur EM, Homs MY, Steyerberg EW, *et al.* (2006). A new esophageal stent design (Niti-S stent) for the prevention of migration: a prospective study in 42 patients. *Gastrointestinal Endoscopy* **63**(1), 134–40.

27 Verschuur EM, Kuipers EJ, Siersema PD (2007). Esophageal stents for malignant strictures close to the upper esophageal sphincter. *Gastrointestinal Endoscopy* **66**, 1082–90.

28 Conio M, Repici A, Battaglia G, *et al.* (2007). A randomized prospective comparison of self-expandable plastic stents and partially covered self-expandable metal stents in the palliation of malignant esophageal dysphagia. *American Journal of Gastroenterology* **102**, 2667e77.

29 Verschuur EM, Repici A, Kuipers EJ, *et al.* (2008). New design esophageal stents for the palliation of dysphagia from esophageal or gastric cardia cancer: a randomized trial. *American Journal of Gastroenterology* **103**, 304e12.

30 Shenfine J, McNamee P, Steen N, *et al.* (2005). A pragmatic randomised controlled trial of the cost-effectiveness of palliative therapies for patients with inoperable oesophageal cancer. *Health Technology Assessment* **9**(5), iii, 1–121.

31 Shenfine J, McNamee P, Steen N, *et al.* (2009). A randomized controlled clinical trial of palliative therapies for patients with inoperable esophageal cancer. *American Journal of Gastroenterology* **104**(7), 1674–85.

32 Hirdes MM, Siersema PD, Houben MH, *et al.* (2011). Stent-in-stent technique for removal of embedded esophageal self-expanding metal stents. *American Journal of Gastroenterology* **106**(2), 286–93.

33 Allum WH, Blazeby JM, Griffin SM, *et al.* (2011). Guidelines for the management of oesophageal and gastric cancer. *Gut* **60**(11), 1449–72.

34 van Boeckel PG, Vleggaar FP, Siersema PD (2013). Biodegradable stent placement in the esophagus. *Expert Review of Medical Devices* **10**(1), 37–43.

35 Hirdes MM, van Hooft JE, Wijrdeman HK, *et al.* (2012). Combination of biodegradable stent placement and single-dose brachytherapy is associated with an unacceptably high complication rate in the treatment of dysphagia from esophageal cancer. *Gastrointestinal Endoscopy* **76**(2), 267–74.

36 Eleftheriadis E, Kotzampassi K (2006). Endoprosthesis implantation at the pharyngoesophageal level: problems, limitations and challenges. *World Journal of Gastroenterology* **12**, 2103–8.

37 Yoon HY, Cheon YK, Choi HJ, Shim CS (2012). Role of photodynamic therapy in the palliation of obstructing esophageal cancer. *Korean Journal of Internal Medicine* **27**, 278–284.

38 Mekhail TM, Adelstein D, Rybicki LA, *et al.* (2001). Enteral nutrition during the treatment of head and neck carcinoma: is a percutaneous endoscopic gastrostomy tube preferable to a nasogastric tube? *Cancer* **91**, 1785–1790.

39 Homann N, Noftz MR, Klingenberg-Noftz RD, *et al.* (2008). Delayed complications after placement of self-expanding stents in malignant esophageal obstruction: treatment strategies and survival rate. *Digestive Diseases and Sciences* **53**, 334e40.

40 Sumiyoshi T, Gotoda T, Muro K, *et al.* (2003). Morbidity and mortality after self-expandable metallic stent placement in patients with progressive or recurrent esophageal cancer after chemoradiotherapy. *Gastrointestinal Endoscopy* **57**(7), 882–5.

41 Lecleire S, Di Fiore F, Ben-Soussan E, *et al.* (2006). Prior chemoradiotherapy is associated with a higher life-threatening complication rate after palliative insertion of

metal stents in patients with oesophageal cancer. *Alimentary Pharmacology & Therapeutics* **23**(12), 1693–702.

42 Qiu G, Tao Y, Du X, *et al.* (2013). The impact of prior radiotherapy on fatal complications after self-expandable metallic stents (SEMS) for malignant dysphagia due to esophageal carcinoma. *Diseases of the Esophagus* **26**(2), 175–81.

43 Homs MY, Hansen BE, van Blankenstein M, *et al.* (2004). Prior radiation and/or chemotherapy has no effect on the outcome of metal stent placement for oesophagogastric carcinoma. *European Journal of Gastroenterology & Hepatology* **16**(2), 163–70.

44 Homs MY, Wahab PJ, Kuipers EJ, *et al.* (2004). Esophageal stents with antireflux valve for tumors of the distal esophagus and gastric cardia: a randomized trial. *Gastrointestinal Endoscopy* **60**, 695e702

45 Steyerberg EW, Homs MY, Stokvis A, *et al.* (2005). Stent placement or brachytherapy for palliation of dysphagia from esophageal cancer: a prognostic model to guide treatment selection. *Gastrointestinal Endoscopy* **62**, 333–340.

46 Shridhar R, Almhanna K, Meredith KL, *et al.* (2013). Radiation therapy and esophageal cancer. *Cancer Control* **20**(2), 97–110.

47 Homs MYV, Steyerberg EW, Eijkenboom WMH, *et al.* (2004). Single-dose brachytherapy versus metal stent placement for the palliation of dysphagia from oesophageal cancer: multicentre randomised trial. *Lancet* **364**, 1497–1504.

48 Bergquist H, Wenger U, Johnsson E, *et al.* (2005). Stent insertion or endoluminal brachytherapy as palliation of patients with advanced cancer of the esophagus and gastroesophageal junction. Results of a randomized, controlled clinical trial. *Diseases of the Esophagus* **18**, 131e9.

49 Wenger U, Johnsson E, Bergquist H, *et al.* (2005). Health economic evaluation of stent or endoluminal brachytherapy as a palliative strategy in patients with incurable cancer of the oesophagus or gastro-oesophageal junction: results of a randomized clinical trial. *European Journal of Gastroenterology & Hepatology* **17**, 1369c77.

50 Bergquist H, Johnsson E, Nyman J, *et al.* (2012). Combined stent insertion and single high-dose brachytherapy in patients with advanced esophageal cancer – results of a prospective safety study. *Diseases of the Esophagus* **25**(5), 410–5.

51 Javed A, Pal S, Dash NR, *et al.* (2012). Palliative stenting with or without radiotherapy for inoperable esophageal carcinoma: a randomized trial. *Journal of Gastrointestinal Cancer* **43**, 63–9.

52 Hirdes MM, van Hooft JE, Wijrdeman HK, *et al.* (2012). Combination of biodegradable stent placement and single-dose brachytherapy is associated with an unacceptably high complication rate in the treatment of dysphagia from esophageal cancer. *Gastrointestinal Endoscopy* **76**(2), 267–74.

53 Guo JH, Teng GJ, Zhu GY, *et al.* (2008). Self-expandable esophageal stent loaded with 125I seeds: initial experience in patients with advanced esophageal cancer. *Radiology* **247**(2), 574–81.

54 Spencer GM, Thorpe SM, Blackman GM, *et al.* (2002). Laser augmented by brachytherapy versus laser alone in the palliation of adenocarcinoma of the oesophagus and cardia: a randomised study. *Gut* **50**(2), 224–7.

55 Lindenmann J, Matzi V, Neuboeck N, *et al.* (2012). Individualized, multimodal palliative treatment of inoperable esophageal cancer: clinical impact of photodynamic therapy resulting in prolonged survival. *Lasers in Surgery and Medicine* **44**(3), 189–98.

56 Rupinski M, Zagorowicz E, Regula J, *et al.* (2011). Randomized comparison of three palliative regimens including brachytherapy, photodynamic therapy, and APC in patients with malignant dysphagia (CONSORT 1a) (Revised II). *American Journal of Gastroenterology* **106**(9), 1612–20.

57 Litle VR, Luketich JD, Christie NA, *et al.* (2003). Photodynamic therapy as palliation for esophageal cancer: experience in 215 patients. *Annals of Thoracic Surgery* **76**(5), 1687–92

58 Moghissi K (2012). Where does photodynamic therapy fit in the esophageal cancer treatment jigsaw puzzle? *Journal of the National Comprehensive Cancer Network* **10**(Suppl 2), S52–5.

59 Dallal HJ, Smith GD, Grieve DC, *et al.* (2001). A randomized trial of thermal ablative therapy versus expandable metal stents in the palliative treatment of patients with esophageal carcinoma. *Gastrointestinal Endoscopy* **54**(5), 549–57.

60 Lightdale CJ, Heier SK, Marcon NE, *et al* (1995). Photodynamic therapy with porfimer sodium versus thermal ablation therapy with Nd:YAG laser for palliation of esophageal cancer: a multicenter randomized trial. *Gastrointestinal Endoscopy* **42**, 507–12.

61 Manner H, May A, Rabenstein T, *et al.* (2007). Prospective evaluation of a new high-power argon plasma coagulation system (hp-APC) in therapeutic gastrointestinal endoscopy. *Scandinavian Journal of Gastroenterology* **42**, 397e405

62 Johnston MH (2003). Cryotherapy and other newer techniques. *Gastrointestinal Endoscopy* **13**, 491–504.

63 Cash BD, Johnston LR, Johnston MH (2007). Cryospray ablation (CSA) in the palliative treatment of squamous cell carcinoma of the esophagus. *World Journal of Surgical Oncology* **5**, 34.

64 Grilo A, Santos CA, Fonseca J (2012). Percutaneous endoscopic gastrostomy for nutritional palliation of upper esophageal cancer unsuitable for esophageal stenting. *Arquivos de Gastroenterologia* **49**(3), 227–31.

65 Harbord M, Dawes RF, Barr H, *et al.* (2002). Palliation of patients with dysphagia due to advanced esophageal cancer by endoscopic injection of cisplatin/epinephrine injectable gel. *Gastrointestinal Endoscopy* **56**(5), 644–51.

Index

Note: Page numbers in *italics* represent figures, those in **bold** represent tables.